Transforming Precision Medicine: The Intersection of Digital Health and AI

Transforming Precision Medicine: The Intersection of Digital Health and AI

Editor

Daniele Giansanti

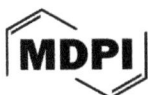 Basel • Beijing • Wuhan • Barcelona • Belgrade • Novi Sad • Cluj • Manchester

Editor
Daniele Giansanti
Centro nazionale per le
tecnologie innovative in
sanità pubblica
ISS
Rome
Italy

Editorial Office
MDPI
St. Alban-Anlage 66
4052 Basel, Switzerland

This is a reprint of articles from the Special Issue published online in the open access journal *Journal of Personalized Medicine* (ISSN 2075-4426) (available at: https://www.mdpi.com/journal/jpm/special_issues/4FMFQUN50A).

For citation purposes, cite each article independently as indicated on the article page online and as indicated below:

Lastname, A.A.; Lastname, B.B. Article Title. *Journal Name* **Year**, *Volume Number*, Page Range.

ISBN 978-3-7258-0874-8 (Hbk)
ISBN 978-3-7258-0873-1 (PDF)
doi.org/10.3390/books978-3-7258-0873-1

© 2024 by the authors. Articles in this book are Open Access and distributed under the Creative Commons Attribution (CC BY) license. The book as a whole is distributed by MDPI under the terms and conditions of the Creative Commons Attribution-NonCommercial-NoDerivs (CC BY-NC-ND) license.

Contents

Preface ix

Daniele Giansanti
Joint Expedition: Exploring the Intersection of Digital Health and AI in Precision Medicine with Team Integration
Reprinted from: *J. Pers. Med.* **2024**, *14*, 388, doi:10.3390/jpm14040388 1

Daniele Giansanti
Precision Medicine 2.0: How Digital Health and AI Are Changing the Game
Reprinted from: *J. Pers. Med.* **2023**, *13*, 1057, doi:10.3390/jpm13071057 10

Ben Allen
The Promise of Explainable AI in Digital Health for Precision Medicine: A Systematic Review
Reprinted from: *J. Pers. Med.* **2024**, *14*, 277, doi:10.3390/jpm14030277 14

Antonio Iannone and Daniele Giansanti
Breaking Barriers—The Intersection of AI and Assistive Technology in Autism Care: A Narrative Review
Reprinted from: *J. Pers. Med.* **2024**, *14*, 41, doi:10.3390/jpm14010041 27

Jing Miao, Charat Thongprayoon, Supawadee Suppadungsuk, Oscar A. Garcia Valencia, Fawad Qureshi and Wisit Cheungpasitporn
Innovating Personalized Nephrology Care: Exploring the Potential Utilization of ChatGPT
Reprinted from: *J. Pers. Med.* **2023**, *13*, 1681, doi:10.3390/jpm13121681 46

Mantapond Ittarat, Wisit Cheungpasitporn and Sunee Chansangpetch
Personalized Care in Eye Health: Exploring Opportunities, Challenges, and the Road Ahead for Chatbots
Reprinted from: *J. Pers. Med.* **2023**, *13*, 1679, doi:10.3390/jpm13121679 67

Vincent W. S. Leung, Curtise K. C. Ng, Sai-Kit Lam, Po-Tsz Wong, Ka-Yan Ng, Cheuk-Hong Tam, et al.
Computed Tomography-Based Radiomics for Long-Term Prognostication of High-Risk Localized Prostate Cancer Patients Received Whole Pelvic Radiotherapy
Reprinted from: *J. Pers. Med.* **2023**, *13*, 1643, doi:10.3390/jpm13121643 98

Diego Morena, Carolina Campos, María Castillo, Miguel Alonso, María Benavent and José Luis Izquierdo
Impact of the COVID-19 Pandemic on the Epidemiological Situation of Pulmonary Tuberculosis–Using Natural Language Processing
Reprinted from: *J. Pers. Med.* **2023**, *13*, 1629, doi:10.3390/jpm13121629 114

Luca Michelutti, Alessandro Tel, Marco Zeppieri, Tamara Ius, Salvatore Sembronio and Massimo Robiony
The Use of Artificial Intelligence Algorithms in the Prognosis and Detection of Lymph Node Involvement in Head and Neck Cancer and Possible Impact in the Development of Personalized Therapeutic Strategy: A Systematic Review
Reprinted from: *J. Pers. Med.* **2023**, *13*, 1626, doi:10.3390/jpm13121626 124

Iqbal M. Lone, Osayd Zohud, Kareem Midlej, Eva Paddenberg, Sebastian Krohn, Christian Kirschneck, et al.
Anterior Open Bite Malocclusion: From Clinical Treatment Strategies towards the Dissection of the Genetic Bases of the Disease Using Human and Collaborative Cross Mice Cohorts
Reprinted from: *J. Pers. Med.* **2023**, *13*, 1617, doi:10.3390/jpm13111617 142

Alaa Fawaz, Alessandra Ferraresi and Ciro Isidoro
Systems Biology in Cancer Diagnosis Integrating Omics Technologies and Artificial Intelligence to Support Physician Decision Making
Reprinted from: *J. Pers. Med.* **2023**, *13*, 1590, doi:10.3390/jpm13111590 169

Bruno Fuchs, Gabriela Studer, Beata Bode-Lesniewska, Philip Heesen and on behalf of the Swiss Sarcoma Network
The Next Frontier in Sarcoma Care: Digital Health, AI, and the Quest for Precision Medicine
Reprinted from: *J. Pers. Med.* **2023**, *13*, 1530, doi:10.3390/jpm13111530 186

Charles Meijer, Hae-Won Uh and Said el Bouhaddani
Digital Twins in Healthcare: Methodological Challenges and Opportunities
Reprinted from: *J. Pers. Med.* **2023**, *13*, 1522, doi:10.3390/jpm13101522 195

Julien Issa, Abanoub Riad, Raphael Olszewski and Marta Dyszkiewicz-Konwińska
The Influence of Slice Thickness, Sharpness, and Contrast Adjustments on Inferior Alveolar Canal Segmentation on Cone-Beam Computed Tomography Scans: A Retrospective Study
Reprinted from: *J. Pers. Med.* **2023**, *13*, 1518, doi:10.3390/jpm13101518 210

Sebastian Griewing, Niklas Gremke, Uwe Wagner, Michael Lingenfelder, Sebastian Kuhn and Jelena Boekhoff
Challenging ChatGPT 3.5 in Senology—An Assessment of Concordance with Breast Cancer Tumor Board Decision Making
Reprinted from: *J. Pers. Med.* **2023**, *13*, 1502, doi:10.3390/jpm13101502 221

Nezar Watted, Iqbal M. Lone, Osayd Zohud, Kareem Midlej, Peter Proff and Fuad A. Iraqi
Comprehensive Deciphering the Complexity of the Deep Bite: Insight from Animal Model to Human Subjects
Reprinted from: *J. Pers. Med.* **2023**, *13*, 1472, doi:10.3390/jpm13101472 236

Iqbal M. Lone, Osayd Zohud, Kareem Midlej, Obaida Awadi, Samir Masarwa, Sebastian Krohn, et al.
Narrating the Genetic Landscape of Human Class I Occlusion: A Perspective-Infused Review
Reprinted from: *J. Pers. Med.* **2023**, *13*, 1465, doi:10.3390/jpm13101465 255

Noppawit Aiumtrakul, Charat Thongprayoon, Supawadee Suppadungsuk, Pajaree Krisanapan, Jing Miao, Fawad Qureshi and Wisit Cheungpasitporn
Navigating the Landscape of Personalized Medicine: The Relevance of ChatGPT, BingChat, and Bard AI in Nephrology Literature Searches
Reprinted from: *J. Pers. Med.* **2023**, *13*, 1457, doi:10.3390/jpm13101457 277

Luís B. Elvas, Miguel Nunes, Joao C. Ferreira, Miguel Sales Dias and Luís Brás Rosário
AI-Driven Decision Support for Early Detection of Cardiac Events: Unveiling Patterns and Predicting Myocardial Ischemia
Reprinted from: *J. Pers. Med.* **2023**, *13*, 1421, doi:10.3390/jpm13091421 291

Christian J. Wiedermann, Angelika Mahlknecht, Giuliano Piccoliori and Adolf Engl
Redesigning Primary Care: The Emergence of Artificial-Intelligence-Driven Symptom Diagnostic Tools
Reprinted from: *J. Pers. Med.* **2023**, *13*, 1379, doi:10.3390/jpm13091379 . . . . **315**

José Pereira, Nuno Antunes, Joana Rosa, João C. Ferreira, Sandra Mogo and Manuel Pereira
Intelligent Clinical Decision Support System for Managing COPD Patients
Reprinted from: *J. Pers. Med.* **2023**, *13*, 1359, doi:10.3390/jpm13091359 . . . . **322**

Preface

Precision medicine is revolutionizing healthcare, reshaping traditional approaches to align with individual patient attributes. This shift is powered by the convergence of digital health technologies and artificial intelligence (AI), offering an unparalleled opportunity to refine and amplify personalized healthcare. Digital health tools, such as electronic health records and wearable devices, provide comprehensive patient data, encompassing genetic profiles, lifestyle choices, and real-time physiological metrics. These data empower healthcare practitioners to craft finely tuned treatment strategies tailored to each patient's unique health profile.

AI plays a crucial role in this evolution, with machine learning algorithms discerning intricate patterns within vast datasets to identify biomarkers and personalized treatment responses. This analytical prowess enhances diagnosis, prognosis, and facilitates a proactive approach to patient care. Together, digital health and AI mark a new era of unprecedented healthcare advancements, extending personalized treatments globally.

The Special Issue "Transforming Precision Medicine: The Intersection of Digital Health and AI" encapsulates these advancements, featuring 21 contributions across various categories, including editorials, scientific articles, reviews, systematic reviews, perspectives, and opinion articles. This collaborative endeavor aims to foster scientific exchange and editorial collaboration, providing a comprehensive environment for scholarly pursuits.

We extend our sincere gratitude to all contributors for their invaluable insights and efforts, which have made this Special Issue possible. It is our hope that the knowledge shared within these pages will inspire further innovation and collaboration, ultimately leading to improved patient care.

Special thanks to Iris Qiao for exceptional support throughout the creation of this collection.

Daniele Giansanti
Editor

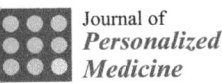 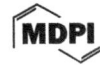

Editorial

Joint Expedition: Exploring the Intersection of Digital Health and AI in Precision Medicine with Team Integration

Daniele Giansanti

Centro Nazionale Tecnologie Innovative in Sanità Pubblica, Istituto Superiore di Sanità, Via Regina Elena 299, 00161 Roma, Italy; daniele.giansanti@iss.it

1. The Joint Expedition Exploring the Intersection of Digital Health and AI in Precision Medicine

Precision medicine stands as a transformative force in the orbit of healthcare, fundamentally reshaping traditional approaches by customizing therapeutic interventions to align with the distinctive attributes of individual patients [1,2]. This revolutionary paradigmatic shift has been propelled forward by the convergence of two pivotal technological frontiers: digital health technologies and the remarkable progress made in artificial intelligence (AI). Together, they forge an unparalleled opportunity to not only refine but also amplify the precision, efficiency, and widespread availability of personalized healthcare. The integration of digital health technologies has played a pivotal role in augmenting the landscape of precision medicine [2,3]. Through the utilization of electronic health records, wearable devices, and other interconnected health monitoring tools, a wealth of patient data has become readily accessible [4]. This important collection of information encompasses genetic profiles, lifestyle choices, environmental factors, and real-time physiological metrics, thereby providing a comprehensive understanding of an individual's health status. The synthesis of these multifaceted, polyhedric, and complex datasets empowers healthcare practitioners with an all-inclusive perspective, enabling them to craft treatment strategies that are finely tuned to the intricate gradations of each patient's unique health profile [5,6]. In tandem with the rise of digital health, AI has emerged as a linchpin in the evolution of precision medicine [7,8]. Machine learning algorithms, powered by vast datasets, can discern intricate patterns and correlations within a diverse range of health information. This analytical prowess facilitates the identification of subtle biomarkers, predictive indicators, and personalized treatment responses that might elude traditional diagnostic methods. By harnessing the predictive capabilities of AI, healthcare professionals can not only refine diagnosis and prognosis but also anticipate potential therapeutic outcomes, fostering a more proactive and preemptive approach to patient care.

The integration of digital health and AI technologies in healthcare enhances efficiency by automating routine tasks, streamlining diagnostics, and allowing more time for nuanced patient care [4,7,8]. The rapid assimilation of vast datasets facilitates quicker, more accurate decision-making, reducing the risk of adverse outcomes. This synergy also democratizes personalized healthcare, extending precision medicine beyond specialized centers through the accessibility of digital tools and scalable AI solutions. Remote patient monitoring, telemedicine, and AI diagnostics overcome geographical barriers, improving healthcare inclusivity and addressing disparities. This convergence marks an era of unprecedented healthcare advancements, refining personalized treatments and extending their global reach, with a vision of placing everyone's unique health profile at the forefront of therapeutic strategies. The initiative to establish a dual opportunity for scientific and editorial collaboration has been initiated with this project's Special Issue (SI), "Transforming Precision Medicine: The Intersection of Digital Health and AI". (available at https://www.mdpi.com/journal/jpm/special_issues/4FMFQUN50A, access on 10 March 2024).

Citation: Giansanti, D. Joint Expedition: Exploring the Intersection of Digital Health and AI in Precision Medicine with Team Integration. *J. Pers. Med.* **2024**, *14*, 388. https://doi.org/10.3390/jpm14040388

Received: 10 March 2024
Accepted: 2 April 2024
Published: 4 April 2024

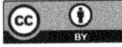

Copyright: © 2024 by the author. Licensee MDPI, Basel, Switzerland. This article is an open access article distributed under the terms and conditions of the Creative Commons Attribution (CC BY) license (https://creativecommons.org/licenses/by/4.0/).

This endeavor aimed to create a platform that not only facilitates scientific exchange but also provides a space for editorial collaboration, fostering a comprehensive environment for both scholarly and publishing pursuits.

This Special Issue has successfully achieved a significant milestone, featuring 20 contributions (Co)s (excluding this editorial) [9–28].

The published papers (see Figure 1), according to the selected categories, encompass 1 introductory editorial [9], 7 full scientific articles [10–16], 5 reviews [17–21], 2 systematic reviews [22,23], 4 perspectives [24–27], and 1 opinion article [28].

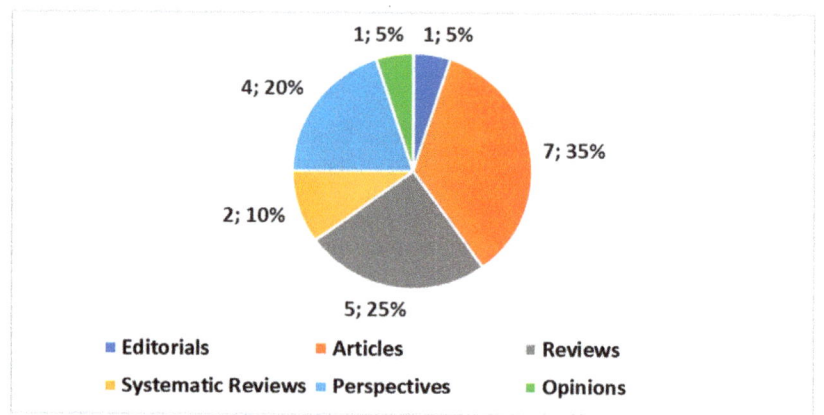

Figure 1. Categories of papers published in this Special Issue.

2. Conclusive Discoveries: A Closer Look at the Contributions

2.1. An Overview of the Contributions

Below, we present a concise overview encapsulating the key points and insights from the contributions featured in this Special Issue. This conclusive list aims to provide a brief yet comprehensive glimpse into the diverse and impactful content published within this specialized collection.

The Editorial by Giansanti [9] introduces the aims of the SI and reflects on the progress and status of the introduction of AI into precision medicine. The focus is on assessing the current state and briefly exploring both its evolution and recent trends. The editorial introduces the need for this initiative as a Special Issue that suggests fields and directions for exploration.

Leung et al. [10] explore the use of planning computed tomography (pCT)-based radiomics for the long-term prognostication of high-risk localized prostate cancer patients who underwent whole pelvic radiotherapy (WPRT). Given the high mortality rate of high-risk prostate cancer and challenges with traditional prognostic markers, the research employed rigorous radiomics methodologies on a cohort of 64 patients. The pCT-based radiomics model demonstrated a consistent and comparable performance to MRI-based studies, predicting six-year progression-free survival with a mean AUC of 0.76 (training) and 0.71 (testing). The radiomics signature, incorporating two texture features, exhibited promising accuracy, sensitivity, and specificity in both training and testing cohorts. This study suggests that pCT-based radiomics could serve as a routine, non-invasive approach for prognostic prediction in high-risk localized prostate cancer cases undergoing WPRT, leveraging the accessibility of CT in standard clinical practices.

The retrospective study proposed by Morena et al. [11] utilizing artificial intelligence aimed to assess the impact of the COVID-19 pandemic on pulmonary tuberculosis (TB). Analyzing electronic health records from Spain's Castilla-La Mancha region, this study compared data from 2015 to 2020. In 2020, pulmonary TB diagnoses decreased by 28% compared to 2019, with 14.2% of patients diagnosed with both TB and COVID-19. Despite a higher risk for coinfection among women, symptoms were no more severe than those with isolated TB. The findings suggest a notable decline in pulmonary TB incidence during the initial year of the COVID-19 pandemic.

Issa et al. [12] investigate the impact of cone-beam computed tomography (CBCT) viewing parameters on the identification of the inferior alveolar nerve (IAC). The study assessed 25 CBCT scans, testing different slice thicknesses, sharpness, and contrast settings. A three-score system evaluated IAC visibility. Optimal parameters were determined, and validation was conducted through semi-automated segmentation and structure overlapping, assessing the mean distance. Inter-rater and intra-rater reliability were significant (69–83%). A 0.25 mm slice thickness, zero sharpness, and contrast of 1200 consistently improved the visibility and accuracy. The consideration of individual patient characteristics is recommended when applying these parameters, including anatomical variations and bone density.

Griewing et al. [13] recall how the rising accessibility of large language models (LLMs) has sparked interest in utilizing generative AI applications for medical purposes. Their observational study addresses the use of LLM ChatGPT 3.5 for treatment recommendations in breast cancer, comparing outcomes with a multidisciplinary tumor board (MTB). Incorporating patient profiles that reflected diverse breast cancer stages, including precancerous lesions and metastasis, the study found an overall concordance of 50%, rising to 58.8% for invasive breast cancer profiles. However, due to occasional fraudulent decisions by the LLM, the study concludes that publicly available LLMs are currently insufficient as support tools for tumor boards. Gynecological oncologists are encouraged to familiarize themselves with LLM capabilities, considering potential risks and limitations while exploring their potential utility.

Aiumtrakul et al. [14] explore the use of AI tools such as ChatGPT, Bing Chat, and Bard AI in the literature through searches on nephrology, specifically evaluating their citation accuracy. The researchers generated prompts to obtain references in Vancouver style for 12 nephrology topics from each AI tool and assessed their validity using PubMed, Google Scholar, and Web of Science. The results reveal varying levels of citation accuracy, with ChatGPT providing 38% accurate references, Bing Chat 30%, and Bard AI only 3%. Common errors included incorrect DOIs. This study underscores the importance of research integrity in medicine and emphasizes the need for refined AI tools before their widespread adoption in medical literature searches.

The work by Elvas et al. [15] addresses the significant global burden of cardiovascular diseases (CVDs), specifically focusing on myocardial infarction, pulmonary thromboembolism, and aortic stenosis. Utilizing data from Hospital Santa Maria, their research employs a comprehensive approach integrating exploratory data analysis (EDA) and predictive machine learning (ML) models. Following the Cross-Industry Standard Process for Data Mining (CRISP-DM) methodology, EDA uncovers intricate patterns and relationships specific to cardiovascular diseases. ML models exhibit accuracies exceeding 80%, providing a 13 min window for predicting myocardial ischemia incidents and enabling proactive interventions. This paper establishes a proof of concept for real-time data and predictive capabilities, offering valuable tools for informed decision making and timely interventions in managing cardiovascular diseases.

Pereira et al. [16] recall how chronic obstructive pulmonary disease (COPD) stands as the third leading cause of global mortality, necessitating effective management strategies. Their study highlights the pivotal role of Health Remote Monitoring Systems (HRMSs) in COPD patient care, employing artificial intelligence (AI) models to predict health deterioration risks by analyzing biometric signs and environmental factors. The research not only reviews recent works in this domain but also introduces an Intelligent Clinical Decision Support System (CIDSS). Comprising vital signs of prediction and early warning score calculation modules, the CIDSS generates early information on patient health evolution and risk analysis. It issues alerts for anomalies in biometric measurements or significant basal value changes, enabling proactive intervention. This system was implemented, assessed in a real case, and validated through an evaluation survey by healthcare professionals, affirming its utility and value in facilitating adjustments to COPD patient treatment. The CIDSS emerges as a valuable tool for medical professionals, supporting proactive healthcare interventions.

The review proposed by Iannone and Giansanti [17] explores the integration of artificial intelligence (AI) with assistive technologies (ATs) in the context of autism, recognizing the need for a multidisciplinary approach to diagnosis and therapy. A systematic review of 22 studies revealed promising interest in AI integration, particularly in AI robotics and wearable automated devices like smart glasses. These innovations hold substantial potential for enhancing communication and social engagement among individuals with autism. However, the emphasis on innovation over establishing a solid presence in healthcare raises concerns about regulatory and acceptance issues. As the field evolves, it becomes evident that integrated ATs with AI play a pivotal role in connecting various domains and addressing the complexities of autism.

Miao et al.'s review [18] discusses the significant impact of artificial intelligence (AI), particularly machine learning, on nephrology and the management of kidney diseases. It specifically focuses on ChatGPT, an innovative language model developed by OpenAI. The article highlights ChatGPT's versatility in engaging in informative conversations and its demonstrated proficiency in medical knowledge assessments. While acknowledging its varying performance across medical subfields, this review provides an overview of ChatGPT's integration in nephrology, exploring its potential benefits in dataset management, diagnostics, treatment planning, patient communication, and medical research. Ethical and legal concerns are discussed, emphasizing the importance of thorough evaluation before implementing AI in real-world medical scenarios. This review aims to be a valuable resource for nephrologists and healthcare professionals interested in utilizing AI for personalized nephrology care.

Ittarat et al. [19] highlight in their review how the integration of ophthalmology chatbots in modern eye care represents a significant technological advancement, offering benefits such as improved access to information, enhanced patient interaction, and streamlined triaging. Evaluations have demonstrated their effectiveness in ophthalmology condition triage and knowledge assessment, highlighting both their potential and areas for improvement. Challenges in integrating these chatbots into healthcare systems include ethical, legal, and integration issues. Future developments, including the synergy of artificial intelligence and machine learning, promise to enhance their diagnostic capabilities globally. This *review* explores the utilization of ophthalmology chatbots, assessing their accuracy, reliability, data protection, security, transparency, potential biases, and ethical considerations. It provides a comprehensive review of their roles in ophthalmology, emphasizing their significance and future potential in the field.

Fawaz et al. [20] propose a review that recalls how cancer is a leading cause of global disease-related death, emphasizing the importance of accurate early diagnosis and intervention. Traditional diagnostic methods include clinical examination, biomarker blood tests, biopsy histopathology, and imaging. The review highlights that the integration of diverse omics data, such as genomic, metabolomic, and microbiomic traits, is challenging and carries a risk of interpretation errors. Systems biology, combining artificial intelligence (AI) with omics technologies, is presented as a solution to analyze and integrate vast patient data, aiding physicians in diagnosis and treatment decisions rapidly and accurately. The article acknowledges the potential of AI in cancer research but highlights the associated risks, including diagnostic and prognostic errors in data interpretation.

Meijer et al.'s review [21] recalls that digital twin technology stands out as a promising advancement in healthcare, offering applications in monitoring, diagnosis, and personalized treatment strategies. It explores digital twins as virtual counterparts of real human patients, aiming to provide an in-depth understanding of the data sources and methodologies contributing to their construction across various healthcare domains. The review covers diverse data sources, such as blood glucose levels, heart MRI and CT scans, cardiac electrophysiology, written reports, and multi-omics data. Each source presents challenges related to standardization, integration, and interpretation, but the review showcases how various datasets and methods are used to overcome these obstacles and generate a digital twin. Despite significant progress, challenges remain in achieving a fully comprehensive patient digital twin. The article discusses critical developments in non-invasive data collection, high-throughput technologies, modeling, and computational power. Overall, while facing challenges, digital twin research holds great promise for personalized patient care and has the potential to shape the future of healthcare innovation.

Allen [22] proposes a systematic review, providing a synthesis of the literature on explaining machine-learning models for digital health data in precision medicine. As healthcare increasingly customizes treatments to individual characteristics, the integration of artificial intelligence with digital health data becomes crucial. Utilizing a topic-modeling approach, this paper distills key themes from 27 journal articles. Topics identified include optimizing patient healthcare through data-driven medicine, predictive modeling with data and algorithms, predicting diseases with the deep learning of biomedical data, and machine learning in medicine. The review explores specific applications of explainable artificial intelligence, emphasizing its role in fostering transparency, accountability, and trust within the healthcare domain. It underscores the need for the further development and validation of explanation methods to advance precision healthcare delivery.

Michelutti et al.'s systematic review [23] aims to analyze the primary reports on the utilization of artificial intelligence algorithms in the medical field, with a specific focus on oncology, particularly in the context of prognostic evaluations for patients with head and neck malignancies. The objective is to comprehensively examine the existing literature pertaining to the application of artificial intelligence in head and neck oncology, specifically for prognostic assessments. The review provides an encompassing overview of how artificial intelligence is employed to derive prognostic information, particularly in predicting survival and recurrence. These findings underscore the potential impact of these prognostic data on tailoring therapeutic strategies to become increasingly personalized.

Lone et al. [24] proposed a perspective focusing on anterior open-bite malocclusion, a dental condition characterized by a lack of contact between the upper and lower front teeth, leading to functional difficulties. Etiology involves genetic, environmental, and developmental factors. Genetic studies have identified genes and pathways related to jaw growth, tooth eruption, and dental occlusion contributing to open-bite development. Orthodontic treatment, including braces and clear aligners, is a primary approach, with adjuvant therapies and, in severe cases, surgical interventions. Technological advancements like 3D printing enhance treatment precision. Genetic research, especially using animal models like the collaborative cross-mouse population, provides insights into the genetic basis of open bite and potential therapeutic targets. Proposing human research using mouse models, including GWAS, EWAS, RNA-seq analysis, and integration of genetic and expression studies, aims to uncover novel genes and factors influencing open bite, paving the way for more precise treatments and preventive strategies.

Fuchs et al.'s perspective article [25] provides an in-depth exploration of the transformative era unfolding in sarcoma care, propelled by the intersection of digital health and artificial intelligence (AI). It examines the multifaceted opportunities and challenges associated with harnessing these technologies for precision and value-based sarcoma care. The article outlines the current state-of-the-art methodologies and technologies in sarcoma care, offering practical insights for healthcare providers, administrators, and policymakers. Emphasis is placed on the limitations of AI and digital health platforms, underscoring the crucial need for high-quality data and ethical considerations.

Watted et al. [26] present a perspective that delves into the malocclusion phenotype known as deep bite, characterized by the excessive overlap of the upper front teeth over the lower front teeth. It discusses current clinical treatment strategies, explores genetic analyses related to the phenotype, and proposes a roadmap for future genetic investigations. The research underscores the potential of understanding genetic and epigenetic factors for developing new preventive and treatment methods, incorporating technological advancements like 3D printing and CAD/CAM. The study suggests conducting comprehensive genomic analyses, including GWAS and RNAseq, in human tissues associated with deep-bite malocclusion. The collaborative cross-mouse model is highlighted as a valuable tool for identifying genetic factors, paving the way for personalized medicine and early prevention strategies.

The study by Lone et al. [27] explores malocclusion, a prevalent condition influenced by genetic, environmental, and oral behavioral factors, impacting oral functionality, aesthetics, and quality of life. Recognizing the significance of managing malocclusion in primary dentition, this review highlights its global prevalence and the use of Angle's classification system. Genetic factors, including variants in genes like MSX1, PAX9, and AXIN2, are associated with an increased risk of Class I occlusion. The review aims to provide insights into clinical strategies, genetic influences from human and murine populations, and RNA alterations in skeletal Class I occlusion. Mouse models are crucial for investigating genetic associations and mandible development.

Wiedermann et al. [28] present an opinion delving into the role of artificial intelligence-driven symptom checkers in addressing the challenges faced by modern healthcare, particularly in the context of an aging population and a decreasing general practitioner workforce. Drawing insights from a study in Italian general practices, the article explores the perspectives of both physicians and patients regarding the efficiency, utility, and challenges of symptom checkers. While these tools are seen as potential solutions, concerns about accuracy and misdiagnosis persist. The article proposes that AI-based symptom checkers can optimize medical history-taking, emphasizing the need for the careful integration of digital innovations while preserving the essential human touch in healthcare. Collaboration among technologists, clinicians, and patients is crucial for the successful evolution of digital tools in healthcare.

2.2. Common Message

All these works have made notable contributions to the field of personalized medicine, particularly at the intersection between AI and digital health. These contributions provide valuable insights and innovative approaches, contributing to our understanding of how AI and digital health can enhance personalized medicine. The integration of the technologies showcased in these studies offers practical implications for patient care, treatment strategies, and medical decision making, contributing to the ongoing progress in this field.

Twenty distinct contributions [9–28] weave through the intricate fields of the health domain focused on the integration of digital health and AI with precision medicine. These studies, spanning diverse medical domains, collectively leverage several AI and digital health approaches to precision medicine.

The scientific articles [10–16] offer a glimpse into the current priorities of scholars, with a distinct focus on the integration of digital health and AI within the realm of precision medicine. These articles illuminate the ongoing efforts of researchers, underscoring the increasing importance of incorporating advanced technologies into healthcare practices.

Transitioning to review studies [17–21], they play a critical role in providing essential scientific insights into the consolidation of themes. Importantly, these reviews highlight the pivotal role of AI in shaping the landscape of precision medicine, emphasizing its significance in guiding the current trajectory of research and knowledge consolidation.

Furthermore, homing in on systematic reviews [22,23], these works systematically identify patterns and scientific questions, offering a focused examination of specific areas where scholars are directing their attention. The thematic emphasis on digital health and AI becomes even more apparent, illustrating their integral role in addressing precise scientific inquiries.

Shifting to perspectives [24–27] and opinions [28], these contributions offer forward-looking insights from various angles, accentuating the dynamic landscape of digital health and AI in precision medicine. By opening up future possibilities, they significantly contribute to our understanding of potential directions and opportunities in this rapidly evolving field.

In essence, this collection not only paints a comprehensive picture of the current scholarly focus [10–28] but also underscores the central role of digital health and AI in advancing precision medicine. The thematic emphasis on these key elements reflects both the present intellectual climate [10–23] and the anticipated trajectories of research in this dynamic domain [24–28].

In this comprehensive exploration of AI in precision medicine, each contribution [9–28] unfolds a distinct facet of the evolving landscape. The focus extends from specialized areas such as radiomics [10] and the TB impact assessment [11] to the meticulous consideration of CBCT parameters [12] and the potential but cautious integration of large language models (LLMs) in breast cancer treatment decisions [13].

The significance of AI tools surfaces in nephrology searches in the literature [14], while the real-time predictive capabilities for cardiovascular diseases (CVDs) [15] promise proactive interventions. Chronic obstructive pulmonary disease (COPD) management [16] and AI's role in autism treatment [17] underscore the transformative impact of healthcare.

The panorama broadens as nephrology's interaction with AI [18] and the integration of ophthalmology chatbots [19] reveal a dynamic diagnostic landscape. AI's potential in cancer research [20] and the promising applications of digital twins in healthcare [21] reflect ongoing advancements and the need for careful ethical considerations.

The narrative unfolds further as we delve into AI's explainable role [22] and the prognostic applications in oncology [23], highlighting transparency and personalized patient care. Dental perspectives offer insights into malocclusions [24,26,27], while sarcoma care's transformation [25] and the role of AI-driven symptom checkers [28] provide a conclusive glance at the future.

This Special Issue not only encapsulates the current state of AI in precision medicine but also lays the foundation for an exciting and dynamic future, emphasizing collaborative efforts between technology, healthcare professionals, and patients.

2.3. Key Emerging Themes and Suggestions for a Broader Investigation

From the overview, it is also possible to detect the emerging themes (Table 1) and the suggestions for a broader investigation.

Table 1. Dominant emerging themes by study.

Themes	Description	Studies	
Cancer Research	Leung et al. [10], Griewing et al. [13], Fuchs et al. [25],	[10,13]	[25]
Pandemic Impact and Disease Dynamics	Morena et al. [11], Issa et al. [12]	[11,12]	
Cardiovascular and Pulmonary Insights	Elvas et al. [15], Pereira et al. [16]	[15,16]	
Neurological Disorders and Autism	Iannone and Giansanti [17]	[17]	
Nephrology and Healthcare Literature	Miao et al. [18], Aiumtrakul et al. [14]	[14,18]	
Ophthalmology Chatbots	Ittarat et al. [19]	[19]	
Cancer Diagnosis and AI Integration	Fawaz et al. [20]	[20]	
Digital Twin Technology in Healthcare	Meijer et al. [21]	[21]	
Dental Research	Lone et al. [24], Watted et al. [26], Lone et al. [27]	[24,26,27]	
Automatic Symptom Checking	Wiedermann et al. [28]	[28]	
Explainable AI in Precision Medicine	Allen [22]	[22]	
Oncology and Prognostic Evaluations	Michelutti et al. [23]	[23]	

The studies also reveal intriguing scientific insights for future research initiatives and expansions. In the exploration of the transformative landscape of precision medicine, interdisciplinary collaborations emerge as a pivotal theme [10–28]. Opportunities abound for AI experts, healthcare professionals, geneticists, and data scientists to forge synergies, fostering a holistic approach to personalized healthcare.

Ethical considerations take a central role in this evolving paradigm [22]. Delving into issues of patient privacy, data security, and equitable access, a thorough examination ensures the responsible integration of AI and digital health in precision medicine. Patient-centricity takes the spotlight [24,27], urging exploration into tailoring precision medicine to individual needs. Active patient involvement in decision making becomes a crucial aspect, aligning treatments with personal preferences and values. A global perspective unfolds [23,26], revealing diverse adoption patterns of precision medicine practices worldwide. Comparative analyses shed light on the challenges and successes within varying healthcare systems driven by AI approaches to personalized care. The long-term impact of AI and digital health reverberates through the discourse [16,28]. Factors such as cost-effectiveness, scalability, and sustainability are scrutinized, offering insights into strategies to overcome barriers and pave the way for widespread adoption. Integration with public health initiatives is a theme of paramount importance [15,21], outlining the potential role of AI-fueled precision medicine in the early detection, prevention, and management of diseases at the population level. Education and training for healthcare professionals come into focus [17,18], prompting an assessment of the current landscape. Strategies for incorporating relevant skills into medical and allied health curricula are proposed, envisioning a workforce that is prepared for the future of healthcare. Unraveling health disparities is a key exploration [11,20], scrutinizing AI-driven precision medicine's impact on existing inequalities. Strategies to ensure equitable access and benefits across diverse populations become integral to the evolving narrative. Regulatory frameworks and policies take center stage [13,19], highlighting the governance needed for the ethical and responsible use of AI in precision medicine. Collaborations on an international scale are investigated to establish common guidelines. The dynamic theme of continuous monitoring and feedback emerges [12,14], advocating real-time data integration into precision medicine models. The adaptation and improvement of treatment strategies over time become integral to the ongoing narrative.

3. Conclusions

In conclusion, the evolution of artificial intelligence technologies and digital health in the field of precision medicine offers promising prospects for enhancing patient outcomes and revolutionizing healthcare practices. The studies presented in this editorial highlight the growing intersection between cutting-edge technologies and personalized medicine. The research emphasizes the transformative potential of AI and digital health in driving precision medicine toward unprecedented levels of accuracy and efficiency.

This Special Issue significantly contributes to various domains, identifying both emerging and established themes and delineating intriguing directions for future advancements in digital health and AI in personalized medicine. This initiative underscores the importance of these editorial collections as a central hub for scholarly exchange and discussions among researchers worldwide, fostering collaboration and innovation in the ever-evolving landscape of precision medicine.

Conflicts of Interest: The authors declare no conflict of interest.

References

1. Available online: https://www.genome.gov/genetics-glossary/Personalized-Medicine (accessed on 10 March 2024).
2. Stefanicka-Wojtas, D.; Kurpas, D. Personalised Medicine—Implementation to the Healthcare System in Europe (Focus Group Discussions). *J. Pers. Med.* **2023**, *13*, 380. [CrossRef]
3. Raghavendran, H.R.B.; Kumaramanickavel, G.; Iwata, T. Editorial: Personalized medicine—Where do we stand regarding bench to bedside translation? *Front. Med.* **2023**, *10*, 1243896. [CrossRef]
4. Bollati, V.; Ferrari, L.; Leso, V.; Iavicoli, I. Personalised Medicine: Implication and perspectives in the field of occupational health. *Med. Lav.* **2020**, *111*, 425–444. [CrossRef] [PubMed]

5. Goetz, L.H.; Schork, N.J. Personalized medicine: Motivation, challenges, and progress. *Fertil. Steril.* **2018**, *109*, 952–963. [CrossRef] [PubMed]
6. Vicente, A.M.; Ballensiefen, W.; Jönsson, J.-I. How personalised medicine will transform healthcare by 2030: The ICPerMed vision. *J. Transl. Med.* **2020**, *18*, 180. [CrossRef] [PubMed]
7. Johnson, K.B.; Wei, W.; Weeraratne, D.; Frisse, M.E.; Misulis, K.; Rhee, K.; Zhao, J.; Snowdon, J.L. Precision Medicine, AI, and the Future of Personalized Health Care. *Clin. Transl. Sci.* **2021**, *14*, 86–93. [CrossRef] [PubMed]
8. Schork, N.J. Artificial Intelligence and Personalized Medicine. *Cancer Treat. Res.* **2019**, *178*, 265–283. [CrossRef] [PubMed]
9. Giansanti, D. Precision Medicine 2.0: How Digital Health and AI Are Changing the Game. *J. Pers. Med.* **2023**, *13*, 1057. [CrossRef] [PubMed]
10. Leung, V.W.S.; Ng, C.K.C.; Lam, S.-K.; Wong, P.-T.; Ng, K.-Y.; Tam, C.-H.; Lee, T.-C.; Chow, K.-C.; Chow, Y.-K.; Tam, V.C.W.; et al. Computed Tomography-Based Radiomics for Long-Term Prognostication of High-Risk Localized Prostate Cancer Patients Received Whole Pelvic Radiotherapy. *J. Pers. Med.* **2023**, *13*, 1643. [CrossRef]
11. Morena, D.; Campos, C.; Castillo, M.; Alonso, M.; Benavent, M.; Izquierdo, J.L. Impact of the COVID-19 Pandemic on the Epidemiological Situation of Pulmonary Tuberculosis–Using Natural Language Processing. *J. Pers. Med.* **2023**, *13*, 1629. [CrossRef]
12. Issa, J.; Riad, A.; Olszewski, R.; Dyszkiewicz-Konwińska, M. The Influence of Slice Thickness, Sharpness, and Contrast Adjustments on Inferior Alveolar Canal Segmentation on Cone-Beam Computed Tomography Scans: A Retrospective Study. *J. Pers. Med.* **2023**, *13*, 1518. [CrossRef] [PubMed]
13. Griewing, S.; Gremke, N.; Wagner, U.; Lingenfelder, M.; Kuhn, S.; Boekhoff, J. Challenging ChatGPT 3.5 in Senology—An Assessment of Concordance with Breast Cancer Tumor Board Decision Making. *J. Pers. Med.* **2023**, *13*, 1502. [CrossRef] [PubMed]
14. Aiumtrakul, N.; Thongprayoon, C.; Suppadungsuk, S.; Krisanapan, P.; Miao, J.; Qureshi, F.; Cheungpasitporn, W. Navigating the Landscape of Personalized Medicine: The Relevance of ChatGPT, BingChat, and Bard AI in Nephrology Literature Searches. *J. Pers. Med.* **2023**, *13*, 1457. [CrossRef] [PubMed]
15. Elvas, L.B.; Nunes, M.; Ferreira, J.C.; Dias, M.S.; Rosário, L.B. AI-Driven Decision Support for Early Detection of Cardiac Events: Unveiling Patterns and Predicting Myocardial Ischemia. *J. Pers. Med.* **2023**, *13*, 1421. [CrossRef] [PubMed]
16. Pereira, J.; Antunes, N.; Rosa, J.; Ferreira, J.C.; Mogo, S.; Pereira, M. Intelligent Clinical Decision Support System for Managing COPD Patients. *J. Pers. Med.* **2023**, *13*, 1359. [CrossRef] [PubMed]
17. Iannone, A.; Giansanti, D. Breaking Barriers—The Intersection of AI and Assistive Technology in Autism Care: A Narrative Review. *J. Pers. Med.* **2024**, *14*, 41. [CrossRef]
18. Miao, J.; Thongprayoon, C.; Suppadungsuk, S.; Garcia Valencia, O.A.; Qureshi, F.; Cheungpasitporn, W. Innovating Personalized Nephrology Care: Exploring the Potential Utilization of ChatGPT. *J. Pers. Med.* **2023**, *13*, 1681. [CrossRef] [PubMed]
19. Ittarat, M.; Cheungpasitporn, W.; Chansangpetch, S. Personalized Care in Eye Health: Exploring Opportunities, Challenges, and the Road Ahead for Chatbots. *J. Pers. Med.* **2023**, *13*, 1679. [CrossRef] [PubMed]
20. Fawaz, A.; Ferraresi, A.; Isidoro, C. Systems Biology in Cancer Diagnosis Integrating Omics Technologies and Artificial Intelligence to Support Physician Decision Making. *J. Pers. Med.* **2023**, *13*, 1590. [CrossRef]
21. Meijer, C.; Uh, H.-W.; el Bouhaddani, S. Digital Twins in Healthcare: Methodological Challenges and Opportunities. *J. Pers. Med.* **2023**, *13*, 1522. [CrossRef]
22. Allen, B. The Promise of Explainable AI in Digital Health for Precision Medicine: A Systematic Review. *J. Pers. Med.* **2024**, *14*, 277. [CrossRef] [PubMed]
23. Michelutti, L.; Tel, A.; Zeppieri, M.; Ius, T.; Sembronio, S.; Robiony, M. The Use of Artificial Intelligence Algorithms in the Prognosis and Detection of Lymph Node Involvement in Head and Neck Cancer and Possible Impact in the Development of Personalized Therapeutic Strategy: A Systematic Review. *J. Pers. Med.* **2023**, *13*, 1626. [CrossRef] [PubMed]
24. Lone, I.M.; Zohud, O.; Midlej, K.; Paddenberg, E.; Krohn, S.; Kirschneck, C.; Proff, P.; Watted, N.; Iraqi, F.A. Anterior Open Bite Malocclusion: From Clinical Treatment Strategies towards the Dissection of the Genetic Bases of the Disease Using Human and Collaborative Cross Mice Cohorts. *J. Pers. Med.* **2023**, *13*, 1617. [CrossRef] [PubMed]
25. Fuchs, B.; Studer, G.; Bode-Lesniewska, B.; Heesen, P.; on behalf of the Swiss Sarcoma Network. The Next Frontier in Sarcoma Care: Digital Health, AI, and the Quest for Precision Medicine. *J. Pers. Med.* **2023**, *13*, 1530. [CrossRef] [PubMed]
26. Watted, N.; Lone, I.M.; Zohud, O.; Midlej, K.; Proff, P.; Iraqi, F.A. Comprehensive Deciphering the Complexity of the Deep Bite: Insight from Animal Model to Human Subjects. *J. Pers. Med.* **2023**, *13*, 1472. [CrossRef]
27. Lone, I.M.; Zohud, O.; Midlej, K.; Awadi, O.; Masarwa, S.; Krohn, S.; Kirschneck, C.; Proff, P.; Watted, N.; Iraqi, F.A. Narrating the Genetic Landscape of Human Class I Occlusion: A Perspective-Infused Review. *J. Pers. Med.* **2023**, *13*, 1465. [CrossRef]
28. Wiedermann, C.J.; Mahlknecht, A.; Piccoliori, G.; Engl, A. Redesigning Primary Care: The Emergence of Artificial-Intelligence-Driven Symptom Diagnostic Tools. *J. Pers. Med.* **2023**, *13*, 1379. [CrossRef]

Disclaimer/Publisher's Note: The statements, opinions and data contained in all publications are solely those of the individual author(s) and contributor(s) and not of MDPI and/or the editor(s). MDPI and/or the editor(s) disclaim responsibility for any injury to people or property resulting from any ideas, methods, instructions or products referred to in the content.

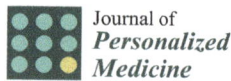

Journal of *Personalized Medicine*

Editorial

Precision Medicine 2.0: How Digital Health and AI Are Changing the Game

Daniele Giansanti

Centre TISP, ISS, 00161 Rome, Italy; daniele.giansanti@iss.it

Citation: Giansanti, D. Precision Medicine 2.0: How Digital Health and AI Are Changing the Game. *J. Pers. Med.* **2023**, *13*, 1057. https://doi.org/10.3390/jpm13071057

Received: 20 June 2023
Accepted: 25 June 2023
Published: 28 June 2023

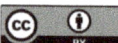

Copyright: © 2023 by the author. Licensee MDPI, Basel, Switzerland. This article is an open access article distributed under the terms and conditions of the Creative Commons Attribution (CC BY) license (https://creativecommons.org/licenses/by/4.0/).

In the era of rapid IT developments, the *health domain* is undergoing a considerable transformation [1]. The integration of *Digital Health* (DH) with *Artificial Intelligence* (AI) has paved the way for Precision Medicine 2.0, a groundbreaking approach that holds the promise of revolutionizing patient care [2–4]. The potential implications of this transformation are widespread, as it empowers healthcare professionals to deliver tailored treatments and improve patient outcomes. It is possible to identify the key contributions of this transformation for both AI and DH.

It can generally be stated that the *medico-biological elements of information* are treated by AI and DH with different roles and approaches. The first, AI, *mainly deals with the intelligent processing of this information, transforming it into decisions and therapeutic activations with the patient at the center* [5–10]; the second, DH, *takes care of its transmission, the taking it (also from the patient through sensors), and transporting/delivering information to the decision-making and activation nodes of the healthcare system, and also by developing innovative devices* [11–18].

AI makes a significant contribution, enabling the processing of large volumes of complex data and producing tailored information about a patient with a predictive capacity for the improvement and fine-tuning of therapeutic path in all phases.

AI enables [5–10]:

-*Data analysis:* Thanks to AI, it is possible to analyze large datasets (e.g.; BIG-DATA) and to extract calibrated intervention models that would otherwise be impossible, through, for example, the identification of more accurate prognostic, diagnostic, and predictive markers for specific diseases.

-*AI-assisted diagnosis:* AI has the potential to provide important support to instrumental diagnosis with specific algorithms, such as in the case of medical diagnostics, in digital pathology, digital radiology, digital dermatology.

-*Personalization of the treatment, monitoring, and management of disease*: AI, through the analysis of clinical and molecular data combined with information obtained from large external electronic data archives, can enable tuning and personalized treatment optimization; the elaboration of physiological parameters derived from wearable devices enables monitoring, and if necessary, adaptation of a patient's care.

-*Predictive medicine:* AI can develop an interoperable data connection from the patient to the healthcare system and vice versa, by applying continuously updated algorithms, which provide and uses distributed *medical knowledge*, and can be used for predictive purposes of pathologies based on risk analysis.

-*Production of medical knowledge:* In all the activities described, AI contributes to the research and development of clinical and medical practice on various scales.

DH plays a fundamental role in precision medicine, enabling the interconnection of medico-biological data and the creation of technological solutions that support the personalization of care that may use AI and/or other decisional approaches based on algorithms [11–18].

DH, for example, enables:

-*Personalized data collection:* DH enables the collection of detailed patient data. Wearable devices allow, by means of specific sensors, the monitoring of physiological parameters, lifestyles, diets, and other useful information. These data can be integrated with further information from other databases.

-*Remote Monitoring:* Digital technologies, such as wearable devices, also enable continuous monitoring of the patient to modify the therapy and/or activate emergency actions when needed.

-*Data Sharing:* DH enables data sharing while respecting cybersecurity. The secure integration of data from many sources, including electronic patient records, diagnostic images, laboratory data, and genomic data, is therefore possible.

-*Clinical Decision Support:* DH can provide the HW/SW base for clinical decision support systems using AI or tools for data analytics.

-*Telemedicine:* Telemedicine enables the remote delivery of healthcare services. Thanks to advanced DH solutions (also using AI), telemedicine can be increasingly tailored to an individual patient.

Targeted searches on PubMed suggest the scale of growth in the volume of studies in this area.

Regarding the studies in precision medicine, searches for the keywords reported in Box 1 *position* 1 highlighted 20,160 studies starting from 1979. Of these studies, 11,646 (57.7%) had been carried out starting from 1 January 2020. In all, there were 8142 reviews (systematic and non-systematic).

Regarding the studies on precision medicine focused on DH, searches for the keywords reported in Box 1 *position* 2 highlighted 94 studies starting from 2013. Of these studies, 65 (69.9%) had been carried out from 1 January 2020. In all, there were 37 reviews (systematic and not).

Regarding the studies on precision medicine focused on AI, searches for the keywords reported in Box 1 *position* 3 highlighted 796 studies starting from 2015. Of these studies, 670 (84, 2%) had been carried out from 1 January 2020. In all, there were 438 reviews (systematic and non-systematic).

This brief overview highlights how, in these sectors, there has been an acceleration of scientific production and interest during the COVID-19 pandemic period; interest in studies on AI and DH is more recent (the 2000s); the comparison between AI and DH indicates greater interest in AI, i.e., a stronger interest in an intelligent IT approach than for the architecture of the information flow; and there is a good proportion of reviews for both AI and DH, indicating good progress in the stabilization of topics of scientific interest (Figure 1).

Box 1. Composite key used for the searches in PubMed.

(precision medicine[Title/Abstract])
(precision medicine[Title/Abstract]) AND (digital health[Title/Abstract])
(precision medicine[Title/Abstract]) AND (artificial intelligence[Title/Abstract])

Precision medicine has an older history than expected; the first studies date back to 1979. Its meaning has evolved [1,19] together with the expectations that scholars have gradually placed on it. Today, it could change healthcare both as we know it and how we evaluate it [20,21].

Emerging technologies, such as AI and DH (both individually and as a whole) are making an important contribution to the developments of this discipline. A real integration with the *health domain* will have to respect all the domains of action, from regulatory to ethical spheres.

There is an urgent need for discussion in this area to exchange and share universal experiences, both on opportunities and on problems and even failures. With this in mind, the Special Issue, entitled "Transforming Precision Medicine: The Intersection of Digital Health and AI" [22] was launched.

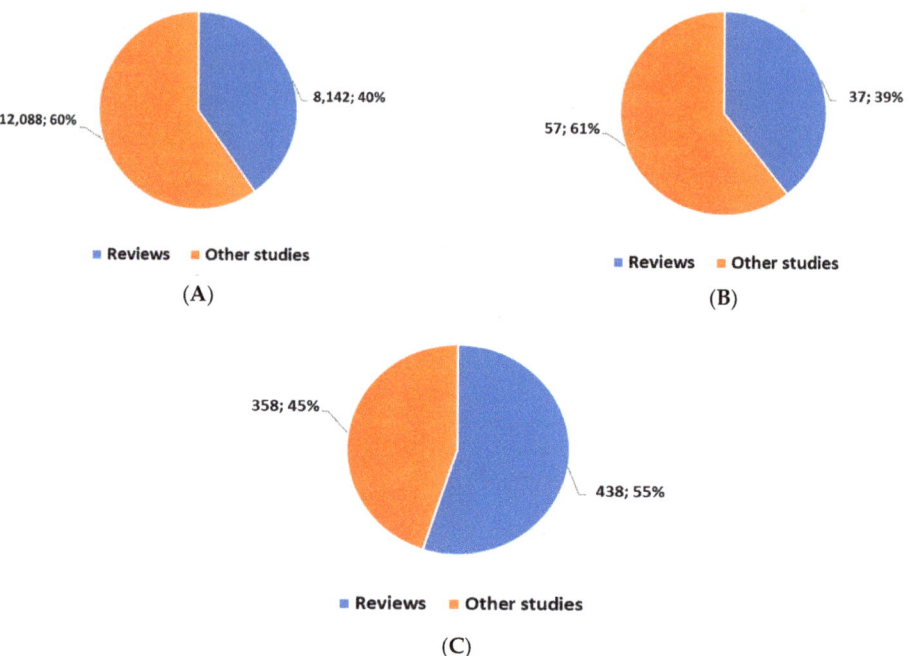

Figure 1. Volume of publications for the field of precision medicine (**A**); for the field of precision medicine and DH (**B**); and for the field of precision medicine and AI (**C**).

Conclusions

The COVID-19 pandemic has led to a considerable acceleration in research and development on the applications of AI and DH in the precision medicine.

Scholars, experts, professionals, and stakeholders in the health domain are working both on the developments and integration on multiple domains. There is an increasing need for studies focused on AI and DH in clinical imaging, as well as synergistic initiatives such as collections or Special Issues which touch on both successes and failures, as well as opportunities and bottlenecks.

Conflicts of Interest: The author declares no conflict of interest.

References

1. Ginsburg, G.S.; Phillips, K.A. Precision Medicine: From Science To Value. *Health Aff.* **2018**, *37*, 694–701. [CrossRef] [PubMed]
2. Yang, Y.C.; Islam, S.U.; Noor, A.; Khan, S.; Afsar, W.; Nazir, S. Influential Usage of Big Data and Artificial Intelligence in Healthcare. *Comput. Math. Methods Med.* **2021**, *2021*, 5812499. [CrossRef] [PubMed]
3. Dhawan, A.P. Collaborative Paradigm of Preventive, Personalized, and Precision Medicine With Point-of-Care Technologies. *IEEE J. Transl. Eng. Health Med.* **2016**, *4*, 2800908. [CrossRef] [PubMed]
4. Huttin, C.C. Global value chains and international pharmaceutical policy. *Technol. Health Care* **2020**, *28*, 337–344. [CrossRef] [PubMed]
5. Bhinder, B.; Gilvary, C.; Madhukar, N.S.; Elemento, O. Artificial Intelligence in Cancer Research and Precision Medicine. *Cancer Discov.* **2021**, *11*, 900–915. [CrossRef] [PubMed]
6. Chen, Z.H.; Lin, L.; Wu, C.F.; Li, C.F.; Xu, R.H.; Sun, Y. Artificial intelligence for assisting cancer diagnosis and treatment in the era of precision medicine. *Cancer Commun.* **2021**, *41*, 1100–1115. [CrossRef] [PubMed]
7. Tunali, I.; Gillies, R.J.; Schabath, M.B. Application of Radiomics and Artificial Intelligence for Lung Cancer Precision Medicine. *Cold Spring Harb. Perspect. Med.* **2021**, *11*, a039537. [CrossRef] [PubMed]
8. Lin, E.; Lin, C.H.; Lane, H.Y. Precision Psychiatry Applications with Pharmacogenomics: Artificial Intelligence and Machine Learning Approaches. *Int. J. Mol. Sci.* **2020**, *21*, 969. [CrossRef] [PubMed]

9. Subramanian, M.; Wojtusciszyn, A.; Favre, L.; Boughorbel, S.; Shan, J.; Letaief, K.B.; Pitteloud, N.; Chouchane, L. Precision medicine in the era of artificial intelligence: Implications in chronic disease management. *J. Transl. Med.* **2020**, *18*, 472. [CrossRef] [PubMed]
10. Bonkhoff, A.K.; Grefkes, C. Precision medicine in stroke: Towards personalized outcome predictions using artificial intelligence. *Brain* **2022**, *145*, 457–475. [CrossRef] [PubMed]
11. Shan, R.; Sarkar, S.; Martin, S.S. Digital health technology and mobile devices for the management of diabetes mellitus: State of the art. *Diabetologia* **2019**, *62*, 877–887. [CrossRef] [PubMed]
12. Barrigon, M.L.; Courtet, P.; Oquendo, M.; Baca-García, E. Precision Medicine and Suicide: An Opportunity for Digital Health. *Curr. Psychiatry Rep.* **2019**, *21*, 131. [CrossRef] [PubMed]
13. Dillenseger, A.; Weidemann, M.L.; Trentzsch, K.; Inojosa, H.; Haase, R.; Schriefer, D.; Voigt, I.; Scholz, M.; Akgün, K.; Ziemssen, T. Digital Biomarkers in Multiple Sclerosis. *Brain Sci.* **2021**, *11*, 1519. [CrossRef] [PubMed]
14. Fernandez-Luque, L.; Al Herbish, A.; Al Shammari, R.; Argente, J.; Bin-Abbas, B.; Deeb, A.; Dixon, D.; Zary, N.; Koledova, E.; Savage, M.O. Digital Health for Supporting Precision Medicine in Pediatric Endocrine Disorders: Opportunities for Improved Patient Care. *Front. Pediatr.* **2021**, *9*, 715705. [CrossRef] [PubMed]
15. Lui, G.Y.; Loughnane, D.; Polley, C.; Jayarathna, T.; Breen, P.P. The Apple Watch for Monitoring Mental Health-Related Physiological Symptoms: Literature Review. *JMIR Ment. Health* **2022**, *9*, e37354. [CrossRef] [PubMed]
16. Espay, A.J.; Bonato, P.; Nahab, F.B.; Maetzler, W.; Dean, J.M.; Klucken, J.; Eskofier, B.M.; Merola, A.; Horak, F.; Lang, A.E.; et al. Movement Disorders Society Task Force on Technology. Technology in Parkinson's disease: Challenges and opportunities. *Mov. Disord.* **2016**, *31*, 1272–1282. [CrossRef] [PubMed]
17. Lee, B.O. Precision Health and Nursing Care in the Digital Age. *Hu Li Za Zhi* **2022**, *69*, 4–6. (In Chinese) [CrossRef] [PubMed]
18. Adamo, J.E.; Bienvenu Ii, R.V.; Dolz, F.; Liebman, M.; Nilsen, W.; Steele, S.J. Translation of Digital Health Technologies to Advance Precision Medicine: Informing Regulatory Science. *Digit. Biomark.* **2020**, *4*, 1–12. [CrossRef] [PubMed]
19. Philisps, jc. Precision Medicine and Its Imprecise History Issue 2.1, Winter 2020 (mit.edu). Available online: https://hdsr.mitpress.mit.edu/pub/y7r65r4k/release/4 (accessed on 19 June 2023).
20. Gameiro, G.R.; Sinkunas, V.; Liguori, G.R.; Auler-Júnior, J.O.C. Precision Medicine: Changing the way we think about healthcare. *Clinics* **2018**, *73*, e723. [CrossRef] [PubMed]
21. Love-Koh, J.; Peel, A.; Rejon-Parrilla, J.C.; Ennis, K.; Lovett, R.; Manca, A.; Chalkidou, A.; Wood, H.; Taylor, M. The Future of Precision Medicine: Potential Impacts for Health Technology Assessment. *Pharmacoeconomics* **2018**, *36*, 1439–1451. [CrossRef] [PubMed]
22. Special Issue: Transforming Precision Medicine: The Intersection of Digital Health and, A.I. Available online: https://www.mdpi.com/journal/jpm/special_issues/4FMFQUN50A (accessed on 20 June 2023).

Disclaimer/Publisher's Note: The statements, opinions and data contained in all publications are solely those of the individual author(s) and contributor(s) and not of MDPI and/or the editor(s). MDPI and/or the editor(s) disclaim responsibility for any injury to people or property resulting from any ideas, methods, instructions or products referred to in the content.

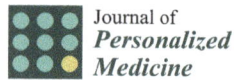

Systematic Review

The Promise of Explainable AI in Digital Health for Precision Medicine: A Systematic Review

Ben Allen

Department of Psychology, University of Kansas, Lawrence, KS 66045, USA; benallen@ku.edu

Abstract: This review synthesizes the literature on explaining machine-learning models for digital health data in precision medicine. As healthcare increasingly tailors treatments to individual characteristics, the integration of artificial intelligence with digital health data becomes crucial. Leveraging a topic-modeling approach, this paper distills the key themes of 27 journal articles. We included peer-reviewed journal articles written in English, with no time constraints on the search. A Google Scholar search, conducted up to 19 September 2023, yielded 27 journal articles. Through a topic-modeling approach, the identified topics encompassed optimizing patient healthcare through data-driven medicine, predictive modeling with data and algorithms, predicting diseases with deep learning of biomedical data, and machine learning in medicine. This review delves into specific applications of explainable artificial intelligence, emphasizing its role in fostering transparency, accountability, and trust within the healthcare domain. Our review highlights the necessity for further development and validation of explanation methods to advance precision healthcare delivery.

Keywords: digital health; explainable artificial intelligence; precision medicine; machine learning

Citation: Allen, B. The Promise of Explainable AI in Digital Health for Precision Medicine: A Systematic Review. *J. Pers. Med.* **2024**, *14*, 277. https://doi.org/10.3390/jpm14030277

Academic Editors: Juergen Hahn and Daniele Giansanti

Received: 18 December 2023
Revised: 14 February 2024
Accepted: 24 February 2024
Published: 1 March 2024

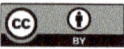

Copyright: © 2024 by the author. Licensee MDPI, Basel, Switzerland. This article is an open access article distributed under the terms and conditions of the Creative Commons Attribution (CC BY) license (https://creativecommons.org/licenses/by/4.0/).

1. Introduction

Precision medicine is a way of personalizing treatments and interventions to the patient's characteristics, such as genetics, environment, and lifestyle [1]. This personalized medicine is a shift in healthcare to the use of information unique to the patient as a guide for diagnosis and prognosis [2]. Precision medicine has the allure of increasing the reach of medical treatment beyond the one-size-fits-all approach, especially when leveraging advanced bioinformatic strategies to interpret and apply clinical data and provide patients with customized medical care [3]. Precision medicine has the potential to make healthcare more efficient and effective [4].

A major catalyst toward the success of personalized medicine is the integration of different forms of digital healthcare data with artificial intelligence to make more accurate interpretations of diagnostic information, reduce medical errors, and improve health system workflow and promote health [5]. A noteworthy example comes from a study of an artificial-intelligence system trained to suggest different chemotherapy treatments based on the predicted treatment response given the patient gene-expression data [6]. The prediction models showed accuracy near 80% and might eventually help cancer patients avoid failing therapies. There are similar studies of artificial-intelligence systems trained to suggest different antidepressant treatments based on digital health records [7]. Overall, these studies suggest that clinical support systems could help personalize healthcare delivery when given the right reservoir of digital health data [8].

Digital health technologies are a rich reservoir of big health data for personalizing medicine. For example, wearable biosensors can measure valuable health-related physiological data for patient monitoring and management [9]. Telemedicine also has the potential to make healthcare more cost-effective while meeting the increasing demand for and insufficient supply of healthcare providers [10]. Overall, artificial-intelligence applications can leverage digital health data to implement personalized treatment strategies [1,5].

One of the key challenges in implementing precision medicine is integrating diverse and comprehensive data sources that encompass genetic, environmental, and lifestyle factors to ensure healthcare systems improve patient outcomes and effectively manage diseases [1,4]. The integration of complex datasets can be an overwhelming task for even a team of humans, but is relatively trivial for artificial-intelligence systems. Evidence of such integration is demonstrated in machine-learning models trained to make breast cancer diagnoses using digital health records along with analysis of mammography images [11]. Notably the prediction model showed a specificity of 77% and sensitivity of 87%, suggesting potential for reducing false-negatives. As artificial-intelligence systems become more prevalent in healthcare, such systems will be able to leverage genetic, environmental, and lifestyle data to help advance a personalized medicine approach [12].

Integrating important health data requires responsible handling and safeguards to prevent misuse of protected health information [13]. More recently, integrating and interpreting complex health data for personalized medicine is becoming the job of artificial intelligence [5]. Yet, developing countries may have limited access to these artificial-intelligence applications, highlighting the importance of open-source code [14]. Moreover, there can be misuse of health information embedded in prediction models used by artificial-intelligence systems to extract patterns from data to inform medical decisions [15]. As artificial-intelligence applications become more prevalent in healthcare, there is a great need to ensure ethical issues are considered along the way [16].

Integrating artificial intelligence into healthcare offers several potential benefits, including more accurate diagnostic/prognostic tools, more efficient personalization of treatment strategies using big data, and overall better optimization of healthcare workflows [5,17]. The sheer volume of patient health data available also makes integration via artificial intelligence into healthcare a necessity. Artificial-intelligence systems can quickly extract meaningful patterns and insights from multiple data sources, enabling better-informed decisions about how to personalize healthcare [15].

But the desire for accurate artificial-intelligence systems must be balanced with the goal of transparency and interpretability to build trust among healthcare practitioners and patients and ensure the responsible integration of insights into clinical decision-making [18]. It is important to foster a collaborative approach between human expertise and machine intelligence by understanding an artificial-intelligence-system's rationale when making medical decisions [5]. The rising field of explainable artificial intelligence centers around the ability to comprehend and interpret artificial-intelligence systems [19]. Explainable artificial intelligence promotes trust through transparency and accountability in artificial-intelligence applications for healthcare [17]. For precision medicine, healthcare practitioners are more likely to trust in the outcome of complex algorithms they can understand, giving explainable methods a position to ensure transparent models for personalized treatment strategies [19,20].

This review is a critical evaluation of the literature on how explainable artificial intelligence can facilitate the pursuit of precision medicine using digital health data. A secondary objective was to offer key strategies and knowledge gaps in addressing the challenges in interpretability and transparency of artificial-intelligence systems for precision medicine using digital health data. The primary inquiry addressed in this review was discerning the core themes and the status of research at the confluence of digital health, precision medicine, and explainable artificial-intelligence methodologies. This systematic review serves to pinpoint the benefits and challenges of applying explainable artificial-intelligence methods with digital health data for precision medicine.

This paper consolidates recent literature and offers a comprehensive synthesis of how to apply explainable artificial-intelligence methods to the utilization of digital health data in precision medicine. Machine learning is an effective approach to identifying treatment targets and accurately predicting treatment outcomes [21]. For example, there is evidence for using an artificial-intelligence-based system to select patients for intervention using the electrocardiograph signal to predict atrial fibrillation [22]. Employing a topic-modeling approach, this study extracted key themes and emerging trends from the literature on using explainable artificial intelligence and digital health data for precision medicine. Topic modeling is an unsupervised learning method for uncovering prevalent themes within a body of text [23,24]. Therefore, this paper provides a compilation for precision medicine of explainable artificial intelligence approaches to digital health.

2. Materials and Methods

2.1. Topic-Modeling-Procedure Overview

Insights derived from a topic-modeling analysis of the relevant literature directed this review. Specifically, the latent Dirichlet allocation (LDA) algorithm helped uncover prevalent themes in a final corpus of journal articles by analyzing the probability patterns of words and word pairs across the documents. The methods outlined in the subsequent sections followed the PRISMA 2020 checklist and were pre-registered on the Open Science Foundation (https://osf.io/tpxh6, registered on 19 September 2023) [25]. The Supplementary Materials include the checklist and code for the data analysis is available at https://zenodo.org/records/10398384, accessed on 19 September 2023.

2.2. Journal Article Search Strategy

A google scholar search (accessed on 19 September 2023) identified 434 journal articles relevant to this review. The search terms included: ("precision medicine" AND "digital health" AND "interpretable machine learning" OR "explainable artificial intelligence"). Inclusion criteria were that the article be written in English and was a peer-reviewed journal article, and full text was available, and included the search terms in the body of the text. The search was not restricted by date, though the earliest article matching our search terms was published in 2018. Citations and full-text articles were imported to the Zotero reference management software (https://www.zotero.org/). Zotero automatically classifies articles by type (i.e., journal article, pre-print, thesis, etc.). Each article's classification was verified by the author. To screen for keywords in the text body, the reference sections were removed from each article, and spelling and grammar were checked through Google Docs. From each journal article, we extracted bigrams (consecutive word pairs). Articles only containing search terms in the reference section were excluded. Figure 1 shows the PRISMA 2020 flowchart which illustrates how the final set of articles was determined [26]. Table 1 shows the resulting 27 articles that directly connected explainable artificial intelligence to digital health and precision medicine.

2.3. Topic Modeling R

All text analysis and pre-processing occurred through the R programming language (version 4.3.1, 16 June 2023). We used the full text of each journal article, with the reference sections deleted; articles were segmented into paragraphs ($n = 1733$). The paragraphs were pre-processed by deleting punctuation, numbers, stop words, and symbols using the *tm* R package (version 0.7-8). Finally, we lemmatized each word and tokenized the text into unigrams, bigrams, and trigrams. This process helped combine counts of similar words with slightly different spellings. We removed 1 paragraph with fewer than 5 terms and removed all terms that occurred in only 1 paragraph ($n = 241{,}027$), resulting in 1732 paragraphs and 262 unique terms.

Using the *ldatuning* R package (version 1.0.2), we calculated coherence metrics for topic models of various sizes to estimate the optimal number of topics inherent to the collection of paragraphs. Next, we randomly split paragraphs into ten subsets, computed coherence metrics for topic models ranging from 2 to 20 topics, and repeated the process ten times to prevent bias. The median coherence scores across iterations suggested that a 5-topic model was optimal based on coherence. Subsequently, we employed the Gibbs algorithm to estimate a 5-topic latent Dirichlet allocation model for the entire corpus.

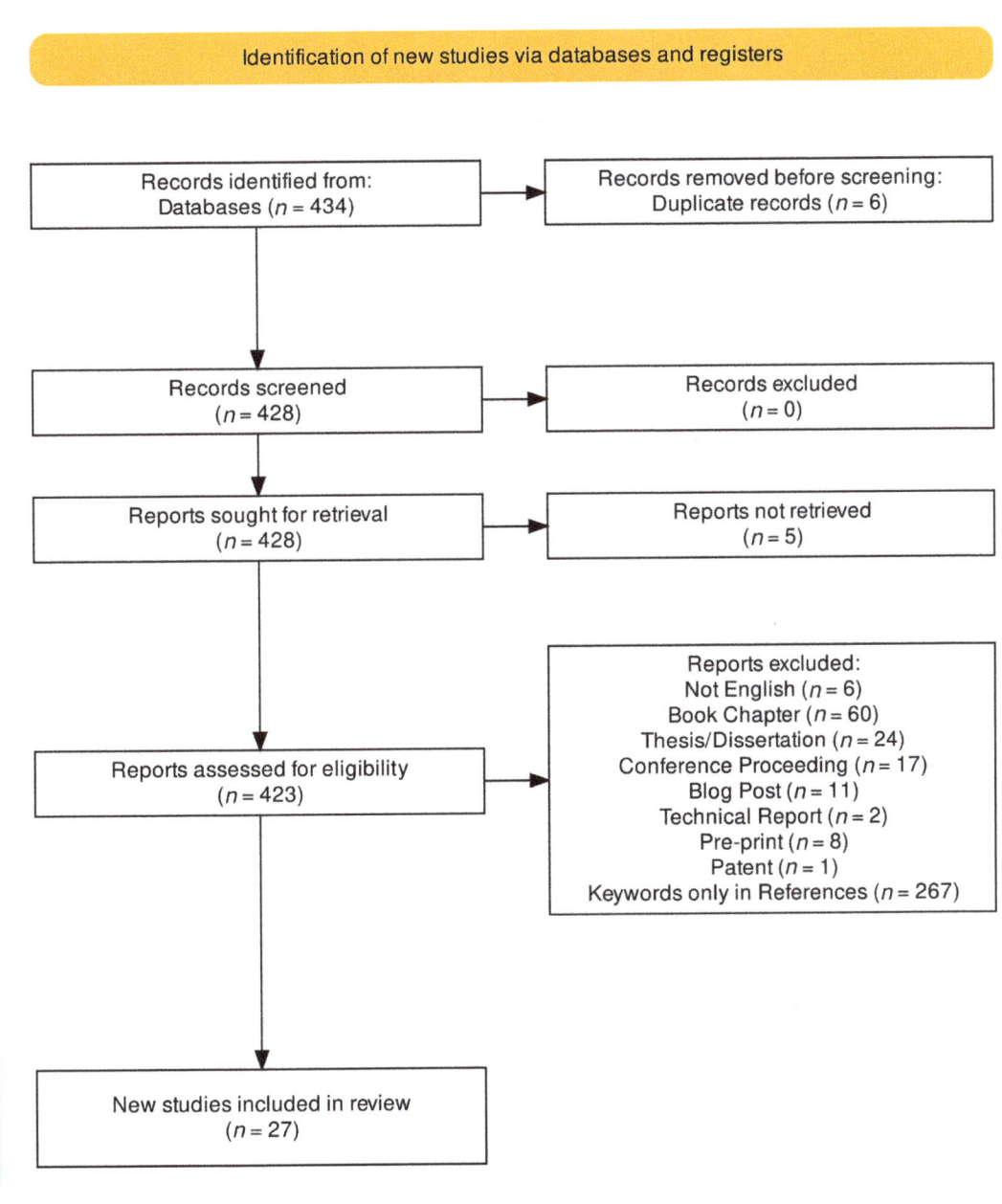

Figure 1. PRISMA 2020 flowchart. https://estech.shinyapps.io/prisma_flowdiagram/ (accessed on 1 January 2024.

Table 1. List of selected journal articles.

Author	Year	Title	Publication Title
Evans et al.	2018	The Challenge of Regulating Clinical Decision Support Software After 21st Century Cures	American Journal of Law & Medicine
Adadi et al.	2019	Gastroenterology Meets Machine Learning: Status Quo and Quo Vadis	Advances in bioinformatics
Shin et al.	2019	Current Status and Future Direction of Digital Health in Korea	The Korean Journal of Physiology & Pharmacology
Ahirwar et al.	2020	Interpretable Machine Learning in Health Care: Survey and Discussions	International Journal of Innovative Research in Technology and Management
Coppola et al.	2021	Human, All Too Human? An All-Around Appraisal of The "Artificial Intelligence Revolution" in Medical Imaging	Frontiers in Psychology
Wickramasinghe et al.	2021	A Vision for Leveraging the Concept of Digital Twins to Support the Provision of Personalized Cancer Care	IEEE Internet Computing
Bhatt et al.	2022	Emerging Artificial Intelligence–Empowered mHealth: Scoping Review	JMIR mHealth and uHealth
Chun et al.	2022	Prediction of Conversion to Dementia Using Interpretable Machine Learning in Patients with Amnestic Mild Cognitive Impairment	Frontiers in Aging Neuroscience
Gerussi et al.	2022	Artificial Intelligence for Precision Medicine in Autoimmune Liver Disease	Frontiers in Immunology
Iqbal et al.	2022	The Use and Ethics of Digital Twins in Medicine	Journal of Law, Medicine & Ethics
Ishengoma et al.	2022	Artificial Intelligence in Digital Health: Issues and Dimensions of Ethical Concerns	Innovación y Software
Khanna et al.	2022	Economics of Artificial Intelligence in Healthcare: Diagnosis vs. Treatment	Healthcare
Kline et al.	2022	Multimodal Machine Learning in Precision Health: A Scoping Review	npj Digital Medicine
Laccourreye et al.	2022	Explainable Machine Learning for Longitudinal Multi-Omic Microbiome	Mathematics
Roy et al.	2022	Demystifying Supervised Learning in Healthcare 4.0: A New Reality of Transforming Diagnostic Medicine	Diagnostics
Shazly et al.	2022	Introduction to Machine Learning in Obstetrics and Gynecology	Obstetrics & Gynecology
Wellnhofer et al.	2022	Real-World and Regulatory Perspectives of Artificial Intelligence in Cardiovascular Imaging	Frontiers in Cardiovascular Medicine
Wesołowski et al.	2022	An Explainable Artificial Intelligence Approach for Predicting Cardiovascular Outcomes Using Electronic Health Records	PLOS digital health
Albahri et al.	2023	A Systematic Review of Trustworthy and Explainable Artificial Intelligence in Healthcare: Assessment of Quality, Bias Risk, and Data Fusion	Information Fusion
Baumgartner et al.	2023	Fair and Equitable AI in Biomedical Research and Healthcare: Social Science Perspectives	Artificial Intelligence in Medicine
Bharati et al.	2023	A Review on Explainable Artificial Intelligence for Healthcare: Why, How, and When?	IEEE Transactions on Artificial Intelligence
Hong et al.	2023	Overcoming the Challenges in the Development and Implementation of Artificial Intelligence in Radiology: A Comprehensive Review of Solutions Beyond Supervised Learning	Korean Journal of Radiology
King et al.	2023	What Works Where and How for Uptake and Impact of Artificial Intelligence in Pathology: Review of Theories for a Realist Evaluation	Journal of Medical Internet Research
Kuwaiti et al.	2023	A Review of the Role of Artificial Intelligence in Healthcare	Journal of Personalized Medicine
Narayan et al.	2023	A Strategic Research Framework for Defeating Diabetes in India: A 21st-Century Agenda	Journal of the Indian Institute of Science
Vorisek et al.	2023	Artificial Intelligence Bias in Health Care: Web-Based Survey	Journal of Medical Internet Research
Zafar et al.	2023	Reviewing Methods of Deep Learning for Intelligent Healthcare Systems in Genomics and Biomedicine	Biomedical Signal Processing and Control

3. Results

Using a latent Dirichlet allocation model, we built a five-topic model based on the corpus of 27 journal articles that matched search terms. As topic modeling is unsupervised machine learning, one of the identified topics did not directly relate to the keywords. It identified a segment of paragraphs that described methods used to conduct literature reviews. That topic is omitted from the results below. The remaining four topics are discussed below based on an evaluation of each topic's most probable n-grams, 100 most probable paragraphs, and their parent paper's findings on precision medicine, digital health, and explainable artificial intelligence. The last two topics are merged under one heading because they are both related to deep learning and explainable artificial-intelligence research.

3.1. AI Explainability Addresses Ethical Challenges in Healthcare

Artificial intelligence (AI) is integral to offering solutions to various challenges in healthcare, including the standardization of digital health applications and ethical concerns related to patient data use [27,28]. Precision medicine, a common application of AI in digital health, involves tailoring healthcare interventions to subgroups of patients by using prediction models trained on patient characteristics and contextual factors [29–31]. However, the reliance on AI in healthcare raises issues regarding transparency and accountability with black-box AI systems whose decision-making processes are opaque [32,33]. Explainable artificial intelligence emerges as a solution to enhance transparency, ensuring that AI-driven decisions are comprehensible to healthcare providers and patients alike [29,34].

Explainable artificial intelligence provides explanations that increase the trustworthiness in the diagnoses and treatments suggested by machine-learning models [32,34–36]. While accuracy is necessary in AI systems, healthcare is a critical domain and requires transparent AI systems that offer reliable explanations [28,37]. When combined with rigorous internal and external validation, explainable artificial intelligence can improve model troubleshooting and system auditing, aligning the AI system with potential regulatory requirements, such as those outlined in the regulations on automated artificial-intelligence systems put forth by the European Union [37–39].

AI is well-suited to help precision medicine by computing mathematical mappings of the connections between patient characteristics and personalized treatment strategies [40–43]. However, challenges persist in the validation of machine-learning models for clinical applications [29,44]. Public and private collaborative efforts involving clinicians, computer scientists, and statisticians are essential to effectively map a machine-learning model onto an explanation that can be understood in the service of precision medicine [40,45].

There are going to be ever-present ethical and social concerns, including issues of accountability, data privacy, and bias [32,46]. Explainable artificial intelligence offers a pathway to addressing these concerns by providing transparent explanations for AI-driven decisions, fostering trust and acceptance among stakeholders [47,48]. Differences between machine-learning models trained on data from practical application vs. proxies make it challenging to have a unitary assessment of interpretability or explainability [49]. As AI continues to grow, there is an ongoing ethical need for the development of explainable artificial-intelligence methods in healthcare [17,50].

3.2. Integrating Explainable AI in Healthcare for Trustworthy Precision Medicine

Integrating explainable artificial intelligence with digital health data is gaining momentum in precision medicine, addressing the need for transparent and understandable models essential for clinical applicability [19,51,52]. As machine-learning models become more complex, interpretability is crucial in clinical contexts such as microbiome research [51,53]. Explainable artificial-intelligence applications can help predict an Alzheimer's disease diagnosis in a pool of patients with mild impairments, showcasing how interpretable machine-learning algorithms can help explain complex patterns that inform individual patient predictions [54,55]. Such models offer patient-level interpretations, aiding clinicians and patients in understanding the patterns of features that predict conversion to dementia, thus enhancing trust in using explainable artificial intelligence as an aid to medical decisions [54,56].

Methods of extracting explanations from complex models can aid in the discovery of new personalized approaches to therapy and new biomarkers [57]. For example, Bayesian networks may serve as a framework for visualizing interactions between biological entities (taxa, genes, metabolites) within a specific environment (human gut) over time [51]. A model agnostic approach to explainability is offered by Shapley additive explanations, which enhance understanding at both global and local levels, improve predictive accuracy, and facilitate informed medical decisions [56,58]. Shapley values can enable visual explanations of how a model makes patient-level predictions and also the impact of changes in training data on model explanations [59]. Yet, a key barrier to advances of AI in healthcare in integrating data across platforms and institutions for precision medicine is the lack of clear governance frameworks for the privacy and security of data [60].

Development of AI systems for disease identification, such as in COVID-19 diagnosis, are underway, highlighting the importance of visual explanations in optimizing diagnostic accuracy [58,61]. For example, a recent study used explainable artificial-intelligence methods to create a multi-modal (visual, text) explanation as an aid in understanding and trusting a melanoma diagnosis [62]. More broadly, explainable artificial intelligence has potential to aid in communicating transparent decision support for healthcare systems that helps healthcare professionals make informed and reliable decisions [58,63]. Moreover, many legal and technological challenges associated with diagnostic models of electronic health records are solved by sharing prediction models and Bayesian networks of comorbidities on health outcomes, rather than the protected health information itself [64]. Overall, explainable artificial-intelligence methods are important for building trustworthiness for AI healthcare systems, supporting advancements in precision medicine and clinical decision-making [49,58,65].

3.3. Advancing Precision Medicine through Deep Learning and Explainable Artificial Intelligence

The great potential of deep learning is as a transformative force in the analysis of health information for precision medicine because of its ability to find patterns in unstructured data, such as images from medical scans, that are important for diagnosis and treatment decisions [66,67]. This ability has advanced the field, enabling the differentiation of medical conditions with high accuracy, as shown in studies comparing benign nevus and melanoma through skin-lesion images [66,68]. Explainable artificial-intelligence approaches to understanding clinical systems using deep learning offer explanatory metrics that can be used in validation studies, and help address ethical considerations and regulatory compliance [56,66].

Deep-learning models combined with explainable artificial intelligence have potential for broad applications in precision medicine, from enhancing disease diagnosis to facilitating drug discovery [69–71]. Deep-learning models offer more exact and efficient diagnosis for diseases requiring analysis of medical images (i.e., cancer, dementia), compared with human experts [72]. Explainable artificial-intelligence approaches to deep-learning models of medical images often include some form of visual explanation highlighting the image segments the model used to make the diagnosis [73,74]. Deep learning can also reduce drug discovery costs by efficiently screening for potential candidates, reducing time compared with traditional methods [29].

Deep-learning models for detecting, segmenting, and classifying biomedical images have accuracy that sometimes meets or exceeds human experts [75,76]. Multimodal data-fusion techniques that combine medical imaging data with other data sources show further improved diagnostic accuracy [77]. Explainable artificial intelligence makes AI algorithms more transparent and controllable, building trust among medical professionals in AI-assisted decisions [78]. Overall, explainable artificial intelligence integration into the healthcare systems can build trust and reliance in deep-learning approaches to diagnosis and drug discovery [56,69,79].

4. Discussion

This review paper gives an overview of key themes in research into digital health using explainable artificial intelligence for precision medicine. We used a topic-modeling approach to extract common themes across 27 full-text journal articles matching search criteria ("precision medicine" AND "digital health" AND "interpretable machine learning" OR "explainable artificial intelligence"). Thus, this review offers a glimpse at the current landscape in explainable artificial-intelligence-driven precision medicine using digital health. Through applying a latent Dirichlet allocation model, the topic model highlights core thematic areas that underscore an emerging focus on explainable artificial intelligence as a key to addressing ethical challenges [27,29,34,58,66,80–82]. These challenges include transparency, trust, and interdisciplinary collaboration in advancing healthcare innovations. Explainable artificial intelligence has many qualities that bridge the gap between complex AI algorithms, such as deep learning, and their practical applications in healthcare, enhancing the acceptability and effectiveness of AI interventions in clinical settings [19,51,52]. By facilitating a better understanding of AI-driven predictions, explainable artificial intelligence enables healthcare professionals to make informed decisions, thus fostering a collaborative environment where AI serves as a supportive tool for opaque decision-making [40,45]. The high-stakes clinical context makes it crucial to integrate explainable artificial intelligence into healthcare systems for advancing personalized treatment strategies that are grounded in an understanding of AI-generated insights.

The alliance between deep learning and explainable artificial intelligence is also critical for advancing precision medicine [66,67]. Deep learning can analyze medical imaging data with electronic health records. Coupled with the explanatory power of explainable artificial intelligence, it offers unprecedented opportunities for diagnosing and treating diseases with greater precision [83]. Explainable artificial intelligence increases accessibility and trust by medical professionals by enhancing the credibility and applicability of deep-learning models in healthcare [56,69,79]. This synergy between deep learning and explainable artificial intelligence can accelerate the pace of medical discoveries and ensure that such advancements are in accordance with the ethical needs of both practitioners and patients.

In sum, this review highlights the ethical importance of explainability when deploying AI systems in healthcare. Precision medicine and patient-centric approaches to healthcare that are driven by AI must be transparent to be trusted. In the future, AI and human expertise will be working in tandem to deliver personalized and ethical healthcare solutions. The implementation of AI systems by physicians is limited by the transparency of the systems and their ability to be understood [68]. However, explainable artificial intelligence can help forge the path towards building trust in precision medicine based on digital health data [84]. The widespread adoption of machine-learning models using digital health data for precision medicine is hindered by the slow progress in developing explainable methods [85]. Thus, integrating explainable artificial-intelligence approaches into healthcare systems is one key to realizing the full potential of AI in precision medicine.

4.1. Limitations

The keywords used to find journal articles limited the topics to interpretable machine learning and/or explainable artificial intelligence. The discovered topics will not necessarily reflect all possible themes in the burgeoning field of artificial intelligence more broadly. The interested reader can see reviews with a broader focus on artificial intelligence and digital health or precision medicine [86,87]. Moreover, five articles in the initial search were published in journals behind a paywall, and not accessible despite contacting authors. The Supplementary Materials include a list of the articles not available, as well as the code for text processing and topic modeling.

As this systematic review was not aimed at quantifying the evidence for a specific effect, traditional risk assessment of bias in individual studies did not directly apply to our topic-modeling synthesis of text from journal articles for a systematic review. The goal of our systematic review was to identify patterns and themes across a body of literature rather than evaluate the methodological quality of individual studies. Nonetheless, our study meets benchmark questions used to assess the overall quality of systematic reviews [88]. There were clear inclusion and exclusion criteria relevant for tapping the appropriate scientific literature, and a comprehensive literature search, unrestricted by time; our topic modeling of journal articles ensured all selected papers were adequately encoded.

4.2. Future Directions

Researchers at the crossroads of digital health and precision medicine should strive to understand their artificial-intelligence applications. For example, explainable artificial-intelligence approaches could help advance biophysical models and understanding of biological processes, as well as improve trust in using artificial-intelligence applications with digital health data to make medical decisions [82]. A barrier to progress is that machine-learning models need big data, yet repositories of publicly available digital health data are limited. Future studies using artificial intelligence should collect a multi-site, nationally representative sample that provides publicly available data from different digital health domains [89]. Ultimately, these endeavors could result in a transparent artificial-intelligence system utilizing digital health data for precision medicine.

The future of personalized medicine appears to be increasing the trustworthiness of AI systems by making them explainable. There are policy implications for how explainable methods can help meet regulations and policies regarding transparency. Future research could include multi-site studies that validate local explaining methods that make reliable predictions at the patient level. The end product of these studies should include some applications for healthcare workers that visualize explanations for diagnostic or treatment planning. Such multi-site studies could also help encourage collaboration across different areas of expertise as the use of artificial intelligence in healthcare grows.

5. Conclusions

This paper provides an up-to-date assessment of themes in research related to explainable artificial intelligence, digital health, and precision medicine. The potential contributions of explainable artificial intelligence to precision medicine span both theoretical and translational aspects. For example, explainable artificial intelligence holds promise for both enhancing our comprehension of disease mechanisms and visualizing regions of medical images important for making a diagnosis. In general, the convergence with digital health is in its early stages, yet precision medicine stands to benefit in many ways by embracing explainable artificial intelligence.

Supplementary Materials: The following supporting information can be downloaded at: https://osf.io/tpxh6. Code can be downloaded at https://zenodo.org/records/10398384.

Funding: This research received no external funding.

Institutional Review Board Statement: Not applicable.

Informed Consent Statement: Not applicable.

Data Availability Statement: The data used in this report came from published articles that are copyrighted. However, the articles used are listed in the report.

Conflicts of Interest: The authors declare no conflicts of interest.

References

1. Collins, F.S.; Varmus, H. A New Initiative on Precision Medicine. *N. Engl. J. Med.* **2015**, *372*, 793–795. [CrossRef]
2. Johnson, K.B.; Wei, W.; Weeraratne, D.; Frisse, M.E.; Misulis, K.; Rhee, K.; Zhao, J.; Snowdon, J.L. Precision Medicine, AI, and the Future of Personalized Health Care. *Clin. Transl. Sci.* **2021**, *14*, 86–93. [CrossRef] [PubMed]
3. Larry Jameson, J.; Longo, D.L. Precision Medicine—Personalized, Problematic, and Promising. *Obstet. Gynecol. Surv.* **2015**, *70*, 612. [CrossRef]
4. Hamburg, M.A.; Collins, F.S. The Path to Personalized Medicine. *N. Engl. J. Med.* **2010**, *363*, 301–304. [CrossRef] [PubMed]
5. Topol, E.J. High-Performance Medicine: The Convergence of Human and Artificial Intelligence. *Nat. Med.* **2019**, *25*, 44–56. [CrossRef] [PubMed]

6. Huang, C.; Clayton, E.A.; Matyunina, L.V.; McDonald, L.D.; Benigno, B.B.; Vannberg, F.; McDonald, J.F. Machine Learning Predicts Individual Cancer Patient Responses to Therapeutic Drugs with High Accuracy. *Sci. Rep.* **2018**, *8*, 16444. [CrossRef] [PubMed]
7. Sheu, Y.; Magdamo, C.; Miller, M.; Das, S.; Blacker, D.; Smoller, J.W. AI-Assisted Prediction of Differential Response to Antidepressant Classes Using Electronic Health Records. *Npj Digit. Med.* **2023**, *6*, 73. [CrossRef] [PubMed]
8. Alowais, S.A.; Alghamdi, S.S.; Alsuhebany, N.; Alqahtani, T.; Alshaya, A.I.; Almohareb, S.N.; Aldairem, A.; Alrashed, M.; Bin Saleh, K.; Badreldin, H.A.; et al. Revolutionizing Healthcare: The Role of Artificial Intelligence in Clinical Practice. *BMC Med. Educ.* **2023**, *23*, 689. [CrossRef]
9. Li, X.; Dunn, J.; Salins, D.; Zhou, G.; Zhou, W.; Rose, S.M.S.-F.; Perelman, D.; Colbert, E.; Runge, R.; Rego, S.; et al. Digital Health: Tracking Physiomes and Activity Using Wearable Biosensors Reveals Useful Health-Related Information. *PLoS Biol.* **2017**, *15*, e2001402. [CrossRef]
10. Kvedar, J.; Coye, M.J.; Everett, W. Connected Health: A Review of Technologies and Strategies to Improve Patient Care with Telemedicine and Telehealth. *Health Aff.* **2014**, *33*, 194–199. [CrossRef]
11. Akselrod-Ballin, A.; Chorev, M.; Shoshan, Y.; Spiro, A.; Hazan, A.; Melamed, R.; Barkan, E.; Herzel, E.; Naor, S.; Karavani, E.; et al. Predicting Breast Cancer by Applying Deep Learning to Linked Health Records and Mammograms. *Radiology* **2019**, *292*, 331–342. [CrossRef]
12. Bohr, A.; Memarzadeh, K. The Rise of Artificial Intelligence in Healthcare Applications. *Artif. Intell. Healthc.* **2020**, 25–60. [CrossRef]
13. McGuire, A.L.; Gibbs, R.A. No Longer De-Identified. *Science* **2006**, *312*, 370–371. [CrossRef]
14. Farhud, D.D.; Zokaei, S. Ethical Issues of Artificial Intelligence in Medicine and Healthcare. *Iran. J. Public Health* **2021**, *50*, i–v. [CrossRef]
15. Obermeyer, Z.; Emanuel, E.J. Predicting the Future—Big Data, Machine Learning, and Clinical Medicine. *N. Engl. J. Med.* **2016**, *375*, 1216–1219. [CrossRef]
16. Obafemi-Ajayi, T.; Perkins, A.; Nanduri, B.; Wunsch, D.C., II; Foster, J.A.; Peckham, J. No-Boundary Thinking: A Viable Solution to Ethical Data-Driven AI in Precision Medicine. *AI Ethics* **2022**, *2*, 635–643. [CrossRef]
17. Rajkomar, A.; Dean, J.; Kohane, I. Machine Learning in Medicine. *N. Engl. J. Med.* **2019**, *380*, 1347–1358. [CrossRef] [PubMed]
18. Char, D.S.; Shah, N.H.; Magnus, D. Implementing Machine Learning in Health Care—Addressing Ethical Challenges. *N. Engl. J. Med.* **2018**, *378*, 981–983. [CrossRef] [PubMed]
19. Barredo Arrieta, A.; Díaz-Rodríguez, N.; Del Ser, J.; Bennetot, A.; Tabik, S.; Barbado, A.; Garcia, S.; Gil-Lopez, S.; Molina, D.; Benjamins, R.; et al. Explainable Artificial Intelligence (XAI): Concepts, Taxonomies, Opportunities and Challenges toward Responsible AI. *Inf. Fusion* **2020**, *58*, 82–115. [CrossRef]
20. Holzinger, A.; Langs, G.; Denk, H.; Zatloukal, K.; Müller, H. Causability and Explainability of Artificial Intelligence in Medicine. *Wiley Interdiscip. Rev. Data Min. Knowl. Discov.* **2019**, *9*, e1312. [CrossRef] [PubMed]
21. Peralta, M.; Jannin, P.; Baxter, J.S.H. Machine Learning in Deep Brain Stimulation: A Systematic Review. *Artif. Intell. Med.* **2021**, *122*, 102198. [CrossRef]
22. Attia, Z.I.; Noseworthy, P.A.; Lopez-Jimenez, F.; Asirvatham, S.J.; Deshmukh, A.J.; Gersh, B.J.; Carter, R.E.; Yao, X.; Rabinstein, A.A.; Erickson, B.J. An Artificial Intelligence-Enabled ECG Algorithm for the Identification of Patients with Atrial Fibrillation during Sinus Rhythm: A Retrospective Analysis of Outcome Prediction. *Lancet* **2019**, *394*, 861–867. [CrossRef] [PubMed]
23. Thakur, K.; Kumar, V. Application of Text Mining Techniques on Scholarly Research Articles: Methods and Tools. *New Rev. Acad. Librariansh.* **2022**, *28*, 279–302. [CrossRef]
24. Abdelrazek, A.; Eid, Y.; Gawish, E.; Medhat, W.; Hassan, A. Topic Modeling Algorithms and Applications: A Survey. *Inf. Syst.* **2023**, *112*, 102131. [CrossRef]
25. Page, M.J.; McKenzie, J.E.; Bossuyt, P.M.; Boutron, I.; Hoffmann, T.C.; Mulrow, C.D.; Shamseer, L.; Tetzlaff, J.M.; Akl, E.A.; Brennan, S.E.; et al. The PRISMA 2020 Statement: An Updated Guideline for Reporting Systematic Reviews. *Int. J. Surg.* **2021**, *88*, 105906. [CrossRef] [PubMed]
26. Haddaway, N.R.; Page, M.J.; Pritchard, C.C.; McGuinness, L.A. PRISMA2020: An R Package and Shiny App for Producing PRISMA 2020-Compliant Flow Diagrams, with Interactivity for Optimised Digital Transparency and Open Synthesis. *Campbell Syst. Rev.* **2022**, *18*, e1230. [CrossRef] [PubMed]
27. Ishengoma, F. Artificial Intelligence in Digital Health: Issues and Dimensions of Ethical Concerns. *Innov. Softw.* **2022**, *3*, 81–108. [CrossRef]
28. Adadi, A.; Berrada, M. Peeking Inside the Black-Box: A Survey on Explainable Artificial Intelligence (XAI). *IEEE Access* **2018**, *6*, 52138–52160. [CrossRef]
29. Roy, S.; Meena, T.; Lim, S. Demystifying Supervised Learning in Healthcare 4.0: A New Reality of Transforming Diagnostic Medicine. *Diagnostics* **2022**, *12*, 2549. [CrossRef]
30. Kosorok, M.R.; Laber, E.B. Precision Medicine. *Annu. Rev. Stat. Its Appl.* **2019**, *6*, 263–286. [CrossRef]
31. Madai, V.I.; Higgins, D.C. Artificial Intelligence in Healthcare: Lost In Translation? *arXiv* **2021**, arXiv:2107.13454.
32. Kuwaiti, A.A.; Nazer, K.; Al-Reedy, A.; Al-Shehri, S.; Al-Muhanna, A.; Subbarayalu, A.V.; Al Muhanna, D.; Al-Muhanna, F.A. A Review of the Role of Artificial Intelligence in Healthcare. *J. Pers. Med.* **2023**, *13*, 951. [CrossRef]

33. Clement, T.; Kemmerzell, N.; Abdelaal, M.; Amberg, M. XAIR: A Systematic Metareview of Explainable AI (XAI) Aligned to the Software Development Process. *Mach. Learn. Knowl. Extr.* **2023**, *5*, 78–108. [CrossRef]
34. Guidotti, R.; Monreale, A.; Ruggieri, S.; Turini, F.; Giannotti, F.; Pedreschi, D. A Survey of Methods for Explaining Black Box Models. *ACM Comput. Surv.* **2019**, *51*, 1–42. [CrossRef]
35. Jadhav, S.; Deng, G.; Zawin, M.; Kaufman, A.E. COVID-View: Diagnosis of COVID-19 Using Chest CT. *IEEE Trans. Vis. Comput. Graph.* **2022**, *28*, 227–237. [CrossRef] [PubMed]
36. Giuste, F.; Shi, W.; Zhu, Y.; Naren, T.; Isgut, M.; Sha, Y.; Tong, L.; Gupte, M.; Wang, M.D. Explainable Artificial Intelligence Methods in Combating Pandemics: A Systematic Review. *IEEE Rev. Biomed. Eng.* **2022**, *16*, 5–21. [CrossRef] [PubMed]
37. Goodman, B.; Flaxman, S. European Union Regulations on Algorithmic Decision-Making and a "Right to Explanation". *AI Mag.* **2017**, *38*, 50–57. [CrossRef]
38. Article 22 GDPR—Automated Individual Decision-Making, Including Profiling. In *General Data Protection Regulation (EU GDPR)*; European Parliament: Strasbourg, France; Council of the European Union: Brussels, Belgium, 2018.
39. Ghassemi, M.; Oakden-Rayner, L.; Beam, A.L. The False Hope of Current Approaches to Explainable Artificial Intelligence in Health Care. *Lancet Digit. Health* **2021**, *3*, e745–e750. [CrossRef] [PubMed]
40. Wellnhofer, E. Real-World and Regulatory Perspectives of Artificial Intelligence in Cardiovascular Imaging. *Front. Cardiovasc. Med.* **2022**, *9*, 890809. [CrossRef] [PubMed]
41. Mayerhoefer, M.E.; Materka, A.; Langs, G.; Häggström, I.; Szczypiński, P.; Gibbs, P.; Cook, G. Introduction to Radiomics. *J. Nucl. Med.* **2020**, *61*, 488–495. [CrossRef]
42. Piccialli, F.; Calabrò, F.; Crisci, D.; Cuomo, S.; Prezioso, E.; Mandile, R.; Troncone, R.; Greco, L.; Auricchio, R. Precision Medicine and Machine Learning towards the Prediction of the Outcome of Potential Celiac Disease. *Sci. Rep.* **2021**, *11*, 5683. [CrossRef] [PubMed]
43. Schork, N.J. Artificial Intelligence and Personalized Medicine. *Cancer Treat. Res.* **2019**, *178*, 265–283. [CrossRef] [PubMed]
44. Kimmelman, J.; Tannock, I. The Paradox of Precision Medicine. *Nat. Rev. Clin. Oncol.* **2018**, *15*, 341–342. [CrossRef]
45. Boehm, K.M.; Khosravi, P.; Vanguri, R.; Gao, J.; Shah, S.P. Harnessing Multimodal Data Integration to Advance Precision Oncology. *Nat. Rev. Cancer* **2021**, *22*, 114–126. [CrossRef] [PubMed]
46. Choudhury, A.; Asan, O. Impact of Accountability, Training, and Human Factors on the Use of Artificial Intelligence in Healthcare: Exploring the Perceptions of Healthcare Practitioners in the US. *Hum. Factors Healthc.* **2022**, *2*, 100021. [CrossRef]
47. Poon, A.I.F.; Sung, J.J.Y. Opening the Black Box of AI-Medicine. *J. Gastroenterol. Hepatol.* **2021**, *36*, 581–584. [CrossRef] [PubMed]
48. Bærøe, K.; Miyata-Sturm, A.; Henden, E. How to Achieve Trustworthy Artificial Intelligence for Health. *Bull. World Health Organ.* **2020**, *98*, 257–262. [CrossRef] [PubMed]
49. Doshi-Velez, F.; Kim, B. Towards A Rigorous Science of Interpretable Machine Learning. *arXiv* **2017**, arXiv:1702.08608.
50. Towards Trustable Machine Learning. *Nat. Biomed. Eng.* **2018**, *2*, 709–710. [CrossRef]
51. Laccourreye, P.; Bielza, C.; Larrañaga, P. Explainable Machine Learning for Longitudinal Multi-Omic Microbiome. *Mathematics* **2022**, *10*, 1994. [CrossRef]
52. Carrieri, A.P.; Haiminen, N.; Maudsley-Barton, S.; Gardiner, L.-J.; Murphy, B.; Mayes, A.E.; Paterson, S.; Grimshaw, S.; Winn, M.; Shand, C.; et al. Explainable AI Reveals Changes in Skin Microbiome Composition Linked to Phenotypic Differences. *Sci. Rep.* **2021**, *11*, 4565. [CrossRef] [PubMed]
53. Wong, C.W.; Yost, S.E.; Lee, J.S.; Gillece, J.D.; Folkerts, M.; Reining, L.; Highlander, S.K.; Eftekhari, Z.; Mortimer, J.; Yuan, Y. Analysis of Gut Microbiome Using Explainable Machine Learning Predicts Risk of Diarrhea Associated with Tyrosine Kinase Inhibitor Neratinib: A Pilot Study. *Front. Oncol.* **2021**, *11*, 604584. [CrossRef] [PubMed]
54. Chun, M.Y.; Park, C.J.; Kim, J.; Jeong, J.H.; Jang, H.; Kim, K.; Seo, S.W. Prediction of Conversion to Dementia Using Interpretable Machine Learning in Patients with Amnestic Mild Cognitive Impairment. *Front. Aging Neurosci.* **2022**, *14*, 898940. [CrossRef] [PubMed]
55. Murdoch, W.J.; Singh, C.; Kumbier, K.; Abbasi-Asl, R.; Yu, B. Definitions, Methods, and Applications in Interpretable Machine Learning. *Proc. Natl. Acad. Sci. USA* **2019**, *116*, 22071–22080. [CrossRef] [PubMed]
56. Lundberg, S.; Lee, S.-I. A Unified Approach to Interpreting Model Predictions. In Proceedings of the Advances in Neural Information Processing Systems 30 (NIPS 2017), Long Beach, CA, USA, 4–9 December 2017.
57. Wang, R.C.; Wang, Z. Precision Medicine: Disease Subtyping and Tailored Treatment. *Cancers* **2023**, *15*, 3837. [CrossRef] [PubMed]
58. Albahri, A.S.; Duhaim, A.M.; Fadhel, M.A.; Alnoor, A.; Baqer, N.S.; Alzubaidi, L.; Albahri, O.S.; Alamoodi, A.H.; Bai, J.; Salhi, A.; et al. A Systematic Review of Trustworthy and Explainable Artificial Intelligence in Healthcare: Assessment of Quality, Bias Risk, and Data Fusion. *Inf. Fusion* **2023**, *96*, 156–191. [CrossRef]
59. Martínez-Agüero, S.; Soguero-Ruiz, C.; Alonso-Moral, J.M.; Mora-Jiménez, I.; Álvarez-Rodríguez, J.; Marques, A.G. Interpretable Clinical Time-Series Modeling with Intelligent Feature Selection for Early Prediction of Antimicrobial Multidrug Resistance. *Future Gener. Comput. Syst.* **2022**, *133*, 68–83. [CrossRef]
60. Ho, C.W.-L.; Caals, K. A Call for an Ethics and Governance Action Plan to Harness the Power of Artificial Intelligence and Digitalization in Nephrology. *Semin. Nephrol.* **2021**, *41*, 282–293. [CrossRef]
61. Rostami, M.; Oussalah, M. A Novel Explainable COVID-19 Diagnosis Method by Integration of Feature Selection with Random Forest. *Inform. Med. Unlocked* **2022**, *30*, 100941. [CrossRef]

62. Lucieri, A.; Bajwa, M.N.; Braun, S.A.; Malik, M.I.; Dengel, A.; Ahmed, S. ExAID: A Multimodal Explanation Framework for Computer-Aided Diagnosis of Skin Lesions. *Comput. Methods Programs Biomed.* **2022**, *215*, 106620. [CrossRef]
63. Müller, H.; Holzinger, A.; Plass, M.; Brcic, L.; Stumptner, C.; Zatloukal, K. Explainability and Causability for Artificial Intelligence-Supported Medical Image Analysis in the Context of the European In Vitro Diagnostic Regulation. *New Biotechnol.* **2022**, *70*, 67–72. [CrossRef] [PubMed]
64. Wesołowski, S.; Lemmon, G.; Hernandez, E.J.; Henrie, A.; Miller, T.A.; Weyhrauch, D.; Puchalski, M.D.; Bray, B.E.; Shah, R.U.; Deshmukh, V.G.; et al. An Explainable Artificial Intelligence Approach for Predicting Cardiovascular Outcomes Using Electronic Health Records. *PLoS Digit. Health* **2022**, *1*, e0000004. [CrossRef] [PubMed]
65. Lucieri, A.; Bajwa, M.N.; Dengel, A.; Ahmed, S. Achievements and Challenges in Explaining Deep Learning Based Computer-Aided Diagnosis Systems. *arXiv* **2020**, arXiv:2011.13169.
66. Shazly, S.A.; Trabuco, E.C.; Ngufor, C.G.; Famuyide, A.O. Introduction to Machine Learning in Obstetrics and Gynecology. *Obstet. Gynecol.* **2022**, *139*, 669–679. [CrossRef] [PubMed]
67. Gerussi, A.; Scaravaglio, M.; Cristoferi, L.; Verda, D.; Milani, C.; De Bernardi, E.; Ippolito, D.; Asselta, R.; Invernizzi, P.; Kather, J.N.; et al. Artificial Intelligence for Precision Medicine in Autoimmune Liver Disease. *Front. Immunol.* **2022**, *13*, 966329. [CrossRef]
68. Reyes, M.; Meier, R.; Pereira, S.; Silva, C.A.; Dahlweid, F.-M.; von Tengg-Kobligk, H.; Summers, R.M.; Wiest, R. On the Interpretability of Artificial Intelligence in Radiology: Challenges and Opportunities. *Radiol. Artif. Intell.* **2020**, *2*, e190043. [CrossRef]
69. Zafar, I.; Anwar, S.; Kanwal, F.; Yousaf, W.; Nisa, F.U.; Kausar, T.; Ain, Q.U.; Unar, A.; Kamal, M.A.; Rashid, S.; et al. Reviewing Methods of Deep Learning for Intelligent Healthcare Systems in Genomics and Biomedicine. *Biomed. Signal Process. Control* **2023**, *86*, 105263. [CrossRef]
70. Lötsch, J.; Kringel, D.; Ultsch, A. Explainable Artificial Intelligence (XAI) in Biomedicine: Making AI Decisions Trustworthy for Physicians and Patients. *BioMedInformatics* **2021**, *2*, 1–17. [CrossRef]
71. Kırboğa, K.K.; Abbasi, S. Explainability and White Box in Drug Discovery. *Chem. Biol. Drug Des.* **2023**, *102*, 217–233. [CrossRef]
72. Selvaraju, R.R.; Cogswell, M.; Das, A.; Vedantam, R.; Parikh, D.; Batra, D. Grad-Cam: Visual Explanations from Deep Networks via Gradient-Based Localization. In Proceedings of the IEEE International Conference on Computer Vision, Venice, Italy, 22–29 October 2017; pp. 618–626.
73. Hong, G.-S.; Jang, M.; Kyung, S.; Cho, K.; Jeong, J.; Lee, G.Y.; Shin, K.; Kim, K.D.; Ryu, S.M.; Seo, J.B.; et al. Overcoming the Challenges in the Development and Implementation of Artificial Intelligence in Radiology: A Comprehensive Review of Solutions Beyond Supervised Learning. *Korean J. Radiol.* **2023**, *24*, e58. [CrossRef]
74. van der Velden, B.H.M.; Kuijf, H.J.; Gilhuijs, K.G.A.; Viergever, M.A. Explainable Artificial Intelligence (XAI) in Deep Learning-Based Medical Image Analysis. *Med. Image Anal.* **2022**, *79*, 102470. [CrossRef]
75. Chorba, J.S.; Shapiro, A.M.; Le, L.; Maidens, J.; Prince, J.; Pham, S.; Kanzawa, M.M.; Barbosa, D.N.; Currie, C.; Brooks, C.; et al. Deep Learning Algorithm for Automated Cardiac Murmur Detection via a Digital Stethoscope Platform. *J. Am. Heart Assoc.* **2021**, *10*, e019905. [CrossRef]
76. Zhou, L.-Q.; Wu, X.-L.; Huang, S.-Y.; Wu, G.-G.; Ye, H.-R.; Wei, Q.; Bao, L.-Y.; Deng, Y.-B.; Li, X.-R.; Cui, X.-W. Lymph Node Metastasis Prediction from Primary Breast Cancer US Images Using Deep Learning. *Radiology* **2020**, *294*, 19–28. [CrossRef]
77. Hassan, R.; Islam, F.; Uddin, Z.; Ghoshal, G.; Hassan, M.M.; Huda, S.; Fortino, G. Prostate Cancer Classification from Ultrasound and MRI Images Using Deep Learning Based Explainable Artificial Intelligence. *Future Gener. Comput. Syst.* **2022**, *127*, 462–472. [CrossRef]
78. Salih, A.; Boscolo Galazzo, I.; Gkontra, P.; Lee, A.M.; Lekadir, K.; Raisi-Estabragh, Z.; Petersen, S.E. Explainable Artificial Intelligence and Cardiac Imaging: Toward More Interpretable Models. *Circ. Cardiovasc. Imaging* **2023**, *16*, e014519. [CrossRef]
79. Ribeiro, M.T.; Singh, S.; Guestrin, C. "Why Should I Trust You?": Explaining the Predictions of Any Classifier. In Proceedings of the 22nd ACM SIGKDD International Conference on Knowledge Discovery and Data Mining, San Francisco, CA, USA, 13–17 August 2016; Association for Computing Machinery: New York, NY, USA, 2016; pp. 1135–1144.
80. Wickramasinghe, N.; Jayaraman, P.P. A Vision for Leveraging the Concept of Digital Twins to Support the Provision of Personalized Cancer Care. *IEEE Internet Comput.* **2021**, *26*, 17–24. [CrossRef]
81. Baumgartner, A.J.; Thompson, J.A.; Kern, D.S.; Ojemann, S.G. Novel Targets in Deep Brain Stimulation for Movement Disorders. *Neurosurg. Rev.* **2022**, *45*, 2593–2613. [CrossRef]
82. Iqbal, J.D.; Krauthammer, M.; Biller-Andorno, N. The Use and Ethics of Digital Twins in Medicine. *J. Law. Med. Ethics* **2022**, *50*, 583–596. [CrossRef] [PubMed]
83. Payrovnaziri, S.N.; Chen, Z.; Rengifo-Moreno, P.; Miller, T.; Bian, J.; Chen, J.H.; Liu, X.; He, Z. Explainable Artificial Intelligence Models Using Real-World Electronic Health Record Data: A Systematic Scoping Review. *J. Am. Med. Inform. Assoc. JAMIA* **2020**, *27*, 1173–1185. [CrossRef] [PubMed]
84. Gunning, D.; Stefik, M.; Choi, J.; Miller, T.; Stumpf, S.; Yang, G.-Z. XAI-Explainable Artificial Intelligence. *Sci. Robot.* **2019**, *4*, eaay7120. [CrossRef] [PubMed]
85. Pinto, M.F.; Leal, A.; Lopes, F.; Pais, J.; Dourado, A.; Sales, F.; Martins, P.; Teixeira, C.A. On the Clinical Acceptance of Black-box Systems for EEG Seizure Prediction. *Epilepsia Open* **2022**, *7*, 247–259. [CrossRef] [PubMed]

86. Gunasekeran, D.V.; Tseng, R.M.W.W.; Tham, Y.-C.; Wong, T.Y. Applications of Digital Health for Public Health Responses to COVID-19: A Systematic Scoping Review of Artificial Intelligence, Telehealth and Related Technologies. *Npj Digit. Med.* **2021**, *4*, 40. [CrossRef] [PubMed]
87. Mesko, B. The Role of Artificial Intelligence in Precision Medicine. *Expert Rev. Precis. Med. Drug Dev.* **2017**, *2*, 239–241. [CrossRef]
88. Kitchenham, B. Procedures for Performing Systematic Reviews. *Keele UK Keele Univ.* **2004**, *33*, 1–26.
89. Casey, B.J.; Cannonier, T.; Conley, M.I.; Cohen, A.O.; Barch, D.M.; Heitzeg, M.M.; Soules, M.E.; Teslovich, T.; Dellarco, D.V.; Garavan, H.; et al. The Adolescent Brain Cognitive Development (ABCD) Study: Imaging Acquisition across 21 Sites. *Dev. Cogn. Neurosci.* **2018**, *32*, 43–54. [CrossRef]

Disclaimer/Publisher's Note: The statements, opinions and data contained in all publications are solely those of the individual author(s) and contributor(s) and not of MDPI and/or the editor(s). MDPI and/or the editor(s) disclaim responsibility for any injury to people or property resulting from any ideas, methods, instructions or products referred to in the content.

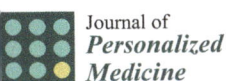

Review

Breaking Barriers—The Intersection of AI and Assistive Technology in Autism Care: A Narrative Review

Antonio Iannone [1] and Daniele Giansanti [2,*]

1. CREA, Italian National Research Body, Via Ardeatina, 546, 00178 Roma, Italy
2. Centro Nazionale TISP, Istituto Superiore di Sanità; Viale Regina Elena 299, 00161 Roma, Italy
* Correspondence: daniele.giansanti@iss.it; Tel.: +39-0649902701

Abstract: (Background) Autism increasingly requires a multidisciplinary approach that can effectively harmonize the realms of diagnosis and therapy, tailoring both to the individual. Assistive technologies (ATs) play an important role in this context and hold significant potential when integrated with artificial intelligence (AI). (Objective) The objective of this study is to analyze the state of integration of AI with ATs in autism through a review. (Methods) A review was conducted on PubMed and Scopus, applying a standard checklist and a qualification process. The outcome reported 22 studies, including 7 reviews. (Key Content and Findings) The results reveal an early yet promising interest in integrating AI into autism assistive technologies. Exciting developments are currently underway at the intersection of AI and robotics, as well as in the creation of wearable automated devices like smart glasses. These innovations offer substantial potential for enhancing communication, interaction, and social engagement for individuals with autism. Presently, researchers are prioritizing innovation over establishing a solid presence within the healthcare domain, where issues such as regulation and acceptance demand increased attention. (Conclusions) As the field continues to evolve, it becomes increasingly clear that AI will play a pivotal role in bridging various domains, and integrated ATs with AI are positioned to act as crucial connectors.

Keywords: assistive technology; accessibility; AAC; autism; AI; artificial intelligence

Citation: Iannone, A.; Giansanti, D. Breaking Barriers—The Intersection of AI and Assistive Technology in Autism Care: A Narrative Review. *J. Pers. Med.* **2024**, *14*, 41. https://doi.org/10.3390/jpm14010041

Academic Editor: Jorge Luis Espinoza

Received: 4 November 2023
Revised: 18 December 2023
Accepted: 23 December 2023
Published: 28 December 2023

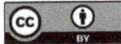

Copyright: © 2023 by the authors. Licensee MDPI, Basel, Switzerland. This article is an open access article distributed under the terms and conditions of the Creative Commons Attribution (CC BY) license (https://creativecommons.org/licenses/by/4.0/).

1. Introduction

1.1. Autism Diagnosis and Therapy

Autism, scientifically known as autism spectrum disorder (ASD), is a neurodevelopmental condition characterized by a wide range of challenges in social communication, language, behavior, and social interaction [1–5]. The manifestations of autism vary widely, giving rise to the concept of the "spectrum", which includes individuals with mild to severe symptoms. Signs of autism can emerge from early childhood but are often identified in preschool or school age, when they become more evident. Symptoms include difficulty with verbal and nonverbal communication, difficulty interacting with others, repetitive and restricted interests and activities, and increased or decreased sensory sensitivity. To diagnose autism, a multidisciplinary approach is used [6–8]. Specialists, such as psychologists, child psychiatrists, and pediatricians, conduct interviews and observations to evaluate the individual's behavior, language, social skills, and cognitive abilities. Diagnosis is often completed through structured questionnaires, developmental assessments, and assessments of communication skills [1–3]. In addition to behavioral assessments and questionnaires, genetic analysis can be an integral part of the diagnosis of autism since there is a genetic component to its etiology [2–5]. Blood tests and genetic tests can identify genetic abnormalities associated with autism [4]. Also, imaging can have a strategic role, as in the case of functional magnetic resonance [9], which is also integrated with AI [10,11]. Therapy is crucial in autism, providing specialized support to address the cognitive, communication, and behavioral challenges associated with the disorder. Through targeted therapeutic interventions, individuals with autism can develop social, communication, and adaptation skills, improving their quality of life and promoting greater inclusion in society [12–16]. Therapy represents an essential foundation for promoting the progress and well-being of people with autism. Multidisciplinary approaches in autism involve different professionals, such as psychologists, occupational therapists, speech therapists, and pediatricians, who collaborate to provide holistic treatment targeted to the specific needs of each individual with autism [12,14,15]. This synergy between experts contributes to a more complete, personalized, and effective intervention, addressing cognitive, communicative, and behavioral challenges in an integrated way and optimizing the progress and well-being of patients. Assistive technology (AT) tools provide personalized technological solutions for people with autism, helping them overcome communication barriers and adapt to their specific needs [16]. These tools amplify skills and improve independence, significantly contributing to the quality of life of people with autism.

1.2. Beyond Communication: The Versatility of Assistive Technology in Autism Care

Assistive technologies [17–21], ranging from robots [17] to sensors [18], particularly Augmentative and Alternative Communications (AAC) [19], play a fundamental role in improving the lives of people with autism by addressing the communication challenges that often accompany this disorder. For many people with autism, verbal communication can be a significant barrier. AAC [19] offers an alternative avenue, allowing these people to express themselves in ways that reflect their individual needs. This customization is critically important, as autism is an extremely heterogeneous disorder, and what works for one individual may not be as effective for another. One of the main benefits of AAC [19,20] is the reduction of frustration. The inability to communicate effectively can lead to high levels of anxiety and stress. AAC reduces this frustration by providing a means to express needs and desires, helping to improve mental health and interpersonal relationships. These technologies also have a significant impact on education. AAC can be used to support learning, helping students with autism develop language and cognitive skills [19]. Furthermore, they improve school inclusion, allowing students with autism to actively participate in educational activities. Another area in which AAC proves essential is improving social interactions. AAC facilitates communication and the establishment of meaningful relationships, which is often challenging for people with autism. These tools help people with autism participate more actively in conversations and social activities, improving the quality of their interactions. Independence is an important goal for many people with autism. AAC contributes to this goal by allowing people to communicate their needs and make autonomous decisions, promoting a greater level of autonomy in daily life. Overall, assistive technologies, such as AAC, are a valuable resource for people with autism. They enable them to overcome communication challenges, improve the quality of social interactions, support learning, and promote independence. These tools are fundamental in the field of autism, contributing significantly to the well-being and inclusion of these people in society.

1.3. AI's Potential in Autism Assistive Technologies

Artificial intelligence (AI) could play a significant role in helping to personalize assistive technologies for individuals with autism [22,23]. From a future perspective, it could be capable of conducting a precise assessment of individual needs. AI, at least potentially, could analyze complex data, such as an individual's behaviors and responses, to determine which tools and supports would be most suitable. This would mean that AI could contribute to designing solutions tailored to each individual, taking specific needs into account. Another potential of AI would be to adapt assistive technologies in real-time. This would mean that devices could automatically adjust settings based on user interactions and behaviors. For instance, if a person with autism were displaying signs of stress or frustration, AI could intervene to offer targeted support. Another important potential aspect of AI is machine learning. AI could learn from the user's progress and challenges over time. This would mean that assistive technologies could continually improve their effectiveness, adapting to the evolving needs of individuals with autism. AI could also be capable of customizing the interfaces of assistive technologies to meet user preferences. This could make the tools more accessible and user-friendly, facilitating interaction and usage by the individual. Finally, AI could contribute to creating personalized learning and communication programs. These programs could take into account the individual's skill level and specific progress, offering targeted support to help them develop their abilities. In summary, AI could play a key role in tailoring and optimizing assistive technologies for individuals with autism, contributing to improving their quality of life and fostering greater engagement and well-being.

1.4. Potential Emerging Questions

Key questions in personalizing assistive technologies with AI in ASD are emerging from the above:

- How can AI precisely assess individual needs for individuals with autism?
- In what ways can AI enable the real-time adaptation of assistive technologies?
- How does machine learning enhance the adaptability of assistive technologies over time?
- To what extent can AI customize interfaces for user preferences in assistive technologies?
- How can AI create personalized learning and communication programs for individuals with autism? What evidence exists regarding the impact of AI-driven personalization on the quality of life for individuals with autism?
- What ethical considerations are crucial when implementing AI in assistive technologies for individuals with autism?
- How can AI contribute to a more user-centered design approach in developing assistive technologies?

These questions suggest the need for a review.

1.5. Purpose of the Study

The purpose of this study is to explore the potential benefits and challenges associated with the integration of AI into assistive technologies for individuals with autism. By overviewing the ways in which AI can personalize and adapt these technologies to meet the specific needs of individuals on the autism spectrum, this article aims to shed light on the opportunities for improved support, communication, and quality of life for this community. Additionally, it seeks to highlight the importance of ongoing research and innovation in this field to ensure that individuals with autism receive the most effective and personalized assistance possible.

2. Methods

This review used the ANDJ standardized checklist designed for the narrative category of reviews [24]. The narrative review was performed based on targeted searches using specific composite keys on PubMed and Scopus.

The overview literature accompanying the main survey was conducted using both a qualification checklist and a qualification methodology based on proposed quality parameters described in [25] to decide the inclusion of the study in the overview.

Algorithm Used in the Literature Overview

1. Set the search query to "defined search query".
2. Conduct a targeted search on PubMed and Scopus using the search query from step 1.
3. Select studies published in peer-reviewed journals that focus on the field.
4. For each study, evaluate the following parameters:
    - N1: Is the rationale for the study in the introduction clear?
    - N2: Is the design of the work appropriate?
    - N3: Are the methods described clearly?

- N4: Are the results presented clearly?
- N5: Are the conclusions based on and justified by the results?
- N6: Did the authors disclose all the conflicts of interest?

5. Assign a graded score to parameters N1–N5, ranging from 1 (minimum) to 5 (maximum).
6. For parameter N6, assign a binary assessment of "Yes" or "No" to indicate if the authors disclosed all the conflicts of interest.
7. Preselect studies that meet the following criteria:
   - Parameter N6 must be "Yes".
   - Parameters N1–N5 must have a score greater than 3.
8. Include the preselected studies in the overview.

Defined search query 1. *"self help devices"[MeSH Terms] OR ("self help"[All Fields] AND "devices"[All Fields]) OR "self help devices"[All Fields] OR ("assistive"[All Fields] AND "technology"[All Fields]) OR "assistive technology"[All Fields] OR ("augmentative"[All Fields] AND ("communicate"[All Fields] OR "communicated"[All Fields] OR "communicates"[All Fields] OR "communicating"[All Fields] OR "communication"[MeSH Terms] OR "communication"[All Fields] OR "communications"[All Fields] OR "communicative"[All Fields] OR "communicational"[All Fields] OR "communicatively"[All Fields] OR "communicativeness"[All Fields] OR "communicator"[All Fields] OR "communicator s"[All Fields] OR "communicators"[All Fields])) AND "autism"[Title/Abstract] AND ("artificial intelligence"[MeSH Terms] OR ("artificial"[All Fields] AND "intelligence"[All Fields]) OR "artificial intelligence"[All Fields] OR ("machine learning"[MeSH Terms] OR ("machine"[All Fields] AND "learning"[All Fields]) OR "machine learning"[All Fields]) OR ("deep learning"[MeSH Terms] OR ("deep"[All Fields] AND "learning"[All Fields]) OR "deep learning"[All Fields]) OR (("neural"[All Fields] OR "neuralization"[All Fields] OR "neuralize"[All Fields] OR "neuralized"[All Fields] OR "neuralizes"[All Fields] OR "neuralizing"[All Fields] OR "neurally"[All Fields]) AND "nework"[All Fields]))*

We applied the defined algorithm for the selection of the articles. In particular, after applying points 3 and 7, we've pinpointed a total of 22 studies [26–47]. It's interesting to highlight that this list precisely matches the number of studies detected in PubMed after excluding one retraction. Scopus, it's important to mention, contained a few conference papers that our algorithm chose to exclude for specific reasons. Out of these 22 studies, seven are comprehensive reviews, encompassing both systematic and non-systematic ones.

The remaining 15 studies are a mix of scientific articles and various other papers.

3. Results

The results have been organized into two parts and presented editorially through two main paragraphs.

In the first part (Section 3.1), a thorough examination is dedicated to the findings extracted from reviews and systematic reviews. Researchers can delve into distilled and structured insights at the crossroads of AI and assistive technologies (ATs) in the context of autism. Reviews and systematic reviews are distinguished from other articles as they offer a broader perspective, functioning as filters that distill the wealth of existing research. This aids researchers in identifying common themes, emerging patterns, and gaps in current knowledge.

The second part (Section 3.2) broadens the research's scope by delving into the outcomes of the remaining studies. This approach captures a more diverse array of perspectives concerning the intersection of AI and ATs in autism. Through a critical examination of these remaining studies, researchers can incorporate various viewpoints and alternative methodologies and potentially discover novel or previously overlooked insights. This holistic understanding of the research landscape promotes a more balanced and nuanced interpretation of the subject, reducing the risk of overlooking valuable contributions to the field.

In essence, this dual approach enhances both the depth and breadth of the research, resulting in a more robust and holistic analysis.

3.1. In-Depth Analysis of the Detected Reviews: A Comprehensive Overview

3.1.1. Analysis in Details

Seven review studies have been detected facing the intersection of AI and ATs in autism.

The review proposed by Muthu et al. [26] emphasizes the significant impact of assistive technology for differently-abled individuals and older adults, covering rehabilitative, adaptive, and assistive devices. It discusses the applications, challenges, and potential for enhancing daily life, with a special focus on AI-powered technologies with reference to autism. The study sheds light on the pros and cons of these technologies, offering valuable insights for rehabilitation engineering.

Focusing on mental disorders with childhood onset, the review by Datta Barua et al. [27] explores the co-morbidity of neurodevelopmental and mental health disorders. It highlights the role of AI-assisted tools in addressing learning challenges in individuals with neurodevelopmental disorders. The review points to the potential of AI tools for improving social interaction and personalized education.

Alabdulkareem et al. [28] delve into the use of interactive robots in autism therapy, utilizing AI technologies. The study analyzes trends in research, showing a significant increase in journal publications in the field, driven by advances in artificial intelligence techniques and machine learning. This highlights the growing role of AI in robot-assisted autism therapy.

Ur Rehman et al. [29] explore in their study the impact of mobile applications, particularly those utilizing AI technologies, on the lives of individuals with autism spectrum disorder (ASD). The study identifies features of highly-rated apps, offering recommendations for enhancing existing applications with AI. Results suggest the potential for progress tracking, personalized content delivery, automated reasoning, image recognition, and natural language processing (NLP) in these AI-powered apps.

Di Pietro et al. [30] focused on computer-assisted and robot-assisted therapies for children with autism spectrum disorder. It aims to identify the types of information technology platforms being used, the professions involved, the outcomes being evaluated, and the benefits to children with autism, with a keen eye on AI-enhanced interventions. The review highlights the promise of these AI-powered interventions while also stressing the need for further research.

Den Brok et al., in their systematic review [31], investigate the use of self-controlled technologies for persons with autism spectrum disorder and intellectual disabilities, some of which leverage AI. The results show that these technologies facilitate the learning of daily living skills and cognitive concepts, with a particular emphasis on AI-powered features. Advanced technologies, such as virtual reality, are effective for learning cognitive concepts. However, more research is needed to assess generalization and the role of AI in effectiveness. Billard et al. [32] dealt with the outcome of a project focused on robotics, the Robota project. This project employs humanoid robots in behavioral studies with low-functioning children with autism, with a focus on the technological aspects, including AI. The review discusses the technological developments and outcomes of these studies, emphasizing the potential for using imitator robots to assess and teach coordinated behaviors and the role of AI in enhancing these interventions. This work informs the future development of robots for children with complex developmental disabilities, incorporating AI-driven innovations.

We have also detected in Table 1 the key elements/points highlighting the intersection of AI with ATs across the studies, showcasing AI's contribution to enhancing assistive technologies for various applications in healthcare, education, and therapy.

Table 1. Key elements/points emerging from the overview of reviews on the intersection of AI and ATs.

Review Study	Key Points on the Intersection of AI and ATs in Autism
Muthu et al. [26]	Integration of AI in ATs for enhanced rehabilitation and independence.
Muthu et al. [26]	AI-driven solutions addressing physical impairments, mobility, education, and more.
Muthu et al. [26]	Insights into AI's role in expanding research areas related to assistive technology.
Datta Barua et al. [27]	AI-assisted tools for improving learning and social interaction in neurodevelopmental disorders.
Datta Barua et al. [27]	Evidence supporting the effectiveness of AI tools in providing personalized education.
Alabdulkareem et al. [28]	Utilization of interactive robots with AI for autism therapy.
Alabdulkareem et al. [28]	Growth in research due to advancements in AI techniques and machine learning.
Ur Rehman et al. [29]	Identification of highly-rated mobile apps for individuals with ASD utilizing AI technologies.
Ur Rehman et al. [29]	Recommendations for enhancing existing applications with AI for personalized support.
Di Pietro et al. [30]	Exploration of AI-driven computer-assisted and robot-assisted therapies for children with autism.
Di Pietro et al. [30]	Focus on identifying AI platforms, professions involved, and outcomes in social skills teaching.
Den Brok et al. [31]	AI-powered self-controlled technologies aiding individuals with autism and intellectual disability.
Den Brok et al. [31]	Use of AI to facilitate the learning of daily living skills and cognitive concepts.
Billard et al. [32]	Application of AI in humanoid robots for assisting low-functioning children with autism.
Billard et al. [32]	AI's role in assessing imitation ability and teaching coordinated behaviors.

It appears that the studies do not extensively cover the limitations and bottlenecks of AI within assistive technologies. The emphasis in these reviews is primarily on the benefits and potential of AI in various applications, while limitations and challenges are not explicitly addressed.

3.1.2. Key Findings

Collectively, the body of research from various studies [26–32] underscores the profound impact and diverse applications of AI within ATs, especially for individuals with neurodevelopmental disorders like autism. The studies collectively reveal a promising landscape where AI-driven solutions are actively contributing to the enhancement of rehabilitation, independence, and overall well-being. These solutions address a spectrum of challenges, ranging from physical impairments and mobility issues to personalized education for individuals with neurodevelopmental disorders. In the realm of autism therapy, the use of interactive robots equipped with AI is a notable trend, reflecting a growing recognition of AI's potential in improving social interaction and engagement. The observed expansion of research in this area attests to the increasing importance and applicability of AI techniques and machine learning within autism therapy.

Additionally, the collective effort in identifying highly-rated mobile apps for individuals with ASD using AI technologies and the subsequent recommendations for enhancing existing applications exemplify a practical approach to leveraging AI for personalized support. This emphasizes the ongoing commitment to tailoring AI-driven tools to the specific needs of individuals with ASD. The exploration of AI-driven computer-assisted and robot-assisted therapies further extends the application of AI into educational contexts for children with autism. The studies shed light on the identification of AI platforms, the involvement of various professions, and the outcomes of social skills teaching, collectively enriching our understanding of how AI can be effectively integrated into educational interventions. Moreover, the use of AI-powered self-controlled technologies for individuals with autism and intellectual disabilities emphasizes the potential of AI to facilitate learning in various domains, including daily living skills and cognitive concepts. The collective findings highlight the adaptability of AI in catering to diverse learning needs within the neurodevelopmental disorder spectrum. In the context of humanoid robots assisting low-functioning children with autism, the studies collectively delve into the intricacies of using AI to assess imitation ability and teach coordinated behaviors. This offers insights into both the challenges and possibilities associated with optimizing the role of AI within humanoid robots for targeted support. Common methodologies across these studies include an interdisciplinary approach, demonstrating collaboration across various professions to integrate AI effectively into ATs. The shared emphasis on developing AI-driven tools for personalized education and support reflects a collective commitment to tailoring interventions to individual needs. However, the challenges identified collectively, such as the ethical considerations associated with privacy, responsible AI use, and the need for interdisciplinary collaboration, underscore the complexities of integrating AI into ATs. These challenges collectively call for a nuanced and thoughtful approach to ensure the responsible and effective use of AI in enhancing the lives of individuals with neurodevelopmental disorders. In summary, the collective view across these studies paints a comprehensive picture of AI's transformative potential in the realm of assistive technologies, showcasing its versatility and adaptability in addressing diverse challenges and providing personalized support for individuals with neurodevelopmental disorders.

3.2. In-Depth Analysis of the Detected Articles: A Comprehensive Overview

3.2.1. Analysis in Details

Fifteen studies have been detected [33–47] in this part of the overview. In some articles, the intersection of AI and ATs is directly faced [33–43,45–47], while in others, it is faced more with an in-perspective overview [44].

Silvera Tawill et al. [33] explore the use of socially-assistive robots, incorporating AI, to support children with autism. The study identifies barriers to implementation and teachers' and therapists' expectations, highlighting the potential of AI-driven robots for teaching support.

Deng et al. [34] introduce a sensory management recommendation system that relies on AI techniques to assist children with ASD in dealing with sensory issues. The system uses sensor fusion and machine learning to identify distractions, anxious situations, and their causes, enabling more effective interventions.

Wan et al. [35] propose an AI-based system for improving emotion recognition in Chinese children with ASD. The system incorporates deep learning algorithms for facial expression recognition and attention analysis, demonstrating its potential in AI-assisted therapies.

Kumar et al. [36] examine the automation of ASD diagnosis using machine learning techniques. The study leverages AI to analyze a dataset of 701 samples, aiming to develop models that can assist in diagnosing ASD automatically.

Jain et al. [37] utilize supervised machine-learning algorithms to model user engagement in long-term, AI-driven, socially-assistive robot interventions for children with ASD. AI models achieve high accuracy in recognizing and responding to user engagement, enhancing human-robot interactions.

Keshav et al. [38] correlate student performance on the Empowered Brain platform with clinical measures of ADHD, demonstrating that AI-driven technologies can aid in monitoring and managing symptoms of co-occurring conditions in students with ASD.

Vahabzadeh et al. [39] explore the feasibility and efficacy of Empowered Brain, an AI-driven smartglasses intervention for students with ASD. It demonstrates the potential of AI in improving socio-emotional behaviors, highlighting its impact in a school-based intervention.

Cooper et al. [40] introduce an AAC software program with an embedded artificial conversational agent, named Alex. The software is designed to assist children with autism who use augmentative and alternative communication (AAC) aids. Alex utilizes symbols and images, can be personalized by therapists, and does not require specialized computer skills. The software emphasizes customization, interoperability, personalization, and considerations for motor skills.

Huijnen et al. [41] focus on the roles, strengths, and challenges of robot KASPAR in interventions for children with ASD, including its use of AI components such as personalization and consistent application of actions.

Keshav et al. [42] assess the tolerability and usability of the Brain Power Autism System (BPAS), which integrates AI and smartglasses. The outcome shows that AI-driven wearable technology is well tolerated and usable by individuals with ASD, emphasizing its role as an assistive technology.

Linstead et al. [43] investigate the influence of treatment intensity and duration on learning in children with autism who are receiving Applied Behavior Analysis (ABA) services. The study assesses the impact of these treatment variables on various domains, such as academic, adaptive, cognitive, executive function, language, motor, play, and social skills. The findings highlight the importance of treatment dosage and provide insights into its varied effects across different domains and the usefulness of AI in perspective.

Desideri et al. [44] explore the potential of a humanoid robot to enhance educational interventions for children with autism spectrum disorders (ASD). Preliminary results indicate that interacting with a humanoid robot can facilitate engagement and goal achievement in educational activities. This highlights the role of advanced technology and AI in improving the effectiveness of educational interventions for children with ASD.

Huijnen et al. [45] aim to practically implement robots, specifically robot KASPAR, into current education and therapy interventions for children with ASD. The study involves focus groups and co-creation sessions with professionals and adults with ASD. It results in requirements for robot-assisted interventions, a template for describing robot interventions, and the generation of new intervention ideas, emphasizing the practical application of robots with AI capabilities in autism therapy and education.

Bekele et al. [46] investigate an AI-driven robot-mediated system to administer joint attention prompts to children with ASD, demonstrating the potential of AI to enhance engagement and learning in educational activities for these children.

Williams et al., in a multicenter study [47], use a computer program with speech synthesizer software and a "virtual" head to investigate audio-visual integration in children with ASD. AI-like systems facilitate speech recognition and training, showcasing the role of AI in improving speech-related skills in individuals with ASD.

For these scientific articles, we have also detected in Table 2 the key points/elements highlighting the intersection of AI with ATs across the studies, showcasing AI's contribution to enhancing assistive technologies for various applications in healthcare, education, and therapy.

Table 2. Key elements/points emerging from the overview of articles on the intersection of AI and ATs.

Article Study	Key Points on the Intersection of AI and ATs in Autism
Silvera Tawill et al. [33]	AI-driven socially-assistive robots for teaching support
Deng et al. [34]	AI-powered sensory management recommendation system for children with ASD.
Wan et al. [35]	AI-based system for improving emotion recognition in children with ASD.
Kumar et al. [36]	Automation of ASD diagnosis using machine learning techniques.
Jain et al. [37]	AI-driven models for recognizing and responding to user engagement in robot interventions.
Keshav et al. [38]	AI-driven models for recognizing and responding to user engagement in robot interventions.
Vahabzadeh et al. [39]	AI-driven smartglasses intervention for improving socio-emotional behaviors in students with ASD.
Cooper et al. [40]	AAC software program with an embedded artificial conversational agent for children with autism.
Huijnen et al. [41]	Roles, strengths, and challenges of AI-equipped robots in interventions for children with ASD.
Keshav et al. [42]	Tolerability and usability of AI-driven smartglasses for individuals with ASD.
Linstead et al. [43]	Usefulness in perspective of AI in the treatment dosage and in providing insights into its varied effects across different domains.
Desideri et al. [44]	Exploration of humanoid robots' potential to enhance educational interventions for children with ASD.
Huijnen et al. [45]	Practical implementation of robots (implementing AI based algorithms), particularly robot KASPAR, in education and therapy interventions for children with ASD.
Bekele et al. [46]	Pilot study on an AI-driven robot-mediated system administering joint attention prompts to children with ASD with a demonstration of AI's potential to enhance engagement and learning in educational activities for children with ASD.
Williams et al. [47]	Highlighting AI-like systems' (with speech synthesizer) role in improving speech recognition and training for individuals with ASD.

3.2.2. Key Findings

The collection of studies [33–47] collectively sheds light on the promising intersection of artificial intelligence (AI) and autism assistive technologies [33–47]. The research landscape reflects a concerted effort to harness AI's capabilities for diverse applications catering to the unique needs of individuals on the autism spectrum.

A recurring theme in these studies is the exploration of AI-driven devices, such as socially-assistive robots, smartglasses, and recommendation systems, to enhance various facets of support for individuals with ASD. This includes teaching support, sensory management, emotion recognition, and even the automation of ASD diagnosis. The integration of AI into AAC software, featuring artificial conversational agents, stands out as a noteworthy endeavor to enhance communication for children with autism.

Common methodologies across these studies include the prevalent use of AI and machine learning techniques. Researchers are leveraging these advanced technologies to develop recommendation systems, models for recognizing and responding to user engagement, and diagnostic tools. Additionally, the implementation of AI-driven devices, particularly in educational interventions, emerges as a consistent approach to improving engagement and learning outcomes for individuals with ASD.

However, amidst the optimism, several challenges are evident. The diversity within the autism spectrum poses a substantial hurdle, requiring nuanced approaches that account for individualized needs. Ethical considerations, ranging from the tolerability and usability of AI-driven devices to broader privacy concerns, are inherent in the integration of AI into assistive technologies. The regulatory landscape and societal acceptance of these innovations within the healthcare domain represent additional challenges that demand careful navigation.

The practical implementation of humanoid robots in education and therapy interventions introduces complexities, with studies highlighting both the strengths and challenges associated with these AI-equipped robots. Moreover, the studies collectively underscore the imperative to strike a balance between pushing the boundaries of technological innovation and addressing the practical and ethical considerations essential for the successful integration of AI into autism assistive technologies.

In essence, this body of research paints a dynamic picture of the evolving relationship between AI and autism assistive technologies. The studies not only showcase the potential of AI to revolutionize support for individuals with ASD but also illuminate the path forward, emphasizing the need for a holistic and ethically grounded approach as these technologies continue to play an increasingly significant role in the lives of those on the autism spectrum.

4. Discussion

The discussion is structured into two parts, which are editorially translated into five paragraphs.

The initial part reported in Section 4.1, sets the stage, delving into the dissemination trends within this field. We examine these trends in contrast to the broader, overarching categories of ATs, which include AAC, both in a general context and, more specifically, within the realm of autism. The second part (Sections 4.2–4.5) delves into: (a) a detailed discussion of the key findings that have emerged in the study results, paying careful attention to the distinctive characteristics of autism. (b) Analyze the limitations and bottlenecks that have come to light within the reviewed studies.

4.1. Numerical Trends in Assistive Technologies for Autism

It is valuable to delve into the analysis of scientific publication trends within this specific field. The key insights encapsulated in Box 1 have been utilized in research conducted on the PubMed platform. Scientific publications pertaining to AAC, as well as other assistive technologies, trace their origins back to the year 1946. In a broader context, as depicted in Figure 1, a cumulative total of 17,607 studies have been brought forth to the scientific community. Notably, a substantial 8500 of these have emerged within the last decade, with a further 3911 publications emerging since the onset of the global COVID-19 pandemic. A significant proportion of these studies, roughly 39%, have seen the light of day in the most recent decade, and particularly noteworthy is the surge in publications following the emergence of the COVID-19 pandemic, accounting for approximately 19% of the total.. The graphical representation in Figure 2 provides a visual insight into the fact that a mere 2% of these studies are centered around the subject of autism. Zooming in on the domain of autism, the data depicted in Figures 3 and 4 reveal that, since 1992, a remarkable 391 studies have been produced on this subject. A considerable majority of these studies, (73%), have been published within the last decade. Furthermore, a significant 129 studies have been generated in the wake of the COVID-19 pandemic, constituting 33% of the total in this time frame. However, when we narrow our focus even further and zero in on those studies that specifically explore the intersection of autism and artificial intelligence (AI), the number is substantially reduced. In its entirety, only 23 studies have been published in this area. Out of these, 10 have emerged in the aftermath of the COVID-19 pandemic, while 21 have surfaced within the last ten years (as presented in Figure 5).

Box 1. The proposed composite keys.

"self help devices"[MeSH Terms] OR ("self help"[All Fields] AND "devices"[All Fields]) OR "self help devices"[All Fields] OR ("assistive"[All Fields] AND "technology"[All Fields]) OR "assistive technology"[All Fields] OR ("augmentative"[All Fields] AND ("communicate"[All Fields] OR "communicated"[All Fields] OR "communicates"[All Fields] OR "communicating"[All Fields] OR "communication"[MeSH Terms] OR "communication"[All Fields] OR "communications"[All Fields] OR "communicative"[All Fields] OR "communicational"[All Fields] OR "communicatively"[All Fields] OR "communicativeness"[All Fields] OR "communicator"[All Fields] OR "communicator s"[All Fields] OR "communicators"[All Fields]))
("self help devices"[MeSH Terms] OR ("self help"[All Fields] AND "devices"[All Fields]) OR "self help devices"[All Fields] OR ("assistive"[All Fields] AND "technology"[All Fields]) OR "assistive technology"[All Fields] OR ("augmentative"[All Fields] AND ("communicate"[All Fields] OR "communicated"[All Fields] OR "communicates"[All Fields] OR "communicating"[All Fields] OR "communication"[MeSH Terms] OR "communication"[All Fields] OR "communications"[All Fields] OR "communicative"[All Fields] OR "communicational"[All Fields] OR "communicatively"[All Fields] OR "communicativeness"[All Fields] OR "communicator"[All Fields] OR "communicator s"[All Fields] OR "communicators"[All Fields]))) AND "autism"[Title/Abstract]
("self help devices"[MeSH Terms] OR ("self help"[All Fields] AND "devices"[All Fields]) OR "self help devices"[All Fields] OR ("assistive"[All Fields] AND "technology"[All Fields]) OR "assistive technology"[All Fields] OR ("augmentative"[All Fields] AND ("communicate"[All Fields] OR "communicated"[All Fields] OR "communicates"[All Fields] OR "communicating"[All Fields] OR "communication"[MeSH Terms] OR "communication"[All Fields] OR "communications"[All Fields] OR "communicative"[All Fields] OR "communicational"[All Fields] OR "communicatively"[All Fields] OR "communicativeness"[All Fields] OR "communicator"[All Fields] OR "communicator s"[All Fields] OR "communicators"[All Fields]))) AND "autism"[Title/Abstract] AND ("artificial intelligence"[MeSH Terms] OR ("artificial"[All Fields] AND "intelligence"[All Fields]) OR "artificial intelligence"[All Fields] OR ("machine learning"[MeSH Terms] OR ("machine"[All Fields] AND "learning"[All Fields]) OR "machine learning"[All Fields]) OR ("deep learning"[MeSH Terms] OR ("deep"[All Fields] AND "learning"[All Fields]) OR "deep learning"[All Fields]) OR (("neural"[All Fields] OR "neuralization"[All Fields] OR "neuralize"[All Fields] OR "neuralized"[All Fields] OR "neuralizes"[All Fields] OR "neuralizing"[All Fields] OR "neurally"[All Fields]) AND "nework"[All Fields]))

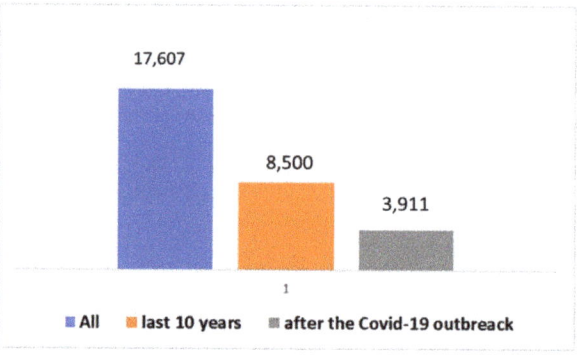

Figure 1. Trends in the studies on ATs (including AAC) over time.

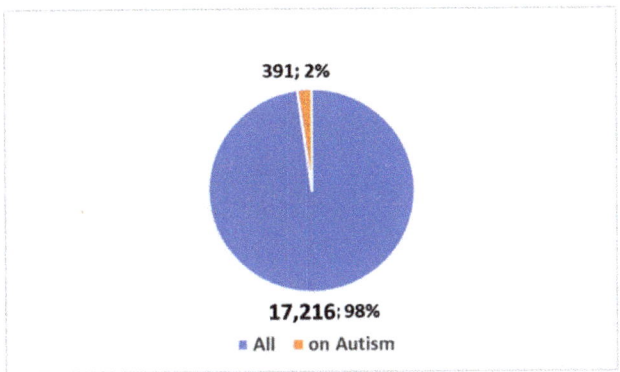

Figure 2. Percentage of studies on AT (including AAC) on autism compared to the total.

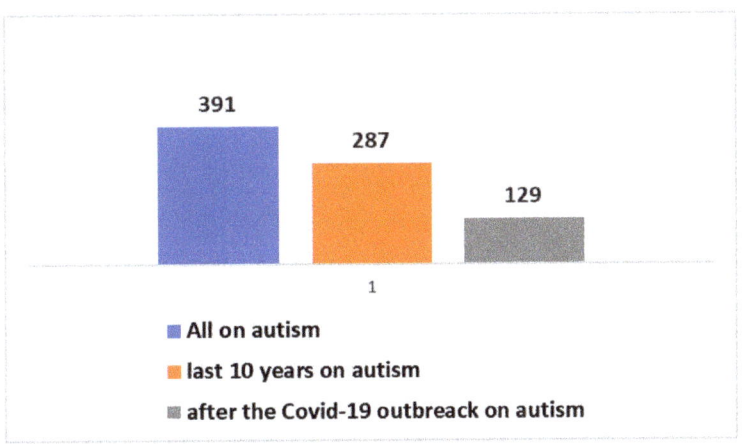

Figure 3. Scientific production of studies dedicated to AT (including AAC) on autism.

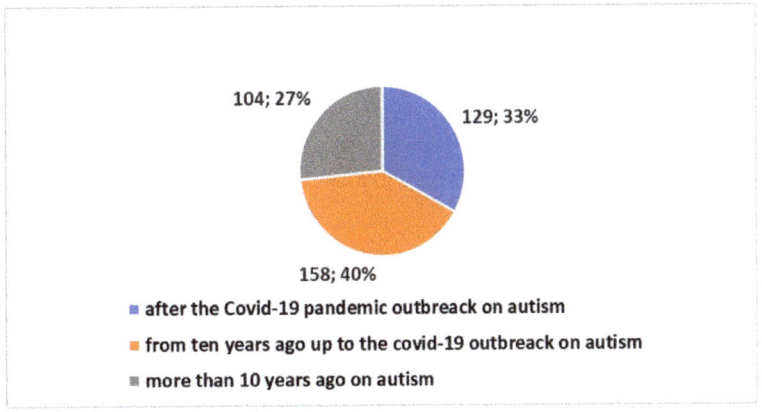

Figure 4. Percentage of studies dedicated to AT (including AAC) on autism over time.

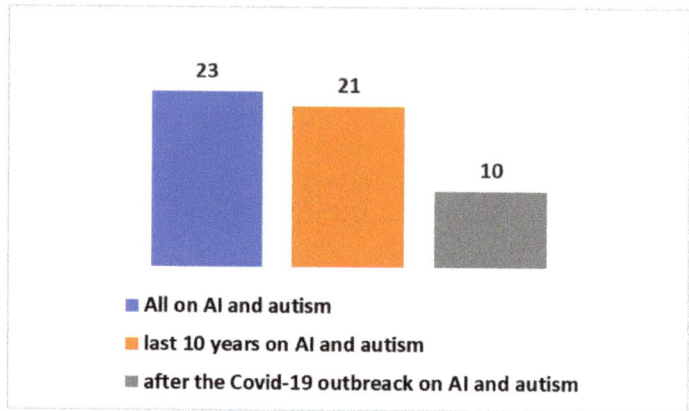

Figure 5. Studies on AI applied to ATs (including AACs) dedicated to autism.

4.2. Interpretation of Results: Findings, Problems

Autism, as a neurodevelopmental disorder, affects social behavior, communication, and interaction. It manifests itself with difficulties in understanding other people's emotions, in verbal and non-verbal communication, in restricted interest in certain topics, and in the repetitiveness of behaviors and routines. Each autistic individual is unique in his or her characteristics and level of functioning [48]. This uniqueness is reflected in the difficulty of diagnosis and therapy [49,50], which requires a multi-faceted approach from different medical disciplines, and in treatment that increasingly highlights the need for personalized medicine dedicated to autism [51,52].

It can unequivocally be asserted that a sound approach to addressing autism hinges upon the seamless interplay between the domains of diagnosis and therapy, encompassing a multitude of key players, ranging from parental associations and diverse professionals to scientific organizations (Figure 6):

- If we focus on the autism diagnosis we can affirm that among the important activities in diagnosis we find [49,50]: -Observation and Interviews: -Physical Exam and Medical History: -Developmental Assessment and Screening: -Psychological and Psychomotor Evaluation: -Assessment of Social Behavior and Social Interactions: -Language and Communication Assessment: -Sensory Assessment-Functional Behavior Assessment. -Genetic, metabolic, biochemical, immunological, neurobiologal assessments-Environmental factors. -Medical Imaging assessment. There are various therapies and interventions used in the treatment of ASD. These therapies aim to address the unique challenges and needs of individuals with autism. Therapies may include medications.

- If we focus on the autism therapy we can affirm that some of the most commonly used non medication therapies include [51]: -Behavioral Therapies: -Communication and Speech Therapies. -Speech-Language Therapy-Occupational Therapy. -Social Skills Training-Sensory Integration Therapy. -Educational Interventions-Medication. -Alternative and Complementary Therapies. It's important to note that the choice of therapy or intervention depends on the individual's specific needs, strengths, and challenges [52,53]. A comprehensive and individualized treatment plan is often the most effective approach, and it should be developed in consultation with healthcare professionals, including speech therapists, occupational therapists, and behavioral specialists, to provide the best possible support for individuals with autism. There are also available programs that provide training and support for parents and caregivers to help them better understand and manage the challenges associated with autism.

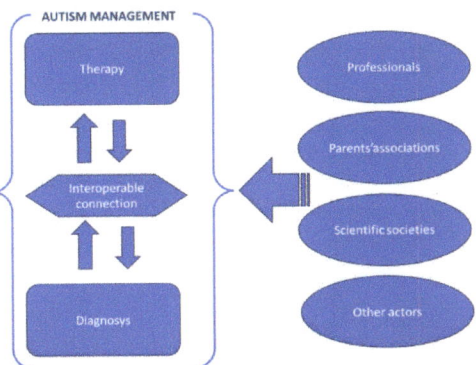

Figure 6. Autism: interoperability between the therapy and the diagnosis domains.

ATs (including AAC) devices occupy a central and strategic position in a multitude of non-medical therapies, as highlighted. However, adhering to the expansive framework established by the WHO [54], which encompasses AT processes and related services, including telemedicine, it becomes evident that ATs possess considerable untapped potential, even within the realm of diagnostic activities.

Our review, through two perspectives (one focused on reviews and the other on scientific articles), has addressed the introduction of AI in assistive technologies for autism.

The initial perspective, cantered on comprehensive reviews, underscores a steadily escalating integration of artificial intelligence (AI) within assistive technologies (ATs) for autism, spanning across fields like robotics [27,30,32], applications [29], and, in a broader context, automated machines such as computers and ICT devices [26–32]. This integration is specifically geared towards the enhancement of communication, interaction, and, most importantly, the overall social development of autistic children. Notably, in the case of mobile applications, a set of valuable recommendations has been proposed as well [29].

The second perspective consistently underscores a fascinating and rapidly growing integration of AI with robotics in the context of autism [33,38,41,44–46]. This integration serves as vital support for enhancing communication, interaction, and social engagement. Furthermore, the strategic aspect of therapy dosage in the realm of autism has been explored across various domains [36]. There's a burgeoning interest in the deployment of customized wearable devices, such as smart glasses [39,42], designed to improve socio-emotional behaviors in students with autism spectrum disorder (ASD), with their tolerability also undergoing assessment.

Across all of these research works, as seen in the perspective on reviews, AI is consistently addressed within the domain of automated machines, including computers and ICT devices [33–47]. In a particular study [36], as we had hoped for, the use of assistive technologies (ATs) in the field of diagnosis is highlighted, specifically the automation of ASD diagnosis through the application of machine learning techniques.

What emerges from the review is undoubtedly an early-phase landscape, particularly highlighted by the modest numbers evident at this stage in the field. Consequently, as expected, researchers are currently dedicating relatively little attention to aspects related to integration with the health domain, such as regulatory and consent issues.

Furthermore, it doesn't seem that there is a strong focus on personalized medicine within the realm of AI in assistive technologies. Personalized medicine, also known as precision medicine or personalized medicine, could represent an innovative approach in the field of autism [55]. This approach would carefully consider individual differences, including genetics, lifestyle, and environment, with the aim of personalizing disease prevention, diagnosis, and treatment with the aim of maximizing therapeutic efficacy and minimizing side effects [56–58], while also integrating with AI [59,60]. In the specific context of autism, personalized medicine could seek to adapt treatments based on the specific genetic and biological characteristics of each individual suffering from ASD [61]. This could mean identifying specific subtypes of autism based on genetic, biochemical, and neurophysiological markers. This customization would allow for a more accurate diagnosis and personalized assessment of each patient's clinical picture, helping to identify the most suitable and effective treatments [62–64].

It will unquestionably be imperative to exert additional efforts in these directions. Undoubtedly, AI is poised to play an ever more pivotal role in interconnecting diverse realms, and the integration of ATs with AI stands to assume an increasingly vital role as a connector of paramount importance (Figure 7).

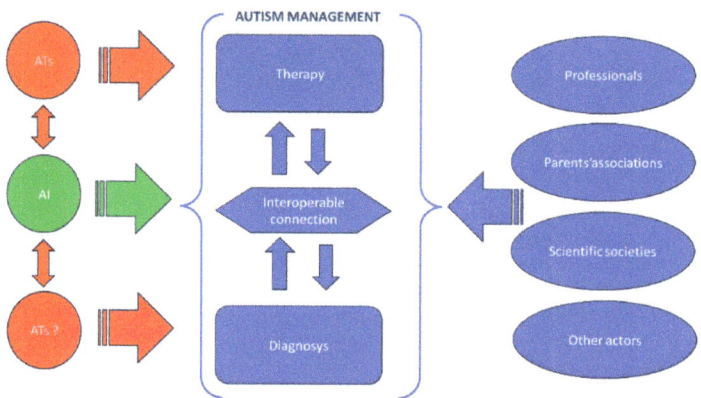

Figure 7. Autism: the potential mediator role of the AI and of the ATs.

4.3. Contextualizing Our Study: A Comparative Analysis with Diverse AI Applications in Autism Interventions

AI's impact on autism research is substantial, with a growing interest in its applications [65–67]. From diagnostics to IoT integrations, AI's transformative influence spans various healthcare facets, marking a remarkable evolution [68,69]. Machine learning (ML) and deep learning, especially in neural networks, play pivotal roles in addressing autism spectrum disorder (ASD) challenges [65]. ML excels in early ASD detection via behavioral and physiological data analysis, while predictive modeling tailors support strategies [66]. Naturalistic behavioral analysis, powered by computer vision and ML, informs interventions by decoding subtle cues [69]. Deep learning contributes to understanding communication challenges and identifying genetic markers associated with autism [65]. AI promises transformative potential in ASD research, from early detection to personalized interventions, exemplifying technology's capacity to improve lives [65–69].

In [70], 11 systematic reviews [28,71–80] focused on the impact of AI on autism. Collectively, these reviews tell a compelling story of AI emerging as a powerful ally in autism research. Themes explored include precision psychiatry [71], virtual reality-based techniques for health improvement [72], bibliometric analysis of AI in autism treatment [73], hybridization of medical tests [74], triage and priority-based healthcare diagnosis [75], mobile and wearable AI in child and adolescent psychiatry [76], robot-assisted therapy [28], machine-learning models in behavioral assessment [77], deep learning in psychiatric disorders classification [78], the impact of technology on ASD [79], and deep learning in neurology [80]. Each systematic review contributes to a nuanced exploration of AI within the realm of autism research, shedding light on technology's intersections with neurodevelopmental disorders. These reviews collectively underscore how AI is becoming integral in understanding and supporting individuals on the autism spectrum, offering diverse insights into tailored interventions, holistic well-being, diagnostic strategies, and advancements in neurology. Some of these themes have connections with assistive technologies

(ATs). The proposed overview can serve as both a valuable contribution and a mediator and connector between some of these fields.

4.4. Reflections on the Limitations

The review indirectly highlights that integration of AI with assistive technologies in the context of autism presents several challenges that merit careful consideration. Firstly, the inherent diversity within the autism spectrum poses a significant limitation. The spectrum encompasses a broad range of characteristics, making it difficult to develop AI solutions that adequately address the unique needs of each individual. A one-size-fits-all approach may fall short in providing meaningful support. Moreover, the highly individualized nature of autism complicates the effectiveness of AI interventions. Each person with autism has distinct preferences, strengths, and challenges that evolve over time. AI technologies may struggle to keep pace with these individualized requirements, potentially limiting their utility. Ethical considerations also loom large in the integration of AI. The collection and analysis of personal information to tailor interventions raises concerns about privacy, consent, and the potential for data misuse. Striking a balance between leveraging data for customization and respecting ethical boundaries is crucial. A fundamental aspect of autism support is human connection and empathetic understanding. AI, by its very nature, lacks the ability to establish genuine emotional connections. This deficit in emotional support may impede the effectiveness of AI-based interventions, particularly for individuals who require a more empathetic touch. Additionally, user acceptance and comfort pose significant challenges. Individuals with autism may face difficulties adapting to or feeling comfortable with AI technologies. Overcoming resistance and ensuring user comfort are paramount to the successful integration of AI with assistive technologies. Overall, while the integration of AI with AT holds promise, navigating the limitations requires a nuanced approach. Addressing the diversity within the spectrum, recognizing the individualized nature of autism, and upholding ethical standards are essential for the meaningful and ethical use of AI in supporting individuals with autism.

4.5. Reflection on the Broader Implications

The review also shows that the integration of AI with ATs for individuals with autism introduces broader implications that encompass issues of bias, ethics, and cybersecurity. Concerns related to bias arise from the potential replication of societal biases within the AI algorithms. If the training data used is not representative or contains inherent biases, the AI systems may inadvertently perpetuate stereotypes and fail to address the diverse needs of individuals on the autism spectrum. Ethical considerations become paramount, particularly concerning privacy and informed consent. The customization of interventions based on personal data necessitates a clear understanding and explicit consent from individuals with autism and their caregivers. Ensuring transparency in decision-making processes and providing individuals with the ability to comprehend and challenge those decisions are ethical imperatives. Equity and accessibility issues emerge as the integration of AI may not guarantee equal access to interventions. This raises ethical concerns about the potential exacerbation of existing disparities, emphasizing the need for ethical considerations that ensure the inclusivity and accessibility of AI benefits for all individuals with autism. Turning to cybersecurity, the sensitive nature of the data involved in autism support systems becomes a focal point. The risk of cyberattacks targeting personal information, communication patterns, and behavioral data underscores the importance of robust data security measures to safeguard the privacy and well-being of individuals with autism. Moreover, vulnerabilities to malicious exploitation of AI systems need careful attention. Tampering with interventions, manipulating data, or using AI tools to harm individuals with autism are potential risks that demand proactive measures to secure AI technologies and prevent exploitation. The interconnected nature of AI and AT systems introduces cybersecurity challenges. A breach in one system could have cascading effects on others, potentially compromising the well-being and privacy of individuals with autism. Establishing a secure and resilient infrastructure becomes imperative to mitigate these interconnected cybersecurity risks. Overall, while the integration of AI with assistive technologies holds promise for individuals with autism, addressing biases, upholding ethical standards, and ensuring robust cybersecurity measures are critical for the responsible and beneficial use of AI in enhancing the lives of those on the autism spectrum. Striking a delicate balance between innovation and ethical considerations is paramount to navigating these complex implications.

5. Brief Summary and Conclusions

5.1. Brief Summary

The amalgamation of findings from 22 studies, encompassing 7 reviews, underscores a burgeoning interest in the integration of AI into autism assistive technologies. The current landscape is marked by promising developments at the intersection of AI and robotics, as well as the creation of wearable automated devices like smart glasses. These technological innovations are poised to significantly improve communication, interaction, and social engagement for individuals with autism, offering a glimpse into a future where AI plays a pivotal role in supporting neurodiversity.

However, as the field progresses, it becomes evident that the emphasis on innovation currently outweighs the establishment of a solid presence within the healthcare domain. Critical issues such as regulation and societal acceptance are demanding increased attention. This underscores the need for a delicate balance between pushing the boundaries of technological advancement and addressing the practicalities of integrating these innovations into mainstream healthcare practices. Despite the exciting prospects, limitations exist on this path towards integrating AI into autism assistive technologies. The diversity within the autism spectrum poses a challenge, as individualized needs vary widely. Ethical concerns, including those related to privacy and data security, emerge as critical considerations that must be carefully navigated. Furthermore, the potential absence of a human touch in AI interventions raises questions about user acceptance, particularly among individuals with autism who may require a more empathetic and personalized approach.

Looking at the broader implications, the innovative fusion of AI with autism assistive technologies opens doors to transformative possibilities. It holds the potential to bridge various domains and act as a crucial connector, facilitating communication and support for individuals with autism. However, as this field evolves, it is imperative to address ethical considerations, establish robust regulatory frameworks, and ensure that these technological advancements are accessible and inclusive for all individuals on the autism spectrum. In navigating this complex landscape, the role of AI in fostering connectivity and support for neurodiverse communities becomes increasingly evident.

5.2. Conclusions

In conclusion, our review highlights an early but promising interest in the integration of artificial intelligence into autism assistive technologies although not without significant problems to face. Particularly fascinating developments are unfolding in the fusion of AI with robotics and the creation of wearable automated devices, such as smart glasses. These advancements hold exciting potential for enhancing communication, interaction, and social activities for individuals with autism. Currently, researchers are dedicating more effort to development than to the establishment of a solid foothold in the health domain, where issues like regulation and acceptance demand increased attention. As the field continues to evolve, it is evident that AI will play an increasingly pivotal role in bridging various domains, and integrated ATs with AI are poised to assume a key role as a vital connector.

Author Contributions: Conceptualization, D.G.; methodology, D.G.; software, D.G.; validation, D.G. and A.I.; formal analysis, All; investigation, All; resources, All; data curation, D.G.; writing—original draft preparation, D.G.; writing—review and editing, All; visualization, A.I.; supervision, D.G.; project administration, D.G.; funding acquisition, D.G. All authors have read and agreed to the published version of the manuscript.

Funding: This research received no external funding.

Conflicts of Interest: The authors declare no conflict of interest.

References

1. Available online: https://www.cdc.gov/ncbddd/autism/facts.html (accessed on 15 December 2023).
2. Available online: https://www.autismspeaks.org/what-autism (accessed on 15 December 2023).
3. Available online: https://www.nhs.uk/conditions/autism/what-is-autism/ (accessed on 15 December 2023).
4. Available online: https://www.nimh.nih.gov/health/topics/autism-spectrum-disorders-asd (accessed on 15 December 2023).
5. Available online: https://www.who.int/news-room/fact-sheets/detail/autism-spectrum-disorders (accessed on 15 December 2023).
6. Available online: https://www.psychiatry.org/patients-families/autism/what-is-autism-spectrum-disorder (accessed on 15 December 2023).
7. Mughal, S.; Faizy, R.M.; Saadabadi, A. *Autism Spectrum Disorder*; StatPearls Publishing: Treasure Island, FL, USA, 2023.
8. Grabrucker, A.M. (Ed.) *Autims Spectrum disor$des Brisbane (AU)*; Exon Publications: Brisbane City, QLD, Australia, 2021.
9. FM Casanova Imaging the Brain in Autism 2013th Edition, Springer 2013. Available online: https://www.amazon.it/Imaging-Brain-Autism-Manuel-Casanova/dp/1489999965 (accessed on 15 December 2023).
10. Liu, M.; Li, B.; Hu, D. Autism Spectrum Disorder Studies Using fMRI Data and Machine Learning: A Review. *Front Neurosci.* **2021**, *15*, 697870. [CrossRef] [PubMed]
11. ElNakieb, Y.; Ali, M.T.; Elnakib, A.; Shalaby, A.; Mahmoud, A.; Soliman, A.; Barnes, G.N.; El-Baz, A. Understanding the Role of Connectivity Dynamics of Resting-State Functional MRI in the Diagnosis of Autism Spectrum Disorder: A Comprehensive Study. *Bioengineering* **2023**, *10*, 56. [CrossRef] [PubMed]
12. Pruneti, C.; Coscioni, G.; Guidotti, S. Evaluation of the effectiveness of behavioral interventions for autism spectrum disorders: A systematic review of randomized controlled trials and quasi-experimental studies. *Clin. Child Psychol. Psychiatry* **2023**, *29*, 13591045231205614. [CrossRef] [PubMed]
13. Hutchinson, J.; Folawemi, O.; Bittla, P.; Kaur, S.; Sojitra, V.; Zahra, A.; Khan, S. The Effects of Risperidone on Cognition in People with Autism Spectrum Disorder: A Systematic Review. *Cureus* **2023**, *15*, e45524. [CrossRef] [PubMed]
14. Yu, Z.; Zhang, P.; Tao, C.; Lu, L.; Tang, C. Efficacy of nonpharmacological interventions targeting social function in children and adults with autism spectrum disorder: A systematic review and meta-analysis. *PLoS ONE.* **2023**, *18*, e0291720. [CrossRef] [PubMed]
15. Watling, R.; Benevides, T.; Robertson, S.M. Family-Centered Interventions for Children on the Autism Spectrum (2013–2021). *Am. J. Occup Ther.* **2023**, *77* (Suppl. S1), 7710393210. [CrossRef]
16. Scarcella, I.; Marino, F.; Failla, C.; Doria, G.; Chilà, P.; Minutoli, R.; Vetrano, N.; Vagni, D.; Pignolo, L.; Di Cara, M.; et al. Information and communication technologies-based interventions for children with autism spectrum conditions: A systematic review of randomized control trials from a positive technology perspective. *Front. Psychiatry* **2023**, *14*, 1212522. [CrossRef]
17. Available online: https://www.nytimes.com/2022/03/29/technology/ai-robots-students-disabilities.html (accessed on 15 December 2023).
18. Qiu, S.; An, P.; Kang, K.; Hu, J.; Han, T.; Rauterberg, M. A Review of Data Gathering Methods for Evaluating Socially Assistive Systems. *Sensors* **2021**, *22*, 82. [CrossRef]
19. Lima Antão, J.Y.F.; Oliveira, A.S.B.; Almeida Barbosa, R.T.; Crocetta, T.B.; Guarnieri, R.; Arab, C.; Massetti, T.; Antunes, T.P.C.; Silva, A.P.D.; Bezerra, Í.M.P.; et al. Instruments for augmentative and alternative communication for children with autism spectrum disorder: A systematic review. *Clinics* **2018**, *73*, e497. [CrossRef]
20. Brignell, A.; Chenausky, K.V.; Song, H.; Zhu, J.; Suo, C.; Morgan, A.T. Communication interventions for autism spectrum disorder in minimally verbal children. *Cochrane Database Syst. Rev.* **2018**, *11*, CD012324. [CrossRef]
21. Smith, D.L.; Atmatzidis, K.; Capogreco, M.; Lloyd-Randolfi, D.; Seman, V. Evidence-Based Interventions for Increasing Work Participation for Persons with Various Disabilities. *OTJR Occup. Particip. Health* **2017**, *37* (Suppl. S2), S3–S13. [CrossRef] [PubMed]
22. Available online: https://www.verywellhealth.com/assistive-technology-for-autism-5076159 (accessed on 15 December 2023).
23. Available online: https://www.atandme.com/contribution-of-artificial-intelligence-on-assistive-technology-innovation/ (accessed on 15 December 2023).
24. ANDJ Checklist. Available online: https://legacyfileshare.elsevier.com/promis_misc/ANDJ%20Narrative%20Review%20Checklist.pdf (accessed on 3 June 2023).
25. Giansanti, D. The Regulation of Artificial Intelligence in Digital Radiology in the Scientific Literature: A Narrative Review of Reviews. *Healthcare* **2022**, *10*, 1824. [CrossRef] [PubMed]
26. Muthu, P.; Tan, Y.; Latha, S.; Dhanalakshmi, S.; Lai, K.W.; Wu, X. Discernment on assistive technology for the care and support requirements of older adults and differently-abled individuals. *Front. Public Health* **2023**, *10*, 1030656. [CrossRef] [PubMed]
27. Barua, P.D.; Vicnesh, J.; Gururajan, R.; Oh, S.L.; Palmer, E.; Azizan, M.M.; Kadri, N.A.; Acharya, U.R. Artificial Intelligence Enabled Personalised Assistive Tools to Enhance Education of Children with Neurodevelopmental Disorders—A Review. *Int. J. Environ. Res. Public Health* **2022**, *19*, 1192. [CrossRef]

28. Alabdulkareem, A.; Alhakbani, N.; Al-Nafjan, A. A Systematic Review of Research on Robot-Assisted Therapy for Children with Autism. *Sensors* **2022**, *22*, 944. [CrossRef]
29. Rehman, I.U.; Sobnath, D.; Nasralla, M.M.; Winnett, M.; Anwar, A.; Asif, W.; Sherazi, H.H.R. Features of Mobile Apps for People with Autism in a Post COVID-19 Scenario: Current Status and Recommendations for Apps Using AI. *Diagnostics* **2021**, *11*, 1923. [CrossRef]
30. DiPietro, J.; Kelemen, A.; Liang, Y.; Sik-Lanyi, C. Computer- and Robot-Assisted Therapies to Aid Social and Intellectual Functioning of Children with Autism Spectrum Disorder. *Medicina* **2019**, *55*, 440. [CrossRef]
31. den Brok, W.L.; Sterkenburg, P.S. Self-controlled technologies to support skill attainment in persons with an autism spectrum disorder and/or an intellectual disability: A systematic literature review. *Disabil. Rehabil. Assist. Technol.* **2015**, *10*, 1–10. [CrossRef]
32. Billard, A.; Robins, B.; Nadel, J.; Dautenhahn, K. Building Robota, a mini-humanoid robot for the rehabilitation of children with autism. *Assist. Technol.* **2007**, *19*, 37–49. [CrossRef]
33. Silvera-Tawil, D.; Bruck, S.; Xiao, Y.; Bradford, D. Socially-Assistive Robots to Support Learning in Students on the Autism Spectrum: Investigating Educator Perspectives and a Pilot Trial of a Mobile Platform to Remove Barriers to Implementation. *Sensors* **2022**, *22*, 6125. [CrossRef]
34. Deng, L.; Rattadilok, P. A Sensor and Machine Learning-Based Sensory Management Recommendation System for Children with Autism Spectrum Disorders. *Sensors* **2022**, *22*, 5803. [CrossRef] [PubMed]
35. Wan, G.; Deng, F.; Jiang, Z.; Song, S.; Hu, D.; Chen, L.; Wang, H.; Li, M.; Chen, G.; Yan, T.; et al. FECTS: A Facial Emotion Cognition and Training System for Chinese Children with Autism Spectrum Disorder. *Comput. Intell. Neurosci.* **2022**, *2022*, 9213526. [CrossRef]
36. Kumar, C.J.; Das, P.R. The diagnosis of ASD using multiple machine learning techniques. *Int. J. Dev. Disabil.* **2021**, *68*, 973–983. [CrossRef] [PubMed]
37. Jain, S.; Thiagarajan, B.; Shi, Z.; Clabaugh, C.; Matarić, M.J. Modeling engagement in long-term, in-home socially assistive robot interventions for children with autism spectrum disorders. *Sci. Robot.* **2020**, *5*, eaaz3791. [CrossRef] [PubMed]
38. Keshav, N.U.; Vogt-Lowell, K.; Vahabzadeh, A.; Sahin, N.T. Digital Attention-Related Augmented-Reality Game: Significant Correlation between Student Game Performance and Validated Clinical Measures of Attention-Deficit/Hyperactivity Disorder (ADHD). *Children* **2019**, *6*, 72. [CrossRef]
39. Vahabzadeh, A.; Keshav, N.U.; Abdus-Sabur, R.; Huey, K.; Liu, R.; Sahin, N.T. Improved Socio-Emotional and Behavioral Functioning in Students with Autism Following School-Based Smartglasses Intervention: Multi-Stage Feasibility and Controlled Efficacy Study. *Behav. Sci.* **2018**, *8*, 85. [CrossRef]
40. Cooper, A.; Ireland, D. Designing a Chat-Bot for Non-Verbal Children on the Autism Spectrum. *Stud. Health Technol. Inform.* **2018**, *252*, 63–68. [PubMed]
41. Huijnen, C.A.G.J.; Lexis, M.A.S.; Jansens, R.; de Witte, L.P. Roles, Strengths and Challenges of Using Robots in Interventions for Children with Autism Spectrum Disorder (ASD). *J. Autism Dev. Disord.* **2019**, *49*, 11–21. [CrossRef]
42. Keshav, N.U.; Salisbury, J.P.; Vahabzadeh, A.; Sahin, N.T. Social Communication Coaching Smartglasses: Well Tolerated in a Diverse Sample of Children and Adults with Autism. *JMIR Mhealth Uhealth* **2017**, *5*, e140. [CrossRef]
43. Linstead, E.; Dixon, D.R.; Hong, E.; Burns, C.O.; French, R.; Novack, M.N.; Granpeesheh, D. An evaluation of the effects of intensity and duration on outcomes across treatment domains for children with autism spectrum disorder. *Transl. Psychiatry* **2017**, *7*, e1234. [CrossRef]
44. Desideri, L.; Negrini, M.; Cutrone, M.C.; Rouame, A.; Malavasi, M.; Hoogerwerf, E.J.; Bonifacci, P.; Di Sarro, R. Exploring the Use of a Humanoid Robot to Engage Children with Autism Spectrum Disorder (ASD). *Stud. Health Technol. Inform.* **2017**, *242*, 501–509.
45. Huijnen, C.A.G.J.; Lexis, M.A.S.; Jansens, R.; de Witte, L.P. How to Implement Robots in Interventions for Children with Autism? A Co-creation Study Involving People with Autism, Parents and Professionals. *J. Autism Dev. Disord.* **2017**, *47*, 3079–3096. [CrossRef]
46. Bekele, E.; Crittendon, J.A.; Swanson, A.; Sarkar, N.; Warren, Z.E. Pilot clinical application of an adaptive robotic system for young children with autism. *Autism* **2014**, *18*, 598–608. [CrossRef] [PubMed]
47. Williams, J.H.; Massaro, D.W.; Peel, N.J.; Bosseler, A.; Suddendorf, T. Visual-auditory integration during speech imitation in autism. *Res. Dev. Disabil.* **2004**, *25*, 559–575. [CrossRef]
48. Available online: https://www.cdc.gov/ncbddd/autism/screening.html#:~:text=Diagnosing%20autism%20spectrum%20disorder%20(ASD,months%20of%20age%20or%20younger (accessed on 15 December 2023).
49. Available online: https://www.cdc.gov/ncbddd/autism/hcp-dsm.html (accessed on 15 December 2023).
50. Lord, C.; Elsabbagh, M.; Baird, G.; Veenstra-Vanderweele, J. Autism spectrum disorder. *Lancet* **2018**, *392*, 508–520. [CrossRef] [PubMed]
51. National Institute of Mental Health. A Parent's Guide to Autism Spectrum Disorder. 2011. Available online: http://www.nimh.nih.gov/health/publications/a-parents-guide-to-autism-spectrum-disorder/index.shtml (accessed on 8 March 2012).
52. Kotte, A.; Joshi, G.; Fried, R.; Uchida, M.; Spencer, A.; Woodworth, K.Y.; Kenworthy, T.; Faraone, S.V.; Biederman, J. Autistic traits in children with and without ADHD. *Pediatrics* **2013**, *132*, e612–e622. [CrossRef]
53. Available online: https://www.nichd.nih.gov/health/topics/autism/conditioninfo/treatments (accessed on 15 December 2023).
54. Available online: https://www.who.int/news-room/fact-sheets/detail/assistive-technology (accessed on 15 December 2023).

55. Goetz, L.H.; Schork, N.J. Personalized medicine: Motivation, challenges, and progress. *Fertil. Steril.* **2018**, *109*, 952–963. [CrossRef] [PubMed]
56. Delpierre, C.; Lefèvre, T. Precision and personalized medicine: What their current definition says and silences about the model of health they promote. Implication for the development of personalized health. *Front. Sociol.* **2023**, *8*, 1112159. [CrossRef]
57. Shlyakhto, E.V. Scientific Basics of Personalized Medicine: Realities and Opportunities. *Her. Russ. Acad. Sci.* **2022**, *92*, 671–682. [CrossRef]
58. Evers, A.W.; Rovers, M.M.; Kremer, J.A.; Veltman, J.A.; Schalken, J.A.; Bloem, B.R.; van Gool, A.J. An integrated framework of personalized medicine: From individual genomes to participatory health care. *Croat. Med. J.* **2012**, *53*, 301–303. [CrossRef]
59. Schork, N.J. Artificial Intelligence and Personalized Medicine. *Cancer Treat. Res.* **2019**, *178*, 265–283. [CrossRef] [PubMed]
60. Johnson, K.B.; Wei, W.Q.; Weeraratne, D.; Frisse, M.E.; Misulis, K.; Rhee, K.; Zhao, J.; Snowdon, J.L. Precision Medicine, AI, and the Future of Personalized Health Care. *Clin. Transl. Sci.* **2021**, *14*, 86–93. [CrossRef] [PubMed]
61. Loth, E.; Murphy, D.G.; Spooren, W. Defining Precision Medicine Approaches to Autism Spectrum Disorders: Concepts and Challenges. *Front. Psychiatry* **2016**, *7*, 188. [CrossRef] [PubMed]
62. Kostic, A.; Buxbaum, J.D. The promise of precision medicine in autism. *Neuron* **2021**, *109*, 2212–2215. [CrossRef]
63. Gabis, L.V.; Gross, R.; Barbaro, J. Editorial: Personalized Precision Medicine in Autism Spectrum-Related Disorders. *Front. Neurol.* **2021**, *12*, 730852. [CrossRef]
64. Frye, R.E.; Boles, R.; Rose, S.; Rossignol, D. A Personalized Medicine Approach to the Diagnosis and Management of Autism Spectrum Disorder. *J. Pers. Med.* **2022**, *12*, 147. [CrossRef]
65. Kautish, S.; Dhiman, G. (Eds.) *Artificial Intelligence for Accurate Analysis and Detection of Autism Spectrum Disorder (Advances in Medical Diagnosis, Treatment, and Care)*; IGI Global Publisher: Hershey, PA, USA, 2021.
66. Mintz, J.; Gyori, M.; Aagaard, M. (Eds.) *Touching the Future Technology for Autism? Lessons from the HANDS Project*; IOS Press: Amsterdam, The Netherlands, 2012.
67. Wu, X.; Deng, H.; Jian, S.; Chen, H.; Li, Q.; Gong, R.; Wu, J. Global trends and hotspots in the digital therapeutics of autism spectrum disorders: A bibliometric analysis from 2002 to 2022. *Front. Psychiatry* **2023**, *14*, 1126404. [CrossRef]
68. Marciano, F.; Venutolo, G.; Ingenito, C.M.; Verbeni, A.; Terracciano, C.; Plunk, E.; Garaci, F.; Cavallo, A.; Fasano, A. Artificial Intelligence: The "Trait D'Union" in Different Analysis Approaches of Autism Spectrum Disorder Studies. *Curr. Med. Chem.* **2021**, *28*, 6591–6618. [CrossRef]
69. Abdel Hameed, M.; Hassaballah, M.; Hosney, M.E.; Alqahtani, A. An AI-Enabled Internet of Things Based Autism Care System for Improving Cognitive Ability of Children with Autism Spectrum Disorders. *Comput. Intell. Neurosci.* **2022**, *2022*, 2247675, Retraction in *Comput. Intell. Neurosci.* **2023**, *2023*, 9878709. [CrossRef]
70. Giansanti, D. An Umbrella Review of the Fusion of fMRI and AI in Autism. *Diagnostics* **2023**, *13*, 3552. [CrossRef]
71. Del Casale, A.; Sarli, G.; Bargagna, P.; Polidori, L.; Alcibiade, A.; Zoppi, T.; Borro, M.; Gentile, G.; Zocchi, C.; Ferracuti, S.; et al. Machine Learning and Pharmacogenomics at the Time of Precision Psychiatry. *Curr. Neuropharmacol.* **2023**, *21*, 2395–2408. [CrossRef] [PubMed]
72. Ali, S.G.; Wang, X.; Li, P.; Jung, Y.; Bi, L.; Kim, J.; Chen, Y.; Feng, D.D.; Magnenat Thalmann, N.; Wang, J.; et al. A systematic review: Virtual-reality-based techniques for human exercises and health improvement. *Front. Public Health* **2023**, *11*, 1143947. [CrossRef] [PubMed]
73. Zhang, S.; Wang, S.; Liu, R.; Dong, H.; Zhang, X.; Tai, X. A bibliometric analysis of research trends of artificial intelligence in the treatment of autistic spectrum disorders. *Front. Psychiatry* **2022**, *13*, 967074. [CrossRef] [PubMed]
74. Alqaysi, M.E.; Albahri, A.S.; Hamid, R.A. Diagnosis-Based Hybridization of Multimedical Tests and Sociodemographic Characteristics of Autism Spectrum Disorder Using Artificial Intelligence and Machine Learning Techniques: A Systematic Review. *Int. J. Telemed. Appl.* **2022**, *2022*, 3551528. [CrossRef] [PubMed]
75. Joudar, S.S.; Albahri, A.S.; Hamid, R.A. Triage and priority-based healthcare diagnosis using artificial intelligence for autism spectrum disorder and gene contribution: A systematic review. *Comput. Biol. Med.* **2022**, *146*, 105553. [CrossRef] [PubMed]
76. Welch, V.; Wy, T.J.; Ligezka, A.; Hassett, L.C.; Croarkin, P.E.; Athreya, A.P.; Romanowicz, M. Use of Mobile and Wearable Artificial Intelligence in Child and Adolescent Psychiatry: Scoping Review. *J. Med. Internet Res.* **2022**, *24*, e33560. [CrossRef] [PubMed]
77. Cavus, N.; Lawan, A.A.; Ibrahim, Z.; Dahiru, A.; Tahir, S.; Abdulrazak, U.I.; Hussaini, A. A Systematic Literature Review on the Application of Machine-Learning Models in Behavioral Assessment of Autism Spectrum Disorder. *J. Pers. Med.* **2021**, *11*, 299. [CrossRef] [PubMed]
78. Quaak, M.; van de Mortel, L.; Thomas, R.M.; van Wingen, G. Deep learning applications for the classification of psychiatric disorders using neuroimaging data: Systematic review and meta-analysis. *Neuroimage Clin.* **2021**, *30*, 102584. [CrossRef]
79. Valencia, K.; Rusu, C.; Quiñones, D.; Jamet, E. The Impact of Technology on People with Autism Spectrum Disorder: A Systematic Literature Review. *Sensors* **2019**, *19*, 4485. [CrossRef]
80. Valliani, A.A.; Ranti, D.; Oermann, E.K. Deep Learning and Neurology: A Systematic Review. *Neurol. Ther.* **2019**, *8*, 351–365. [CrossRef]

Disclaimer/Publisher's Note: The statements, opinions and data contained in all publications are solely those of the individual author(s) and contributor(s) and not of MDPI and/or the editor(s). MDPI and/or the editor(s) disclaim responsibility for any injury to people or property resulting from any ideas, methods, instructions or products referred to in the content.

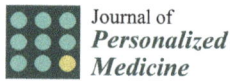

Review

Innovating Personalized Nephrology Care: Exploring the Potential Utilization of ChatGPT

Jing Miao [1], Charat Thongprayoon [1], Supawadee Suppadungsuk [1,2], Oscar A. Garcia Valencia [1], Fawad Qureshi [1] and Wisit Cheungpasitporn [1,*]

[1] Division of Nephrology and Hypertension, Department of Medicine, Mayo Clinic, Rochester, MN 55905, USA; miao.jing@mayo.edu (J.M.); thongprayoon.charat@mayo.edu (C.T.); supawadee.sup@mahidol.ac.th (S.S.); garciavalencia.oscar@mayo.edu (O.A.G.V.); qureshi.fawad@mayo.edu (F.Q.)

[2] Chakri Naruebodindra Medical Institute, Faculty of Medicine Ramathibodi Hospital, Mahidol University, Samut Prakan 10540, Thailand

* Correspondence: cheungpasitporn.wisit@mayo.edu

Abstract: The rapid advancement of artificial intelligence (AI) technologies, particularly machine learning, has brought substantial progress to the field of nephrology, enabling significant improvements in the management of kidney diseases. ChatGPT, a revolutionary language model developed by OpenAI, is a versatile AI model designed to engage in meaningful and informative conversations. Its applications in healthcare have been notable, with demonstrated proficiency in various medical knowledge assessments. However, ChatGPT's performance varies across different medical subfields, posing challenges in nephrology-related queries. At present, comprehensive reviews regarding ChatGPT's potential applications in nephrology remain lacking despite the surge of interest in its role in various domains. This article seeks to fill this gap by presenting an overview of the integration of ChatGPT in nephrology. It discusses the potential benefits of ChatGPT in nephrology, encompassing dataset management, diagnostics, treatment planning, and patient communication and education, as well as medical research and education. It also explores ethical and legal concerns regarding the utilization of AI in medical practice. The continuous development of AI models like ChatGPT holds promise for the healthcare realm but also underscores the necessity of thorough evaluation and validation before implementing AI in real-world medical scenarios. This review serves as a valuable resource for nephrologists and healthcare professionals interested in fully utilizing the potential of AI in innovating personalized nephrology care.

Keywords: artificial intelligence; chatbot; ChatGPT; nephrology; kidney disease; application

1. Introduction

Advancements in artificial intelligence (AI) technologies have notably influenced the landscape of various fields, including finance, transportation, and healthcare [1], leading to remarkable improvements in efficiency and productivity. AI is characterized by its capability to handle diverse tasks that traditionally need human intelligence. As AI applications become more integrated across different fields, the technology has grown to include major subsets like machine learning and deep learning. In medical research, machine learning has become particularly valuable for its ability to analyze and draw meaningful conclusions from the extensive data generated in healthcare. Specifically, in nephrology, a medical specialty focused on kidney diseases, machine learning has proven effective in classifying different patient subgroups across various kidney conditions, such as acute kidney injury (AKI), chronic kidney disease (CKD), end-stage kidney disease (ESKD), and kidney transplants [2–5]. Additionally, since 2018, there has been a surge in the utilization of machine learning-powered medical devices in healthcare. A thorough study revealed that a significant majority (77%) of these FDA-approved devices are predominantly used in radiology, with cardiovascular applications coming in second at 10% [6]. The most commonly approved types of these devices are radiological image processing and computer-assisted triage and notification systems [6]. However, it is noteworthy that in nephrology, the use of FDA-approved AI-enhanced medical devices is still an unexplored area.

ChatGPT, a significant language model introduced by OpenAI on 30 November 2022, is noted for generating human-like responses in a conversational style to user input [7,8]. Currently, ChatGPT has two primary versions: the broadly available GPT-3.5 and the more sophisticated, subscription-based GPT-4 [9]. ChatGPT exhibits its potential in various healthcare areas, including medical practices, research, and education [10,11]. Particularly notable is its remarkable proficiency in medical knowledge, which has been demonstrated to approach or even exceed the passing threshold (approximately 60%) for the United States Medical Licensing Examination (USMLE) [12,13]. In another study, ChatGPT nearly passed a radiology board-style examination with an accuracy of 69% [14]. In a third study, ChatGPT achieved an accuracy of approximately 80% in answering the questions from the competency-based medical education curriculum of microbiology [15]. However, it is important to consider the outcomes of an observational study that utilized the General Practitioners Applied Knowledge Test (GPAKT). The study revealed that ChatGPT's overall performance was 60%, falling below the average passing threshold of 70% [16].

In our initial investigation, we observed that GPT-3.5's performance was very limited when it came to responding to 150 questions related to glomerular disease from the Nephrology Self-Assessment Program (NephSAP) and Kidney Self-Assessment Program (KSAP). On the first and second runs, GPT-3.5 achieved an overall accuracy of only 44% and 41%, respectively. These results fell significantly below the required passing threshold of 75% set by the American Society of Nephrology (ASN) for nephrologists [17]. Subsequently, we conducted a comprehensive assessment using a larger set of 975 nephrology test questions, consisting of 508 questions from NephSAP and 467 from KSAP (Figure 1) [18]. GPT-3.5 obtained a total accuracy rate of 51% and a total concordance rate of 78%. Although GPT-4 showed improvement with a total accuracy rate of 74% and a total concordance rate of 83%, it still fell short of both the passing threshold and the average score of 77% achieved by nephrology examinees [18].

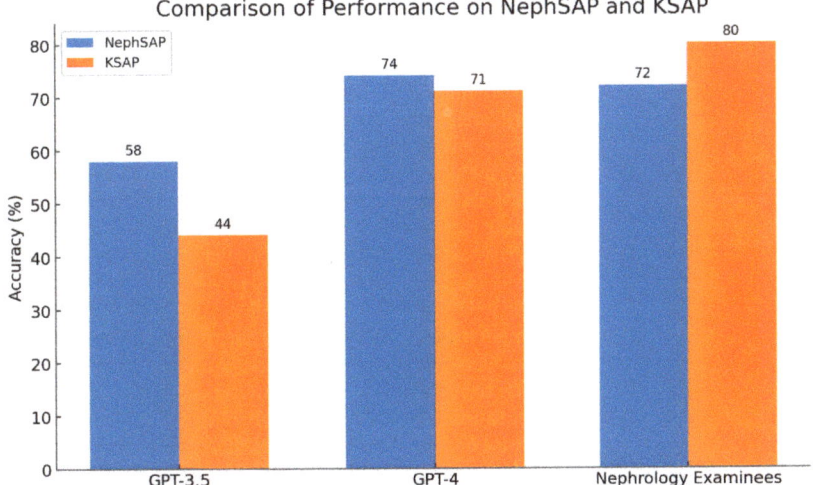

Figure 1. The performance of GPT-3.5, GPT-4, and nephrology examinees on NephSAP and KSAP test questions.

This comprehensive assessment also highlighted that ChatGPT's performance varied notably across different subfields (Figure 2). As we observed, accuracy rates were relatively lower in areas such as electrolyte and acid–base disorders, glomerular diseases, and renal-related bone and stone disorders [18]. These subjects were more likely to require higher-level cognitive engagement, which ChatGPT is documented to be weaker at performing. For instance, clinical questions related to electrolyte and acid–base disorders require more complex calculations. This was also evident in glomerular diseases, where questions often require a detailed understanding of kidney pathology, physiology, and various treatment options, spanning a broad range of topics including immunology, genetics, and pharmacology. These results indicate that the AI model struggles more with tasks requiring in-depth understanding, analytical skills, and precise calculations.

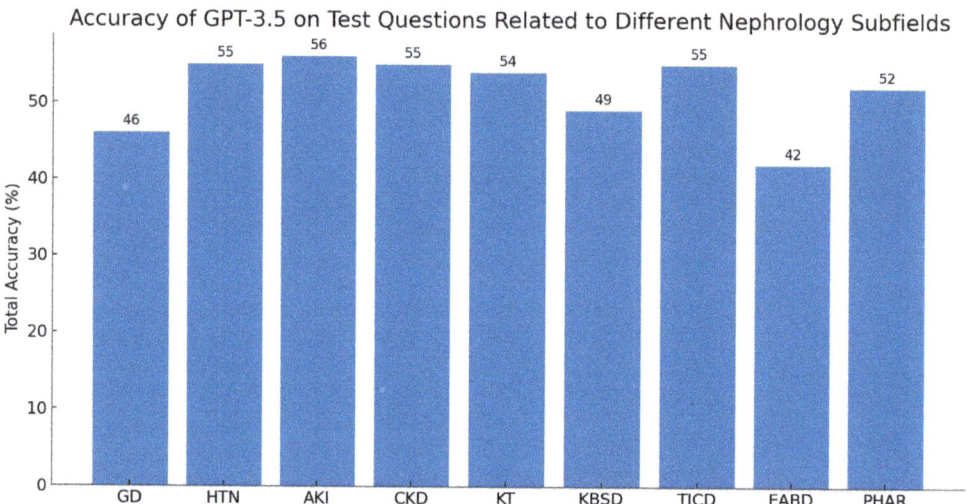

Figure 2. The performance of GPT-3.5 on test questions related to different nephrology subfields: GD: glomerular disease; HTN: gypertension; AKI: acute kidney injury; CKD: chronic kidney disease; KT: kidney transplant; KBSD: kidney-related bone and stone disorders; TICD: tubulointerstitial and cystic disorders; EABD: electrolytes and acid–base disorders; PHAR: pharmacology.

There has been a surge of interest in examining and discussing the potential practical uses of ChatGPT in various domains, which has mostly focused on its impact on medical education, scientific research, medical writing, ethical considerations, diagnostic or treatment decision making, automated data analysis, and criticisms [10,19–24], with over 1000 papers in PubMed dedicated to this subject. Yet, as far as our understanding goes, there is still a noticeable lack of a review consolidating the potential applications of ChatGPT, specifically within the field of nephrology, aiming to innovate personalized nephrology care.

2. Potential Applications of ChatGPT in Nephrology

In nephrology, mastering the core principles and having access to appropriate datasets are vital elements for optimizing personalized patient outcomes and facilitating substantial research contributions. The following discussion will focus on the practical implications of integrating ChatGPT into nephrological clinical settings, as shown in (Figure 3). It is important to note that the GPT Builder represents a key feature of ChatGPT models [25]. One of the most significant advantages of the GPT Builder is its user-friendly interface, which does not require extensive programming knowledge. This accessibility means that nephrologists, researchers, and healthcare providers can directly involve themselves in the development and adaptation of AI models to suit their specific clinical and research requirements. The GPT Builder not only simplifies the creation and configuration of GPT models but also ensures that these models are more aligned with the specific needs of nephrology, thereby maximizing their effectiveness and utility in both clinical and research settings.

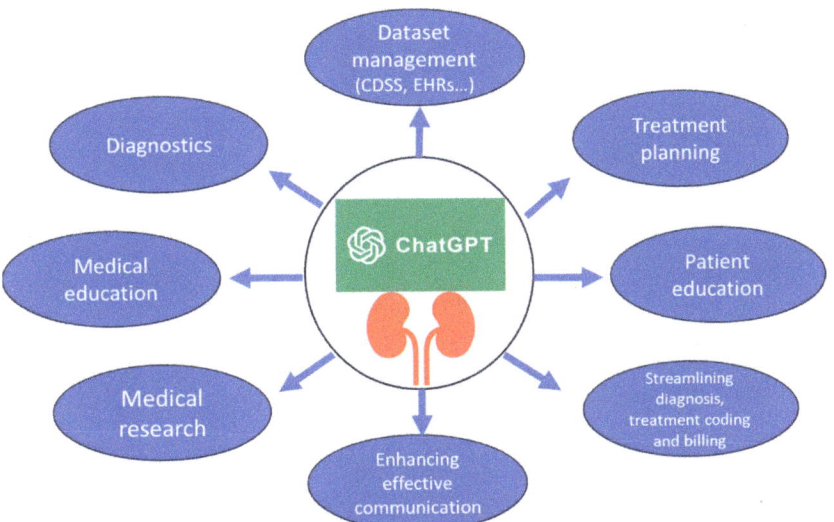

Figure 3. Potential applications of ChatGPT in the field of nephrology.

2.1. Integration of ChatGPT with Nephrology Datasets

2.1.1. Current Datasets in Nephrology

Electronic health records (EHRs) have revolutionized healthcare by providing a comprehensive digital repository of patient information [26]. In nephrology, EHRs capture clinical data related to kidney health, including laboratory results, imaging studies, medication history, and progress notes. EHRs offer several advantages, such as real-time availability of patient data, facilitating clinical decision making, and supporting research endeavors. By harnessing the wealth of information stored within EHRs, researchers and clinicians can conduct retrospective analyses, identify patterns, and generate evidence-based guidelines for optimal management of kidney diseases.

Besides EHRs, several datasets specifically curated for nephrology research also provide valuable information on patient characteristics, disease profiles, treatment modalities, and outcomes [27]. Examples of widely used nephrology datasets (Figure 4) include the United States Renal Data System (USRDS), the United Network for Organ Sharing (UNOS), the Organ Procurement and Transplantation Network (OPTN), and the Nephrotic Syndrome Study Network (NEPTUNE). In addition to these databases in the United States, other countries worldwide also have big datasets within nephrology for researchers, such as the European Renal Association-European Dialysis and Transplant Association (ERA-EDTA) Registry, the National Kidney Disease Surveillance Program in Ireland, the surveillance project on CKD management in Canada, and the China Kidney Disease Network (CK-NET). These datasets offer valuable insights into diverse aspects of kidney disease, such as CKD progression, dialysis outcomes, and kidney transplantation.

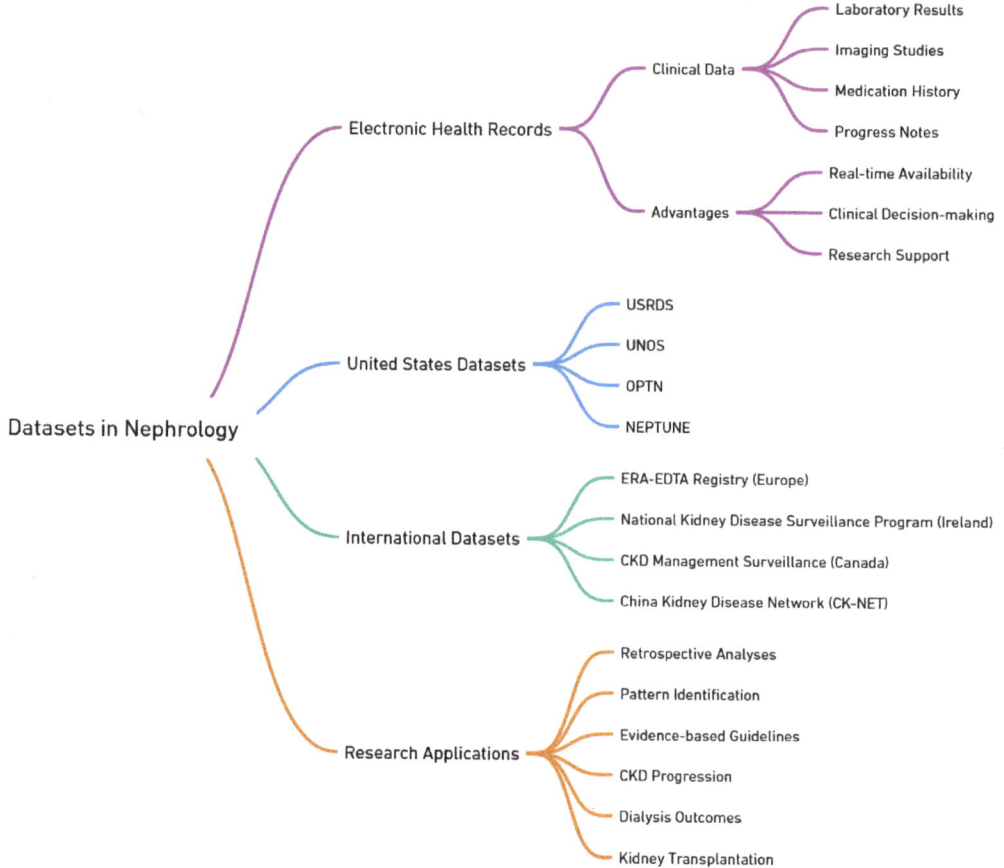

Figure 4. Overview of the datasets available for nephrology research.

2.1.2. Implications for ChatGPT Integration

While nephrology data sources offer immense potential, they are not without challenges and limitations. First and foremost is how to manage, handle, and process such a great amount of data that increased rapidly over time. Data quality and completeness can also be a significant concern. Inaccurate or missing data elements may limit the validity and generalizability of research findings. Furthermore, data interoperability and standardization issues across different healthcare systems can pose challenges in data integration and analysis.

Machine learning and other AI techniques possess the ability to handle intricate datasets and vast numbers of variables, surpassing the capabilities of classical statistical methods [28]. By leveraging AI tools like ChatGPT, the management of databases becomes significantly more feasible [29]. ChatGPT can be specifically fine-tuned to operate with a particular dataset and generate commands capable of executing various operations on that database. When incorporating ChatGPT or any other AI tool into nephrology data, it is essential to acknowledge and tackle potential biases and limitations associated with the model. Language models heavily rely on their training data, which can introduce inherent biases.

However, when applied appropriately, using ChatGPT for database management offers several advantages. Firstly, it saves valuable time and effort by automatically generating complex queries and commands, eliminating the need for manual and error-prone writing. Additionally, the fine-tuned model can be seamlessly integrated into larger applications, such as chatbots, enabling users to interact with the database using natural language. To ensure the accuracy and reliability of results, it is crucial to thoroughly evaluate and validate ChatGPT-generated outputs against expert knowledge and diverse patient populations. This evaluation helps mitigate potential biases. By addressing these challenges and leveraging available data effectively, researchers and healthcare professionals can lead to significant advancements in nephrology practice.

2.2. Applying ChatGPT in Nephrology Diagnostics

Accurate diagnosis is crucial for effective treatment and patient well-being. Human error can impede precise diagnostics due to the complexity and cognitive challenges of interpreting medical information. The advent of AI and natural language processing (NLP) technologies offers promising opportunities to revolutionize diagnostics [30].

2.2.1. Integration of CDSS with ChatGPT in Nephrology

Clinical decision support systems (CDSSs) are computer-based tools designed to assist healthcare professionals in making clinical decisions and providing patient care [31,32]. These systems utilize patient-specific data, medical knowledge, and algorithms to provide recommendations, alerts, and reminders at the point of care. Although CDSSs offer numerous advantages, they also come with some drawbacks [31]. For instance, CDSSs can disrupt clinician workflows, especially in the case of stand-alone systems. Excessive and inappropriate alerts can burden clinicians with additional verification tasks and result in alert fatigue. Limited technological proficiency can hinder the effective utilization of CDSSs. A study indicated that ChatGPT-generated suggestions have the potential to serve as a valuable complement in the optimization of CDSS alerts [22,33]. They could play a significant role in assisting experts in developing their own suggestions for enhancing CDSS effectiveness.

Additionally, many CDSSs lack transportability and interoperability, limiting their seamless integration into existing systems. While ChatGPT has limited ability to directly execute specific algorithms, it plays a valuable role in facilitating algorithm design for intelligent CDSS at the textual level [34]. One key aspect of integrating ChatGPT with CDSS is the seamless integration of the language model into the existing CDSS infrastructure. To optimize integration, ChatGPT should undergo fine-tuning specifically for nephrology-related tasks and queries. Real-time data integration from EHRs is also essential in the CDSS-ChatGPT system. By accessing up-to-date patient information such as laboratory results, medication history, and clinical notes, ChatGPT can generate more precise recommendations and assist clinicians in making informed decisions. Moreover, the integration can enhance clinical education and knowledge sharing by providing access to relevant literature, clinical guidelines, and case studies.

2.2.2. Development of ChatGPT Diagnostic Model for Kidney Disease

Building a ChatGPT diagnostic model specifically for kidney disease classification involves several crucial steps and considerations. Nephrology experts and data scientists need to collaborate to gather and curate diverse data from various sources like EHRs. These data include a wide range of kidney diseases, their associated symptoms, and relevant diagnostic criteria, as well as individual patient information (e.g., demographics, medical histories, laboratory results, imaging findings, and diagnostic outcomes). The dataset can be used to train ChatGPT to learn the relationships between input features and the corresponding kidney disease classifications, thus recognizing patterns and making accurate predictions. During the training process, the model's performance is evaluated and adjusted by partitioning the dataset into training and validation subsets and further enhanced through techniques like transfer learning and fine-tuning. This ChatGPT diagnostic tool has the potential to assist healthcare providers in accurately identifying and classifying various kidney diseases, contributing to timely and effective treatment decisions [35].

2.2.3. Assessing Performance of ChatGPT in Nephrology Diagnostics

Evaluating the performance, including the accuracy and repeatability, of ChatGPT in nephrology diagnostics is crucial for assessing its reliability for clinical use. During an assessment involving a typical clinical scenario of acute organophosphate poisoning, ChatGPT-3 demonstrated commendable performance in addressing all inquiries, including making a diagnosis [36]. In a research study, the diagnostic accuracy of ChatGPT-3 was evaluated for ten common clinical cases with typical symptoms. The study showed that ChatGPT generated differential diagnosis lists with a high accuracy of 93%, although this accuracy rate was slightly lower compared to the physicians' rate of 98% [37]. In another examination focused on evaluating the diagnostic capabilities of ChatGPT-3.5 in relation to kidney disease, the system exhibited an impressive accuracy rate of 91%, outperforming human physicians in both accuracy and speed [38]. ChatGPT, particularly GPT-4, showed the potential to provide faster responses to routine clinical laboratory questions. The study reported a correct rate of 76% (completely correct 51% and partially correct 23%), but the correct answers were most frequently seen in questions related to basic medical or technical knowledge [39].

Several important considerations should be taken into account during these evaluations to ensure robust and valid results. Firstly, a benchmark must be established for comparison. This can be achieved by using existing diagnostic methods or expert opinions as a reference standard. By comparing ChatGPT's diagnostic performance against established standards, we can evaluate its accuracy, sensitivity, specificity, and overall diagnostic usefulness. To ensure generalizability and minimize bias, a comprehensive evaluation should involve a diverse range of patient cases covering various nephrological conditions and different patient demographics. Secondly, to quantitatively evaluate and compare the diagnostic accuracy of ChatGPT, it is recommended to employ performance metrics such as precision, recall, F1 score (combination of the precision and recall scores), and receiver operating characteristic (ROC) curves. These metrics offer objective measures of the model's performance, enabling a comprehensive assessment of its strengths and limitations [40,41]. Prospective studies can be conducted to compare the diagnostic accuracy and treatment decisions made with and without the assistance of ChatGPT.

2.3. Applying ChatGPT in Treatment Planning

2.3.1. ChatGPT-Powered Treatment Recommendations and Personalized Care

A significant benefit of incorporating ChatGPT into treatment strategies lies in its capacity for crafting individualized medical guidance [42–44]. Research shows that ChatGPT-4 has demonstrated proficiency in pinpointing medications adhering to established guidelines for treating advanced solid tumors [45]. By processing diverse patient data, including medical histories, lab test results, and coexisting health issues, ChatGPT can formulate personalized treatment options. These may involve specific drug dosages, recommended dietary changes, alterations in daily habits, and tailored monitoring protocols [46]. Right now, there exist two main types of leading chatbot models. One type revolves around OpenAI's versions like ChatGPT-3.5, ChatGPT-4, and Bing Chat. Microsoft introduced Bing Chat in February 2023 as part of its search engine, utilizing OpenAI's GPT-4 model for conversational AI features [47]. The other notable model is Bard AI from Google, which is based on the Pathways Language Model 2 (PaLM2), a transformer language model [48]. In a recent study evaluating the capability of ChatGPT-3.5, ChatGPT-4, Bard AI, and Bing Chat in discerning potassium and phosphorus content in foods for CKD patients, distinct levels of accuracy were observed (Figure 5). Using 240 food items from the Mayo Clinic Renal Diet Handbook, each model categorized foods as high or low in potassium and phosphorus, and their results were compared to the handbook's guidelines. ChatGPT-4 led in potassium identification with 81% accuracy, excelling notably over ChatGPT-3.5, which had a 66% accuracy rate. In phosphorus identification, Bard AI achieved perfect accuracy, while ChatGPT-4 lagged with 77%. These findings highlight the burgeoning role of AI in facilitating renal dietary planning, though improvements are needed for maximum effectiveness.

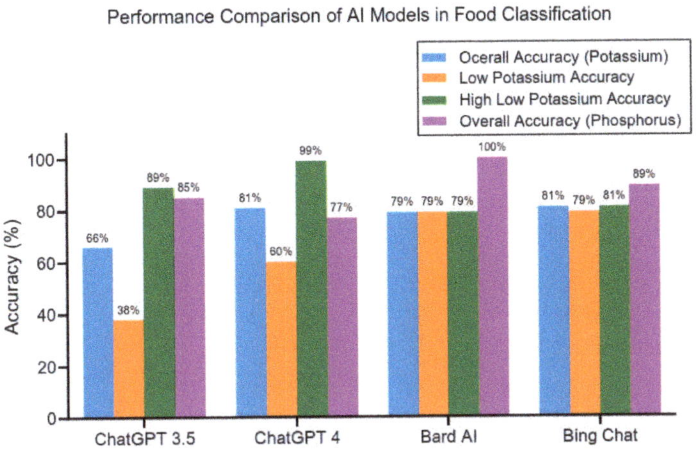

Figure 5. The performance of the four AI models in classifying food items based on their potassium and phosphorus content.

2.3.2. ChatGPT-Powered Decision Support for Medication Management

Medication management is a critical aspect of nephrology care, considering the complexity of drug regimens and the potential for medication-related complications. By integrating with EHRs and leveraging its vast knowledge base, ChatGPT can assist in drug–drug interaction checks, dosage adjustments based on renal function, and adherence monitoring. Furthermore, ChatGPT can facilitate communication between healthcare professionals and patients regarding medication-related queries, side effects, and treatment goals. The utilization of ChatGPT in a case report regarding a delayed diagnosis for a 27-year-old woman who reported chest pain and shortness of breath to the emergency department suggests its potential for clinical decision making, including improved diagnostic accuracy and addressing human factors contributing to medical errors [49]. Another study was conducted to see how well ChatGPT can answer medical questions [50]. The authors tested it with a case of a 22-year-old man who has a condition called treatment-resistant schizophrenia (TRS) and compared ChatGPT's recommendations for assessment and treatment with the current standards used by doctors. The results showed that ChatGPT correctly identified the patient's condition as TRS. It also suggested a thorough examination to find out the possible medical and psychiatric causes of the symptoms. Additionally, ChatGPT provided a comprehensive treatment plan, including medication and non-medication options, which matched the usual care provided by healthcare professionals for TRS.

2.4. Integrating Patient Education and Counseling with ChatGPT

Patient education and counseling are critical components of healthcare, aimed at empowering patients to actively participate in their treatment and manage their condition effectively. ChatGPT can serve as a valuable tool for integrating patient education and counseling into the nephrological treatment planning process [51], such as enhancing kidney transplant care [52].

Firstly, ChatGPT can provide accessible and personalized educational materials to patients. With its vast knowledge base, ChatGPT can offer comprehensive information on kidney diseases, treatment options, lifestyle modifications, and self-care practices [53]. Patients can engage in interactive conversations with ChatGPT, asking questions and seeking clarification on complex medical concepts. By delivering information in a conversational and user-friendly manner, ChatGPT can enhance patient comprehension and engagement with educational content. A study indicated that ChatGPT answered all queries well and offered good explanations of the underlying reasons regarding a typical clinical toxicology case of acute organophosphate poisoning retrieved from an online presentation [36]. The accuracy and reproducibility of ChatGPT were also examined in answering questions regarding knowledge, management, and emotional support for cirrhosis and hepatocellular carcinoma. While approximately 75% of the questions were answered with reliable information, the information regarding treatment recommendations such as decision-making cut-offs and treatment durations did not always align with the United States guidelines [54,55].

Secondly, ChatGPT can support counseling sessions by providing empathetic and supportive interactions. Patients living with kidney disease often face emotional and psychosocial challenges, including anxiety, depression, and uncertainty about the future. ChatGPT can act as a virtual companion, offering emotional support and guidance during counseling sessions. Patients can express their concerns, fears, and frustrations to ChatGPT, which can respond with empathy, validation, and practical advice. By facilitating open and non-judgmental conversations, ChatGPT can help patients navigate their emotional well-being and improve their overall quality of life. A cross-sectional study showed that ChatGPT generated quality and empathetic responses to patient questions posed in an online forum [56]. Moreover, ChatGPT can also help patients set realistic goals, develop personalized action plans, and track their progress. By providing reminders, motivational messages, and accountability, ChatGPT can support patients in making sustainable lifestyle changes and adhering to their prescribed treatment regimens [46]. The interactive nature of ChatGPT allows for ongoing communication, enabling patients to seek guidance and discuss challenges they encounter in their self-management journey.

2.5. Streamlining Diagnosis, Treatment Coding, and Billing with ChatGPT

ChatGPT presents the opportunity to enhance productivity and reduce expenses, thereby streamlining overall operations in healthcare services [57]. Proper coding and billing are essential for documenting diagnoses, procedures, and services provided to patients accurately. They enable healthcare providers to communicate essential information to payers, government agencies, and other stakeholders involved in reimbursement processes. Moreover, accurate coding and billing contribute to transparent and ethical financial practices in healthcare settings.

2.5.1. Enhancing ICD-10 Diagnosis Coding with ChatGPT

ICD-10 coding is a complex process that requires adherence to specific guidelines and conventions for accurate diagnosis coding. The extensive range of kidney diseases, their variations, and associated comorbidities pose challenges in selecting the appropriate diagnosis codes. A study was conducted to develop an automated ICD-10 coding system using a deep neural network based on supervised learning. The researchers' model demonstrated a notable improvement in the F1 score; however, it did not result in a reduction in the time required for disease coders to perform coding tasks [58]. ChatGPT's NLP capabilities enable it to analyze patient information, laboratory results, imaging reports, and clinical notes in real-time, and provide immediate suggestions for diagnosis codes. Through continuous feedback and suggestions, ChatGPT can enhance coding accuracy, reduce the need for retrospective code correction, and minimize the potential for claim denials or payment delays. ChatGPT's real-time coding assistance can also save time for healthcare providers, allowing them to focus more on patient care and reducing the administrative burden associated with coding tasks [59].

2.5.2. Enhancing Treatment Coding with ChatGPT

Current procedural terminology (CPT) codes provide a standardized system for identifying and reporting medical procedures and services. Nephrologists encounter various procedures in their practice, such as dialysis, kidney transplantation, vascular access placement, and kidney biopsies. Each procedure has a specific CPT code associated with it, reflecting the nature and complexity of the intervention. ChatGPT can provide coding support for these procedures by offering guidance on the appropriate CPT codes, documentation requirements, and coding modifiers that may be necessary [10]. For example, in the case of dialysis, ChatGPT can assist nephrologists in selecting the correct CPT codes for various dialysis modalities (e.g., hemodialysis, peritoneal dialysis, etc.) and associated services (e.g., vascular access management, dialysis catheter insertion, etc.). Similarly, in kidney transplantation, ChatGPT can aid in coding the transplant procedure, immunosuppressive therapy, and post-transplant follow-up care. Moreover, ChatGPT can offer real-time coding suggestions, ensuring that the appropriate CPT codes are assigned for the procedures performed. This can reduce the potential for coding errors and minimize the need for retrospective code corrections.

2.5.3. Improving Billing Efficiency with ChatGPT

ChatGPT can analyze the clinical data within the EHR and assist in generating accurate billing codes, such as diagnosis-related group (DRG) codes, CPT codes, and evaluation and management (E/M) codes. This integration eliminates the need for manual code selection and reduces the potential for coding errors, leading to improved billing accuracy and efficiency [60]. In addition, this integration can offer the potential for enhanced communication between healthcare providers and insurance companies [60]. Through the generation of precise and standardized codes, the AI model enables smoother information exchange, leading to expedited claim processing and reimbursements. Furthermore, the integration of ChatGPT into billing processes can maximize revenue cycle efficiency by automating repetitive billing tasks, such as code generation, charge capture, and claims submission and identifying potential coding and billing discrepancies. This not only saves time but also reduces the risk of errors and improves overall billing accuracy [60]. Consequently, this can alleviate the administrative workload on healthcare providers, enabling them to dedicate more attention to patient care.

Utilizing ChatGPT and similar AI tools built on extensive large language models (LLMs) provides remarkable assistance in programming tasks, although their application necessitates careful consideration [61]. It is crucial to assess the influence of ChatGPT on coding accuracy, billing efficiency, and reimbursement to effectively determine its effectiveness in the field of nephrology practice.

2.6. Enhancing Effective Communication with ChatGPT

Effective communication is a cornerstone of quality healthcare delivery. Written communication plays a crucial role in conveying important information, facilitating collaboration, and advocating for patients. By utilizing ChatGPT, the field of medical writing has the potential to undergo a revolutionary transformation [62]. A systematic review indicated that the benefits of ChatGPT were most frequently cited in the context of academic and/or scientific writing, such as efficiency and versatility in writing with text of high quality, improved language, and good readability [10].

2.6.1. Significance of Written Communication in Nephrology

Written communication serves as a vital means of transmitting crucial information in nephrology practice [63]. It enables nephrologists to deliver comprehensive and well-organized messages, ensuring clarity and minimizing misinterpretation [64]. Letters are particularly valuable in conveying complex medical information to patients, referring providers, and payers, promoting understanding, collaboration, and continuity of care. Well-documented letters serve as a permanent record of patient assessments, treatment plans, and progress updates. These records not only support clinical decision making but also provide a legal and professional framework for healthcare providers to justify their actions and decisions.

2.6.2. Utilizing ChatGPT for Crafting Patient Correspondence

When writing letters to patients, it is crucial to use language that is easily understandable and free of medical jargon. In the United States, it is recommended that patient-facing health literature be written at or below a sixth-grade level [65]. In addition, patient letters should provide educational resources (i.e., websites, brochures, or educational videos) to empower patients in self-management and address common questions and concerns that patients may have regarding their condition or treatment. ChatGPT can help craft patient-friendly letters to explain the diagnosis, treatment plans, and lifestyle recommendations using plain language and visual aids whenever possible. A pilot study showed that it is possible to generate clinic letters with a high overall correctness and humanness score with ChatGPT in a series of different clinical communication scenarios that covered the remit of a clinician's skin cancer practice. Furthermore, these letters were written at a reading level that is broadly similar to current real-world human-generated letters [66,67].

2.6.3. Leveraging ChatGPT for Communicating with Referring Providers

When communicating with referring providers, referral letters play a vital role in ensuring a seamless transition of care. Referral letters should provide a concise summary of the patient's medical history, current condition, and the reason for referral and include relevant test results, imaging findings, and any specific questions or concerns that require attention.

In the context of referring letters, integrating ChatGPT can offer several benefits in updating referring providers on patient progress and recommendations. Firstly, ChatGPT can be utilized to automatically generate concise summaries of patient progress, extracting key information from EHRs and clinical notes. Secondly, ChatGPT can seamlessly integrate with CDSS to provide evidence-based treatment suggestions and recommendations. This integration ensures that referring providers receive accurate and up-to-date information regarding the patient's progress. The suggestions can be included in the follow-up and consultation letters, ensuring that referring providers are informed about the most appropriate management strategies based on the latest medical knowledge. Thirdly, ChatGPT can assist in enhancing the language and clarity of the follow-up and consultation letters. By refining the language, ChatGPT can help nephrologists convey complex medical information in a more understandable and concise manner, facilitating better communication and comprehension for referring providers. In addition, ChatGPT can provide real-time assistance and feedback to nephrologists as they draft follow-up and consultation letters. By analyzing the content being written, ChatGPT can suggest additional details to include, prompt for clarification, or identify potential gaps in information. This interactive feedback helps nephrologists ensure that the letters are comprehensive and accurate before finalizing and sending them to referring providers. Furthermore, ChatGPT can support the implementation of shared decision making between nephrologists and referring providers. It can provide educational resources and relevant literature to facilitate discussions about treatment options, potential risks and benefits, and patient preferences. Ultimately, ChatGPT promotes a patient-centered approach and strengthens the therapeutic alliance between nephrologists and referring providers.

2.6.4. Utilizing ChatGPT for Medication Approval Appeals

Medication approval appeals are essential when patients require specific medications that may not be initially approved by insurance providers or healthcare organizations. Writing medication approval appeal letters is a critical aspect of nephrology practice, as it involves advocating for patients' therapeutic needs and ensuring that patients receive timely access to the medications required for managing their kidney disease and related conditions.

ChatGPT can provide valuable assistance in writing medication approval appeal letters. It can offer healthcare providers access to a vast array of medical literature, research articles, and clinical guidelines, enabling them to incorporate the most up-to-date and relevant information into their appeals. Additionally, ChatGPT can help refine the language, suggest alternative phrases, and ensure that the appeal letter adheres to the conventions of academic writing. By leveraging ChatGPT's capabilities, healthcare providers can enhance the persuasiveness and effectiveness of their medication approval appeals, ultimately advocating for patients' therapeutic needs.

2.7. Enhancing Nephrology Research with ChatGPT

2.7.1. Leveraging ChatGPT for Data Analysis

ChatGPT, as a powerful language model, can be used to gather data from large numbers of patients and extract valuable insights from unstructured textual data sources such as EHRs, clinical trial reports, and the scientific literature, streamlining the process of data collection and analysis [19,68]. This can be particularly useful in longitudinal studies, where ChatGPT can be used to track patient outcomes over time. One specific application of ChatGPT in nephrology research is the analysis of EHRs. By training ChatGPT on large-scale EHR datasets, researchers can develop models that can extract and analyze specific data elements relevant to nephrology, such as kidney function indicators, disease progression markers, and treatment outcomes. This enables researchers to gain deeper insights into the factors influencing kidney diseases, develop predictive models, and identify potential interventions for improved patient outcomes.

In addition, ChatGPT can generate commands and syntax for various statistical software packages, enabling researchers, even those with limited programming experience, to explore and analyze their data efficiently.

2.7.2. Enhancing Articles Writing with ChatGPT

ChatGPT excels in accelerating the writing process, generating outlines, incorporating additional details, and enhancing the overall writing style [69–75]. The assistance of ChatGPT can be instrumental in identifying discussion points and clarifying language for the readers of medical literature reports [76,77]. However, it is important to acknowledge its limitations. As a precautionary measure, it is crucial to carefully review and edit the generated text to ensure that it adheres to ethical standards, avoiding issues like plagiarism and fabrication.

2.7.3. Assisting Nephrology Literature Analysis with ChatGPT

The vast amount of publications makes it challenging for researchers to keep up with the latest findings and integrate the existing knowledge effectively. Traditional literature review methods are time consuming and prone to human error. ChatGPT can aid in literature mining and analysis by automatically extracting relevant information from scientific articles, summarizing key findings and evidence, and identifying potential biases of relevant studies and relationships between different concepts. By leveraging ChatGPT's capabilities, researchers can streamline the literature review process, identify knowledge gaps, and accelerate the discovery of new insights [78]. Its ability to handle large volumes of data and extract meaningful insights makes it a valuable tool for conducting rigorous systematic reviews and meta-analyses.

We conducted an initial evaluation of ChatGPT's performance in recognizing references related to literature reviews in the field of nephrology [79]. Our results showed that out of a total of 610 references, only 62% were accurately sourced by ChatGPT, while 31% were fabricated references, and 7% were incomplete citations (Figure 6).

Furthermore, approximately 70% of the provided links and half of the Digital Object Identifiers (DOIs) were found to be inaccurate (Figure 7). Notably, when we examined specific topics such as electrolyte balance, hemodialysis, and kidney stones, we found that over 60% of the references were either incorrect or misleading, often containing unreliable authorship and links.

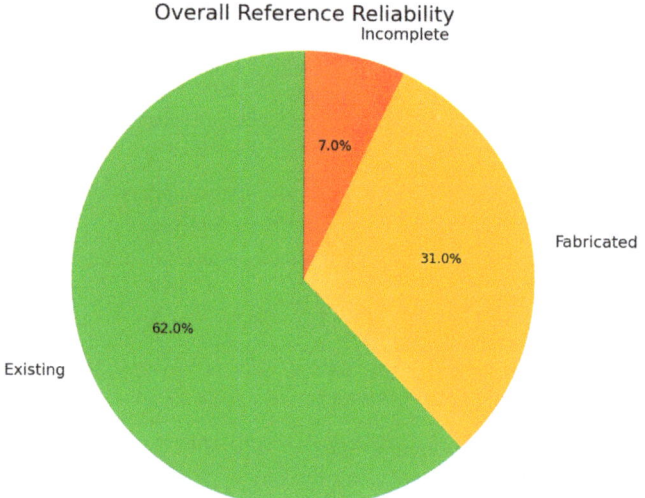

Figure 6. Overall Reference Reliability by ChatGPT 3.5.

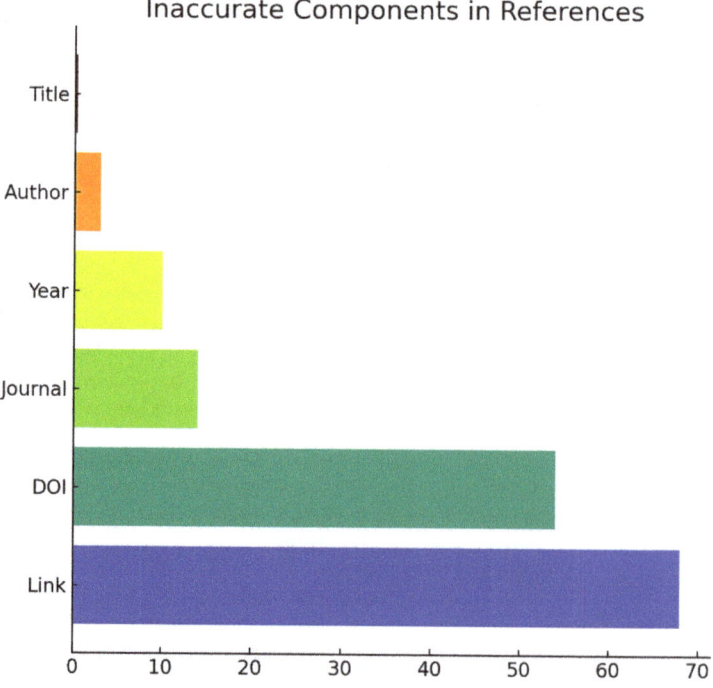

Figure 7. Inaccurate Components in References by ChatGPT 3.5.

Moreover, we recently evaluated the citation accuracy of AI tools, specifically ChatGPT, Bing Chat, and Bard AI, in the field of nephrology [80]. The evaluation involved generating prompts for each tool to provide 20 references in Vancouver style across 12 topics, followed by validation through PubMed, Google Scholar, and Web of Science. The findings reveal that Bard AI was the least accurate, providing only 3% accurate references along with a high percentage of fabricated (63%) and incomplete (11%) citations (Figure 8). Bing Chat performed marginally better but was still inadequate, with 30% accurate, 49% inaccurate, 13% fabricated, and 8% incomplete references. The most frequent error across platforms was incorrect DOIs.

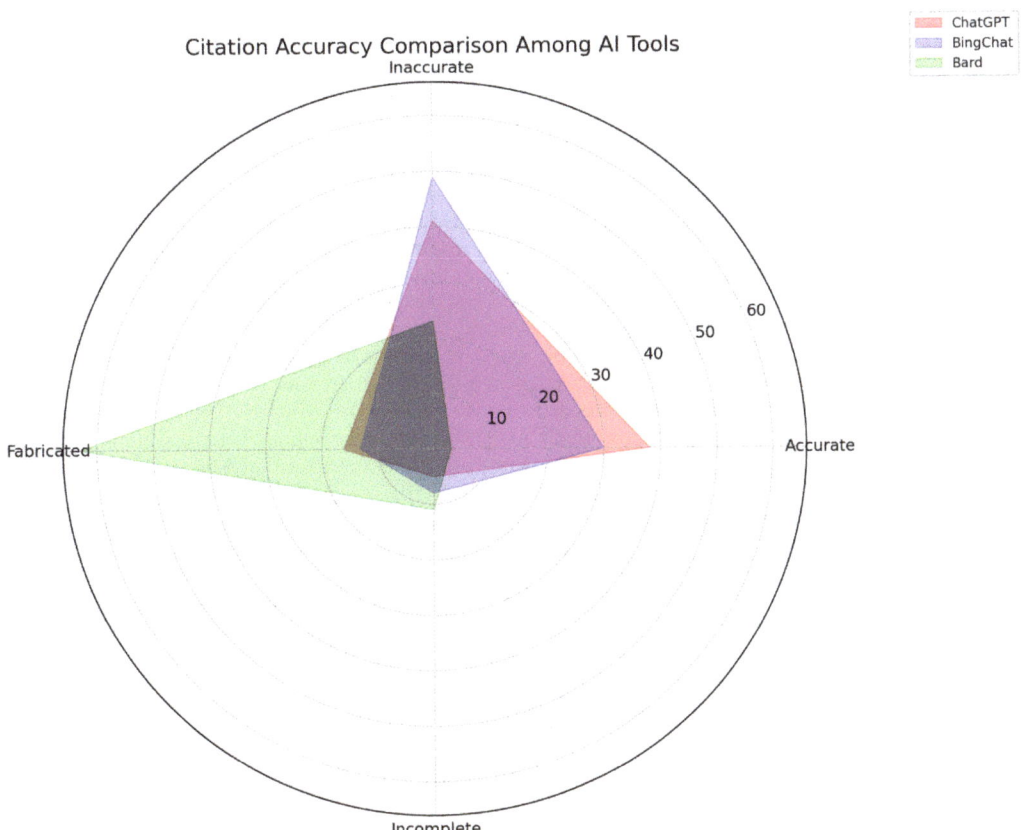

Figure 8. The radar plot provides a visual comparison of the citation accuracy of ChatGPT 3.5, BingChat, and Bard AI as of 1 August 2023.

In light of our findings, it is advisable not to solely rely on ChatGPT for identifying references to literature reviews in the nephrology field at this time. Therefore, as with any automated tool, evaluating the reliability and accuracy of ChatGPT for literature review is of utmost importance. Researchers and developers need to assess its performance against established benchmarks and human reviewers. This involves conducting comparative studies to evaluate its ability to identify relevant articles, extract key information accurately, and provide reliable summaries. Additionally, assessing the robustness of ChatGPT in handling different study designs, languages, and data sources is crucial for determining its generalizability and applicability in the field of nephrology.

2.8. Enhancing Nephrology Education with ChatGPT

The successful completion of examinations like the USMLE by ChatGPT brings attention to certain shortcomings within medical education, particularly its heavy reliance on memorization rather than the analysis of intricate health and disease models. This accomplishment serves as a crucial reminder to re-evaluate the methods used to train and evaluate our medical students [81]. It is important to acknowledge that ChatGPT lacks the nuanced reasoning abilities possessed by humans. Consequently, it is imperative to recognize that AI can never replace the invaluable role played by nurses, doctors, and other healthcare professionals on the frontlines. However, there is no denying that AI and LLMs will revolutionize all aspects of our work, spanning from research and writing to medical diagnosis, treatment, and education across various fields [81–84].

2.8.1. ChatGPT as an Educational Tool: Facilitating Learning and Knowledge Dissemination

With its ability to generate human-like responses and engage in interactive conversations, ChatGPT can simulate real-time interactions between students and virtual tutors or instructors. This enables learners to ask questions, seek explanations, and receive instant feedback, thereby enhancing their understanding of complex nephrological concepts. Moreover, ChatGPT can adapt its responses based on the learner's level of knowledge, providing personalized and tailored explanations to address individual learning needs.

Traditional educational materials, such as textbooks and lectures, may have limitations in terms of availability and accessibility. However, ChatGPT can be deployed as a web-based or mobile application, allowing learners to access educational content anytime and anywhere. Learners can engage in interactive discussions, explore case studies, and receive guidance on nephrology topics, ultimately fostering a self-directed and flexible learning experience. Furthermore, ChatGPT can also assist in knowledge dissemination within the nephrology community. It can be used to develop virtual educational platforms where nephrology experts can share their expertise, engage in discussions, and disseminate the latest research findings. By leveraging ChatGPT's natural language generation capabilities, educational content such as question banks, tutorials, case studies, and guidelines can be generated and shared with a wider audience [85]. This not only promotes collaboration and knowledge exchange among healthcare professionals but also ensures that the most up-to-date information is readily available to support evidence-based practice.

2.8.2. Integration of ChatGPT into Continuing Medical Education (CME) Programs

By incorporating ChatGPT into CME platforms, clinicians can access up-to-date research findings, summaries, and interactive discussions on relevant nephrology topics. This integration allows for personalized and on-demand learning experiences, enabling clinicians to stay informed about the latest advancements in the field. Moreover, ChatGPT can serve as a virtual assistant during CME activities, answering questions, providing clarification, and facilitating case-based discussions. The ability of ChatGPT to optimize and summarize the medical conference panel recommendations was assessed in the first Pan-Arab Pediatric Palliative Critical Care Hybrid Conference [86]. The results suggest that ChatGPT-4 effectively facilitated complex do-not-resuscitate (DNR) conflict resolution by summarizing key themes such as effective communication, collaboration, patient- and family-centered care, trust, and ethical considerations and demonstrated its potential benefits for enhancing critical thinking among medical professionals [86].

3. Ethical and Legal Implications of ChatGPT Integration in Nephrology

Adherence to secure data exchange protocols and privacy regulations is crucial for ensuring patient confidentiality during clinical practices [87,88]. It is important to identify and address any potential ethical or regulatory concerns regarding the use of ChatGPT. At present, the norms and protocols governing the clinical implementation of AI are inadequately defined or non-existent [89]. Even so, the integration of ChatGPT in nephrology firstly requires compliance with existing regulatory frameworks and ethical guidelines, such as the Health Insurance Portability and Accountability Act (HIPAA) in the United States. Secondly, obtaining informed consent is imperative to ensuring that patients willingly consent to the utilization of AI-assisted healthcare (i.e., diagnostics or treatment planning) and have the autonomy to decline participation if they choose [90] (Figure 9).

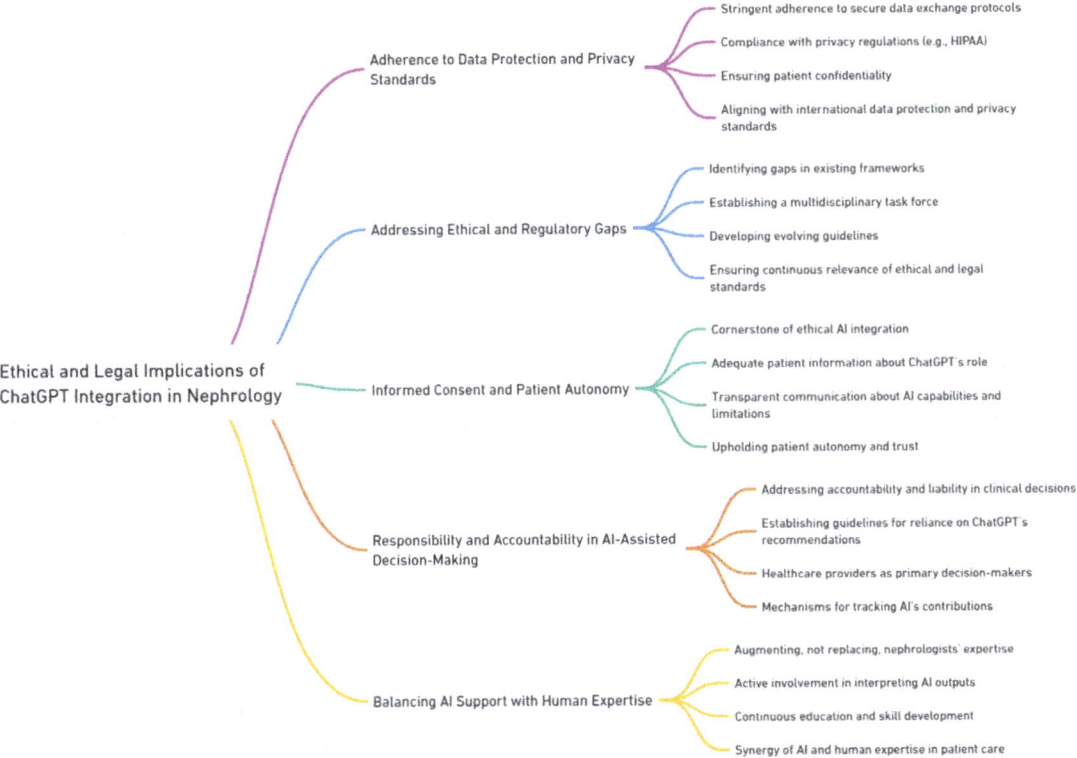

Figure 9. Ethical and legal implications of ChatGPT integration in nephrology.

Additionally, integrating ChatGPT in nephrology raises questions about accountability and liability in decision-making processes [91,92]. While ChatGPT can provide valuable insights and recommendations, the ultimate responsibility for patient care lies with healthcare providers. Clear guidelines should be established to outline the roles and responsibilities of healthcare providers when using ChatGPT in clinical practice. It is crucial to define the extent to which healthcare providers rely on ChatGPT recommendations and how they integrate these recommendations with their own clinical expertise and judgment. Mechanisms for tracking and documenting ChatGPT's contributions to clinical decision making should be established to ensure transparency and accountability.

Moreover, the integration of ChatGPT should aim to enhance, rather than replace, the expertise of nephrologists. Healthcare providers must maintain an active role in interpreting ChatGPT outputs, critically evaluating recommendations, and making informed decisions based on the patient's unique clinical context. Nephrologists should continuously update their knowledge and skills to effectively utilize ChatGPT as a supportive tool. The ethical integration of ChatGPT requires striking a balance between AI support and human expertise [24,93], ensuring that patients receive the highest quality of care that combines the benefits of AI technology and the human touch.

4. Future Directions and Challenges in Nephrology with ChatGPT

ChatGPT explores the latest developments in NLP, machine learning, and AI algorithms that have the potential to revolutionize nephrology practice in various ways [10,24,94]. In the future, collaboration between nephrologists and AI specialists is essential for optimizing the performance and impact of ChatGPT in nephrology practice, where nephrologists provide domain expertise and clinical insights while AI specialists contribute technical expertise in machine learning and NLP. By working together, these professionals can refine ChatGPT's algorithms, develop specialized models tailored to nephrology-specific tasks, and integrate feedback mechanisms for continuous improvement. Collaboration also enables the customization of ChatGPT to address the unique challenges and complexities of nephrology, ultimately enhancing its clinical utility and effectiveness to provide personalized patient care. Additionally, we emphasize the importance of developing strong protocols for data collection, storage, and sharing to protect privacy and guarantee the security of data [95,96]. Furthermore, regulatory bodies, such as medical boards and professional associations, should start to establish the guidelines and ensure that ChatGPT applications meet the required standards for safety, accuracy, and reliability.

5. Conclusions

ChatGPT holds immense potential to revolutionize nephrology practice by facilitating clinical decision making, enhancing patient communication, streamlining research, and improving operational efficiency. By embracing a multidisciplinary approach, fostering collaboration between nephrologists and AI specialists, and prioritizing ethical considerations, the future of ChatGPT in nephrology appears promising. Continued research, development, and evaluation will shape the evolution of ChatGPT, leading to its wider adoption and integration into routine nephrology care and ultimately improving patient outcomes and advancing personalized patient care in the field. However, it is essential to acknowledge that with the ongoing evolution of AI, it becomes particularly vital for the upcoming generation of physicians to adeptly navigate these challenges. They must weigh the potential benefits and risks to effectively determine how extensively AI should be integrated into medical practice.

Author Contributions: Conceptualization, J.M. and W.C.; writing—original draft preparation, J.M., C.T., F.Q. and W.C.; writing—review and editing, J.M., C.T., S.S., O.A.G.V., F.Q. and W.C.; supervision J.M., C.T., F.Q. and W.C.; project administration W.C. The mind map showcased in this manuscript was designed using Whimsical. All authors have read and agreed to the published version of the manuscript.

Funding: This research received no external funding.

Institutional Review Board Statement: Not applicable.

Informed Consent Statement: Not applicable.

Data Availability Statement: The data used in this study can be obtained upon reasonable request to the corresponding author.

Conflicts of Interest: The authors declare no conflict of interest.

References

1. Moshawrab, M.; Adda, M.; Bouzouane, A.; Ibrahim, H.; Raad, A. Reviewing Federated Machine Learning and Its Use in Diseases Prediction. *Sensors* **2023**, *23*, 2112. [CrossRef] [PubMed]
2. Thongprayoon, C.; Vaitla, P.; Jadlowiec, C.C.; Leeaphorn, N.; Mao, S.A.; Mao, M.A.; Pattharanitima, P.; Bruminhent, J.; Khoury, N.J.; Garovic, V.D.; et al. Use of Machine Learning Consensus Clustering to Identify Distinct Subtypes of Black Kidney Transplant Recipients and Associated Outcomes. *JAMA Surg.* **2022**, *157*, e221286. [CrossRef] [PubMed]
3. Krisanapan, P.; Tangpanithandee, S.; Thongprayoon, C.; Pattharanitima, P.; Cheungpasitporn, W. Revolutionizing Chronic Kidney Disease Management with Machine Learning and Artificial Intelligence. *J. Clin. Med.* **2023**, *12*, 3018. [CrossRef] [PubMed]

4. Ravizza, S.; Huschto, T.; Adamov, A.; Bohm, L.; Busser, A.; Flother, F.F.; Hinzmann, R.; Konig, H.; McAhren, S.M.; Robertson, D.H.; et al. Predicting the early risk of chronic kidney disease in patients with diabetes using real-world data. *Nat. Med.* **2019**, *25*, 57–59. [CrossRef] [PubMed]
5. Abdel-Fattah, M.A.; Othman, N.A.; Goher, N. Predicting Chronic Kidney Disease Using Hybrid Machine Learning Based on Apache Spark. *Comput. Intell. Neurosci.* **2022**, *2022*, 9898831. [CrossRef] [PubMed]
6. Joshi, G.; Jain, A.; Araveeti, S.R.; Adhikari, S.; Garg, H.; Bhandari, M. FDA approved Artificial Intelligence and Machine Learning (AI/ML)-Enabled Medical Devices: An updated landscape. *medRxiv* **2023**. [CrossRef]
7. Models. Available online: https://platform.openai.com/docs/models (accessed on 3 June 2023).
8. Introducing ChatGPT. Available online: https://openai.com/blog/chatgpt (accessed on 18 April 2023).
9. Ecoffet, A. GPT-4 Technical Report. *arXiv* **2023**. [CrossRef]
10. Sallam, M. ChatGPT Utility in Healthcare Education, Research, and Practice: Systematic Review on the Promising Perspectives and Valid Concerns. *Healthcare* **2023**, *11*, 887. [CrossRef]
11. Eysenbach, G. The Role of ChatGPT, Generative Language Models, and Artificial Intelligence in Medical Education: A Conversation with ChatGPT and a Call for Papers. *JMIR Med. Educ.* **2023**, *9*, e46885. [CrossRef]
12. Kung, T.H.; Cheatham, M.; Medenilla, A.; Sillos, C.; De Leon, L.; Elepano, C.; Madriaga, M.; Aggabao, R.; Diaz-Candido, G.; Maningo, J.; et al. Performance of ChatGPT on USMLE: Potential for AI-assisted medical education using large language models. *PLoS Digit. Health* **2023**, *2*, e0000198. [CrossRef]
13. Gilson, A.; Safranek, C.W.; Huang, T.; Socrates, V.; Chi, L.; Taylor, R.A.; Chartash, D. How Does ChatGPT Perform on the United States Medical Licensing Examination? The Implications of Large Language Models for Medical Education and Knowledge Assessment. *JMIR Med. Educ.* **2023**, *9*, e45312. [CrossRef] [PubMed]
14. Bhayana, R.; Krishna, S.; Bleakney, R.R. Performance of ChatGPT on a Radiology Board-style Examination: Insights into Current Strengths and Limitations. *Radiology* **2023**, *307*, e230582. [CrossRef] [PubMed]
15. Das, D.; Kumar, N.; Longjam, L.A.; Sinha, R.; Deb Roy, A.; Mondal, H.; Gupta, P. Assessing the Capability of ChatGPT in Answering First- and Second-Order Knowledge Questions on Microbiology as per Competency-Based Medical Education Curriculum. *Cureus* **2023**, *15*, e36034. [CrossRef] [PubMed]
16. Thirunavukarasu, A.J.; Hassan, R.; Mahmood, S.; Sanghera, R.; Barzangi, K.; El Mukashfi, M.; Shah, S. Trialling a Large Language Model (ChatGPT) in General Practice with the Applied Knowledge Test: Observational Study Demonstrating Opportunities and Limitations in Primary Care. *JMIR Med. Educ.* **2023**, *9*, e46599. [CrossRef] [PubMed]
17. Miao, J.; Thongprayoon, C.; Cheungpasitporn, W. Assessing the Accuracy of ChatGPT on Core Questions in Glomerular Disease. *Kidney Int. Rep.* **2023**, *8*, 1657–1659. [CrossRef] [PubMed]
18. Miao, J.; Thongprayoon, C.; Garcia Valencia, O.A.; Krisanapan, P.; Sheikh, M.S.; Davis, P.W.; Mekraksakit, P.; Gonzalez Suarez, M.; Craici, I.M.; Cheungpasitporn, W. Performance of ChatGPT on nephrology test questions. *Clin. J. Am. Soc. Nephrol.* **2023**. [CrossRef] [PubMed]
19. Lu, Y.; Wu, H.; Qi, S.; Cheng, K. Artificial Intelligence in Intensive Care Medicine: Toward a ChatGPT/GPT-4 Way? *Ann. Biomed. Eng.* **2023**, *51*, 1898–1903. [CrossRef]
20. Cheng, K.; Guo, Q.; He, Y.; Lu, Y.; Gu, S.; Wu, H. Exploring the Potential of GPT-4 in Biomedical Engineering: The Dawn of a New Era. *Ann. Biomed. Eng.* **2023**, *51*, 1645–1653. [CrossRef]
21. Biswas, S.S. Role of Chat GPT in Public Health. *Ann. Biomed. Eng.* **2023**, *51*, 868–869. [CrossRef]
22. Liu, S.; Wright, A.P.; Patterson, B.L.; Wanderer, J.P.; Turer, R.W.; Nelson, S.D.; McCoy, A.B.; Sittig, D.F.; Wright, A. Using AI-generated suggestions from ChatGPT to optimize clinical decision support. *J. Am. Med Inform. Assoc.* **2023**, *30*, 1237–1245. [CrossRef]
23. Temsah, O.; Khan, S.A.; Chaiah, Y.; Senjab, A.; Alhasan, K.; Jamal, A.; Aljamaan, F.; Malki, K.H.; Halwani, R.; Al-Tawfiq, J.A.; et al. Overview of Early ChatGPT's Presence in Medical Literature: Insights from a Hybrid Literature Review by ChatGPT and Human Experts. *Cureus* **2023**, *15*, e37281. [CrossRef] [PubMed]
24. Lee, P.; Bubeck, S.; Petro, J. Benefits, Limits, and Risks of GPT-4 as an AI Chatbot for Medicine. *N. Engl. J. Med.* **2023**, *388*, 1233–1239. [CrossRef] [PubMed]
25. GPT Builder. Available online: https://chat.openai.com/gpts/editor (accessed on 30 November 2023).
26. Evans, R.S. Electronic Health Records: Then, Now, and in the Future. *Yearb. Med. Inform.* **2016**, *25* (Suppl. S1), S48–S61. [CrossRef] [PubMed]
27. Thongprayoon, C.; Kaewput, W.; Kovvuru, K.; Hansrivijit, P.; Kanduri, S.R.; Bathini, T.; Chewcharat, A.; Leeaphorn, N.; Gonzalez-Suarez, M.L.; Cheungpasitporn, W. Promises of Big Data and Artificial Intelligence in Nephrology and Transplantation. *J. Clin. Med.* **2020**, *9*, 1107. [CrossRef] [PubMed]
28. Xie, G.; Chen, T.; Li, Y.; Chen, T.; Li, X.; Liu, Z. Artificial Intelligence in Nephrology: How Can Artificial Intelligence Augment Nephrologists' Intelligence? *Kidney Dis.* **2020**, *6*, 1–6. [CrossRef] [PubMed]
29. Adeojo, O. How to Connect ChatGPT to Your Database. Available online: https://docs.kanaries.net/articles/chatgpt-database (accessed on 8 June 2023).
30. Mirbabaie, M.; Stieglitz, S.; Frick, N.R.J. Artificial intelligence in disease diagnostics: A critical review and classification on the current state of research guiding future direction. *Health Technol.* **2021**, *11*, 693–731. [CrossRef]

31. Sutton, R.T.; Pincock, D.; Baumgart, D.C.; Sadowski, D.C.; Fedorak, R.N.; Kroeker, K.I. An overview of clinical decision support systems: Benefits, risks, and strategies for success. *NPJ Digit. Med.* **2020**, *3*, 17. [CrossRef]
32. Kawamoto, K.; Houlihan, C.A.; Balas, E.A.; Lobach, D.F. Improving clinical practice using clinical decision support systems: A systematic review of trials to identify features critical to success. *BMJ* **2005**, *330*, 765. [CrossRef]
33. Liu, S.; Wright, A.P.; Patterson, B.L.; Wanderer, J.P.; Turer, R.W.; Nelson, S.D.; McCoy, A.B.; Sittig, D.F.; Wright, A. Assessing the Value of ChatGPT for Clinical Decision Support Optimization. *medRxiv* **2023**. [CrossRef]
34. Liao, Z.; Wang, J.; Shi, Z.; Lu, L.; Tabata, H. Revolutionary Potential of ChatGPT in Constructing Intelligent Clinical Decision Support Systems. *Ann. Biomed. Eng.* **2023**. [CrossRef]
35. Alhasan, K.; Raina, R.; Jamal, A.; Temsah, M.H. Combining human and AI could predict nephrologies future, but should be handled with care. *Acta Paediatr.* **2023**, *112*, 1844–1848. [CrossRef] [PubMed]
36. Sabry Abdel-Messih, M.; Kamel Boulos, M.N. ChatGPT in Clinical Toxicology. *JMIR Med. Educ.* **2023**, *9*, e46876. [CrossRef] [PubMed]
37. Hirosawa, T.; Harada, Y.; Yokose, M.; Sakamoto, T.; Kawamura, R.; Shimizu, T. Diagnostic Accuracy of Differential-Diagnosis Lists Generated by Generative Pretrained Transformer 3 Chatbot for Clinical Vignettes with Common Chief Complaints: A Pilot Study. *Int. J. Environ. Res. Public Health* **2023**, *20*, 3378. [CrossRef] [PubMed]
38. Frackiewicz, M. ChatGPT for Diagnosis of Kidney Diseases: Advancements and Limitations. Available online: https://ts2.space/en/chatgpt-for-diagnosis-of-kidney-diseases-advancements-and-limitations/ (accessed on 17 April 2023).
39. Munoz-Zuluaga, C.; Zhao, Z.; Wang, F.; Greenblatt, M.B.; Yang, H.S. Assessing the Accuracy and Clinical Utility of ChatGPT in Laboratory Medicine. *Clin. Chem.* **2023**, *69*, 939–940. [CrossRef] [PubMed]
40. Brinch, M.L.; Hald, T.; Wainaina, L.; Merlotti, A.; Remondini, D.; Henri, C.; Njage, P.M.K. Comparison of Source Attribution Methodologies for Human Campylobacteriosis. *Pathogens* **2023**, *12*, 786. [CrossRef]
41. Munir, K.; Elahi, H.; Ayub, A.; Frezza, F.; Rizzi, A. Cancer Diagnosis Using Deep Learning: A Bibliographic Review. *Cancers* **2019**, *11*, 1235. [CrossRef]
42. Arslan, S. Exploring the Potential of Chat GPT in Personalized Obesity Treatment. *Ann. Biomed. Eng.* **2023**, *51*, 1887–1888. [CrossRef]
43. Ismail, A.M.A. Chat GPT in Tailoring Individualized Lifestyle-Modification Programs in Metabolic Syndrome: Potentials and Difficulties? *Ann. Biomed. Eng.* **2023**, *51*, 2634–2635. [CrossRef]
44. Cheng, K.; Li, Z.; He, Y.; Guo, Q.; Lu, Y.; Gu, S.; Wu, H. Potential Use of Artificial Intelligence in Infectious Disease: Take ChatGPT as an Example. *Ann. Biomed. Eng.* **2023**, *51*, 1130–1135. [CrossRef]
45. Schulte, B. Capacity of ChatGPT to Identify Guideline-Based Treatments for Advanced Solid Tumors. *Cureus* **2023**, *15*, e37938. [CrossRef]
46. Qarajeh, A.; Tangpanithandee, S.; Thongprayoon, C.; Suppadungsuk, S.; Krisanapan, P.; Aiumtrakul, N.; Garcia Valencia, O.A.; Miao, J.; Qureshi, F.; Cheungpasitporn, W. AI-Powered Renal Diet Support: Performance of ChatGPT, Bard AI, and Bing Chat. *Clin. Pract.* **2023**, *13*, 1160–1172. [CrossRef] [PubMed]
47. Bing Chat with GPT-4. Available online: https://www.microsoft.com/en-us/bing?form=MA13FV (accessed on 14 October 2023).
48. Anil, R.; Dai, A.M.; Firat, O.; Johnson, M.; Lepikhin, D.; Passos, A.; Shakeri, S.; Taropa, E.; Bailey, P.; Chen, Z.; et al. PaLM 2 Technical Report. *arXiv* **2023**. [CrossRef]
49. Brown, C.; Nazeer, R.; Gibbs, A.; Le Page, P.; Mitchell, A.R. Breaking Bias: The Role of Artificial Intelligence in Improving Clinical Decision-Making. *Cureus* **2023**, *15*, e36415. [CrossRef] [PubMed]
50. Galido, P.V.; Butala, S.; Chakerian, M.; Agustines, D. A Case Study Demonstrating Applications of ChatGPT in the Clinical Management of Treatment-Resistant Schizophrenia. *Cureus* **2023**, *15*, e38166. [CrossRef] [PubMed]
51. Khan, R.A.; Jawaid, M.; Khan, A.R.; Sajjad, M. ChatGPT—Reshaping medical education and clinical management. *Pak. J. Med. Sci.* **2023**, *39*, 605–607. [CrossRef] [PubMed]
52. Garcia Valencia, O.A.; Thongprayoon, C.; Jadlowiec, C.C.; Mao, S.A.; Miao, J.; Cheungpasitporn, W. Enhancing Kidney Transplant Care through the Integration of Chatbot. *Healthcare* **2023**, *11*, 2518. [CrossRef] [PubMed]
53. Sharma, S.; Pajai, S.; Prasad, R.; Wanjari, M.B.; Munjewar, P.K.; Sharma, R.; Pathade, A. A Critical Review of ChatGPT as a Potential Substitute for Diabetes Educators. *Cureus* **2023**, *15*, e38380. [CrossRef]
54. Benyon, B. ChatGPT Can Answer Cancer Questions, But Clinician Input Still Vital. Available online: https://www.curetoday.com/view/chatgpt-can-answer-cancer-questions-but-clinician-input-still-vital (accessed on 10 April 2023).
55. Yeo, Y.H.; Samaan, J.S.; Ng, W.H.; Ting, P.S.; Trivedi, H.; Vipani, A.; Ayoub, W.; Yang, J.D.; Liran, O.; Spiegel, B.; et al. Assessing the performance of ChatGPT in answering questions regarding cirrhosis and hepatocellular carcinoma. *Clin. Mol. Hepatol.* **2023**, *29*, 721–732. [CrossRef]
56. Ayers, J.W.; Poliak, A.; Dredze, M.; Leas, E.C.; Zhu, Z.; Kelley, J.B.; Faix, D.J.; Goodman, A.M.; Longhurst, C.A.; Hogarth, M.; et al. Comparing Physician and Artificial Intelligence Chatbot Responses to Patient Questions Posted to a Public Social Media Forum. *JAMA Intern. Med.* **2023**, *183*, 589–596. [CrossRef]
57. ChatGPT's Potential Impact on the Delivery of Healthcare Services. Available online: https://abcsrcm.com/chatgpts-potential-impact-on-the-delivery-of-healthcare-services/ (accessed on 28 February 2023).
58. Chen, P.F.; Wang, S.M.; Liao, W.C.; Kuo, L.C.; Chen, K.C.; Lin, Y.C.; Yang, C.Y.; Chiu, C.H.; Chang, S.C.; Lai, F. Automatic ICD-10 Coding and Training System: Deep Neural Network Based on Supervised Learning. *JMIR Med. Inform.* **2021**, *9*, e23230. [CrossRef]

59. DiGiorgio, A.M.; Ehrenfeld, J.M. Artificial Intelligence in Medicine & ChatGPT: De-Tether the Physician. *J. Med. Syst.* **2023**, *47*, 32. [CrossRef]
60. Frackiewicz, M. The Impact of ChatGPT on Medical Coding and Billing Accuracy. Available online: https://ts2.space/en/the-impact-of-chatgpt-on-medical-coding-and-billing-accuracy/ (accessed on 2 May 2023).
61. Perkel, J.M. Six tips for better coding with ChatGPT. *Nature* **2023**, *618*, 422–423. [CrossRef] [PubMed]
62. Biswas, S. ChatGPT and the Future of Medical Writing. *Radiology* **2023**, *307*, e223312. [CrossRef] [PubMed]
63. Payton, J. Improving Communication Skills within the Nephrology Unit. *Nephrol. Nurs. J.* **2018**, *45*, 269–280. [PubMed]
64. Geetha, D.; Lee, S.K.; Srivastava, A.J.; Kraus, E.S.; Wright, S.M. Clinical excellence in nephrology: Examples from the published literature. *BMC Nephrol.* **2015**, *16*, 141. [CrossRef] [PubMed]
65. National Action Plan to Improve Health Literacy. Available online: https://health.gov/sites/default/files/2019-09/Health_Literacy_Action_Plan.pdf (accessed on 3 July 2023).
66. Ali, S.R.; Dobbs, T.D.; Hutchings, H.A.; Whitaker, I.S. Using ChatGPT to write patient clinic letters. *Lancet Digit. Health* **2023**, *5*, e179–e181. [CrossRef] [PubMed]
67. Drury, D.J.; Kaur, A.; Dobbs, T.; Whitaker, I.S. The Readability of Outpatient Plastic Surgery Clinic Letters: Are We Adhering to Plain English Writing Standards? *Plast. Surg. Nurs.* **2021**, *41*, 27–33. [CrossRef] [PubMed]
68. D'Amico, R.S.; White, T.G.; Shah, H.A.; Langer, D.J. I Asked a ChatGPT to Write an Editorial About How We Can Incorporate Chatbots into Neurosurgical Research and Patient Care. *Neurosurgery* **2023**, *92*, 663–664. [CrossRef]
69. Benichou, L.; ChatGpt. Role de l'utilisation de l'intelligence artificielle ChatGPT dans la redaction des articles scientifiques medicaux The Role of Using ChatGPT AI in Writing Medical Scientific Articles. *J. Stomatol. Oral Maxillofac. Surg.* **2023**, *124*, 101456. [CrossRef]
70. Huang, J.; Tan, M. The role of ChatGPT in scientific communication: Writing better scientific review articles. *Am. J. Cancer Res.* **2023**, *13*, 1148–1154.
71. Verhoeven, F.; Wendling, D.; Prati, C. ChatGPT: When artificial intelligence replaces the rheumatologist in medical writing. *Ann. Rheum. Dis.* **2023**, *82*, 1015–1017. [CrossRef]
72. Athaluri, S.A.; Manthena, S.V.; Kesapragada, V.; Yarlagadda, V.; Dave, T.; Duddumpudi, R.T.S. Exploring the Boundaries of Reality: Investigating the Phenomenon of Artificial Intelligence Hallucination in Scientific Writing Through ChatGPT References. *Cureus* **2023**, *15*, e37432. [CrossRef] [PubMed]
73. Salvagno, M.; Taccone, F.S.; Gerli, A.G. Can artificial intelligence help for scientific writing? *Crit. Care* **2023**, *27*, 75. [CrossRef] [PubMed]
74. Lubowitz, J.H. ChatGPT, An Artificial Intelligence Chatbot, Is Impacting Medical Literature. *Arthroscopy* **2023**, *39*, 1121–1122. [CrossRef] [PubMed]
75. Dergaa, I.; Chamari, K.; Zmijewski, P.; Ben Saad, H. From human writing to artificial intelligence generated text: Examining the prospects and potential threats of ChatGPT in academic writing. *Biol. Sport* **2023**, *40*, 615–622. [CrossRef] [PubMed]
76. Zhou, Z. Evaluation of ChatGPT's Capabilities in Medical Report Generation. *Cureus* **2023**, *15*, e37589. [CrossRef] [PubMed]
77. Schuppe, K.; Burke, S.; Cohoe, B.; Chang, K.; Lance, R.S.; Mroch, H. Atypical Nelson Syndrome Following Right Partial and Left Total Nephrectomy with Incidental Bilateral Total Adrenalectomy of Renal Cell Carcinoma: A Chat Generative Pre-Trained Transformer (ChatGPT)-Assisted Case Report and Literature Review. *Cureus* **2023**, *15*, e36042. [CrossRef] [PubMed]
78. Gilat, R.; Cole, B.J. How Will Artificial Intelligence Affect Scientific Writing, Reviewing and Editing? The Future is Here. *Arthroscopy* **2023**, *39*, 1119–1120. [CrossRef] [PubMed]
79. Suppadungsuk, S.; Thongprayoon, C.; Krisanapan, P.; Tangpanithandee, S.; Garcia Valencia, O.; Miao, J.; Mekraksakit, P.; Kashani, K.; Cheungpasitporn, W. Examining the Validity of ChatGPT in Identifying Relevant Nephrology Literature: Findings and Implications. *J. Clin. Med.* **2023**, *12*, 5550. [CrossRef]
80. Aiumtrakul, N.; Thongprayoon, C.; Suppadungsuk, S.; Krisanapan, P.; Miao, J.; Qureshi, F.; Cheungpasitporn, W. Navigating the Landscape of Personalized Medicine: The Relevance of ChatGPT, BingChat, and Bard AI in Nephrology Literature Searches. *J. Pers. Med.* **2023**, *13*, 1457. [CrossRef]
81. Mbakwe, A.B.; Lourentzou, I.; Celi, L.A.; Mechanic, O.J.; Dagan, A. ChatGPT passing USMLE shines a spotlight on the flaws of medical education. *PLoS Digit. Health* **2023**, *2*, e0000205. [CrossRef]
82. Miao, H.; Ahn, H. Impact of ChatGPT on Interdisciplinary Nursing Education and Research. *Asian Pac. Isl. Nurs. J.* **2023**, *7*, e48136. [CrossRef] [PubMed]
83. Fatani, B. ChatGPT for Future Medical and Dental Research. *Cureus* **2023**, *15*, e37285. [CrossRef] [PubMed]
84. Lee, H. The rise of ChatGPT: Exploring its potential in medical education. *Anat. Sci. Educ.* **2023**. ahead of print. [CrossRef] [PubMed]
85. Biswas, S. Passing is Great: Can ChatGPT Conduct USMLE Exams? *Ann. Biomed. Eng.* **2023**, *51*, 1885–1886. [CrossRef] [PubMed]
86. Almazyad, M.; Aljofan, F.; Abouammoh, N.A.; Muaygil, R.; Malki, K.H.; Aljamaan, F.; Alturki, A.; Alayed, T.; Alshehri, S.S.; Alrbiaan, A.; et al. Enhancing Expert Panel Discussions in Pediatric Palliative Care: Innovative Scenario Development and Summarization with ChatGPT-4. *Cureus* **2023**, *15*, e38249. [CrossRef]
87. Price, W.N., 2nd; Cohen, I.G. Privacy in the age of medical big data. *Nat. Med.* **2019**, *25*, 37–43. [CrossRef]
88. Kayaalp, M. Patient Privacy in the Era of Big Data. *Balk. Med. J.* **2018**, *35*, 8–17. [CrossRef]

89. Crossnohere, N.L.; Elsaid, M.; Paskett, J.; Bose-Brill, S.; Bridges, J.F.P. Guidelines for Artificial Intelligence in Medicine: Literature Review and Content Analysis of Frameworks. *J. Med. Internet Res.* **2022**, *24*, e36823. [CrossRef]
90. Kavian, J.A.; Wilkey, H.L.; Patel, P.A.; Boyd, C.J. Harvesting the Power of Artificial Intelligence for Surgery: Uses, Implications, and Ethical Considerations. *Am. Surg.* **2023**, 31348231175454. [CrossRef]
91. Kleebayoon, A.; Wiwanitkit, V. Assessing the performance of ChatGPT: Comment. *Clin. Mol. Hepatol.* **2023**, *29*, 815–816. [CrossRef]
92. Dave, T.; Athaluri, S.A.; Singh, S. ChatGPT in medicine: An overview of its applications, advantages, limitations, future prospects, and ethical considerations. *Front. Artif. Intell.* **2023**, *6*, 1169595. [CrossRef] [PubMed]
93. Fernandes, A.C.; Souto, M. Benefits, Limits, and Risks of GPT-4 as an AI Chatbot for Medicine. *N. Engl. J. Med.* **2023**, *388*, 2399–2400. [CrossRef] [PubMed]
94. Ruksakulpiwat, S.; Kumar, A.; Ajibade, A. Using ChatGPT in Medical Research: Current Status and Future Directions. *J. Multidiscip. Healthc.* **2023**, *16*, 1513–1520. [CrossRef] [PubMed]
95. Garcia Valencia, O.A.; Suppadungsuk, S.; Thongprayoon, C.; Miao, J.; Tangpanithandee, S.; Craici, I.M.; Cheungpasitporn, W. Ethical Implications of Chatbot Utilization in Nephrology. *J. Pers. Med.* **2023**, *13*, 1363. [CrossRef]
96. Mello, M.M.; Guha, N. ChatGPT and Physicians' Malpractice Risk. *JAMA Health Forum* **2023**, *4*, e231938. [CrossRef]

Disclaimer/Publisher's Note: The statements, opinions and data contained in all publications are solely those of the individual author(s) and contributor(s) and not of MDPI and/or the editor(s). MDPI and/or the editor(s) disclaim responsibility for any injury to people or property resulting from any ideas, methods, instructions or products referred to in the content.

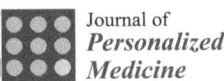

Review

Personalized Care in Eye Health: Exploring Opportunities, Challenges, and the Road Ahead for Chatbots

Mantapond Ittarat [1], Wisit Cheungpasitporn [2,*] and Sunee Chansangpetch [3,4]

1. Surin Hospital and Surin Medical Education Center, Suranaree University of Technology, Surin 32000, Thailand; mantapond.sur@cpird.in.th
2. Department of Medicine, Mayo Clinic, Rochester, MN 55905, USA
3. Center of Excellence in Glaucoma, Chulalongkorn University, Bangkok 10330, Thailand; sunee.ch@chula.ac.th
4. Department of Ophthalmology, Faculty of Medicine, Chulalongkorn University and King Chulalongkorn Memorial Hospital, Thai Red Cross Society, Bangkok 10330, Thailand
* Correspondence: wcheungpasitporn@gmail.com

Abstract: In modern eye care, the adoption of ophthalmology chatbots stands out as a pivotal technological progression. These digital assistants present numerous benefits, such as better access to vital information, heightened patient interaction, and streamlined triaging. Recent evaluations have highlighted their performance in both the triage of ophthalmology conditions and ophthalmology knowledge assessment, underscoring their potential and areas for improvement. However, assimilating these chatbots into the prevailing healthcare infrastructures brings challenges. These encompass ethical dilemmas, legal compliance, seamless integration with electronic health records (EHR), and fostering effective dialogue with medical professionals. Addressing these challenges necessitates the creation of bespoke standards and protocols for ophthalmology chatbots. The horizon for these chatbots is illuminated by advancements and anticipated innovations, poised to redefine the delivery of eye care. The synergy of artificial intelligence (AI) and machine learning (ML) with chatbots amplifies their diagnostic prowess. Additionally, their capability to adapt linguistically and culturally ensures they can cater to a global patient demographic. In this article, we explore in detail the utilization of chatbots in ophthalmology, examining their accuracy, reliability, data protection, security, transparency, potential algorithmic biases, and ethical considerations. We provide a comprehensive review of their roles in the triage of ophthalmology conditions and knowledge assessment, emphasizing their significance and future potential in the field.

Keywords: ophthalmology; artificial intelligence; machine learning; language processing; large language models; chatbot; ChatGPT

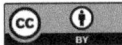

1. Introduction to the Utilization of Chatbots for Ophthalmology

1.1. Overview of Chatbot Technology

The rise of chatbot technology, as showcased by industry leaders like ChatGPT by OpenAI, Google's Bard AI, Microsoft's BingChat, and Anthropic's Claude AI, has been a focal point of interest across myriad sectors, notably within the healthcare domain [1–6]. These chatbots are applications powered by artificial intelligence, meticulously designed to simulate human conversation through either text or voice interactions [4,7–10]. Utilizing cutting-edge natural language processing algorithms, these advanced systems can discern and address user inquiries with precision, delivering bespoke and pertinent information [1,2,11].

In the context of ophthalmology, chatbots introduce a fresh and innovative approach to delivering healthcare services, engaging with patients, and providing support to healthcare professionals [12–14]. Through harnessing the potential of chatbot technology, ophthalmology practices have the opportunity to augment accessibility, operational efficiency, and overall patient experience. For instance, integrating chatbots into their systems enables ophthalmology practices to deliver round-the-clock support, address common inquiries regarding eye health, facilitate appointment scheduling, and even offer preliminary guidance concerning eye conditions.

In the expansive landscape of ophthalmology, ChatGPT and chatbots of its ilk have heralded an era of uninterrupted communication, instantaneous information retrieval, and tailor-made interactions. These tools equip patients with the means to secure immediate help, while empowering healthcare practitioners to dispense proficient support. In streamlining the triage of patient queries, providing educational materials, and shepherding patients through both pre- and post-operative care directions, these chatbots have carved an indispensable niche for themselves. A clear demonstration of the influence of ChatGPT, which was developed by OpenAI, is found in the domain of medical pedagogy. Within this scope, it functions as an enhancer of search efficiency and a rectifier of manuscript inconsistencies. ChatGPT has emerged as an invaluable asset, especially in accessing specialized literature germane to renal transplant care. Equally impactful are other AI-driven conversational platforms, such as Microsoft's BingChat and Google's Bard AI. These technologically adept interfaces excel in enhancing search capabilities, remedying typographical and grammatical oversights, and enhancing the scrutiny of academic content [15]. Bard AI, with its rich foundational training in a myriad of texts and coding paradigms, is poised to craft context-sensitive textual interpretations [16]. This prowess positions it as an invaluable asset in healthcare, ranging from buttressing decisions anchored in evidence to honing the quality of communication (Figure 1).

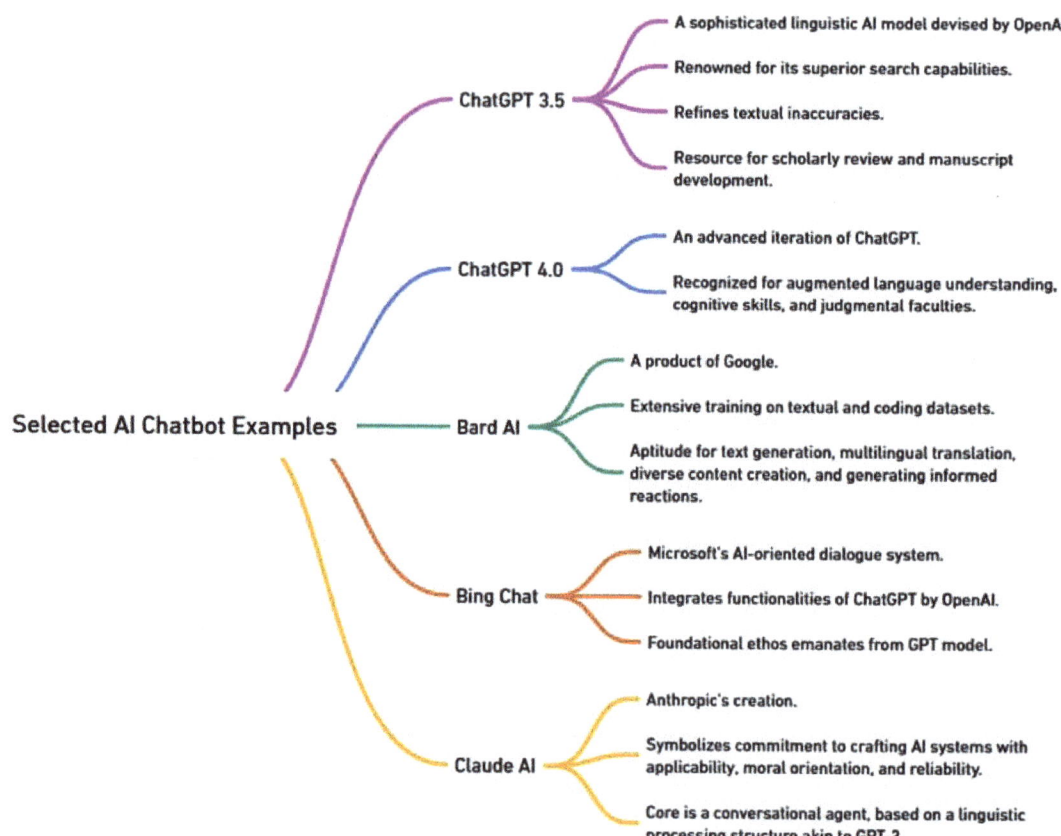

Figure 1. Examples of notable AI chatbots.

The incorporation of chatbot technology in ophthalmology represents a promising advancement, capable of reshaping the provision of eye care by improving accessibility, operational efficiency, and patient satisfaction. Utilizing the capabilities of chatbots enables ophthalmology practices to provide a higher standard of care, improve patient outcomes, and furnish individuals with essential information and support.

The scoping review methodology used in our study has provided a detailed panorama of the current and potential applications of chatbot technology in ophthalmology, underscoring its role in enhancing patient engagement and improving care delivery. This comprehensive understanding is vital for formulating strategies that effectively incorporate chatbots into ophthalmological practices, thereby meeting the dynamic needs of patients and healthcare professionals in this field.

1.2. The Growing Need for Innovative Solutions in Ophthalmology

As the incidence of eye conditions increases, so does the demand for eye care services. This upswing highlights the urgent need for innovative solutions that can enhance healthcare delivery in the field of ophthalmology. The traditional methods, while effective, may not be sufficient to cater for the increasing number of patients requiring attention, especially in a timely manner. This is where technology, particularly chatbots, can make a significant difference [17,18], Figure 2.

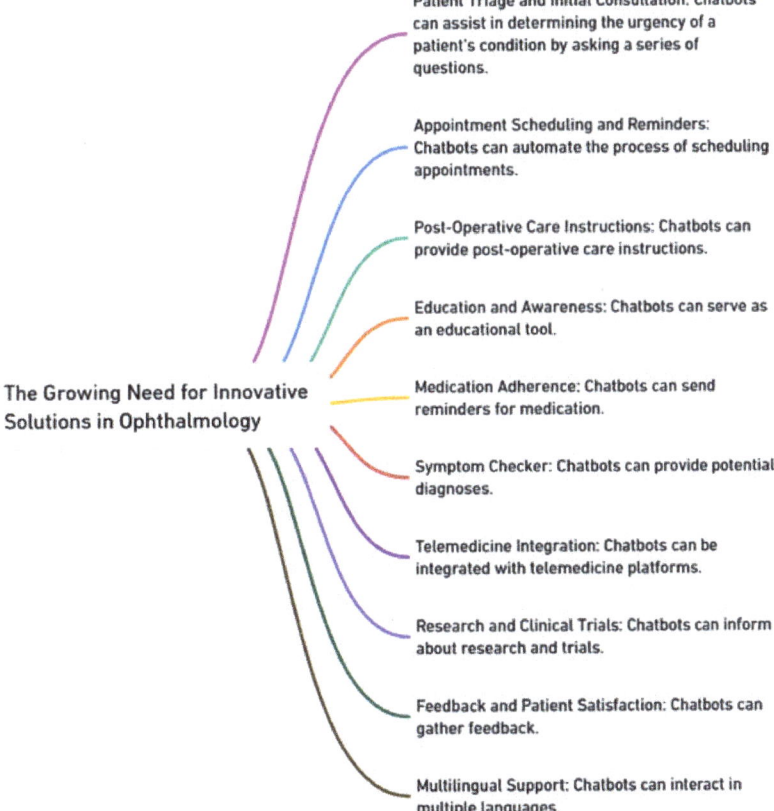

Figure 2. The growing need for innovative solutions in ophthalmology.

Chatbots have the potential to play a pivotal role in ophthalmology by providing instantaneous access to information. One of their primary uses lies in patient triage and initial consultation. By asking a series of targeted questions, chatbots can assist in determining the urgency of a patient's condition, thereby helping to prioritize those who need immediate attention. Additionally, these intelligent systems can automate the process of scheduling appointments, send timely reminders, and provide pre-appointment instructions. This ensures that patients are well-prepared for their visit, reducing wait times and enhancing the overall efficiency of the healthcare system.

Post-operative care is crucial in ophthalmology, especially after procedures like cataract surgery or LASIK. Chatbots can step in to provide patients with detailed post-operative care instructions, significantly reducing the risk of complications. Beyond this, they serve as an invaluable educational tool. Patients can receive information on common eye conditions, preventive measures, and general eye health tips directly from chatbots. This not only improves awareness but also empowers patients to take proactive steps in their healthcare journey. Furthermore, for chronic conditions where medication adherence is crucial, chatbots can send reminders, ensuring consistent medication use.

The integration of chatbots extends beyond basic patient interactions and doctor–patient consultations. They can be seamlessly integrated with various telemedicine platforms, facilitating a range of services such as medical video consultations for patient benefit, tele-reporting, administrative medical-health tele-consultancy, and tele-assistance for data transmission from ambulances to hospitals. This versatility enhances the efficiency and accessibility of healthcare services, making telemedicine more responsive to patient needs and healthcare dynamics. This is particularly beneficial in remote areas where immediate physical consultation might not be feasible. Additionally, chatbots can inform patients about ongoing research and clinical trials, aiding in participant recruitment and preliminary data gathering. They can also play a role in gathering feedback post-consultation or post-surgery, offering ophthalmologists insights into areas for improvement. Lastly, with multilingual support, chatbots ensure that language barriers do not impede the provision of quality care, making healthcare more inclusive and accessible.

2. Design and Development of Ophthalmology Chatbots

2.1. Understanding User Needs and Requirements

When designing and developing chatbots for ophthalmology, it is critical to have an extensive understanding of the unique needs and requirements of users specific to the ophthalmology practice [19]. This includes considering the particular challenges faced in ophthalmology and adhering to user-centered design principles to ensure the creation of effective chatbots. The development process should also incorporate the collection and analysis of user feedback, to confirm that the chatbot meets the expectations and requirements of both patients and professionals in the discipline. Importantly, this entails creating two distinct paths in chatbot development: one tailored for doctors, using scientific and medical terminologies, and another for patients, employing non-medical, layperson-friendly language. This bifurcation ensures that the chatbot effectively communicates and engages with each group according to their specific knowledge levels and communication preferences (Figure 3).

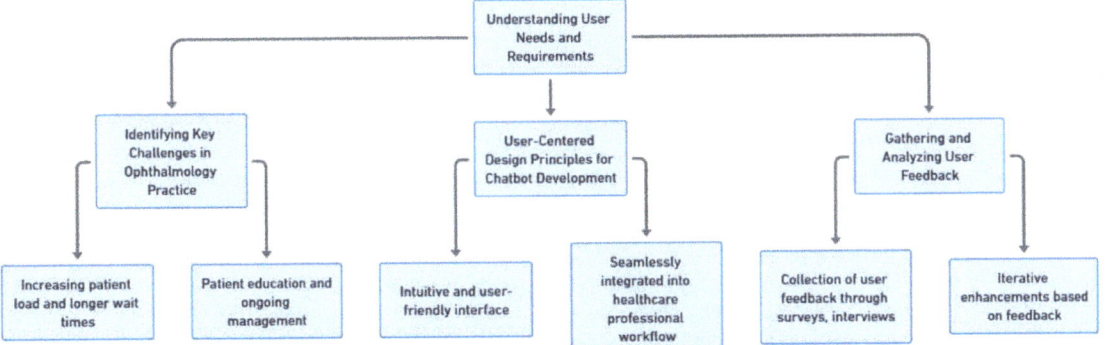

Figure 3. Understanding user needs and requirements.

2.1.1. Identifying Key Challenges in Ophthalmology Practice

The practice of ophthalmology is confronted with a variety of unique challenges that can be effectively addressed through the integration of chatbot technology. One notable challenge lies in the increasing patient load stemming from the escalating prevalence of eye conditions, [17] resulting in longer wait times and limited availability of consultations [20–22]. Chatbots offer a potential solution to this challenge by providing automated symptom assessment and triage capabilities, enabling patients to promptly receive initial guidance concerning their conditions. However, it is crucial to underline that automatic triage systems have limitations and should not replace professional medical evaluation, especially in complex cases. For instance, distinguishing between initial herpetic keratitis, where cortisone is contraindicated, and conjunctivitis, where cortisone may be prescribed, requires precise symptom assessment and medical expertise that a chatbot may not reliably provide. Therefore, while chatbots can assist in preliminary guidance, they should be used in conjunction with, and not as a substitute for, professional medical advice.

Another significant challenge pertains to patient education. Many eye conditions necessitate ongoing management and patient compliance, which can be improved through the provision of effective education and information [23–26]. Ophthalmology chatbots have the ability to dispense general eye health information, elucidate common ophthalmic procedures and treatments, and offer guidance regarding pre- and post-operative care. This empowers patients to take an active role in their eye health, leading to improved adherence and better treatment outcomes.

2.1.2. User-Centered Design Principles for Chatbot Development

The development of chatbots for ophthalmology necessitates adherence to user-centered design principles. This approach entails gaining a deep understanding of the specific needs, preferences, and behaviors of both patients and healthcare professionals operating within the field of ophthalmology.

Regarding patients, it is essential for the chatbot interface to be intuitive and user-friendly, featuring clear instructions and prompts, and avoiding complex medical terminology. Moreover, visual design elements should be optimized with ophthalmology in mind, taking into consideration factors such as color contrast, font size, and readability, to ensure inclusivity and accessibility for users with visual impairments [27].

As for healthcare professionals, the chatbot should be seamlessly integrated into their workflow. It should provide relevant and concise information, assist in the process of decision-making, and grant access to reference materials. Additionally, the chatbot should facilitate tasks such as appointment scheduling and reminders, streamlining the administrative responsibilities of healthcare professionals.

2.1.3. Gathering and Analyzing User Feedback

The collection of user feedback plays a critical role in refining and enhancing the design and functionality of ophthalmology chatbots. User feedback can be obtained through various channels, such as surveys, interviews, and user testing sessions. This valuable input provides insights into UX, challenges encountered, and areas in need of improvement.

The analysis of user feedback enables iterative enhancements of the chatbot's performance. It aids in the identification of common issues, understanding user preferences, and more importantly, uncovering any gaps in the chatbot's capabilities. This is achieved by systematically analyzing feedback for patterns of misunderstandings, incorrect responses, or inadequate information provided by the chatbot. For instance, if multiple users report confusion over a particular set of symptoms or express dissatisfaction with the guidance provided, this indicates a gap in the chatbot's knowledge or in its ability to interpret user inputs accurately. Additionally, feedback can highlight areas where the chatbot's communication style is not effective or user-friendly. This iterative process ensures that the chatbot aligns with user needs, ultimately enhancing its effectiveness and overall user satisfaction.

2.2. Chatbot Architecture and Functionality

In the context of ophthalmology chatbots, it is of importance to have a well-designed and functional architecture that specifically caters to the unique requirements of the field. This section thoroughly examines three pivotal aspects: natural language processing (NLP) tailored for ophthalmology, the integration of the knowledge base and medical databases, and conversational flow and dialogue management (Figure 4).

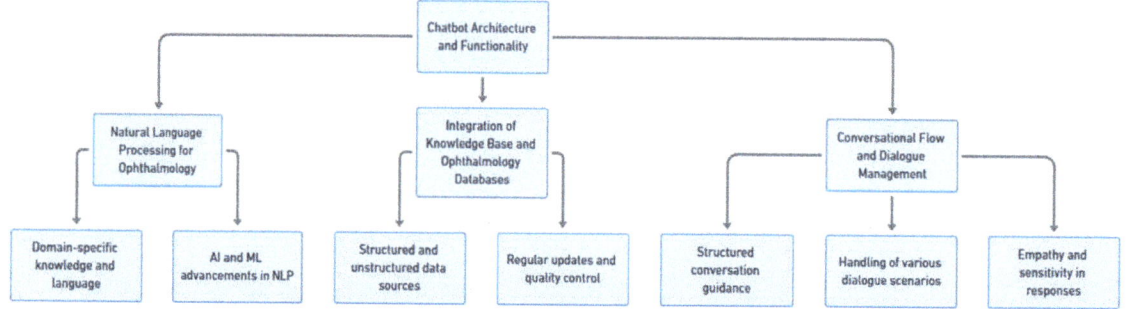

Figure 4. Chatbot architecture and functionality.

2.2.1. Natural Language Processing for Ophthalmology

Within the ophthalmology domain, NLP technology must be tailored to the specific language and terminology used. Accurate recognition and comprehension of ophthalmic terms, medical abbreviations, and anatomical references by the chatbot are essential. Moreover, NLP algorithms must be equipped to handle the complexity of ophthalmic queries, which often involve specific symptoms, laterality, and ophthalmic investigations. The chatbot should possess the capability to extract pertinent information from user inputs and generate appropriate responses. Additionally, it should demonstrate an understanding of the context of the conversation, thereby facilitating more meaningful interactions.

To attain these capabilities, the development of ophthalmology chatbots necessitates an in-depth understanding of domain-specific knowledge and language. Incorporating domain-specific ontologies, medical literature, and expert knowledge can significantly enhance the accuracy and effectiveness of the employed NLP algorithms. With the development of AI and ML, NLP in ophthalmology has evolved significantly in recent years, encompassing text data extraction, part-of-speech tagging, indexing, tokenization, classification, entity recognition, and word embeddings [28]. This has enabled Chatbot development to achieve desirable features.

2.2.2. Integration of Knowledge Base and Ophthalmology Databases

The integration of the knowledge base and ophthalmology databases is pivotal for ophthalmology chatbots to provide accurate and up-to-date information. It is imperative that this information be readily accessible to the chatbot, facilitating the delivery of reliable responses and recommendations.

The knowledge base can encompass structured information such as clinical guidelines, best practices, and standardized treatment protocols. These protocols are typically derived from clinical trials and the consensus among medical experts. However, it is important to acknowledge that clinical trials can sometimes yield conflicting results. In such cases, the role of comprehensive databases like PubMed becomes crucial. PubMed serves as a repository of diverse medical literature, allowing chatbots to access a wide range of research articles, case studies, and meta-analyses. This enables the chatbot to incorporate the most current and widely accepted medical knowledge, while also considering differing viewpoints and emerging research. Additionally, the integration of medical databases enables the chatbot to access patient-specific data, empowering it to provide personalized recommendations based on individual patient characteristics and specific eye conditions.

To ensure the accuracy and reliability of the information, regular updates and quality control measures should be implemented. Collaboration with ophthalmology experts, clinicians, and researchers is essential to validate and maintain the data sources.

2.2.3. Conversational Flow and Dialogue Management

An effective ophthalmology chatbot should possess the ability to manage conversational flow and dialogue in a seamless and natural manner. The dialogue management system orchestrates the interaction between the chatbot and the user, ensuring smooth transitions and relevant responses.

A chatbot is designed to engage in comprehensive conversations with patients, effectively addressing a wide range of concerns and queries. This includes guiding users through structured dialogues to gather necessary medical information; handling various dialogue scenarios, such as clarifying ambiguous queries; asking pertinent follow-up questions; and providing clear, detailed explanations. Importantly, the chatbot should be equipped to discuss treatment options and medical advice, tailoring its responses to the individual's medical history and current health status.

In addition to general inquiries, the chatbot must be adept at managing interruptions, context switches, and multi-turn conversations, thereby enabling a more natural and user-friendly interaction. It should exhibit empathy and sensitivity in its responses, considering the emotional aspects of patients' discussions, which is crucial in conversations about treatment and health concerns. The utilization of advanced language generation techniques aids in creating responses that are not only informative and compassionate, but also easily comprehensible to patients from diverse backgrounds. Continuous testing and analysis of user feedback are essential for optimizing conversational flow and dialogue management, ensuring that the chatbot remains effective in both general and treatment-specific discussions.

2.3. Chatbot User Interface and User Experience Design

The creation of an effective user interface (UI) and the provision of a positive user experience (UX) are imperative for achieving optimal engagement and usability. This section emphasizes three fundamental aspects: visual design elements tailored specifically for ophthalmology chatbots, interactive and intuitive UI design, and the optimization of UX with regard to accessibility and inclusivity (Figure 5).

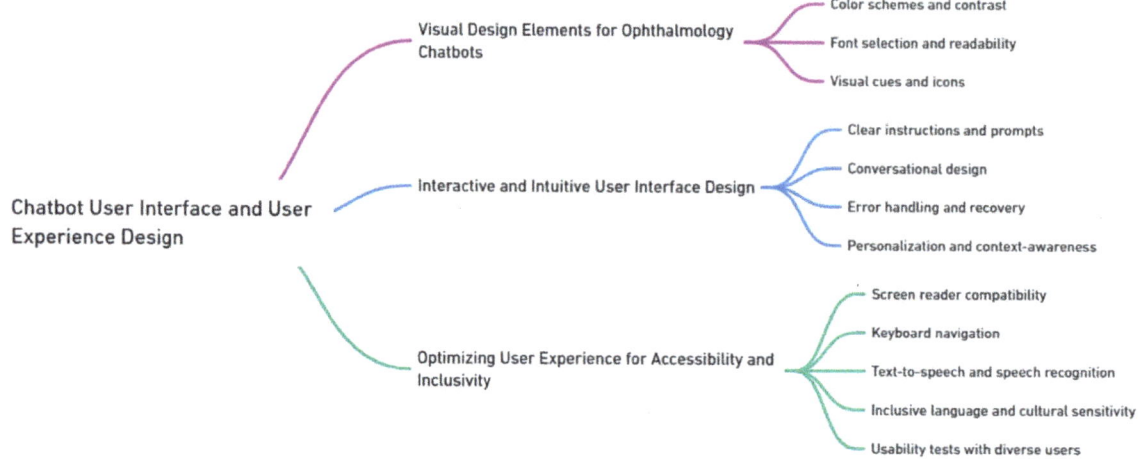

Figure 5. Chatbot user interface.

2.3.1. Visual Design Elements for Ophthalmology Chatbots

Visual design elements play a pivotal role in the development of an engaging and user-friendly UI for ophthalmology chatbots. To ensure these elements are effectively customized, it is imperative that the chatbot first gathers and understands the distinctive characteristics and requirements of each patient in the ophthalmology practice.

Color schemes and contrast are key aspects of this customization. Selecting appropriate color schemes and ensuring suitable contrast levels are vital for enhancing readability and visual comfort, especially for users with visual impairments. The chatbot must be capable of adapting its interface based on the specific visual needs of the patient. For example, utilizing high-contrast colors for text and background elements can significantly improve readability for individuals with low vision. This adaptive approach ensures that the chatbot's UI is not only visually appealing but also tailored to meet the unique needs of each patient, thereby providing a more personalized and effective user experience [27].

Font selection and readability: Employing clear and easily readable fonts facilitates effortless navigation for users of the chatbot interface. Additionally, incorporating font sizes that can be easily adjusted enables users to customize the display according to their specific needs.

Visual cues and icons: The integration of visual cues and icons contributes to an enhanced UX overall. Utilizing intuitive icons and symbols that are specific to ophthalmology, such as eye-related illustrations or medical symbols, assists in quickly conveying information and guiding users through the chatbot interface.

2.3.2. Interactive and Intuitive User Interface Design

Creating an interactive and intuitive UI is pivotal for ophthalmology chatbots to effectively engage and assist users. The UI design should enable seamless navigation and provide a user-friendly experience [29].

Clear instructions and prompts: Chatbots should employ explicit instructions and prompts to guide users throughout their interactions. Offering step-by-step guidance and clear instructions on how to interact with the chatbot facilitates a smooth flow of conversation.

Conversational design: Emulating natural conversation in a chatbot interface is crucial for enhancing user engagement. The chatbot should provide a conversational tone, mimicking human-like interactions, and appropriate responses to user inputs, including variations in language, phrasing, and sentence structure.

Error handling and recovery: To maintain a positive user UX, the chatbot should adeptly handle user errors or misunderstandings, provide suggestions for correcting or rephrasing queries, and offer help options for users to recover from errors or confusion.

Personalization and context-awareness: Personalization and context-awareness in UI design can enhance the UX by allowing chatbot to remember user preferences, past interactions, and relevant information. This facilitates a more personalized and tailored conversation, providing users with a sense of continuity and familiarity.

2.3.3. Optimizing User Experience for Accessibility and Inclusivity

Ensuring accessibility and inclusivity in the design of ophthalmology chatbots is of importance. The UI must be designed to accommodate the diverse needs of users, including those with visual impairments or disabilities.

Ensuring the compatibility of the chatbot interface with screen readers and other assistive technologies is a critical aspect of our design, particularly for users with visual impairments. To achieve this, a chatbot should be regularly evaluated and updated by a dedicated accessibility team, which includes experts in assistive technology, user experience designers, and representatives from the visually impaired community. This team is responsible for providing text alternatives for visual elements and incorporating appropriate semantic markup, enabling screen readers to effectively interpret and convey information.

Another key feature of chatbot accessibility is enabling keyboard navigation, which is essential for users who rely solely on keyboard interactions. The chatbot interface should be designed to allow users to navigate through the conversation and access all functionalities using keyboard commands. Modifications to keyboard navigation are also overseen by an accessibility team, which bases changes on user feedback, technological advancements, and best practices in digital accessibility.

Text-to-speech and speech recognition: Integration of text-to-speech and speech recognition capabilities enhances accessibility for users with visual or motor impairments. This feature enables users to interact with the chatbot through voice commands and receive audio responses.

Inclusive language and cultural sensitivity: The language used by the chatbot should be inclusive and culturally sensitive. It should avoid biased language and be designed to cater to users from diverse cultural and linguistic backgrounds. The utilization of natural language generation techniques assists in generating inclusive and respectful responses.

To optimize UX for accessibility and inclusivity, it is crucial to conduct usability tests with a diverse group of users, including individuals with disabilities. Gathering feedback and incorporating suggested improvements ensures that the chatbot interface meets the needs of a wide range of users.

By adhering to these design principles and focusing on visual elements, interactive UI, and accessibility, ophthalmology chatbots can provide a seamless and inclusive UX.

3. Applications and Benefits of Chatbots in Ophthalmology

3.1. Remote Patient Monitoring and Triage

In the field of ophthalmology, chatbots have emerged as valuable tools for remote patient monitoring and triage, providing numerous advantages for both patients and healthcare providers. This section explores three primary applications of chatbots in ophthalmology, namely automated symptom assessment and triage, remote monitoring of eye conditions and treatment adherence, and facilitating telemedicine consultations (Figure 6).

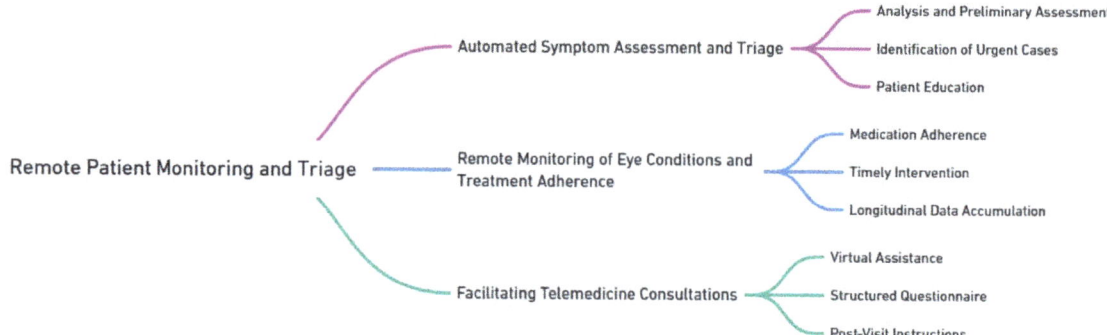

Figure 6. Remote patient monitoring and triage in ophthalmology.

3.1.1. Automated Symptom Assessment and Triage

Chatbots equipped with advanced NLP capabilities can assess and triage ophthalmic symptoms. Patients can interact with the chatbot, describing their symptoms and providing relevant information. The chatbot then analyzes this input and generates preliminary assessments based on established medical guidelines and protocols.

An ophthalmology chatbot is designed to perform automated symptom assessment and triage, enabling the timely identification of urgent cases, such as acute vision loss or severe eye pain. This system utilizes a sophisticated algorithm, developed in collaboration with ophthalmology experts, which assesses the severity and nature of symptoms reported by the patient. Urgent cases are identified based on predefined criteria, such as the sudden onset of symptoms, intensity of pain, or risk factors for serious eye conditions.

For non-urgent cases, the chatbot provides appropriate care recommendations. These may include self-care advice for minor symptoms or guidance to schedule a routine appointment with an ophthalmologist. These recommendations are based on established clinical guidelines and tailored to the individual's reported symptoms. This prioritization not only helps in preventing irreversible vision impairment or complications in urgent cases but also ensures that patients with less severe symptoms receive the most suitable care advice. This approach optimizes healthcare resources and reduces unnecessary visits to ophthalmology clinics or emergency departments.

Furthermore, the automated symptom assessment and triage conducted through chatbots contribute to patient education. The chatbot can provide information about common ophthalmic conditions, preventive measures, and self-management strategies. This empowers patients to make informed decisions about their eye health and promotes active participation in their own care.

3.1.2. Remote Monitoring of Eye Conditions and Treatment Adherence

Ophthalmology chatbots can assist in the remote monitoring of eye conditions and ensuring treatment adherence in patients with chronic eye conditions. Through regular interactions with patients, chatbots can gather information about visual symptoms, medication usage, and lifestyle factors that may impact eye health. Chatbots can improve medication adherence for patients with complex eye medication regimens. By sending reminders, educational messages, and addressing common concerns, chatbots can improve understanding and compliance, ensuring better treatment outcomes.

The remote monitoring capabilities of ophthalmology chatbots are crucial for timely intervention in cases of disease progression or non-adherence to treatment. In this context, "high-risk situations" refer to scenarios where there is a significant risk of rapid disease progression, potential vision loss, or other serious complications. These situations may include, but are not limited to, sudden changes in vision, symptoms indicating potential retinal detachment, or signs of acute glaucoma.

Healthcare providers, including ophthalmologists, can be alerted by the chatbot to these high-risk situations, allowing for proactive management and prevention of complications. This feature is particularly beneficial for patients in remote areas or those with limited access to healthcare, as it reduces the need for travel and associated costs. Furthermore, remote monitoring facilitates the accumulation of longitudinal data on patients' eye health, which can be invaluable for research purposes, population health management, and the improvement of treatment protocols.

3.1.3. Facilitating Telemedicine Consultations

The integration of chatbots in ophthalmology facilitates telemedicine consultations, enabling remote access to specialized eye care. While telemedicine has gained prominence, especially in situations where physical visits are challenging, it is important to recognize the current limitations of chatbots in this context. Chatbots may serve as virtual assistants during telemedicine consultations, providing support to ophthalmologists and enhancing the patient experience. Patients can engage with the chatbot for tasks like providing medical history and addressing preliminary concerns. However, we acknowledge that in the current implementation, chatbots do not support the sharing of images, which is a significant aspect of telemedicine in ophthalmology. For instance, a patient describing symptoms of a red eye could provide much more diagnostic value through an image, which a chatbot currently cannot process.

Prior to the telemedicine consultation, the chatbot can guide patients through a structured questionnaire to collect essential information. However, the integration of image-sharing capabilities in future iterations could greatly enhance the diagnostic process. After the consultation, the chatbot provides post-visit instructions and resources, but the addition of image analysis could further personalize and improve post-visit care. We recognize the importance of image exchange in ophthalmology and anticipate future advancements in chatbot technology that will enable this functionality, thereby significantly enhancing the effectiveness of telemedicine consultations in this field.

3.2. Patient Education and Information Provision

Within the field of ophthalmology, chatbots have emerged as effective tools for providing patient education and information (Table 1). This section examines three key aspects of patient education and information provision facilitated by ophthalmology chatbots, namely the dispensing of general eye health information, the explanation of common ophthalmic procedures and treatments, and the provision of guidance on pre- and post-operative care.

Table 1. Ophthalmology chatbots for patient education and information provision.

Case Scenario	Description	Advantages
1. Glaucoma Diagnosis	The chatbot assists patients in comprehending the diagnostic process for glaucoma, elucidating various tests such as tonometry and visual field tests. It imparts knowledge to patients regarding the condition, its symptoms, and available treatment options.	– Enhances patient awareness regarding glaucoma. – Provides precise and consistent information. – Empowers patients to make informed decisions regarding their treatment.
2. Prevention of Diabetic Retinopathy	The chatbot educates diabetic patients about the significance of regular eye examinations, early indicators of diabetic retinopathy, and risk factors. It offers recommendations on maintaining optimal blood sugar levels and lifestyle adjustments to minimize the risk.	– Encourages proactive eye care among individuals with diabetes. – Raises awareness regarding the connection between diabetes and ocular health. – Promotes preventive measures to mitigate complications.

Table 1. Cont.

Case Scenario	Description	Advantages
3. Preparation for Cataract Surgery	The chatbot guides patients through the pre-operative process of cataract surgery, elucidating the procedure, potential intraocular lens options, and post-operative care. It addresses common concerns such as anesthesia, recovery time, and potential risks.	– Reduces anxiety and uncertainty associated with surgery. – Provides comprehensive guidance for pre and post-operative care. – Ensures patients possess realistic expectations and are well-prepared.
4. Management of Age-related Macular Degeneration (AMD)	The chatbot furnishes information about AMD, encompassing risk factors, symptoms, and treatment options. It assists patients in understanding the significance of regular monitoring, lifestyle modifications, and available support resources.	– Empowers patients to actively manage their AMD. – Offers resources for emotional support and coping strategies. – Promotes adherence to treatment plans.
5. Pediatric Eye Conditions	The chatbot educates parents about prevalent pediatric eye conditions such as amblyopia (lazy eye) and strabismus (crossed eyes). It elucidates the importance of early intervention, available treatment options, and the role of regular eye examinations for children.	– Enhances parental awareness regarding pediatric eye health. – Encourages timely diagnosis and intervention. – Addresses common concerns and dispels misconceptions.

3.2.1. Dispensing General Eye Health Information

Ophthalmology chatbots can serve as interactive platforms that grant patients access to accurate and up-to-date information [30]. Through engagement with the chatbot, patients can obtain tailored information based on their individual needs and concerns. Moreover, it can educate patients on the significance of regular eye examinations and lifestyle factors such as protection from ultraviolet (UV) radiation.

Chatbots can address frequently asked questions, debunk myths and misconceptions, and clarify doubts related to eye health. They can offer guidance on topics such as proper eye hygiene, contact lens care, and vision correction options (Figure 7). The chatbot is capable of adapting its responses to accommodate the patient's level of understanding and of delivering information in a concise and comprehensible manner.

Dispensing general eye health information through chatbots fosters patient engagement and active participation in eye care. They encourage proactive measures and reduce reliance on traditional sources such as pamphlets or websites. Patients can receive personalized information and engage in interactive conversations with the chatbot, thereby enhancing their overall learning experience.

ChatGPT: Hello! How can I assist you today with your eye care?

Patient: Hi there! I've been experiencing some discomfort in my eyes lately. I want to know if there's anything I can do to improve my eye hygiene.

ChatGPT: I'm sorry to hear that you're experiencing discomfort. Proper eye hygiene is essential for maintaining healthy eyes. Here are some tips for you:

1. Wash your hands thoroughly before touching your eyes or handling your contact lenses.
2. Avoid rubbing your eyes, as it can cause irritation and potential infections.
3. Use a clean, lint-free towel to gently dry your face and eyes after washing.
4. If you wear makeup, make sure to remove it before going to bed to prevent any residue from getting into your eyes.
5. Avoid sharing eye cosmetics or contact lenses with others, as this can spread infections.
6. Replace your contact lens case regularly, and never use water to clean or store your lenses.

Patient: Thanks for the tips! That's really helpful. Is there anything specific I should do for my contact lenses?

ChatGPT: You're welcome! Proper care of your contact lenses is crucial for your eye health. Here are some steps to follow:

1. Wash your hands thoroughly with soap and water before handling your contact lenses.
2. Use the recommended contact lens solution to clean and disinfect your lenses. Never use water or saliva as these can introduce harmful bacteria.
3. Rub your contact lenses gently with your fingers while cleaning them to remove any debris or protein deposits.
4. Store your lenses in a clean, dry case when you're not wearing them, and replace the solution every day.
5. Follow the recommended wearing schedule provided by your eye care professional. Avoid wearing your lenses while swimming or sleeping, unless they are approved for extended wear.

Figure 7. This figure illustrates a two-way conversation between a patient and ChatGPT, a language model designed to offer guidance on eye care topics. The patient seeks advice regarding discomfort in their eyes and ways to improve eye hygiene. ChatGPT responds by providing concise and comprehensible information, including tips on proper eye hygiene and steps for the care of contact lenses. The chatbot adapts its responses to accommodate the patient's level of understanding, making the conversation informative and helpful for the patient's eye health.

3.2.2. Explanation of Common Ophthalmic Procedures and Treatments

Ophthalmology chatbots serve as valuable tools for elucidating common ophthalmic procedures and treatments to patients. They provide detailed information about diagnostic tests, surgical interventions, and medical treatments in a user-friendly and accessible manner.

Patients can interact with the chatbot to acquire knowledge about the purpose, process, and potential outcomes of various ophthalmic procedures. The chatbot can guide them through the steps involved in diagnostic tests such as visual acuity assessments, tonometry, and fundoscopy. Moreover, it can guide them in understanding surgical procedures like cataract surgery, LASIK, or corneal transplant, including the associated benefits, risks, and recovery process.

Chatbots help bridge the communication gap between patients and healthcare provider, allowing patients to review and reinforce their understanding of procedures and treatments at their own pace. They can educate patients about different treatment modalities for specific eye conditions. They can also elucidate the mechanisms of action and potential side effects of medications used in ophthalmology. Additionally, the explanation of common ophthalmic procedures and treatments enhances patient comprehension and reduces anxiety, by offering clear and accurate information. Patients gain a better understanding of the procedures or treatments they may undergo, thereby promoting informed decision-making and alleviating fears or uncertainties.

3.2.3. Guidance on Pre- and Post-Operative Care

Adequate preparation of patients for the surgical experience and the provision of appropriate post-operative care are essential for optimizing outcomes and minimizing complications.

Prior to surgery, chatbots can recommend to patients the necessary preparations, which may include fasting requirements and medication adjustments. They can provide advice on what to expect during the procedure, address common concerns, and offer reassurance and support. It is important to note that while chatbots can provide these recommendations based on standard pre-surgical protocols, the final preparation plan may be modified by the surgeon as necessary, tailored to the individual patient's condition. This ensures that patients receive personalized care, while also benefiting from the convenience and support offered by the chatbot.

Following the surgery, chatbots can offer comprehensive guidance on post-operative care, medication regimens, proper wound care, and the use of protective measures such as eye shields or patches. They can educate patients about common post-operative symptoms, signs of complications, and the need for follow-up appointments.

Gathering guidance on pre- and post-operative care through chatbots ensures that patients are well-informed, leading to improved compliance and better surgical outcomes. Clear instructions and guidance make patients more likely to adhere to the recommended care plans, thereby reducing the risk of complications and promoting successful recoveries. Additionally, chatbots can offer ongoing support and accessibility to patients during the post-operative period, reducing the need for unnecessary emergency visits and fostering continuity of care.

3.3. Support for Ophthalmology Professionals

Ophthalmology chatbots provide assistance in diagnosis and decision-making, delivery of clinical guidelines and reference materials, as well as in managing appointment scheduling and reminders. This section offers a detailed examination of these key areas, emphasizing the benefits and enhancements they bring to healthcare professionals in ophthalmology (Figure 8).

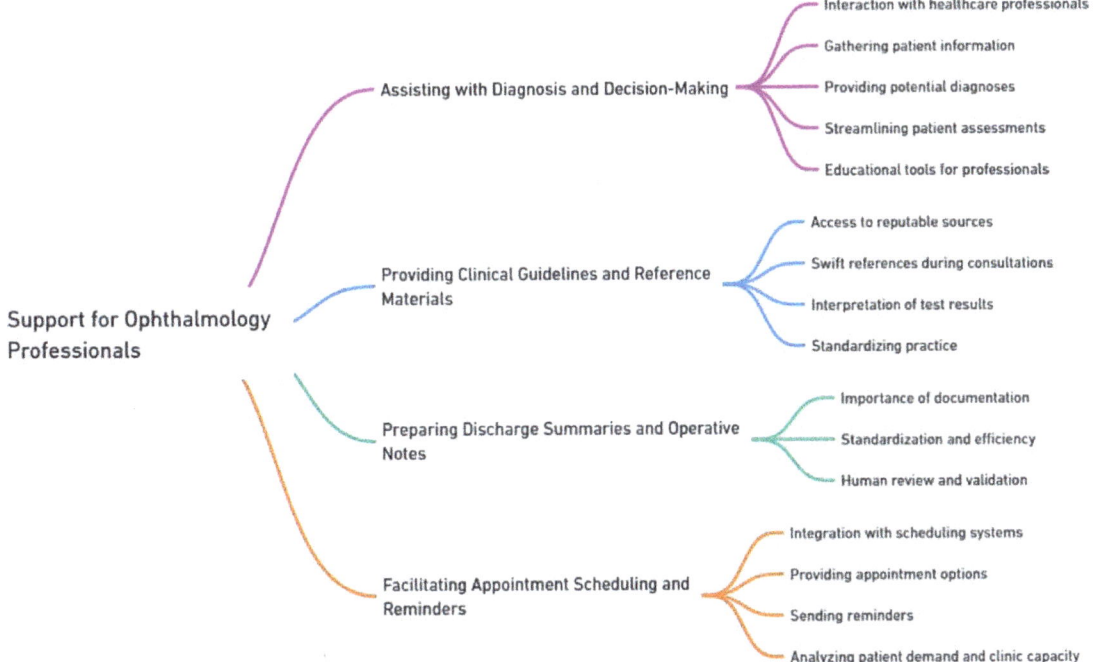

Figure 8. Support for ophthalmology professionals.

3.3.1. Assisting with Diagnosis and Decision-Making

Ophthalmology chatbots can assume a pivotal role in assisting healthcare professionals with diagnosis and decision-making processes. By utilizing their conversational and data processing capabilities, these chatbots interact with healthcare professionals, assisting in the collection of pertinent information related to patients' ocular conditions.

Chatbots can be programmed to pose targeted questions regarding patients' symptoms, medical history, ocular examinations, and other factors that may relate to certain diseases. By assimilating this information, chatbots assist healthcare professionals in developing a comprehensive understanding of the patient's condition, which can facilitate accurate diagnoses and informed treatment decisions. Additionally, chatbots can analyze the collected data and furnish healthcare professionals with potential diagnoses or differential diagnoses based on established clinical guidelines and algorithms, as well as integrating preexisting risk calculation tools, such as the age-related macular degeneration (AMD) risk calculator and the ocular hypertension treatment study (OHTS) risk calculator [31–35].

This serves as a valuable reference point for healthcare professionals, enabling them to make well-grounded and timely decisions. Ophthalmology chatbots can save healthcare professionals time by streamlining patient assessments and gathering relevant information. They also serve as valuable educational tools, providing up-to-date information on research findings, treatment options, and emerging trends, contributing to professional growth and enhancing expertise in the field.

3.3.2. Providing Clinical Guidelines and Reference Materials

Ophthalmology chatbots possess the capability to furnish healthcare professionals with clinical guidelines and reference materials. These chatbots can be programmed to access and retrieve information from reputable sources, such as medical databases, clinical practice guidelines, and research articles.

By having access to an extensive array of information, healthcare professionals can employ chatbots as swift references during patient consultations. Chatbots provide evidence-based recommendations for the diagnosis, treatment, and management of various ocular conditions. They also offer guidelines for monitoring and follow-up care, ensuring that healthcare professionals remain abreast of best practices in ophthalmology. Moreover, chatbots assist healthcare professionals in interpreting test results and imaging studies. They provide explanations for various ophthalmic tests, such as visual field testing, optical coherence tomography (OCT), or fundus photography. This aids healthcare professionals in accurately interpreting results and making well-informed decisions regarding patient care.

The provision of clinical guidelines and reference materials by ophthalmology chatbots confers numerous benefits. First, it ensures that healthcare professionals have immediate access to reliable and evidence-based information. This supports the decision-making process and facilitates the delivery of high-quality care to patients.

Second, chatbots aid in standardizing practice and fostering consistency in care delivery. By providing guidelines and recommendations, chatbots assist healthcare professionals in adhering to established protocols and best practices. This fosters improved patient outcomes and enhances the quality of care across various healthcare settings.

3.3.3. Preparing Discharge Summaries and Operative Notes

Discharge summaries and operative notes are of importance in ophthalmology for maintaining continuity of care, facilitating effective communication among healthcare providers, serving as legal documentation, supporting research and education, and promoting patient safety and quality improvement. While the significance of these factors is recognized, variations in content and the time-consuming process pose the greatest challenges in achieving excellence [36–38].

Using a chatbot for writing discharge summaries and operative notes can offer several advantages in terms of standardization, efficiency, accuracy, and convenience [39]. With proper training and the improvement of AI libraries, chatbots can be seen as tools to assist ophthalmology healthcare in generating comprehensive and efficient discharge summary and operative notes. It is important to note that human review and validation are crucial to ensure accuracy, especially in complex cases and for handling situations that require clinical judgement and empathy.

3.3.4. Facilitating Appointment Scheduling and Reminders

Ophthalmology chatbots possess the capability to facilitate appointment scheduling and reminders for healthcare professionals. They can seamlessly integrate with existing scheduling systems and electronic health records, enabling patients to conveniently book appointments and receive timely reminders about their upcoming visits.

Chatbots provide patients with options for available appointment slots, assisting them in finding suitable times that align with their schedules. They also automatically send reminders to patients, reducing the likelihood of missed appointments and enhancing overall clinic efficiency. Patients can access the chatbot at their convenience, obviating the need for phone calls or waiting on hold to schedule appointments, thus enhancing patient satisfaction and engagement.

Furthermore, chatbots can aid healthcare professionals in managing their schedules by optimizing appointment bookings. Through analyzing patient demand and clinic capacity, chatbots suggest optimal scheduling strategies that minimize wait times and maximize clinic utilization. This enables healthcare professionals to streamline their workflow, for reduced administrative burden and increased productivity, to provide timely care to their patients.

3.4. Ophthalmology Training

Chatbots hold immense potential as valuable educational tools in medical training, offering accessible and interactive resources to learners [40]. In the context of ophthalmology training, chatbots can play a crucial role in various aspects, including providing the fundamentals of ophthalmology, facilitating case studies and diagnostic support, offering adaptive assessment, and even simulating surgical procedures. Furthermore, they can assist with administrative tasks and personalized course organization, tailoring the learning experience to individual needs. One of the most significant advantages of chatbots in this domain is their ability to provide comprehensive knowledge and reference materials essential for ophthalmology training. By harnessing AI's continuous updating capabilities, these chatbots can ensure that learners access the most up-to-date information, thereby enhancing the overall learning experience.

Through incorporating simulated patient interactions, chatbots enable learners to practice and refine their clinical skills effectively. By presenting realistic case scenarios, students can engage in diagnostic decision-making and treatment proposals. The chatbot can then offer valuable feedback on their decisions, guiding them throughout the process. This feedback mechanism not only helps learners identify areas for improvement but also provides specific recommendations for additional study or practice, which can be invaluable for their professional growth. However, it is essential to acknowledge that there are still areas for improvement in the utilization of chatbots in ophthalmology training. One such aspect is the need to focus on enhancing accuracy. Ensuring that the chatbot's responses are consistently reliable and aligned with established medical knowledge is crucial for the success of such educational tools.

4. Availability and Performance of Current Ophthalmology Chatbots

Chatbots have emerged as innovative tools in the field of ophthalmology. Chatbots, such as ChatGPT, can be integrated into various platforms such as web-based platforms, mobile applications, messaging applications, and virtual reality platforms. The following sections present examples of chatbot use in ophthalmology and summarize the current performance of chatbots employed in various ophthalmology-related contexts.

4.1. Chatbot Performance in Triage Ophthalmology Conditions

In a study performed by Tsui, J.C. et al., ten prompts reflecting common patient complaints related to common ophthalmology conditions were used to determine the suitability of ChatGPT 3.0 responses. The study also evaluated the precision of the responses by comparing the responses to the same questions from three individual chats. The study found a majority of responses were precise and suitable; however, 20% of responses were considered imprecise or unsuitable [41].

A more recent study by Lyons, R.J. and associates also evaluated the triage performance of 44 vignettes representing common emergency room ophthalmologic diagnosis using three publicly available AI chatbots, namely ChatGPT 4.0, Bing Chat (Microsoft Corporation, Redmond, WA, USA), and WebMD Symptom Checker (WebMD Inc., New York, NY, USA). The responses from the chatbots were compared with physician respondents. The study found that ChatGPT using GPT-4 model yielded the highest diagnostic (93%) and triage (98%) accuracy (Figure 9). Although Bing resulted in a high accuracy of diagnosis, there were incorrect responses in 14% of cases, whereas none were discovered for ChatGPT [42].

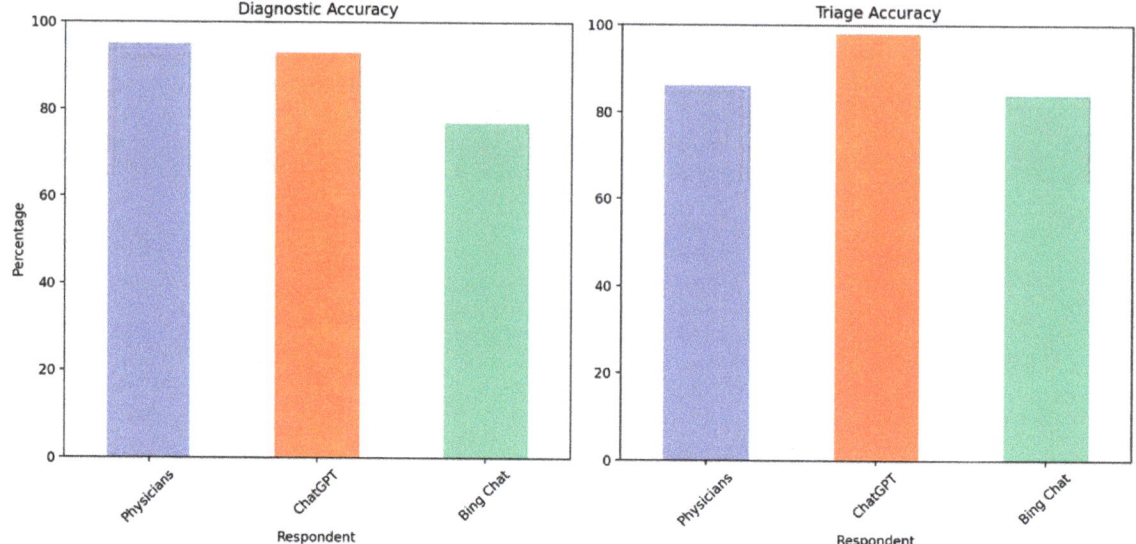

Figure 9. Chatbot performance in triage ophthalmology conditions. On the left, "correct diagnosis accuracy" bar chart; and on the right, "correct triage accuracy" bar chart.

4.2. ChatGPT Performance in Patient Education and Information Provision

A study from Potapenko et al. assessed the accuracy of patient information for five common retinal diseases (i.e., age-related macular degeneration, diabetic retinopathy, retinal vein occlusion, retinal artery occlusion, and central serous chorioretinopathy) using ChatGPT 3.0. They evaluated accuracies in disease summary, prevention, treatment options, and prognosis. Most responses showed high accuracy, with median ratings ranging from "good/only minor non-harmful inaccuracies" to "very good/no inaccuracies." However, treatment options had "moderate/potentially misinterpretable inaccuracies", with 12 of 100 treatment responses showing "potentially harmful inaccuracies" [7].

Similarly, another study focusing on patient information from ChatGPT 3.0 on vernal keratoconjunctivitis (VKC) also found that current ChatGPT responses, while relevant to typical questions, are still imperfect. The responses related to treatment and prevention received considerably lower accuracy ratings from the experts than VKC general, prognosis, and allergy-related questions. Inaccuracies such as missing essential information regarding potentially serious steroid side effects and harmful suggestions such as removal of conjunctiva were discovered [30].

4.3. Chatbots Examples in Supporting for Healthcare Professionals

A preliminary work utilizing ChatGPT 3.0 to generate discharge summaries across subspecialties found that the AI-constructed documents were able to shorten the processes; however, their quality was based on the completeness of the prompts given and required training and adjustment [39]. Table 2 shows an example of a discharge summary generated by ChatGPT.

Table 2. Example of an ophthalmology discharge summary generated by ChatGPT 3.5.

Prompt	Please write discharge summary for Mr. Somchai Jade, who had a left eye superior retinal detachment involving macular and underwent 25G pars plana vitrectomy with fluid air exchange and endolaser and C3F8 injection, 3 days ago. On the day of discharge, the retina is attached, wound is secure, ac cell is 2+, gas filled 100%, but the intraocular pressure is 25 mm of Hg. He is now initiated on anti-glaucoma medication, Timolol twice a day, in the left eye, instructed to keep face down position and need a follow-up after 5 days at the retina clinic, outpatient clinic with Dr. Ray.
ChatGPT's response	Patient Name: Mr. Somchai Jade Date of Discharge: [Date] Admitting Physician: [Physician's Name] Discharging Physician: [Physician's Name] Diagnosis: Left eye superior retinal detachment involving macular Procedure: Mr. Somchai Jade underwent a 25G pars plana vitrectomy with fluid air exchange and endolaser, followed by C3F8 injection, three days ago. Condition on Discharge: On the day of discharge, the following observations were made: 1. Retina: The retina is attached after the surgical procedure. 2. Wound: The wound is secure and healing well. 3. Anterior Chamber: Anterior chamber cell (ac cell) count is 2+. 4. Gas Fill: The eye is filled with 100% C3F8 gas. 5. Intraocular Pressure (IOP): The intraocular pressure is currently elevated at 25 mm of Hg. Treatment and Medication: Mr. Jade has been initiated on anti-glaucoma medication, Timolol, to manage the elevated intraocular pressure. He is instructed to administer Timolol twice a day in the left eye, as prescribed. Detailed instructions on the proper administration technique and potential side effects of the medication have been provided to the patient. Additionally, Mr. Jade is instructed to maintain a face-down position as much as possible during his recovery period. This position aids in the proper positioning of the gas bubble in the eye, ensuring optimal healing and attachment of the retina. The patient is advised to follow the specific instructions provided by the surgeon regarding the duration and frequency of the face-down position. Follow-up: Mr. Somchai Jade is advised to follow up with Dr. Ray, a retina specialist, at the retina clinic in the outpatient department after five days. The purpose of the follow-up visit is to assess the progress of the retinal attachment, monitor the intraocular pressure, and evaluate the need for further treatment or adjustment of the medication regimen. Instructions: 1. The patient should continue with the prescribed anti-glaucoma medication, Timolol, as instructed. 2. Mr. Jade should maintain a face-down position as directed by the surgeon. Specific instructions regarding the duration and frequency of this position should be followed strictly. 3. It is important to protect the eye from any trauma or injury. 4. The patient should maintain good hygiene and avoid rubbing or touching the eye unnecessarily. 5. In case of any sudden changes in vision, severe pain, or worsening symptoms, Mr. Jade should seek immediate medical attention. Summary: Mr. Somchai Jade underwent a successful 25G pars plana vitrectomy with fluid gas exchange and endolaser, along with C3F8 injection, for a left eye superior retinal detachment involving macular. On the day of discharge, the retina was found to be attached, the wound secure, and the anterior chamber showing a moderate cell reaction. The intraocular pressure was elevated, and the patient was initiated on Timolol eye drops for glaucoma management. In addition, Mr. Jade has been instructed to maintain a face-down position during the recovery period to optimize retinal healing. A follow-up appointment has been scheduled after five days with Dr. Ray at the retina clinic to monitor the patient's progress and adjust the treatment plan if necessary.

Note: This discharge summary is a simulated case created for demonstration purposes only and has not been derived from an actual patient case. It is intended to showcase the capabilities of ChatGPT 3.5 in generating medical content.

GlauCUTU is another example of a chatbot designed to aid with glaucoma diagnosis. This chatbot utilizes a deep learning algorithm to provides real-time response to help in screening glaucoma based on optic disc photo [43]. GlauCUTU operates on the mobile and desktop social messaging service LINE (Figure 10). With the integration of a messaging application, it provides a convenient and readily accessible mode of communication and can be considered an example of an ophthalmologist virtual assistant [43].

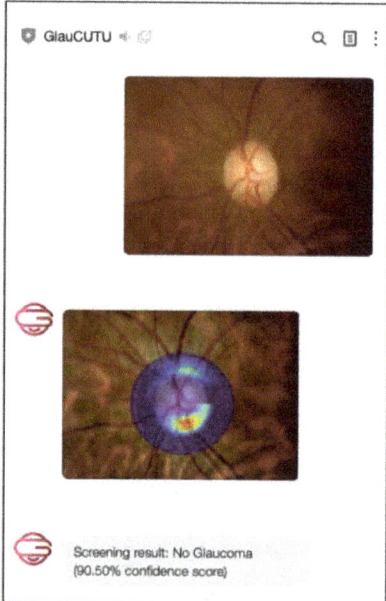 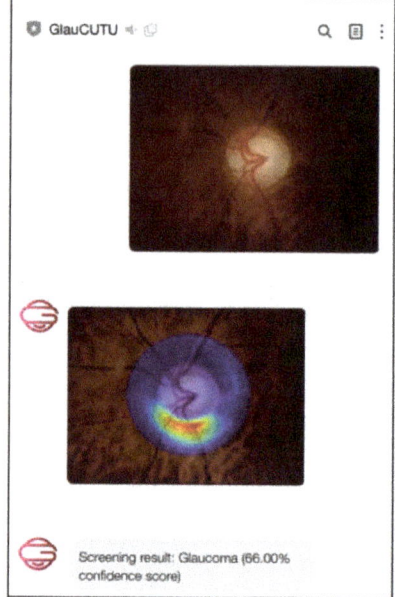

Figure 10. Example of responses generated by GlauCUTU illustrating glaucoma risk assessment from an optic disc photo.

4.4. Chatbot Performance in Ophthalmology Knowledge Assessment

The performance of chatbots can vary across disciplines and different subspecialties (Table 3). While ChatGPT answered a majority of general medicine licensing examination questions correctly [44], the present version of ChatGPT did not correctly answer multiple-choice questions (MCQ) for the US board certification preparation (i.e., Ophthalmic Knowledge Assessment Program (OKAP) and Written Qualifying Exam (WQE) from the OphthoQuestions) to a desirable level. A study indicated that ChatGPT 3.0 correctly answered only 46% of 125 multiple-choice questions intended to prepare for board certification examinations [45] Figure 11.

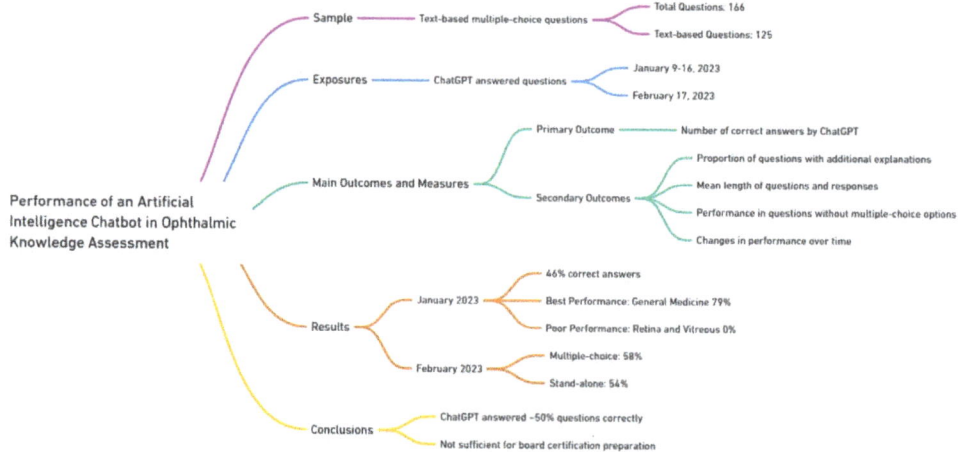

Figure 11. Performance of an artificial intelligence chatbot in ophthalmic knowledge assessment.

Table 3. Studies assessing chatbot performance in ophthalmology knowledge assessment.

Study	Mihalache et al. [45]	Raimondi et al. [46]	Bernstein et al. [47]
Study Designs and Population	Cross-sectional study assessing ChatGPT's performance on ophthalmology board certification practice questions.	Comparative analysis of LLM chatbots on the Fellowship of Royal College of Ophthalmologists (FRCOphth) postgraduate exams.	Cross-sectional study evaluating the quality of ophthalmology advice by ChatGPT compared to ophthalmologists.
Methods	125 text-based multiple-choice questions from OphthoQuestions were used.	Tested on 48 Part 1 and 43 Part 2 multiple choice questions from the FRCOphth curriculum.	200 online forum posts with patient eye care questions and responses were analyzed.
Key Results	- Correct answers: 58 of 125 questions (46%) in January 2023. - Correct answers: 73 of 125 multiple-choice questions (58%) and 42 of 78 stand-alone questions (54%) without multiple-choice options in February 2023.	- Accuracies for chatbots: Part 1 ranged from 55.1–78.9% and Part 2 ranged from 49.6–82.9%. - Bing Chat had the highest scores of 78.9% and 82.9% for Part 1 and Part 2, respectively.	- Expert reviewers identified chatbot vs. human responses with 61% accuracy. - Incorrect information: chatbot 21% vs. human 19%. - Likelihood of harm: chatbot 13% vs. human 15%. - Extent of harm: chatbot 3% vs. human 3%.
Conclusion	ChatGPT answered approximately half of the questions correctly. It may not provide substantial assistance in preparing for board certification currently.	LLM chatbots can achieve high accuracy on ophthalmology specialty exams without specific tuning. They have potential to advance ophthalmic education and care but issues like validation, transparency, biases, and accessibility need addressing.	Chatbot's ophthalmology advice was not significantly different from ophthalmologists' advice. LLMs may be capable of providing appropriate responses to patient eye care questions. Further research is needed.

Abbreviations: LLM—large language model; FRCOphth—Fellowship of Royal College of Ophthalmologists.

Another study compared more update versions of ChatGPT (ChatGPT 3.5 and 4.0) with Bing Chat and Google Bard (Alphabet Inc., CA, US) in their accuracy in answering the UK's postgraduate MCQ exam for the Fellowship of Royal College of Ophthalmologists (FRCOphth) [46]. The study found accuracy rates of 49.6%, 51.9%, 82.9%, and 79.1% for ChatGPT 3.5, Google Bard, Bing Chat, and ChatGPT 4.0, respectively. However, the accuracy of ChatGPT 4.0 increased to 88.4% with prompting or tuning strategies. It should be noted that the accuracy varied widely across subspecialty topics with the lowest for trauma (accuracy 38.5%) and the highest for cornea and external eye (accuracy 96.2%), Figure 12.

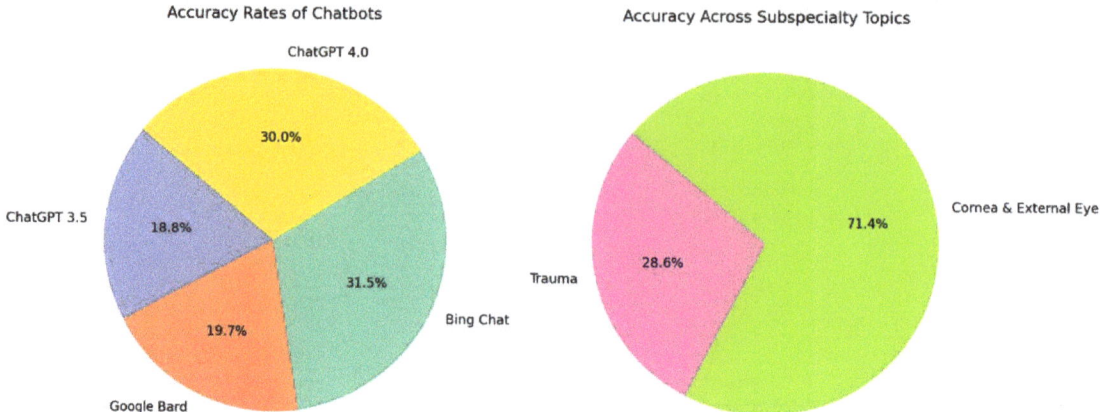

Figure 12. Comparative analysis of large language models in the Royal College of Ophthalmologists fellowship exams.

Recently, Bernstein et al. [47] conducted a cross-sectional study evaluating the quality of ophthalmology advice generated by ChatGPT, a large language model (LLM) chatbot, compared to advice written by ophthalmologists (Figure 13). The authors analyzed 200 pairs of online forum posts with patient eye care questions and responses by American Academy of Ophthalmology physicians. A panel of eight masked ophthalmologists were asked to distinguish between chatbot and human answers. The expert reviewers correctly identified chatbot vs. human responses with 61% accuracy on average (Figure 13A). However, the ratings of chatbot and human answers were comparable regarding the inclusion of incorrect information (21% vs. 19%), likelihood to cause harm (13% vs. 15%), and extent of harm (3% vs. 3%), (Figure 13B). The quality of chatbot answers was not rated as significantly inferior to human answers. The results suggest large language models may be capable of providing appropriate responses to patient eye care questions across a range of complexity. Further research is needed to evaluate the performance, ethics, and optimal clinical integration of chatbots in ophthalmology.

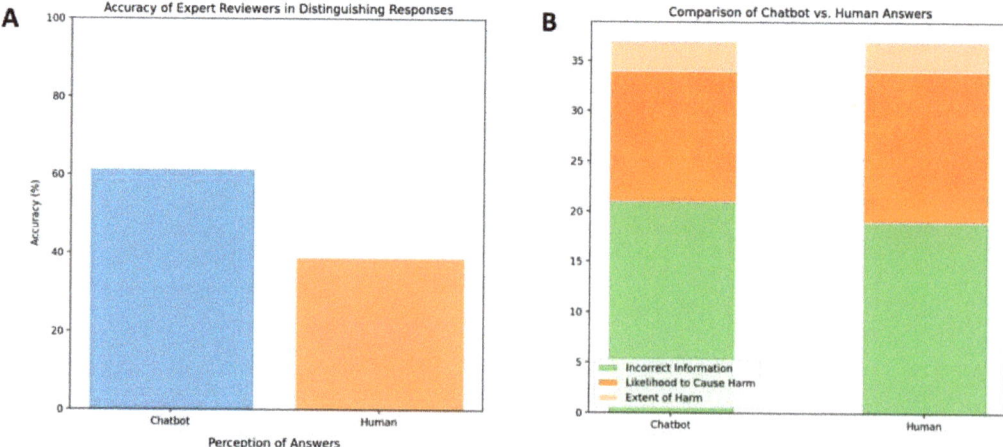

Figure 13. (**A**) Accuracy of expert reviewers in distinguishing responses. (**B**) Comparison of chatbot vs. human answers.

In ophthalmology, chatbots have the potential to be useful tools. The currently available chatbots are restricted in their availability and performance. Generally, they are able to provide acceptably broad knowledge and initial guidance. However, users must be mindful of their limitations, particularly in complicated settings where the proportion of incorrect chatbots' responses is high. New versions tend to perform better than the older ones. Future chatbot advancements may rectify these deficiencies.

5. Challenges and Future Directions in Ophthalmology Chatbots

5.1. Ethical and Legal Considerations

5.1.1. Privacy and Data Security

Privacy and data security are critical concerns in the context of ophthalmology chatbots, particularly when considering the diverse legal frameworks across different nations. These chatbots gather and process sensitive patient information and personal identifiers, necessitating robust security measures to safeguard these data from unauthorized access, breaches, or misuse.

Ensuring adherence to industry standards and best practices for data encryption and storage is fundamental. Employing encryption techniques, such as secure socket layer (SSL) encryption, can protect the transmission of data. However, developers must also navigate the complexities of varying national laws, which often include additional rules in the field of transmissions, servers, administration, and telecommunication standards. This necessitates a flexible approach to compliance, ensuring that chatbots meet the specific legal requirements of each jurisdiction in which they operate.

Healthcare organizations and developers should establish explicit protocols for data access and sharing, considering different legal landscapes. Transparency in data handling practices is crucial to foster trust among patients, healthcare professionals, and chatbot providers.

To mitigate potential privacy risks and comply with diverse legal standards, privacy-by-design principles should be integrated into the development process. This involves incorporating privacy features from the outset, such as anonymization and data minimization techniques, which are essential in addressing the varied legal requirements across nations (Table 4).

5.1.2. Informed Consent and Confidentiality

Obtaining informed consent and ensuring confidentiality are pivotal ethical considerations when utilizing ophthalmology chatbots. Patients should be fully informed about the purpose, capabilities, and limitations of the chatbot, as well as the type of data it collects and how that data will be used. Informed consent should be sought before engaging patients in chatbot interactions and data collection.

Furthermore, ophthalmology chatbots should provide patients with explicit options to opt in or out of data collection and sharing. Patients should have the ability to withdraw their consent and request the deletion of their data at any time. This empowers patients to exercise control over their personal information, fostering transparency and respecting patient autonomy.

Confidentiality is equally crucial in maintaining patient trust and complying with ethical and legal standards. Ophthalmology chatbots must adhere to stringent confidentiality protocols to ensure that patient data are accessible only to authorized individuals involved in healthcare provision. Measures such as encryption, secure data transmission, and restricted data access help preserve the confidentiality of patient information.

Table 4. Privacy and data security: case scenarios and suggested solutions in ophthalmology chatbots.

Case Scenario: Unauthorized Access to Patient Data	Suggested Solutions
Privacy and data security breach occurs when unauthorized individuals access patient data in the ophthalmology chatbot system.	– Implement strong authentication methods, such as multi-factor authentication. – Encrypt patient data both at rest and in transit using strong encryption algorithms. – Implement role-based access control mechanisms to restrict access based on job roles. – Conduct regular security audits and penetration testing to identify vulnerabilities. – Provide comprehensive training to personnel on privacy and data security best practices.
Case Scenario: Data Breach during Data Transfer	**Suggested Solutions**
Data breach occurs when patient data are compromised during transmission in ophthalmology chatbots.	– Use secure protocols (e.g., HTTPS, SSL/TLS) for data transmission. – Implement data loss prevention mechanisms to monitor and control data transfers. – Keep software and systems up to date with the latest security patches and updates. – Use secure and well-tested APIs for data exchange with external systems. – Encrypt patient data during transmission for an additional layer of protection.
Case Scenario: Inadequate Data Retention Policies	**Suggested Solutions**
The ophthalmology chatbot system retains patient data for longer than necessary.	– Implement data minimization practices to collect and store only necessary patient data. – Regularly review and delete outdated or unnecessary patient data from the system. – Consider anonymizing or de-identifying patient data to protect privacy. – Establish clear data retention policies and guidelines for different types of data. – Stay updated with privacy laws and regulations and ensure compliance with data retention policies.

Additionally, chatbots should be programmed to provide appropriate disclaimers and warnings regarding the limitations of their capabilities. Patients should be aware that chatbots do not replace in-person consultations with healthcare professionals and that they should seek medical advice when necessary. This ensures that patients understand the boundaries of chatbot interactions and prompt them to seek appropriate care when needed.

5.1.3. Compliance with Regulatory Standards

Compliance with regulatory standards is essential for ophthalmology chatbots, to ensure patient safety, quality of care, and legal compliance. These chatbots must adhere to relevant regulations and guidelines, such as the Health Insurance Portability and Accountability Act (HIPAA) in the United States and the General Data Protection Regulation (GDPR) in the European Union.

Thorough assessments should be conducted by healthcare organizations and developers of ophthalmology chatbots to ensure compliance with these regulations. This involves reviewing and aligning data handling practices, security measures, and consent procedures with the requirements stipulated in the regulations. Regular audits and assessments can identify any gaps in compliance and facilitate necessary adjustments.

Moreover, collaboration among healthcare organizations, chatbot developers, and regulatory bodies is pivotal in establishing guidelines and standards specific to ophthalmology chatbots. These guidelines should address concerns such as data privacy, informed consent, and the ethical use of chatbots in ophthalmology. By working together, stakeholders can ensure that chatbots meet the necessary ethical and legal standards, while maximizing their potential benefits.

Looking to the future, the development of standardized frameworks and guidelines for ophthalmology chatbots can provide a roadmap for ethical and legal compliance. These frameworks should address the unique challenges and considerations associated with ophthalmology, guaranteeing that chatbots align with the specific needs and requirements of the field. Additionally, ongoing research and evaluation of ophthalmology chatbots can help identify and address emerging ethical and legal issues. Regular monitoring of the evolving regulatory landscape and continuous improvements in chatbot technology can facilitate the development of adaptable and ethically sound solutions.

5.2. Integration with Existing Healthcare Systems

5.2.1. Interoperability and Integration Challenges

Ophthalmology chatbots require seamless interoperability and integration with diverse healthcare systems, including electronic medical records, diagnostic devices, and telehealth systems, for efficient usage and effective usage.

One of the primary challenges lies in the diversity of existing healthcare systems, each with its own compatibility level. In addition, diagnosis in the field of ophthalmology frequently requires the integration of multimodality instruments, such as tonometry, perimetry, fundus photography, and optical coherence tomography. Ophthalmology chatbots need to be designed in a way that enables communication and data exchange with various software applications and databases. This necessitates adherence to standardized data formats and protocols that facilitate smooth interoperability.

Ophthalmology chatbots should also be compatible with a variety of devices and operating systems (e.g., desktops, mobile devices). Compatibility across a wide range of devices ensures accessibility and usability for healthcare professionals in clinics, hospitals, and remote sites.

To overcome these challenges, collaboration among healthcare organizations, chatbot developers, and technology providers becomes imperative. The development of standardized application programming interfaces (APIs) and protocols specifically tailored to ophthalmology can expedite the seamless integration of chatbots with existing healthcare systems. The establishment of common standards helps minimize interoperability barriers, thereby enabling efficient data exchange and communication between chatbots and other healthcare tools.

5.2.2. Collaboration with Electronic Health Records

Collaboration with electronic health records (EHR) that contain comprehensive patient information allows chatbots to access and update information in real time. This enhances their capacity to provide personalized and accurate care. However, challenges arise when it comes to EHR integration. Different healthcare organizations may utilize diverse EHR systems, each characterized by a unique data structure and interface. This variability poses a challenge in developing chatbots capable of seamlessly interacting with a wide range of EHR systems.

One potential solution is the development of standardized data exchange formats such as fast healthcare interoperability resources (FHIR), which promote interoperability between EHRs and chatbots. FHIR facilitates the exchange of structured health data, enabling chatbots to retrieve and update patient information from EHR systems in a standardized and consistent manner. Furthermore, collaboration between developers of ophthalmology chatbots and EHR vendors plays a crucial role. Close cooperation can lead to the development of specific interfaces and integration solutions tailored to the field of ophthalmology, thereby ensuring smooth data exchange and seamless connectivity between chatbots and EHR systems.

5.2.3. Seamless Communication with Healthcare Providers

Effective care requires seamless communication between ophthalmology chatbots and healthcare providers. Chatbots should facilitate easy and efficient information exchange, enabling healthcare professionals to review patient data, provide guidance, and make well-informed decisions.

One challenge in achieving seamless communication lies in presenting information in a format that is easily comprehensible and actionable for healthcare providers. Chatbots should present patient data and clinical recommendations concisely and in an organized manner, allowing healthcare providers to quickly grasp the relevant information. The incorporation of NLP capabilities can assist in understanding and presenting complex medical information. Moreover, ophthalmology chatbots should enable bidirectional communication between healthcare providers and the chatbot system. This allows healthcare providers to provide additional context, clarify patient information, and request specific actions from the chatbot. The seamless integration of chatbots with the messaging platforms utilized by healthcare professionals, such as secure messaging applications, can facilitate real-time communication and collaboration.

Ensuring the security and privacy of communications is also of utmost importance. Chatbot systems should employ secure communication channels and encryption techniques to safeguard sensitive patient information during interactions with healthcare providers. Compliance with relevant privacy regulations, such as HIPAA, is essential in upholding patient confidentiality and meeting legal requirements.

To address these challenges, collaboration between chatbot developers and healthcare providers is indispensable. Employing user-centered design methodologies can facilitate the gathering of feedback and insights from healthcare professionals, ensuring that chatbots are designed with their workflow and communication needs in mind. Regular feedback loops and iterative improvements can enhance the usability and effectiveness of chatbot communication with healthcare providers.

5.3. Advancements and Future Innovations

5.3.1. Artificial Intelligence and Machine Learning in Chatbots

AI and ML are driving advancements in ophthalmology chatbots, enabling them to learn and improve from interactions with patients and healthcare providers. This leads to more accurate and effective diagnostic capabilities (Figure 14).

Through the analysis of vast amounts of patient data, chatbots can provide valuable insights and assist healthcare professionals in making informed decisions regarding patient care. AI and ML also enhance the NLP capabilities of chatbots. This allows them to understand and interpret patient queries and responses more effectively, facilitating improved communication and interaction. As AI and ML algorithms continue to advance, chatbots have the potential to provide increasingly accurate and personalized recommendations, leading to improved patient outcomes.

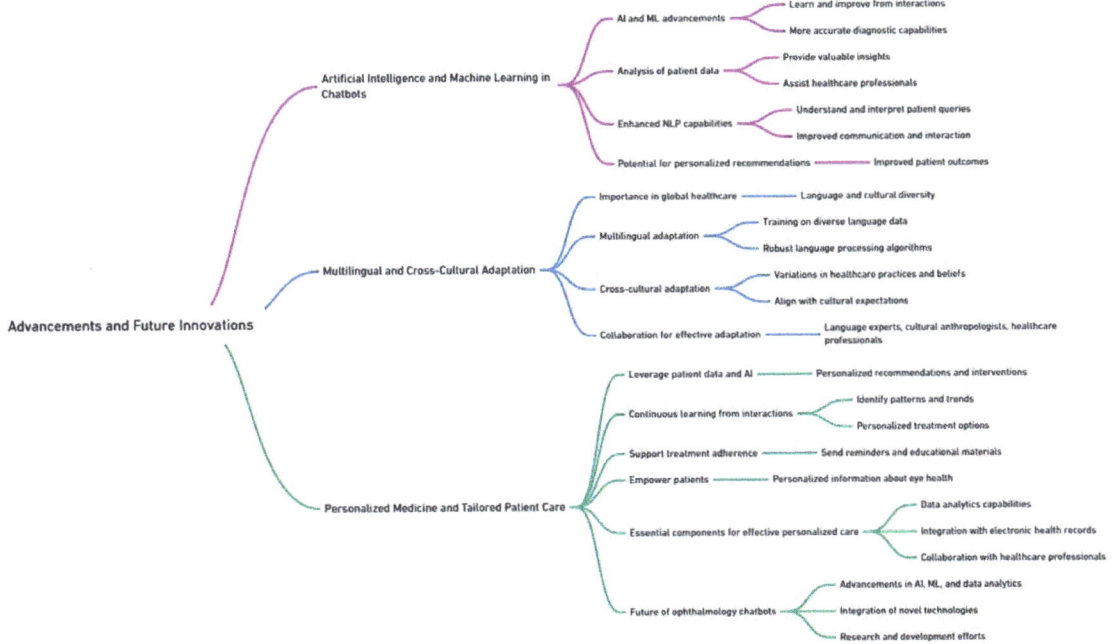

Figure 14. Future studies in the utilization of ophthalmology chatbots.

5.3.2. Multilingual and Cross-Cultural Adaptation

Multilingual and cross-cultural adaptation is a significant advancement in ophthalmology chatbots, particularly in the context of global healthcare, where language and cultural diversity are prevalent. Chatbots that can effectively communicate and interact with patients from different linguistic and cultural backgrounds improve access to care and enhance patient satisfaction (Table 5).

Table 5. Gaps and Research Opportunities in Ophthalmology Chatbots.

Area of Advancement	Current Gaps	Research Opportunities
AI and Machine Learning in Chatbots.	Limited accuracy in diagnosing eye diseases and conditions; challenges in interpreting ophthalmic data.	Developing advanced AI algorithms for precise diagnosis of eye conditions; enhancing ML capabilities for interpreting complex ophthalmic imaging and data.
Multilingual and Cross-Cultural Adaptation.	Difficulty in addressing language barriers and cultural differences in patient interactions, especially in diverse ophthalmology practices.	Creating chatbots capable of understanding and responding in multiple languages; incorporating cultural sensitivity in patient interactions for global ophthalmology care.
Personalized Medicine and Tailored Patient Care	Lack of personalized treatment recommendations based on individual eye health profiles; limited integration with ophthalmology-specific electronic health records.	Utilizing patient-specific data, to offer personalized eye care recommendations; improving chatbot integration with ophthalmology EHR systems for tailored patient management.

Abbreviations: AI—artificial intelligence; ML—machine learning; EHR—electronic health records.

Developing chatbots capable of multilingual adaptation involves training them on diverse language data and implementing robust language processing algorithms. This enables chatbots to understand and respond to patient inquiries in multiple languages, breaking down language barriers and enabling effective communication.

In addition to language diversity, cross-cultural adaptation is crucial to account for variations in healthcare practices, beliefs, and cultural norms. Chatbots can be programmed to adapt their responses and recommendations based on cultural considerations, ensuring they align with patients' cultural expectations and preferences. This promotes trust and engagement, ultimately leading to better patient experiences.

Successful multilingual and cross-cultural adaptation requires collaboration with language experts, cultural anthropologists, and healthcare professionals from diverse backgrounds. Such collaboration helps identify specific linguistic and cultural nuances that should be incorporated into chatbot design and development, ensuring cultural sensitivity and effectiveness in different contexts.

5.3.3. Personalized Medicine and Tailored Patient Care

Personalized medicine and tailored patient care hold great promise in the field of ophthalmology chatbots. By utilizing patient data and AI algorithms, chatbots can offer personalized recommendations and interventions tailored to individual patient characteristics, preferences, and medical history.

Through continuous learning from patient interactions, chatbots can gather and analyze data to identify patterns, trends, and personalized treatment options. Chatbots can also support treatment adherence by sending reminders and tailored educational materials, to meet the needs individual of patients. Moreover, chatbots empower patients by providing personalized information about eye health, treatment options, and lifestyle modifications, promoting active participation in their care.

To realize effective personalized medicine and tailored patient care, it is essential to possess robust data analytics capabilities, integrate with electronic health records, and collaborate with healthcare professionals. Developing advanced algorithms that can process and interpret large volumes of patient data, while simultaneously ensuring privacy and security, is of critical importance. Collaborative efforts between chatbot developers and ophthalmologists can refine algorithms and ensure that personalized recommendations align with clinical guidelines and best practices. Looking ahead, advancements in AI, ML, and data analytics will continue to shape the future of ophthalmology chatbots. Integration of novel technologies like computer vision and deep learning holds potential for more accurate and efficient diagnosis of eye conditions. Ongoing research and development efforts are focused on improving chatbots' ability to handle complex medical scenarios and provide comprehensive and personalized patient care.

In conclusion, advancements and future innovations in ophthalmology chatbots offer exciting opportunities for transforming eye care delivery. Integration of AI and ML can enhance diagnostic capabilities, while multilingual and cross-cultural adaptation can enable effective communication with diverse patient populations. Personalized medicine and tailored patient care promote improved patient outcomes. Continuous research, collaboration, and technological advancements will drive the evolution of ophthalmology chatbots, ultimately benefiting both patients and healthcare providers in the field of ophthalmology.

Author Contributions: Conceptualization, M.I., W.C. and S.C.; methodology, M.I.; software, M.I.; validation, M.I., W.C. and S.C.; formal analysis, S.C.; investigation, S.C.; resources, S.C.; data curation, S.C.; writing—original draft preparation, M.I.; writing—review and editing, S.C. and W.C.; visualization, S.C.; supervision, S.C.; project administration, S.C.; funding acquisition, S.C. All authors have read and agreed to the published version of the manuscript.

Funding: This research received no external funding.

Institutional Review Board Statement: Not applicable.

Informed Consent Statement: Not applicable.

Data Availability Statement: Data supporting this study are available in the original publication, reports, and preprints that are cited in the reference citation.

Acknowledgments: The responses, demonstrations, and figures presented in this manuscript were created using AI chatbots, including ChatGPT (GPT-3.5), an AI language model developed by OpenAI, Bing Chat (GPT-4.0) generated by Microsoft, and Bard AI built on PaLM operated by Google. The flow diagram and mind map showcased in this manuscript were designed using Whimsical.

Conflicts of Interest: The authors declare no conflict of interest.

References

1. Biswas, S.S. Role of Chat GPT in Public Health. *Ann. Biomed. Eng.* **2023**, *51*, 868–869. [CrossRef]
2. Miao, J.; Thongprayoon, C.; Cheungpasitporn, W. Assessing the Accuracy of ChatGPT on Core Questions in Glomerular Disease. *Kidney Int Rep* **2023**, *8*, 1657–1659. [CrossRef]
3. Panch, T.; Pearson-Stuttard, J.; Greaves, F.; Atun, R. Artificial intelligence: Opportunities and risks for public health. *Lancet Digit. Health* **2019**, *1*, e13–e14. [CrossRef]
4. Bressler, N.M. What Artificial Intelligence Chatbots Mean for Editors, Authors, and Readers of Peer-Reviewed Ophthalmic Literature. *JAMA Ophthalmol.* **2023**, *141*, 514–515. [CrossRef]
5. Suppadungsuk, S.; Thongprayoon, C.; Krisanapan, P.; Tangpanithandee, S.; Garcia Valencia, O.; Miao, J.; Mekraksakit, P.; Kashani, K.; Cheungpasitporn, W. Examining the Validity of ChatGPT in Identifying Relevant Nephrology Literature: Findings and Implications. *J. Clin. Med.* **2023**, *12*, 5550. [CrossRef]
6. Miao, J.; Thongprayoon, C.; Garcia Valencia, O.A.; Krisanapan, P.; Sheikh, M.S.; Davis, P.W.; Mekraksakit, P.; Suarez, M.G.; Craici, I.M.; Cheungpasitporn, W. Performance of ChatGPT on Nephrology Test Questions. *Clin. J. Am. Soc. Nephrol.* **2023**; *online ahead of print*. [CrossRef]
7. Potapenko, I.; Boberg-Ans, L.C.; Stormly Hansen, M.; Klefter, O.N.; van Dijk, E.H.C.; Subhi, Y. Artificial intelligence-based chatbot patient information on common retinal diseases using ChatGPT. *Acta Ophthalmol.* **2023**, *101*, 829–831. [CrossRef] [PubMed]
8. Ayers, J.W.; Poliak, A.; Dredze, M.; Leas, E.C.; Zhu, Z.; Kelley, J.B.; Faix, D.J.; Goodman, A.M.; Longhurst, C.A.; Hogarth, M.; et al. Comparing Physician and Artificial Intelligence Chatbot Responses to Patient Questions Posted to a Public Social Media Forum. *JAMA Intern. Med.* **2023**, *183*, 589–596. [CrossRef]
9. Tam, W.; Huynh, T.; Tang, A.; Luong, S.; Khatri, Y.; Zhou, W. Nursing education in the age of artificial intelligence powered Chatbots (AI-Chatbots): Are we ready yet? *Nurse Educ. Today* **2023**, *129*, 105917. [CrossRef] [PubMed]
10. Garcia Valencia, O.A.; Thongprayoon, C.; Jadlowiec, C.C.; Mao, S.A.; Miao, J.; Cheungpasitporn, W. Enhancing Kidney Transplant Care through the Integration of Chatbot. *Healthcare* **2023**, *11*, 2518. [CrossRef]
11. Fayed, A.M.; Mansur, N.S.B.; de Carvalho, K.A.; Behrens, A.; D'Hooghe, P.; de Cesar Netto, C. Artificial intelligence and ChatGPT in Orthopaedics and sports medicine. *J. Exp. Orthop.* **2023**, *10*, 74. [CrossRef] [PubMed]
12. Hua, H.U.; Kaakour, A.H.; Rachitskaya, A.; Srivastava, S.; Sharma, S.; Mammo, D.A. Evaluation and Comparison of Ophthalmic Scientific Abstracts and References by Current Artificial Intelligence Chatbots. *JAMA Ophthalmol.* **2023**, *141*, 819–824. [CrossRef] [PubMed]
13. Moshirfar, M.; Altaf, A.W.; Stoakes, I.M.; Tuttle, J.J.; Hoopes, P.C. Artificial Intelligence in Ophthalmology: A Comparative Analysis of GPT-3.5, GPT-4, and Human Expertise in Answering StatPearls Questions. *Cureus* **2023**, *15*, e40822. [CrossRef] [PubMed]
14. Mihalache, A.; Huang, R.S.; Popovic, M.M.; Muni, R.H. Performance of an Upgraded Artificial Intelligence Chatbot for Ophthalmic Knowledge Assessment. *JAMA Ophthalmol.* **2023**, *141*, 798–800. [CrossRef] [PubMed]
15. Aiumtrakul, N.; Thongprayoon, C.; Suppadungsuk, S.; Krisanapan, P.; Miao, J.; Qureshi, F.; Cheungpasitporn, W. Navigating the Landscape of Personalized Medicine: The Relevance of ChatGPT, BingChat, and Bard AI in Nephrology Literature Searches. *J. Pers. Med.* **2023**, *13*, 1457. [CrossRef] [PubMed]
16. Qarajeh, A.; Tangpanithandee, S.; Thongprayoon, C.; Suppadungsuk, S.; Krisanapan, P.; Aiumtrakul, N.; Garcia Valencia, O.A.; Miao, J.; Qureshi, F.; Cheungpasitporn, W. AI-Powered Renal Diet Support: Performance of ChatGPT, Bard AI, and Bing Chat. *Clin. Pract.* **2023**, *13*, 1160–1172. [CrossRef]
17. Trends in prevalence of blindness and distance and near vision impairment over 30 years: An analysis for the Global Burden of Disease Study. *Lancet Glob. Health* **2021**, *9*, e130–e143. [CrossRef]
18. Li, J.O.; Liu, H.; Ting, D.S.J.; Jeon, S.; Chan, R.V.P.; Kim, J.E.; Sim, D.A.; Thomas, P.B.M.; Lin, H.; Chen, Y.; et al. Digital technology, tele-medicine and artificial intelligence in ophthalmology: A global perspective. *Prog. Retin. Eye Res.* **2021**, *82*, 100900. [CrossRef]
19. Bhattacharyya, O.; Mossman, K.; Gustafsson, L.; Schneider, E.C. Using Human-Centered Design to Build a Digital Health Advisor for Patients With Complex Needs: Persona and Prototype Development. *J. Med. Internet Res.* **2019**, *21*, e10318. [CrossRef]

20. Ajibode, H.; Jagun, O.; Bodunde, O.; Fakolujo, V. Assessment of barriers to surgical ophthalmic care in South-Western Nigeria. *J. West. Afr. Coll. Surg.* **2012**, *2*, 38–50.
21. Parikh, D.; Armstrong, G.; Liou, V.; Husain, D. Advances in Telemedicine in Ophthalmology. *Semin. Ophthalmol.* **2020**, *35*, 210–215. [CrossRef]
22. Dorsey, E.R.; Topol, E.J. State of Telehealth. *N. Engl. J. Med.* **2016**, *375*, 154–161. [CrossRef] [PubMed]
23. Frank, T.; Rosenberg, S.; Talsania, S.; Yeager, L. Patient education in pediatric ophthalmology: A systematic review. *J. Am. Assoc. Pediatr. Ophthalmol. Strabismus* **2022**, *26*, 287–293. [CrossRef] [PubMed]
24. Wang, E.; Kalloniatis, M.; Ly, A. Assessment of patient education materials for age-related macular degeneration. *Ophthalmic Physiol. Opt.* **2022**, *42*, 839–848. [CrossRef] [PubMed]
25. McMonnies, C.W. Improving patient education and attitudes toward compliance with instructions for contact lens use. *Cont. Lens Anterior Eye* **2011**, *34*, 241–248. [CrossRef] [PubMed]
26. Ooms, A.; Shaikh, I.; Patel, N.; Kardashian-Sieger, T.; Srinivasan, N.; Zhou, B.; Wilson, L.; Szirth, B.; Khouri, A.S. Use of Telepresence Robots in Glaucoma Patient Education. *J. Glaucoma* **2021**, *30*, e40–e46. [CrossRef] [PubMed]
27. Xiong, Y.Z.; Lei, Q.; Calabrèse, A.; Legge, G.E. Simulating Visibility and Reading Performance in Low Vision. *Front. Neurosci.* **2021**, *15*, 671121. [CrossRef] [PubMed]
28. Chen, J.S.; Baxter, S.L. Applications of natural language processing in ophthalmology: Present and future. *Front. Med.* **2022**, *9*, 906554. [CrossRef]
29. Islam, A.; Chaudhry, B.M. Design Validation of a Relational Agent by COVID-19 Patients: Mixed Methods Study. *JMIR Hum. Factors* **2023**, *10*, e42740. [CrossRef]
30. Rasmussen, M.L.R.; Larsen, A.C.; Subhi, Y.; Potapenko, I. Artificial intelligence-based ChatGPT chatbot responses for patient and parent questions on vernal keratoconjunctivitis. *Graefes Arch. Clin. Exp. Ophthalmol.* **2023**, *261*, 3041–3043. [CrossRef]
31. Gordon, M.O.; Torri, V.; Miglior, S.; Beiser, J.A.; Floriani, I.; Miller, J.P.; Gao, F.; Adamsons, I.; Poli, D.; D'Agostino, R.B.; et al. Validated prediction model for the development of primary open-angle glaucoma in individuals with ocular hypertension. *Ophthalmology* **2007**, *114*, 10–19. [CrossRef]
32. Seddon, J.M.; Rosner, B. Validated Prediction Models for Macular Degeneration Progression and Predictors of Visual Acuity Loss Identify High-Risk Individuals. *Am. J. Ophthalmol.* **2019**, *198*, 223–261. [CrossRef]
33. Manoharan, M.K.; Thakur, S.; Dhakal, R.; Gupta, S.K.; Priscilla, J.J.; Bhandary, S.K.; Srivastava, A.; Marmamula, S.; Poigal, N.; Verkicharla, P.K. Myopia progression risk assessment score (MPRAS): A promising new tool for risk stratification. *Sci. Rep.* **2023**, *13*, 8858. [CrossRef] [PubMed]
34. Delcourt, C.; Souied, E.; Sanchez, A.; Bandello, F. Development and Validation of a Risk Score for Age-Related Macular Degeneration: The STARS Questionnaire. *Invest. Ophthalmol. Vis. Sci.* **2017**, *58*, 6399–6407. [CrossRef] [PubMed]
35. UMass Chan Medical School. AMD Risk Score Calculator. Available online: https://www.umassmed.edu/seddonlab/research-amd/our-work/amd-risk-calculator/ (accessed on 19 July 2023).
36. Craig, J.; Callen, J.; Marks, A.; Saddik, B.; Bramley, M. Electronic discharge summaries: The current state of play. *Health Inf. Manag.* **2007**, *36*, 30–36. [CrossRef] [PubMed]
37. Silver, A.M.; Goodman, L.A.; Chadha, R.; Higdon, J.; Burton, M.; Palabindala, V.; Jonnalagadda, N.; Thomas, A.; O'Donnell, C. Optimizing Discharge Summaries: A Multispecialty, Multicenter Survey of Primary Care Clinicians. *J. Patient Saf.* **2022**, *18*, 58–63. [CrossRef] [PubMed]
38. Tremoulet, P.D.; Shah, P.D.; Acosta, A.A.; Grant, C.W.; Kurtz, J.T.; Mounas, P.; Kirchhoff, M.; Wade, E. Usability of Electronic Health Record-Generated Discharge Summaries: Heuristic Evaluation. *J. Med. Internet Res.* **2021**, *23*, e25657. [CrossRef] [PubMed]
39. Singh, S.; Djalilian, A.; Ali, M.J. ChatGPT and Ophthalmology: Exploring Its Potential with Discharge Summaries and Operative Notes. *Semin. Ophthalmol.* **2023**, *38*, 503–507. [CrossRef]
40. Mokmin, N.A.M.; Ibrahim, N.A. The evaluation of chatbot as a tool for health literacy education among undergraduate students. *Educ. Inf. Technol.* **2021**, *26*, 6033–6049. [CrossRef]
41. Tsui, J.C.; Wong, M.B.; Kim, B.J.; Maguire, A.M.; Scoles, D.; VanderBeek, B.L.; Brucker, A.J. Appropriateness of ophthalmic symptoms triage by a popular online artificial intelligence chatbot. *Eye* **2023**, *37*, 3692–3693. [CrossRef]
42. Lyons, R.J.; Arepalli, S.R.; Fromal, O.; Choi, J.D.; Jain, N. Artificial Intelligence Chatbot Performance in Triage of Ophthalmic Conditions. *medRxiv* **2023**. [CrossRef]
43. Phasuk, S.; Tantibundhit, C.; Poopresert, P.; Yaemsuk, A.; Suvannachart, P.; Itthipanichpong, R.; Chansangpetch, S.; Manassakorn, A.; Tantisevi, V.; Rojanapongpun, P. Automated Glaucoma Screening from Retinal Fundus Image Using Deep Learning. *Annu. Int. Conf. IEEE Eng. Med. Biol. Soc.* **2019**, *2019*, 904–907. [CrossRef]
44. Gilson, A.; Safranek, C.W.; Huang, T.; Socrates, V.; Chi, L.; Taylor, R.A.; Chartash, D. How Does ChatGPT Perform on the United States Medical Licensing Examination? The Implications of Large Language Models for Medical Education and Knowledge Assessment. *JMIR Med. Educ.* **2023**, *9*, e45312. [CrossRef]
45. Mihalache, A.; Popovic, M.M.; Muni, R.H. Performance of an Artificial Intelligence Chatbot in Ophthalmic Knowledge Assessment. *JAMA Ophthalmol.* **2023**, *141*, 589–597. [CrossRef] [PubMed]

46. Raimondi, R.; Tzoumas, N.; Salisbury, T.; Di Simplicio, S.; Romano, M.R.; North East Trainee Research in Ophthalmology Network. Comparative analysis of large language models in the Royal College of Ophthalmologists fellowship exams. *Eye* **2023**, *37*, 3530–3533. [CrossRef] [PubMed]
47. Bernstein, I.A.; Zhang, Y.V.; Govil, D.; Majid, I.; Chang, R.T.; Sun, Y.; Shue, A.; Chou, J.C.; Schehlein, E.; Christopher, K.L.; et al. Comparison of Ophthalmologist and Large Language Model Chatbot Responses to Online Patient Eye Care Questions. *JAMA Netw. Open* **2023**, *6*, e2330320. [CrossRef] [PubMed]

Disclaimer/Publisher's Note: The statements, opinions and data contained in all publications are solely those of the individual author(s) and contributor(s) and not of MDPI and/or the editor(s). MDPI and/or the editor(s) disclaim responsibility for any injury to people or property resulting from any ideas, methods, instructions or products referred to in the content.

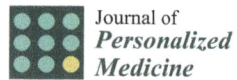

Article

Computed Tomography-Based Radiomics for Long-Term Prognostication of High-Risk Localized Prostate Cancer Patients Received Whole Pelvic Radiotherapy

Vincent W. S. Leung [1,*], Curtise K. C. Ng [2,3], Sai-Kit Lam [4], Po-Tsz Wong [1], Ka-Yan Ng [1], Cheuk-Hong Tam [1], Tsz-Ching Lee [1], Kin-Chun Chow [1], Yan-Kate Chow [1], Victor C. W. Tam [1], Shara W. Y. Lee [1], Fiona M. Y. Lim [5], Jackie Q. Wu [6] and Jing Cai [1]

[1] Department of Health Technology and Informatics, Faculty of Health and Social Sciences, The Hong Kong Polytechnic University, Hong Kong SAR, China; abi_potsz@yahoo.com.hk (P.-T.W.); victorcw.tam@connect.polyu.hk (V.C.W.T.); shara.lee@polyu.edu.hk (S.W.Y.L.); jing.cai@polyu.edu.hk (J.C.)

[2] Curtin Medical School, Curtin University, GPO Box U1987, Perth, WA 6845, Australia; curtise.ng@curtin.edu.au or curtise_ng@yahoo.com

[3] Curtin Health Innovation Research Institute (CHIRI), Faculty of Health Sciences, Curtin University, GPO Box U1987, Perth, WA 6845, Australia

[4] Department of Biomedical Engineering, Faculty of Engineering, The Hong Kong Polytechnic University, Hong Kong SAR, China; saikit.lam@polyu.edu.hk

[5] Department of Oncology, Princess Margaret Hospital, Hong Kong SAR, China; lmy084@ha.org.hk

[6] Department of Radiation Oncology, Duke University Medical Center, Durham, NC 27708, USA; jackie.wu@duke.edu

* Correspondence: wsv.leung@polyu.edu.hk; Tel.: +852-3400-8655

Abstract: Given the high death rate caused by high-risk prostate cancer (PCa) (>40%) and the reliability issues associated with traditional prognostic markers, the purpose of this study is to investigate planning computed tomography (pCT)-based radiomics for the long-term prognostication of high-risk localized PCa patients who received whole pelvic radiotherapy (WPRT). This is a retrospective study with methods based on best practice procedures for radiomics research. Sixty-four patients were selected and randomly assigned to training ($n = 45$) and testing ($n = 19$) cohorts for radiomics model development with five major steps: pCT image acquisition using a Philips Big Bore CT simulator; multiple manual segmentations of clinical target volume for the prostate ($CTV_{prostate}$) on the pCT images; feature extraction from the $CTV_{prostate}$ using PyRadiomics; feature selection for overfitting avoidance; and model development with three-fold cross-validation. The radiomics model and signature performances were evaluated based on the area under the receiver operating characteristic curve (AUC) as well as accuracy, sensitivity and specificity. This study's results show that our pCT-based radiomics model was able to predict the six-year progression-free survival of the high-risk localized PCa patients who received the WPRT with highly consistent performances (mean AUC: 0.76 (training) and 0.71 (testing)). These are comparable to findings of other similar studies including those using magnetic resonance imaging (MRI)-based radiomics. The accuracy, sensitivity and specificity of our radiomics signature that consisted of two texture features were 0.778, 0.833 and 0.556 (training) and 0.842, 0.867 and 0.750 (testing), respectively. Since CT is more readily available than MRI and is the standard-of-care modality for PCa WPRT planning, pCT-based radiomics could be used as a routine non-invasive approach to the prognostic prediction of WPRT treatment outcomes in high-risk localized PCa.

Keywords: artificial intelligence; biomarker; machine learning; malignancy; medical imaging; prognosis; progression-free survival; radiation therapy; recurrence; tumor

Citation: Leung, V.W.S.; Ng, C.K.C.; Lam, S.-K.; Wong, P.-T.; Ng, K.-Y.; Tam, C.-H.; Lee, T.-C.; Chow, K.-C.; Chow, Y.-K.; Tam, V.C.W.; et al. Computed Tomography-Based Radiomics for Long-Term Prognostication of High-Risk Localized Prostate Cancer Patients Received Whole Pelvic Radiotherapy. *J. Pers. Med.* **2023**, *13*, 1643. https://doi.org/10.3390/jpm13121643

Academic Editor: Daniele Giansanti

Received: 3 November 2023
Revised: 21 November 2023
Accepted: 23 November 2023
Published: 24 November 2023

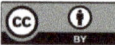

Copyright: © 2023 by the authors. Licensee MDPI, Basel, Switzerland. This article is an open access article distributed under the terms and conditions of the Creative Commons Attribution (CC BY) license (https://creativecommons.org/licenses/by/4.0/).

1. Introduction

According to Global Cancer Statistics, prostate cancer (PCa) was the third most common cancer accounting for 7.3% of all cancer deaths in 2020 [1]. In 2023, the most common male cancer in USA was PCa causing an estimated 34,700 deaths, which is the second highest cancer death rate of 11% [2]. As per the European Society for Medical Oncology (ESMO) [3] and American Cancer Society (ACS) [4] guidelines, patients with localized prostate cancer can be classified into three main risk groups based on T category, Gleason score (GS) and prostate-specific antigen (PSA) representing low, intermediate and high risks, respectively: T1-T2a and GS $\leq$ 6 and PSA $\leq$ 10; T2b and/or GS 7 and/or PSA 10–20; and T3a or GS 8–10 or PSA > 20. More than one third of PCa patients belong to the high-risk group [5].

Low- and intermediate-risk patients may only need active surveillance. However, either long-term androgen deprivation therapy (ADT) plus radical radiotherapy (RT) or radical prostatectomy (RP) and pelvic lymphadenectomy are required for treating high-risk patients [3]. Whole pelvic RT (WPRT) and prostate-only RT (PORT) are the two typical radical RT options used for treating high-risk prostate cancer patients [6–8]. Usually, the Roach formula is used to estimate involvement of pelvic nodes based on GS and PSA, with 15% or greater nodal risk as an indicator for adopting WPRT despite its increased acute and late gastrointestinal toxicity compared to PORT [6,7,9]. Nonetheless, a recent literature review on the identification and prediction of prostate cancer indicated that PSA and GS may not be reliable prognostic markers. This is because PSA can increase without PCa, and intermediate- and high-risk patients may have low PSA levels. Also, the variation of GS determined from pre- and post-RP specimens is common [10]. It is noted that more than 40% of high-risk patients die from PCa, which is 10 times greater than for low-risk patients [5]. Hence, better approaches to PCa risk stratification, treatment selection and outcome assessment have been explored over the years, and radiomics is considered one of the potential candidates [10,11].

Radiomics refers to quantitative feature extraction from medical images as imaging biomarkers for clinical decision support with the aim of improving the accuracy of diagnosis, prognosis and outcome prediction, which are essential in personalized medicine (also known as precision medicine) and include diagnosis and treatment [10,12]. Although the concept of radiomics has only emerged over the last decade, numerous studies have explored its potential in precision medicine including for the prognostication of prostate cancer [10–38]. So far, the benefits of radiomics have not been translated into clinical practice because of its limited reproducibility as a result of a lack of process standardization [10,12]. Typically, five major steps are involved in the radiomics workflow including medical image acquisition and segmentation, feature extraction and selection, and model development [10–14]. However, the approaches involved in each step varied across studies in terms of different scanning protocols for image acquisition and the use of manual, semi-automatic or fully automatic segmentation. These have subsequent impacts on the reproducibility of results because features determined as clinically relevant to one setting become irrelevant to another setting when images are acquired and segmentation is performed in varying ways [10–12,17–38]. Commonly, magnetic resonance imaging (MRI) [17–22], positron emission tomography (PET) [23–35] and computed tomography (CT) [36–38] are used for PCa diagnosis and management [10]. However, CT is the standard-of-care modality for PCa RT planning, while the other modalities may not be available in some clinical settings [39]. Also, the use of MRI for radiomics appears problematic due to its non-standardized voxel intensity values, which are greatly influenced by the variation in scanning protocols [10,17–22]. Although planning CT (pCT)-based radiomics allows seamless integration into existing RT workflow, there is a paucity of studies on this for high-risk PCa. These include that published in 2019 on PCa risk stratification and our latest study published in 2023 on pCT-based radiomics for the long-term prognostication of high-risk localized PCa patients who received PORT [10–13,39]. To the best of our knowledge, no study has explored the potential of pCT-based radiomics with its counterpart, WPRT. Given the high death rate of high-risk PCa (>40%) and the reliability issues associated with traditional prognostic markers [5,10], the purpose of this study is to investigate pCT-based radiomics for the long-term prognostication of high-risk localized PCa patients who received WPRT. We hypothesized that pCT-based radiomics could be used as a routine non-invasive approach for the prognostic prediction of WPRT treatment outcomes in high-risk localized PCa.

2. Materials and Methods

This is a retrospective study with methods based on Lambin et al.'s [12] best practice procedures for radiomics research derived from their radiomics quality score instrument. The best practice procedures employed in our radiomics workflow included multiple segmentations, feature reduction to avoid overfitting, cutoff analyses, use of discrimination statistics such as receiver operating characteristic curve (ROC) and area under the ROC curve (AUC), and a three-fold cross-validation resampling method [12,13]. This study was conducted in accordance with the Declaration of Helsinki, and approved by the Institutional Review Board of The Hong Kong Polytechnic University (approval number: HSEARS20200902001 and date of approval: 20 September 2020), and Clinical & Research Ethics Committee of New Territories East Cluster of Hospital Authority of Government of Hong Kong Special Administrative Region (approval number: NTEC-2020-0633 and date of approval: 9 December 2020).

2.1. Patient Selection

Eighty-four high-risk localized PCa patients, who received treatments between May 2009 and October 2014, and met the following inclusion criteria were identified through the electronic health record system of Princess Margaret Hospital, Hong Kong Special Administrative Region. The inclusion criteria were as follows: those with risk of pelvic lymph node involvement estimated by the Roach formula $\geq 15\%$; and whose WPRT were received [7,9]. The identified patients were excluded for the following reasons: second malignancies other than PCa; previous PCa treatment; unavailability of pre-treatment biopsy results; or death unrelated to PCa. Eventually, sixty-four patients were selected and randomly assigned to training (n = 45) and testing (n = 19) cohorts for the radiomics model development. Their clinical and WPRT treatment data such as age, pre-treatment TNM stage, GS, PSA, WPRT technique, dose fractionation, ADT drug regimen, follow-up duration and clinical outcome and Digital Imaging and Communications in Medicine (DICOM) datasets (pCT images and structure sets) were collected accordingly [36–38]. Figure 1 summarizes the patient selection procedures.

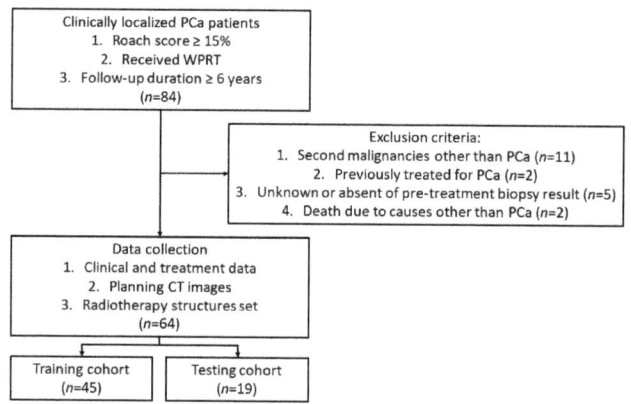

Figure 1. Patient selection procedures for radiomics model development. CT, computed tomography; PCa, prostate cancer; WPRT, whole pelvic radiotherapy.

2.2. ADT and WPRT Treatment

All selected patients were given neoadjuvant ADT (2 weeks of flutamide and 2 injections of 3-month luteinising hormone-releasing hormone agonist (LHRHa)) prior to WPRT. The WPRT's clinical target volume (CTV) for the prostate ($CTV_{prostate}$) was given 70–76 Gy in 2 Gy per fraction over 7–8 weeks with static field intensity-modulated radiotherapy or volumetric modulated arc therapy (VMAT). CTV for whole pelvic lymph nodes (CTV_{LN}) was given 44 or 50 Gy with three-dimensional (3D) conformal radiotherapy or VMAT. All treatment plans were computed to meet acceptance criteria and organs at risk (OARs) constraints. Details on CTV, planning target volume (PTV), acceptance criteria and OARs constraints are given in Tables S1 and S2. After completion of WPRT, patients were prescribed adjuvant LHRHa for up to 3 years, and there were follow-ups at intervals of 3–6 months for disease monitoring. The PSA levels were determined and evaluated at each visit. Imaging tests were performed when an increase of PSA was found [6,7,9,40].

2.3. Clinical Endpoint

This study's clinical endpoint was the six-year progression-free survival (PFS) of patients after WPRT. This referred to patients not having any distant metastasis, local recurrence, regional recurrence and/or chemical recurrence for six years after completing the WPRT course. Patient deaths unrelated to PCa were censored [9].

2.4. Radiomics Workflow

2.4.1. Medical Image Acquisition

Non-contrast pCT scans were performed on all selected patients using the Koninklijke Philips N.V. Brilliance Big Bore CT simulator (Amsterdam, The Netherlands) as per in-house protocol. Patients were required to empty their bladders and then drink 400 cc of water an hour before the scans to achieve comparable bladder status. The images were taken with the patients in the treatment position (both hands on the chest in the supine position and the use of customized foam for immobilization) and the following scan parameters—tube voltage: 120 kV; tube current: 350–450 mAs; slice thickness: 1.5 or 3 mm; field of view: 60 cm; matrix size: 512 × 512; pixel spacing: 1.18; and a standard convolution kernel for image reconstruction [41].

2.4.2. Medical Image Segmentation

All the collected DICOM structure sets including OARs (bladder, bowel, femoral head, penile bulb and rectum), CTV and PTV (prostate and lymph nodes) were manually contoured by a radiation oncologist experienced in prostate cancer radiotherapy using the 'Draw Planar Contour' function of the 'Contouring' interface on the Eclipse version 13 treatment planning system (Varian Medical Systems, Palo Alto, CA, USA). These were subsequently reviewed and approved by another radiation oncologist with associate consultant grade or above on the same system for original clinical use. To adhere to Lambin et al.'s [12] best practice procedure for segmentation, an additional consultant radiation oncologist was involved in reviewing and approving these DICOM structure sets, including the $CTV_{prostate}$ as volume of interest (VOI), on the Eclipse version 13 treatment planning system based on the European Society for Therapeutic Radiology and Oncology (ESTRO) consensus guideline for this study [39,42]. The definitions of level of apex, lateral, anterior and posterior borders and the base of the prostate as well as seminal vesicles stated in the ESTRO consensus guideline were used to check the accuracy and consistency of the $CTV_{prostate}$ manual segmentation to minimize intra- and inter-observer variabilities. For example, the level of prostate apex was defined as about 1 cm above the upper border of the penile bulb. Complete details on these definitions are available in the ESTRO consensus guideline [42]. The average number of consecutive pCT slices segmented for the $CTV_{prostate}$ was 21 (standard deviation [SD]: 3 and range: 15–28). Figure 2 shows pCT image examples with the manually delineated $CTV_{prostate}$ contours included in the study.

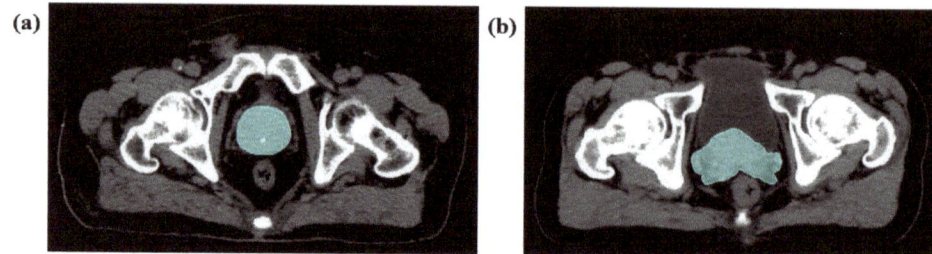

Figure 2. Axial planning computed tomography images with manually delineated CTV$_{prostate}$ contours (green overlay). (**a**) CTV$_{prostate}$ covering the entire prostate gland. (**b**) CTV$_{prostate}$ including the entire prostate gland with a proximal two-thirds of the seminal vesicles.

2.4.3. Feature Extraction

The pCT image pre-processing and feature extraction procedures used in this study were based on those of the Image Biomarker Standardization Initiative (IBSI) [43], and were performed using the open-source Python-based radiomics feature extraction package, PyRadiomics version 2.2.0 [10,44]. Uniform volumetric spacing was achieved through isotropic resampling by resizing the images to $1 \times 1 \times 1$ mm^3 based on linear interpolation. Subsequently, a constant intensity resolution was attained by discretizing the images to a fixed bin width of 10 Hounsfield units (HU) to extract texture features. Also, the Laplacian of Gaussian (LoG) filter with 0.5, 2, 3, 4, 4.5 and 5 mm sigma values was used to reconstruct the images for feature extraction from various scales of edge detection and image smoothing. Shape features ($n = 14$), first-order features ($n = 126$) and texture features ($n = 511$) of the CTV$_{prostate}$ were extracted after the pre-processing of images as per Figure S1 and Table S3. The shape, first-order and texture features described the 3D size and shape and voxel intensity distribution of the CTV$_{prostate}$ and voxel intensity relationship within the CTV$_{prostate}$ sub-regions, respectively. For every pCT dataset, 651 radiomic features were extracted in total [43].

2.4.4. Feature Selection

Statistical approaches were used to consecutively select a smaller set of features for our model from the training data. The training cohort features were scaled and centered to avoid under- or over-presentation of individual ones. Additionally, the mean and SD of the scaled and centered training data were used to normalize the testing cohort features. A Mann–Whitney U test was conducted to determine the clinical association of every radiomic feature for its selection. Features having no statistically significant differences across the outcome groups ($p > 0.05$) were removed. Also, redundant features were identified based on the pair-wise correlation of the features using Spearman's rank correlation coefficient. When the absolute correlation coefficient of two features was greater than or equal to 0.4, the feature with the greater mean absolute correlation was removed. The model was then developed based on all remaining features [12,39,45–48]. A correlation coefficient of 0.4 was selected as the threshold because previous radiomics studies used it to indicate moderate correlation with promising outcomes for feature reduction [49,50].

2.4.5. Model Development

The model development was based on logistic regression with a least absolute shrinkage and selection operator (LASSO) penalty as well as three-fold cross-validation. The LASSO penalty was used for prediction error reduction and model simplification. It enabled the most predictive feature selection through the penalization of the sum of feature coefficient absolute values. Features that had minor contributions to the model were forced to undergo coefficient reduction to become zero and subsequently being removed. The three-fold cross-validation involved randomly dividing the training data into three groups. Two out of three groups were employed to train with the other reserved for validation.

This process was repeated three times to involve each group once in the validation. In addition to the model testing and bias minimization, the three-fold cross-validation was also responsible for identifying the optimal regularization parameter for LASSO (lambda). Finally, 1000 models were developed as a result of repeating the process of model training a 1000 times [12,39,45–48].

2.4.6. Statistical Analysis

The statistical analysis was performed using R version 3.6.3 (The R Foundation, Indianapolis, IN, USA). The R packages used include the following: base package for randomization and normalization; stats package for chi-squared test, Fisher's exact test, Mann–Whitney U test and Spearman's rank correlation coefficients; caret package for pair-wise correlations; glmnet package for logistic regression with the three-fold cross-validation and LASSO penalty; and ROCR and cvAUC packages for ROC analysis and AUC calculation. A p-value of less than 0.05 represented statistical significance [12,39,45–48].

Models with the lowest number of selected features were used for radiomics signature development. Every feature coefficient (β) and intercept within the radiomics signature was determined by taking the average of those values of the included models. Equation (1) illustrates the radiomics signature and was used to calculate the radiomics score (Rad-score) for every patient [51,52].

$$Rad - score = \sum_{i=1}^{n} \beta_i \times feature_i + intercept \tag{1}$$

The cutoff of the Rad-score was determined based on the evaluation of model accuracy, sensitivity and specificity. The cutoff was used to classify whether a patient was more likely to have six-year PFS based on their Rad-score. The performance of the derived radiomics signature was evaluated in terms of accuracy, sensitivity and specificity. Additionally, the average AUC values of the training and testing cohorts were calculated [12,39,45–48]. Figure 3 summarizes the feature selection, model development and statistical analysis processes.

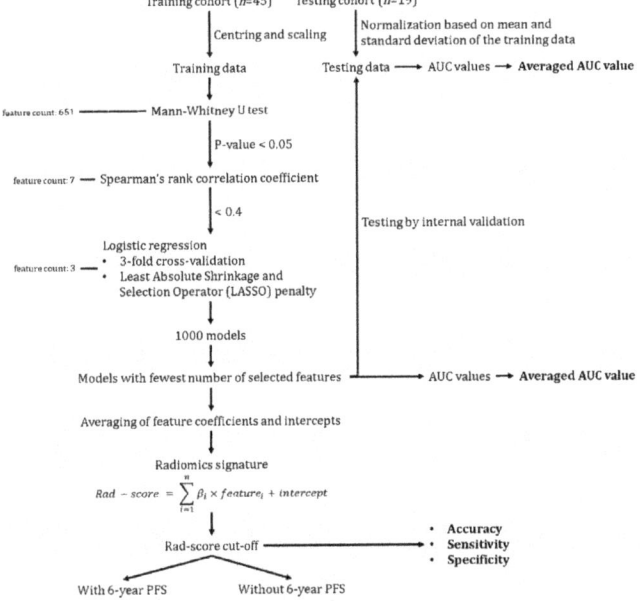

Figure 3. Feature selection, model development and statistical analysis workflow. AUC, area under receiver operating characteristic curve; PFS, progression-free survival.

3. Results

Table 1 shows the clinicopathological characteristics of the included patients. There was no statistically significant difference found between the characteristics of the training and testing cohorts. Regarding the clinical endpoint, 81.5 months was the median PFS of all patients, and 80.0% and 78.9% of patients in the training and testing cohorts had six-year PFS, respectively. There were 13 included patients (20.3%) with metastasis and/or recurrence in six years after completing the WPRT course, constituting 20.0% of the training and 21.1% of the testing cohorts.

Table 1. Patients' clinicopathological characteristics.

Characteristic	All Included Patients ($n = 64$)	Training Cohort ($n = 45$)	Testing Cohort ($n = 19$)	p-Value
Median age at start of radiotherapy (years)	70	71	70	0.691 [1]
Histology				
Adenocarcinoma	49 (76.6%)	31 (68.9%)	17 (89.5%)	
Acinar adenocarcinoma	14 (21.9%)	13 (28.9%)	2 (10.5%)	0.160 [2]
Unknown	1 (1.6%)	1 (2.2%)	0 (0%)	
Stage				
T1	8 (12.5%)	6 (13.3%)	2 (10.5%)	
T2	20 (31.3%)	11 (24.4%)	9 (47.4%)	
T3	33 (51.6%)	25 (55.6%)	8 (42.1%)	0.189 [2]
Unknown	3 (4.7%)	3 (6.7%)	0 (0%)	
Pre-treatment PSA level (ng/mL)				
<10	5 (7.8%)	2 (4.4%)	3 (15.8%)	
10–20	18 (28.1%)	16 (35.6%)	2 (10.5%)	0.052 [2]
>20	41 (64.1%)	27 (60.0%)	14 (73.7%)	
Pre-treatment GS				
≤6	16 (25.0%)	10 (22.2%)	6 (31.6%)	
7	17 (26.6%)	11 (24.4%)	6 (31.6%)	0.476 [2]
≥8	31 (48.4%)	24 (53.3%)	7 (36.8%)	
Median pre-treatment Roach score	32.8	33.6	27.9	0.130 [1]
Median $CTV_{prostate}$ volume (mm^3)	39951.5	41695.0	38943.0	0.797 [1]
CTV_{LN} dose (Gy)				
44	11 (17.2%)	7 (15.6%)	4 (21.1%)	0.719 [3]
50	53 (82.8%)	38 (84.4%)	15 (78.9%)	
$CTV_{prostate}$ dose (Gy)				
<76	12 (18.8%)	8 (17.8%)	4 (21.1%)	0.739 [3]
≥76	52 (81.3%)	37 (82.2%)	15 (78.9%)	
Treatment modality for PTV_{LN}				
3DCRT	10 (15.6%)	6 (13.3%)	4 (21.1%)	0.466 [3]
VMAT	54 (84.4%)	39 (86.7%)	15 (78.9%)	
Treatment modality for $PTV_{prostate}$				
IMRT	9 (14.1%)	5 (11.1%)	4 (21.1%)	0.432 [3]
VMAT	55 (85.9%)	40 (88.9%)	15 (78.9%)	
Patients received neoadjuvant ADT	62 (96.9%)	44 (97.8%)	18 (94.7%)	0.509 [3]
Patients received adjuvant ADT	52 (81.3%)	36 (80.0%)	16 (84.2%)	1.000 [3]
Median follow-up time (months)	88.0	91.0	88.0	0.872 [1]
Median progression-free survival (months)	81.5	81.0	85.0	0.659 [1]
Patients with six-year disease progression	13 (20.3%)	9 (20.0%)	4 (21.1%)	1.000 [3]
Events				
Biochemical recurrence	12	10	2	
Local failure	3	2	1	-
Regional failure	1	0	1	
Distant failure	5	5	0	

[1] Mann–Whitney U test; [2] Chi-squared test; [3] Fisher's exact test. 3DCRT, three-dimensional conformal radiotherapy; ADT, androgen deprivation therapy; CTV_{LN}, clinical target volume for whole pelvic lymph nodes; $CTV_{prostate}$, clinical target volume for prostate; GS, Gleason score; IMRT, intensity-modulated radiotherapy; PSA, prostate-specific antigen; PTV_{LN}, planning target volume for whole pelvic lymph nodes; $PTV_{prostate}$, planning target volume for prostate; VMAT, volumetric modulated arc therapy.

Among the 1000 developed models, 799 models with the fewest (two) selected features were used for radiomics signature development. Both selected features were textural:

run entropy of grey level run length matrix after LoG filtering with a sigma value of 2 mm (RE-GLRLM$_{\sigma 2mm}$); and small area emphasis of grey level size zone matrix after LoG filtering with a sigma value of 4.5 mm (SAE-GLSZM$_{\sigma 4.5mm}$). Both RE-GLRLM$_{\sigma 2mm}$ and SAE-GLSZM$_{\sigma 4.5mm}$ had statistically significant differences in the feature values between patients with and without six-year PFS (p-values: 0.0208 and 0.0191), respectively. The developed radiomics signature is illustrated in Equation (2).

$$\text{Rad-score} = 0.291 \, (\text{RE-GLRLM}_{\sigma 2mm}) + 0.358 \, (\text{SAE-GLSZM}_{\sigma 4.5mm}) - 1.47 \quad (2)$$

The average AUC values of the developed model for the training and testing cohorts were 0.756 (95% confidence interval (CI): 0.756–0.757) and 0.707 (95% CI: 0.706–0.707), respectively (Figure 4). With the cutoff determined as a third-quartile value (i.e., −1.11), patients were stratified into high- (Rad-score ≥ −1.11) and low- (Rad-score < −1.11) risk groups, which refer to unlikely and more likely to have six-year PFS, respectively (Figure 5). The respective accuracy, sensitivity and specificity of the radiomics signature were 0.778, 0.833 and 0.556 in the training cohort and 0.842, 0.867 and 0.750 in the testing cohort.

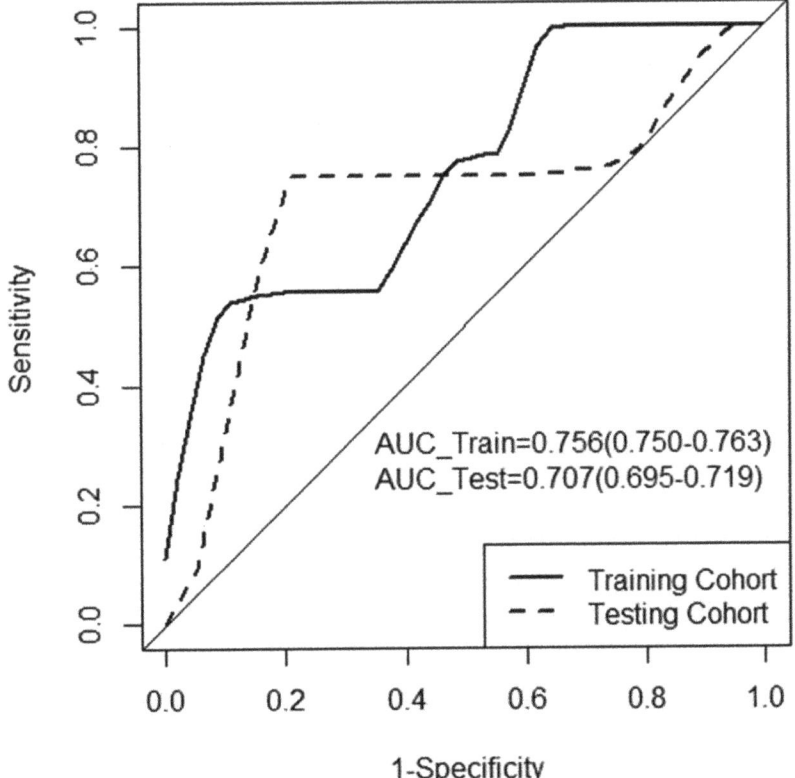

Figure 4. Receiver operating characteristic (ROC) curves of the developed model for training and testing cohorts. Figures in parentheses are 95% confidence intervals. AUC_Train, area under ROC curve (AUC) of training cohort; AUC_Test, AUC of testing cohort.

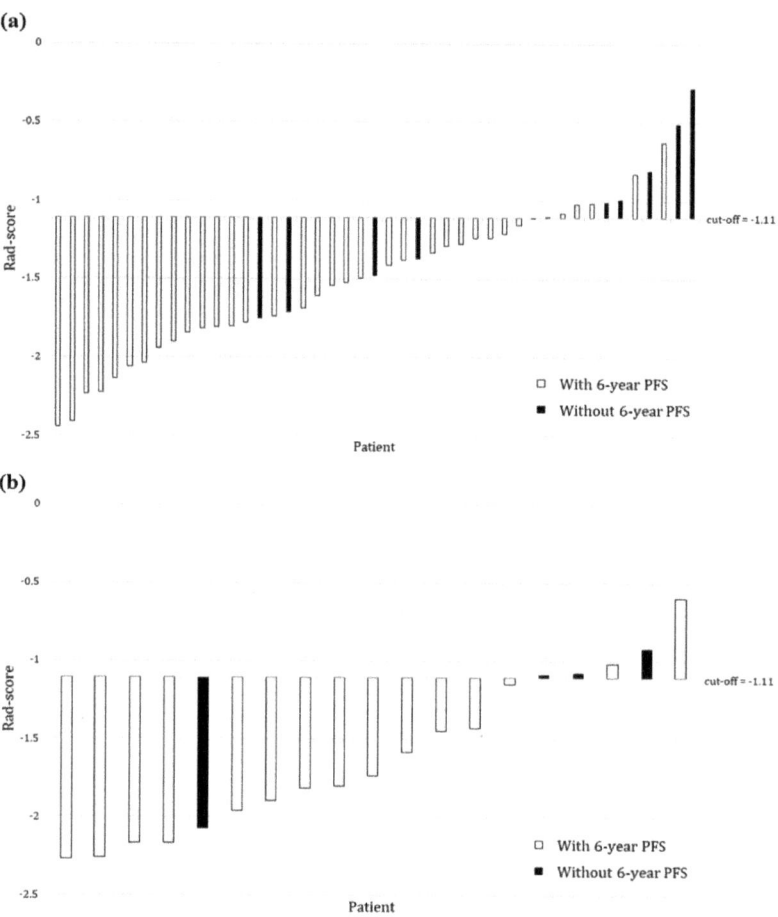

Figure 5. Rad-score charts for (**a**) training and (**b**) testing cohorts. PFS, progression-free survival.

4. Discussion

In our study, the key radiomic features among the large arrays of data extracted from the $CTV_{prostate}$ of the pre-treatment pCT images were selected to develop a two-feature radiomics signature to predict the six-year PFS in high-risk localized PCa patients with WPRT as the primary treatment. Highly consistent predictive performances were achieved by our model with average AUC values of 0.76 and 0.71 in the training and testing cohorts, respectively. The consistent performances could be attributed to the fact that the pCT for the external beam RT is highly standardized and calibrated for dose calculation, hence improving results reproducibility [10–12,17–38]. This potentially addresses one of the major issues associated with radiomics, which is the inability to translate benefits into clinical practice [10,12].

According to the review on the radiomics used for the identification and prediction of PCa published in 2021, most studies have focused on PET radiomics because PET is a functional imaging modality that provides detailed information on cell metabolism and proliferation, morphology, perfusion, receptor density and tumor viability, which are important for this identification and prediction task [10,23–35]. Although MRI might not be available in some settings, it is suggested that MRI should be a standard-of-care modality for PCa diagnosis [53,54]. Hence, there are more studies on MRI radiomics than CT for PCa identification and prediction [10,17–22,36–38]. However, a review on MRI radiomics for PCa risk stratification published in 2023 showed that only three studies used MRI to predict biochemical failure after receiving RT, with two reporting the AUC values of their models [55–58]. In Dinis Fernandes et al.'s study, their model achieved an AUC value of 0.63 [57]. Although Zhong et al.'s model was able to attain a mean AUC value of 0.99 during training, it reduced to 0.73 in testing [58]. This highlights one main limitation of the use of MRI in radiomics: its non-standardized voxel intensity values are greatly affected by scanning protocol variations, resulting in less reproducible results [10,17–22]. In contrast, our study's model attained average training and testing AUC values of 0.76 and 0.71, demonstrating higher reproducibility despite the training AUC value of 0.71 being a little lower than that of Zhong et al.'s model at 0.73 [58]. Similarly reproducible model performance results were also shown in our previous study on CT radiomics for long-term prognostication of high-risk localized PCa patients who received PORT (mean training and testing AUC: 0.798 and 0.795, respectively) [39]. Additionally, CT is more readily available than MRI and PET and the standard-of-care modality for PCa RT planning, which allows for seamless integration into the existing RT workflow. These could be considered as other merits of CT radiomics for long-term prognostication of high-risk localized PCa patients who received RT [11,39,53].

Our developed radiomics signature with the determined cutoff of −1.11 again achieved consistent accuracy, sensitivity and specificity between training (0.778, 0.833 and 0.556) and testing (0.842, 0.867 and 0.750) cohorts to stratify patients into high- (Rad-score $\geq$ −1.11) and low- (Rad-score < −1.11) risk groups. Our radiomics signature consists of two texture features: GLRLM Run Entropy (RE-GLRLM$_{\sigma 2mm}$) and SAE-GLSZM Small Area Emphasis (GLSZM$_{\sigma 4.5mm}$). RE-GLRLM$_{\sigma 2mm}$ quantifies the heterogeneous texture pattern within the CTV$_{prostate}$ by representing the variations in the allocations of run lengths and grey levels. SAE-GLSZM$_{\sigma 4.5mm}$ measures the quantities of smaller-sized zones and fine textures within the CTV$_{prostate}$ by representing the distribution of consecutive voxels that share identical intensity values. As these two features have positive weightings in our radiomic signature with higher values of RE-GLRLM$_{\sigma 2mm}$ and SAE-GLSZM$_{\sigma 4.5mm}$, the Rad-score becomes greater and indicates the CTV$_{prostate}$ of patients showing more heterogeneous 3D patterns. Also, a higher Rad-score represents a higher possibility of disease progression within six years after completing WPRT, which is in line with a previous study's findings that a more heterogenous PCa tumor has greater resistance to therapies [59]. Similar investigations have been conducted on other malignancies showing a variety of texture features correlating with angiogenesis and hypoxia, which could be used to indicate the aggressiveness of breast cancer [60,61] and distant metastasis for nasopharyngeal carcinomas [62]. Hence, these show that radiomics is a viable approach to extract the distinctive characteristics of a malignant mass and quantify the respective heterogeneity to determine the prognosis and therapeutic response to oncological diseases [63].

Clinical failure or biochemical failure after primary RT is common in PCa patients. About 30–50% of patients are affected by biochemical failure within 10 years after RT [64]. Clinical failure occurs in approximately 25% of patients with biochemical failure within eight years with symptoms because of disease recurrency [65–67]. Palliative approaches, such as observation and ADT, are eventually employed to manage many of these patients [68–70]. However, curative intent salvage treatments—e.g., salvage prostatectomy, brachytherapy, stereotactic body radiotherapy, etc.—can be applied to selected patients with biochemical failure or isolated local recurrences without coexisting metastatic lesions [71–73]. Our radiomics model would be useful for the pretreatment identification of patients with a higher likelihood of disease progression after treatment, resulting in better clinical decision making and patient management, e.g., the use of state-of-the-art imaging examination to follow-up with these patients, increasing opportunities to offer salvage treatments to them when still applicable. In this way, personalized or precision medicine could be realized [10,12,74].

Our study has several limitations. It is a retrospective study with a relatively small sample size of 64 patients from one single center. According to Lambin et al.'s [12] radiomics quality score instrument, a prospective study with data collected from multiple sites would be a better design as this allows for model external validation [12,75,76]. However, our arrangement should be considered acceptable because some recent CT radiomics studies on identification and prediction of PCa also retrospectively collected patient datasets from one single site with comparable sample sizes of 69–80 patients [36–38]. Despite multiple manual segmentations of the $CTV_{prostate}$ as per the ESTRO consensus guideline to address the potential intra- and inter-observer variability issues and the selection of ≥ 0.4 Spearman's rank correlation coefficient for feature reduction based on previous radiomics studies, our model's generalizability needs to be confirmed by assessing the intra- and inter-observer variability and the effect of other correlation coefficient threshold settings in future studies [12,42,49,50]. Nonetheless, this is the first study on pCT radiomics for the long-term prognostication of high-risk localized PCa patients who received WPRT, which could further justify our study design. Given the promising results of this study, future studies with a larger number of datasets collected prospectively from multiple centers with assessments on the intra- and inter-observer variability and the effect of various correlation coefficient settings is warranted for our model's external validation and to confirm its generalizability. It is noted that deep learning (DL) has become popular in medical imaging [75–80]. Hence, another direction for further study is to develop a DL-based radiomics model for the long-term prognostication of high-risk localized PCa patients after WPRT [10].

5. Conclusions

This study's results show that our pCT-based radiomics model was able to predict six-year PFS in high-risk localized PCa patients who received WPRT as the primary treatment with highly consistent performances (mean AUC: 0.76 (training) and 0.71 (testing)) and was comparable to other similar studies including those on MRI-based radiomics. The accuracy, sensitivity and specificity of our radiomics signature that consists of two texture features, namely GLRLM Run Entropy ($RE-GLRLM_{\sigma 2mm}$) and SAE-GLSZM Small Area Emphasis ($GLSZM_{\sigma 4.5mm}$), were 0.778, 0.833 and 0.556 (training) and 0.842, 0.867 and 0.750 (testing), respectively. Since CT is more readily available than MRI and PET and is the standard-of-care modality for PCa RT planning, pCT-based radiomics can be used as a routine non-invasive approach to the prognostic prediction of WPRT treatment outcomes in high-risk localized PCa. Nonetheless, further study on the external validation of our model is warranted to ensure that its benefits can be realized in clinical settings to achieve personalized or precision medicine.

Supplementary Materials: The following supporting information can be downloaded at: https://www.mdpi.com/article/10.3390/jpm13121643/s1. Table S1: Definitions of clinical target volumes (CTVs) and planning target volumes (PTVs); Table S2: Acceptance criteria and organs at risk constraints; Table S3. Number of extracted radiomic features. Figure S1. Shape features, first-order features and texture features extracted from the $CTV_{prostate}$.

Author Contributions: Conceptualization, V.W.S.L., C.K.C.N., J.Q.W. and J.C.; methodology, V.W.S.L., S.-K.L., P.-T.W., K.-Y.N., V.C.W.T., S.W.Y.L. and F.M.Y.L.; software, V.W.S.L. and S.-K.L.; validation, V.W.S.L. and S.-K.L.; formal analysis, P.-T.W., K.-Y.N., C.-H.T., T.-C.L., K.-C.C. and Y.-K.C.; investigation, V.W.S.L. and S.-K.L.; resources, V.W.S.L. and S.-K.L.; data curation, S.-K.L.; writing—original draft preparation, V.W.S.L., C.K.C.N., S.-K.L., P.-T.W., K.-Y.N., C.-H.T., T.-C.L., K.-C.C., Y.-K.C., V.C.W.T., S.W.Y.L., F.M.Y.L., J.Q.W. and J.C.; writing—review and editing, V.W.S.L., C.K.C.N., S.-K.L., P.-T.W., K.-Y.N., C.-H.T., T.-C.L., K.-C.C., Y.-K.C., V.C.W.T., S.W.Y.L., F.M.Y.L., J.Q.W. and J.C.; visualization, P.-T.W., K.-Y.N., C.-H.T., T.-C.L., K.-C.C. and Y.-K.C.; supervision, V.W.S.L.; project administration, V.W.S.L.; funding acquisition, V.W.S.L. and J.C. All authors have read and agreed to the published version of the manuscript.

Funding: This research was funded by Government of Hong Kong Special Administrative Region Health and Medical Research Fund Research Fellowship Scheme 2021, grant number 06200137; and The Hong Kong Polytechnic University Project of Strategic Importance Fund 2021, grant number P0035421.

Institutional Review Board Statement: The study was conducted in accordance with the Declaration of Helsinki, and approved by the Institutional Review Board of The Hong Kong Polytechnic University (approval number: HSEARS20200902001 and date of approval: 20 September 2020), and Clinical & Research Ethics Committee of New Territories East Cluster of Hospital Authority of Government of Hong Kong Special Administrative Region (approval number: NTEC-2020-0633 and date of approval: 9 December 2020).

Informed Consent Statement: Patient consent was waived due to the retrospective nature.

Data Availability Statement: The datasets used and/or analyzed in this study are available from the corresponding author on reasonable request.

Acknowledgments: The authors would like to thank Virginia Kwong (Senior Radiation Therapist) and Ben Chiu (Radiation Therapist) for their assistance with the collection of data from Department of Clinical Oncology, Prince of Wales Hospital, Hong Kong Special Administrative Region.

Conflicts of Interest: The authors declare no conflict of interest. The funders had no role in the design of the study; in the collection, analyses, or interpretation of data; in the writing of the manuscript; or in the decision to publish the results.

References

1. Sung, H.; Ferlay, J.; Siegel, R.L.; Laversanne, M.; Soerjomataram, I.; Jemal, A.; Bray, F. Global cancer statistics 2020: GLOBOCAN estimates of incidence and mortality worldwide for 36 cancers in 185 countries. *CA Cancer J. Clin.* **2021**, *71*, 209–249. [CrossRef] [PubMed]
2. Siegel, R.L.; Miller, K.D.; Wagle, N.S.; Jemal, A. Cancer statistics, 2023. *CA Cancer J. Clin.* **2023**, *73*, 17–48. [CrossRef] [PubMed]
3. Parker, C.; Castro, E.; Fizazi, K.; Heidenreich, A.; Ost, P.; Procopio, G.; Tombal, B.; Gillessen, S.; ESMO Guidelines Committee. Prostate cancer: ESMO Clinical Practice Guidelines for diagnosis, treatment and follow-up. *Ann. Oncol.* **2020**, *31*, 1119–1134. [CrossRef] [PubMed]
4. Risk Groups for Localized Prostate Cancer. Available online: https://www.cancer.org/cancer/types/prostate-cancer/detection-diagnosis-staging/risk-groups.html (accessed on 5 September 2023).
5. Roy, S.; Morgan, S.C. Who dies from prostate cancer? An analysis of the surveillance, epidemiology and end results database. *Clin. Oncol.* **2019**, *31*, 630–636. [CrossRef] [PubMed]
6. Wang, S.; Tang, W.; Luo, H.; Jin, F.; Wang, Y. Efficacy and toxicity of whole pelvic radiotherapy versus prostate-only radiotherapy in localized prostate cancer: A systematic review and meta-analysis. *Front. Oncol.* **2022**, *11*, 796907. [CrossRef] [PubMed]
7. Murthy, V.; Maitre, P.; Kannan, S.; Panigrahi, G.; Krishnatry, R.; Bakshi, G.; Prakash, G.; Pal, M.; Menon, S.; Phurailatpam, R.; et al. Prostate-only versus whole-pelvic radiation therapy in high-risk and very high-risk prostate cancer (POP-RT): Outcomes from phase III randomized controlled trial. *J. Clin. Oncol.* **2021**, *39*, 1234–1242. [CrossRef] [PubMed]
8. Burgess, L.; Roy, S.; Morgan, S.; Malone, S. A review on the current treatment paradigm in high-risk prostate cancer. *Cancers* **2021**, *13*, 4257. [CrossRef]
9. Roach, M.; Moughan, J.; Lawton, C.A.F.; Dicker, A.P.; Zeitzer, K.L.; Gore, E.M.; Kwok, Y.; Seider, M.J.; Hsu, I.C.; Hartford, A.C.; et al. Sequence of hormonal therapy and radiotherapy field size in unfavourable, localised prostate cancer (NRG/RTOG 9413): Long-term results of a randomised, phase 3 trial. *Lancet Oncol.* **2018**, *19*, 1504–1515. [CrossRef]
10. Kendrick, J.; Francis, R.; Hassan, G.M.; Rowshanfarzad, P.; Jeraj, R.; Kasisi, C.; Rusanov, B.; Ebert, M. Radiomics for identification and prediction in metastatic prostate cancer: A review of studies. *Front. Oncol.* **2021**, *11*, 771787. [CrossRef]
11. Osman, S.O.S.; Leijenaar, R.T.H.; Cole, A.J.; Lyons, C.A.; Hounsell, A.R.; Prise, K.M.; O'Sullivan, J.M.; Lambin, P.; McGarry, C.K.; Jain, S. Computed tomography-based radiomics for risk stratification in prostate cancer. *Int. J. Radiat. Oncol. Biol. Phys.* **2019**, *105*, 448–456. [CrossRef]
12. Lambin, P.; Leijenaar, R.T.H.; Deist, T.M.; Peerlings, J.; de Jong, E.E.C.; van Timmeren, J.; Sanduleanu, S.; Larue, R.T.H.M.; Even, A.J.G.; Jochems, A.; et al. Radiomics: The bridge between medical imaging and personalized medicine. *Nat. Rev. Clin. Oncol.* **2017**, *14*, 749–762. [CrossRef] [PubMed]
13. Stanzione, A.; Cuocolo, R.; Ugga, L.; Verde, F.; Romeo, V.; Brunetti, A.; Maurea, S. Oncologic imaging and radiomics: A walkthrough review of methodological challenges. *Cancers* **2022**, *14*, 4871. [CrossRef] [PubMed]
14. Coppola, F.; Giannini, V.; Gabelloni, M.; Panic, J.; Defeudis, A.; Lo Monaco, S.; Cattabriga, A.; Cocozza, M.A.; Pastore, L.V.; Polici, M.; et al. Radiomics and magnetic resonance imaging of rectal cancer: From engineering to clinical practice. *Diagnostics* **2021**, *11*, 756. [CrossRef] [PubMed]
15. Lambin, P.; Rios-Velazquez, E.; Leijenaar, R.; Carvalho, S.; van Stiphout, R.G.; Granton, P.; Zegers, C.M.; Gillies, R.; Boellard, R.; Dekker, A.; et al. Radiomics: Extracting more information from medical images using advanced feature analysis. *Eur. J. Cancer* **2012**, *48*, 441–446. [CrossRef] [PubMed]
16. Kumar, V.; Gu, Y.; Basu, S.; Berglund, A.; Eschrich, S.A.; Schabath, M.B.; Forster, K.; Aerts, H.J.; Dekker, A.; Fenstermacher, D.; et al. Radiomics: The process and the challenges. *Magn. Reason. Imaging* **2012**, *30*, 1234–1248. [CrossRef] [PubMed]

17. Damascelli, A.; Gallivanone, F.; Cristel, G.; Cava, C.; Interlenghi, M.; Esposito, A.; Brembilla, G.; Briganti, A.; Montorsi, F.; Castiglioni, I.; et al. Advanced imaging analysis in prostate MRI: Building a radiomic signature to predict tumor aggressiveness. *Diagnostics* **2021**, *11*, 594. [CrossRef] [PubMed]
18. Hou, Y.; Bao, J.; Song, Y.; Bao, M.L.; Jiang, K.W.; Zhang, J.; Yang, G.; Hu, C.H.; Shi, H.B.; Wang, X.M.; et al. Integration of clinicopathologic identification and deep transferrable image feature representation improves predictions of lymph node metastasis in prostate cancer. *eBioMedicine* **2021**, *68*, 103395. [CrossRef] [PubMed]
19. Li, L.; Shiradkar, R.; Leo, P.; Algohary, A.; Fu, P.; Tirumani, S.H.; Mahran, A.; Buzzy, C.; Obmann, V.C.; Mansoori, B.; et al. A novel imaging based nomogram for predicting post-surgical biochemical recurrence and adverse pathology of prostate cancer from pre-operative bi-parametric MRI. *eBioMedicine* **2021**, *68*, 103163. [CrossRef]
20. Reischauer, C.; Patzwahl, R.; Koh, D.M.; Froehlich, J.M.; Gutzeit, A. Texture analysis of apparent diffusion coefficient maps for treatment response assessment in prostate cancer bone metastases-A pilot study. *Eur. J. Radiol.* **2018**, *101*, 184–190. [CrossRef]
21. Wang, Y.; Yu, B.; Zhong, F.; Guo, Q.; Li, K.; Hou, Y.; Lin, N. MRI-based texture analysis of the primary tumor for pre-treatment prediction of bone metastases in prostate cancer. *Magn. Reason. Imaging* **2019**, *60*, 76–84. [CrossRef]
22. Zhang, W.; Mao, N.; Wang, Y.; Xie, H.; Duan, S.; Zhang, X.; Wang, B. A radiomics nomogram for predicting bone metastasis in newly diagnosed prostate cancer patients. *Eur. J. Radiol.* **2020**, *128*, 109020. [CrossRef] [PubMed]
23. Alongi, P.; Stefano, A.; Comelli, A.; Laudicella, R.; Scalisi, S.; Arnone, G.; Barone, S.; Spada, M.; Purpura, P.; Bartolotta, T.V.; et al. Radiomics analysis of 18F-Choline PET/CT in the prediction of disease outcome in high-risk prostate cancer: An explorative study on machine learning feature classification in 94 patients. *Eur. Radiol.* **2021**, *31*, 4595–4605. [CrossRef] [PubMed]
24. Cysouw, M.C.F.; Jansen, B.H.E.; van de Brug, T.; Oprea-Lager, D.E.; Pfaehler, E.; de Vries, B.M.; van Moorselaar, R.J.A.; Hoekstra, O.S.; Vis, A.N.; Boellaard, R. Machine learning-based analysis of [18F]DCFPyL PET radiomics for risk stratification in primary prostate cancer. *Eur. J. Nucl. Med. Mol. Imaging* **2021**, *48*, 340–349. [CrossRef] [PubMed]
25. Khurshid, Z.; Ahmadzadehfar, H.; Gaertner, F.C.; Papp, L.; Zsóter, N.; Essler, M.; Bundschuh, R.A. Role of textural heterogeneity parameters in patient selection for 177Lu-PSMA therapy via response prediction. *Oncotarget* **2018**, *9*, 33312–33321. [CrossRef] [PubMed]
26. Lin, C.; Harmon, S.; Bradshaw, T.; Eickhoff, J.; Perlman, S.; Liu, G.; Jeraj, R. Response-to-repeatability of quantitative imaging features for longitudinal response assessment. *Phys. Med. Biol.* **2019**, *64*, 025019. [CrossRef] [PubMed]
27. Moazemi, S.; Khurshid, Z.; Erle, A.; Lütje, S.; Essler, M.; Schultz, T.; Bundschuh, R.A. Machine learning facilitates hotspot classification in PSMA-PET/CT with nuclear medicine specialist accuracy. *Diagnostics* **2020**, *10*, 622. [CrossRef] [PubMed]
28. Moazemi, S.; Erle, A.; Lütje, S.; Gaertner, F.C.; Essler, M.; Bundschuh, R.A. Estimating the potential of radiomics features and radiomics signature from pretherapeutic PSMA-PET-CT scans and clinical data for prediction of overall survival when treated with 177Lu-PSMA. *Diagnostics* **2021**, *11*, 186. [CrossRef]
29. Perk, T.; Bradshaw, T.; Chen, S.; Im, H.J.; Cho, S.; Perlman, S.; Liu, G.; Jeraj, R. Automated classification of benign and malignant lesions in 18F-NaF PET/CT images using machine learning. *Phys. Med. Biol.* **2018**, *63*, 225019. [CrossRef]
30. Zamboglou, C.; Carles, M.; Fechter, T.; Kiefer, S.; Reichel, K.; Fassbender, T.F.; Bronsert, P.; Koeber, G.; Schilling, O.; Ruf, J.; et al. Radiomic features from PSMA PET for non-invasive intraprostatic tumor discrimination and characterization in patients with intermediate- and high-risk prostate cancer—A comparison study with histology reference. *Theranostics* **2019**, *9*, 2595–2605. [CrossRef]
31. Borrelli, P.; Larsson, M.; Ulén, J.; Enqvist, O.; Trägårdh, E.; Poulsen, M.H.; Mortensen, M.A.; Kjölhede, H.; Høilund-Carlsen, P.F.; Edenbrandt, L. Artificial intelligence-based detection of lymph node metastases by PET/CT predicts prostate cancer-specific survival. *Clin. Physiol. Funct. Imaging* **2021**, *41*, 62–67. [CrossRef]
32. Lee, J.J.; Yang, H.; Franc, B.L.; Iagaru, A.; Davidzon, G.A. Deep learning detection of prostate cancer recurrence with 18F-FACBC (fluciclovine, Axumin®) positron emission tomography. *Eur. J. Nucl. Med. Mol. Imaging* **2020**, *47*, 2992–2997. [CrossRef] [PubMed]
33. Hartenstein, A.; Lübbe, F.; Baur, A.D.J.; Rudolph, M.M.; Furth, C.; Brenner, W.; Amthauer, H.; Hamm, B.; Makowski, M.; Penzkofer, T. Prostate cancer nodal staging: Using deep learning to predict 68Ga-PSMA-positivity from CT imaging alone. *Sci. Rep.* **2020**, *10*, 3398. [CrossRef] [PubMed]
34. Masoudi, S.; Mehralivand, S.; Harmon, S.A.; Lay, N.; Lindenberg, L.; Mena, E.; Pinto, P.A.; Citrin, D.E.; Gulley, J.L.; Wood, B.J.; et al. Deep learning based staging of bone lesions from computed tomography scans. *IEEE Access.* **2021**, *9*, 87531–87542. [CrossRef] [PubMed]
35. Zhao, Y.; Gafita, A.; Vollnberg, B.; Tetteh, G.; Haupt, F.; Afshar-Oromieh, A.; Menze, B.; Eiber, M.; Rominger, A.; Shi, K. Deep neural network for automatic characterization of lesions on 68Ga-PSMA-11 PET/CT. *Eur. J. Nucl. Med. Mol. Imaging* **2020**, *47*, 603–613. [CrossRef]
36. Acar, E.; Leblebici, A.; Ellidokuz, B.E.; Başbınar, Y.; Kaya, G.Ç. Machine learning for differentiating metastatic and completely responded sclerotic bone lesion in prostate cancer: A retrospective radiomics study. *Br. J. Radiol.* **2019**, *92*, 20190286. [CrossRef] [PubMed]
37. Hayakawa, T.; Tabata, K.I.; Tsumura, H.; Kawakami, S.; Katakura, T.; Hashimoto, M.; Watanabe, Y.; Iwamura, M.; Hasegawa, T.; Ishiyama, H. Size of pelvic bone metastasis as a significant prognostic factor for metastatic prostate cancer patients. *Jpn. J. Radiol.* **2020**, *38*, 993–996. [CrossRef] [PubMed]

38. Peeken, J.C.; Shouman, M.A.; Kroenke, M.; Rauscher, I.; Maurer, T.; Gschwend, J.E.; Eiber, M.; Combs, S.E. A CT-based radiomics model to detect prostate cancer lymph node metastases in PSMA radioguided surgery patients. *Eur. J. Nucl. Med. Mol. Imaging* **2020**, *47*, 2968–2977. [CrossRef] [PubMed]
39. Ching, J.C.F.; Lam, S.; Lam, C.C.H.; Lui, A.O.Y.; Kwong, J.C.K.; Lo, A.Y.H.; Chan, J.W.H.; Cai, J.; Leung, W.S.; Lee, S.W.Y. Integrating CT-based radiomic model with clinical features improves long-term prognostication in high-risk prostate cancer. *Front. Oncol.* **2023**, *13*, 1060687. [CrossRef]
40. Artibani, W.; Porcaro, A.B.; De Marco, V.; Cerruto, M.A.; Siracusano, S. Management of biochemical recurrence after primary curative treatment for prostate cancer: A review. *Urol. Int.* **2018**, *100*, 251–262. [CrossRef]
41. Chan, Y.; Li, M.; Parodi, K.; Belka, C.; Landry, G.; Kurz, C. Feasibility of CycleGAN enhanced low dose CBCT imaging for prostate radiotherapy dose calculation. *Phys. Med. Biol.* **2023**, *68*, 105014. [CrossRef]
42. Harris, V.A.; Staffurth, J.; Naismith, O.; Esmail, A.; Gulliford, S.; Khoo, V.; Lewis, R.; Littler, J.; McNair, H.; Sadoyze, A.; et al. Consensus guidelines and contouring atlas for pelvic node delineation in prostate and pelvic node intensity modulated radiation therapy. *Int. J. Radiat. Oncol. Biol. Phys.* **2015**, *92*, 874–883. [CrossRef] [PubMed]
43. Zwanenburg, A.; Vallières, M.; Abdalah, M.A.; Aerts, H.J.W.L.; Andrearczyk, V.; Apte, A.; Ashrafinia, S.; Bakas, S.; Beukinga, R.J.; Boellaard, R.; et al. The image biomarker standardization initiative: Standardized quantitative radiomics for high-throughput image-based phenotyping. *Radiology* **2020**, *295*, 328–338. [CrossRef] [PubMed]
44. van Griethuysen, J.J.M.; Fedorov, A.; Parmar, C.; Hosny, A.; Aucoin, N.; Narayan, V.; Beets-Tan, R.G.H.; Fillion-Robin, J.C.; Pieper, S.; Aerts, H.J.W.L. Computational radiomics system to decode the radiographic phenotype. *Cancer Res.* **2017**, *77*, e104–e107. [CrossRef] [PubMed]
45. Zhang, J.; Lam, S.K.; Teng, X.; Ma, Z.; Han, X.; Zhang, Y.; Cheung, A.L.Y.; Chau, T.C.; Ng, S.C.Y.; Lee, F.K.H.; et al. Radiomic feature repeatability and its impact on prognostic model generalizability: A multi-institutional study on nasopharyngeal carcinoma patients. *Radiother Oncol.* **2023**, *183*, 109578. [CrossRef] [PubMed]
46. Ho, L.M.; Lam, S.K.; Zhang, J.; Chiang, C.L.; Chan, A.C.Y.; Cai, J. Association of Multi-Phasic MR-Based Radiomic and Dosimetric Features with Treatment Response in Unresectable Hepatocellular Carcinoma Patients following Novel Sequential TACE-SBRT-Immunotherapy. *Cancers* **2023**, *15*, 1105. [CrossRef] [PubMed]
47. Teng, X.; Zhang, J.; Han, X.; Sun, J.; Lam, S.K.; Ai, Q.Y.H.; Ma, Z.; Lee, F.K.H.; Au, K.H.; Yip, C.W.Y.; et al. Explainable machine learning via intra-tumoral radiomics feature mapping for patient stratification in adjuvant chemotherapy for locoregionally advanced nasopharyngeal carcinoma. *Radiol. Medica* **2023**, *128*, 828–838. [CrossRef] [PubMed]
48. Zheng, X.; Guo, W.; Wang, Y.; Zhang, J.; Zhang, Y.; Cheng, C.; Teng, X.; Lam, S.K.; Zhou, T.; Ma, Z.; et al. Multi-omics to predict acute radiation esophagitis in patients with lung cancer treated with intensity-modulated radiation therapy. *Eur. J. Med. Res.* **2023**, *28*, 126. [CrossRef]
49. Wei, W.; Hu, X.W.; Cheng, Q.; Zhao, Y.M.; Ge, Y.Q. Identification of common and severe COVID-19: The value of CT texture analysis and correlation with clinical characteristics. *Eur. Radiol.* **2020**, *30*, 6788–6796. [CrossRef]
50. Zhang, J.; Qiu, Q.; Duan, J.; Gong, G.; Jiang, Q.; Sun, G.; Yin, Y. Variability of radiomic features extracted from multi-b-value diffusion-weighted images in hepatocellular carcinoma. *Transl. Cancer Res.* **2019**, *8*, 130–140. [CrossRef]
51. Ligero, M.; Garcia-Ruiz, A.; Viaplana, C.; Villacampa, G.; Raciti, M.V.; Landa, J.; Matos, I.; Martin-Liberal, J.; Ochoa-de-Olza, M.; Hierro, C.; et al. A CT-based radiomics signature is associated with response to immune checkpoint inhibitors in advanced solid tumors. *Radiology* **2021**, *299*, 109–119. [CrossRef]
52. Papanikolaou, N.; Matos, C.; Koh, D.M. How to develop a meaningful radiomic signature for clinical use in oncologic patients. *Cancer Imaging* **2020**, *20*, 33. [CrossRef] [PubMed]
53. Diagnostic Imaging Pathways: Prostate Cancer (Suspected and Staging). Available online: https://radiologyacrossborders.org/diagnostic_imaging_pathways/imaging-pathways/urological/staging-of-prostate-cancer#pathway (accessed on 26 October 2023).
54. Stabile, A.; Giganti, F.; Rosenkrantz, A.B.; Taneja, S.S.; Villeirs, G.; Gill, I.S.; Allen, C.; Emberton, M.; Moore, C.M.; Kasivisvanathan, V. Multiparametric MRI for prostate cancer diagnosis: Current status and future directions. *Nat. Rev. Urol.* **2020**, *17*, 41–61. [CrossRef]
55. Huynh, L.M.; Hwang, Y.; Taylor, O.; Baine, M.J. The use of MRI-derived radiomic models in prostate cancer risk stratification: A critical review of contemporary literature. *Diagnostics* **2023**, *13*, 1128. [CrossRef] [PubMed]
56. Gnep, K.; Fargeas, A.; Gutiérrez-Carvajal, R.E.; Commandeur, F.; Mathieu, R.; Ospina, J.D.; Rolland, Y.; Rohou, T.; Vincendeau, S.; Hatt, M.; et al. Haralick textural features on T2-weighted MRI are associated with biochemical recurrence following radiotherapy for peripheral zone prostate cancer. *J. Magn. Reason. Imaging* **2017**, *45*, 103–117. [CrossRef] [PubMed]
57. Dinis Fernandes, C.; Dinh, C.V.; Walraven, I.; Heijmink, S.W.; Smolic, M.; van Griethuysen, J.J.M.; Simões, R.; Losnegård, A.; van der Poel, H.G.; Pos, F.J.; et al. Biochemical recurrence prediction after radiotherapy for prostate cancer with T2w magnetic resonance imaging radiomic features. *Phys. Imaging Radiat. Oncol.* **2018**, *7*, 9–15. [CrossRef] [PubMed]
58. Zhong, Q.Z.; Long, L.H.; Liu, A.; Li, C.M.; Xiu, X.; Hou, X.Y.; Wu, Q.H.; Gao, H.; Xu, Y.G.; Zhao, T.; et al. Radiomics of multiparametric MRI to predict biochemical recurrence of localized prostate cancer after radiation therapy. *Front. Oncol.* **2020**, *10*, 731. [CrossRef] [PubMed]

59. Varghese, B.; Chen, F.; Hwang, D.; Palmer, S.L.; De Castro Abreu, A.L.; Ukimura, O.; Aron, M.; Aron, M.; Gill, I.; Duddalwar, V.; et al. Objective risk stratification of prostate cancer using machine learning and radiomics applied to multiparametric magnetic resonance images. *Sci. Rep.* **2019**, *9*, 1570. [CrossRef]
60. Park, H.; Lim, Y.; Ko, E.S.; Cho, H.H.; Lee, J.E.; Han, B.K.; Ko, E.Y.; Choi, J.S.; Park, K.W. Radiomics signature on magnetic resonance imaging: Association with disease-free survival in patients with invasive breast cancer. *Clin. Cancer Res.* **2018**, *24*, 4705–4714. [CrossRef]
61. Tsougos, I.; Vamvakas, A.; Kappas, C.; Fezoulidis, I.; Vassiou, K. Application of radiomics and decision support systems for breast MR differential diagnosis. *Comput. Math. Methods Med.* **2018**, *2018*, 7417126. [CrossRef]
62. Zhang, Y.; Lam, S.; Yu, T.; Teng, X.; Zhang, J.; Lee, F.K.; Au, K.; Yip, C.W.; Wang, S.; Cai, J. Integration of an imbalance framework with novel high-generalizable classifiers for radiomics-based distant metastases prediction of advanced nasopharyngeal carcinoma. *Knowl.-Based Syst.* **2022**, *235*, 107649. [CrossRef]
63. Bailly, C.; Bodet-Milin, C.; Bourgeois, M.; Gouard, S.; Ansquer, C.; Barbaud, M.; Sébille, J.C.; Chérel, M.; Kraeber-Bodéré, F.; Carlier, T. Exploring tumor heterogeneity using PET imaging: The big picture. *Cancers* **2019**, *11*, 1282. [CrossRef] [PubMed]
64. Harsini, S.; Wilson, D.; Saprunoff, H.; Allan, H.; Gleave, M.; Goldenberg, L.; Chi, K.N.; Kim-Sing, C.; Tyldesley, S.; Bénard, F. Outcome of patients with biochemical recurrence of prostate cancer after PSMA PET/CT-directed radiotherapy or surgery without systemic therapy. *Cancer Imaging* **2023**, *23*, 27. [CrossRef] [PubMed]
65. Cornford, P.; Bellmunt, J.; Bolla, M.; Briers, E.; De Santis, M.; Gross, T.; Henry, A.M.; Joniau, S.; Lam, T.B.; Mason, M.D.; et al. EAU-ESTRO-SIOG guidelines on prostate cancer. Part II: Treatment of relapsing, metastatic, and castration-resistant prostate cancer. *Eur. Urol.* **2017**, *71*, 630–642. [CrossRef] [PubMed]
66. Van den Broeck, T.; van den Bergh, R.C.N.; Briers, E.; Cornford, p.; Cumberbatch, M.; Tilki, D.; De Santis, M.; Fanti, S.; Fossati, N.; Gillessen, S.; et al. Biochemical Recurrence in Prostate Cancer: The European Association of Urology Prostate Cancer Guidelines Panel Recommendations. *Eur. Urol. Focus* **2020**, *6*, 231–234. [CrossRef] [PubMed]
67. Freedland, S.J.; de Almeida Luz, M.; Giorgi, U.D.; Gleave, M.; Gotto, G.T.; Pieczonka, C.M.; Haas, G.P.; Kim, C.S.; Ramirez-Backhaus, M.; Rannikko, A.; et al. Improved outcomes with enzalutamide in biochemically recurrent prostate cancer. *N. Engl. J. Med.* **2023**, *389*, 1453–1465. [CrossRef] [PubMed]
68. Ong, W.L.; Koh, T.L.; Lim Joon, D.; Chao, M.; Farrugia, B.; Lau, E.; Khoo, V.; Lawrentschuk, N.; Bolton, D.; Foroudi, F. Prostate-specific membrane antigen-positron emission tomography/computed tomography (PSMA-PET/CT)-guided stereotactic ablative body radiotherapy for oligometastatic prostate cancer: A single-institution experience and review of the published literature. *BJU Int.* **2019**, *124*, 19–30. [CrossRef] [PubMed]
69. Kesavan, M.; Meyrick, D.; Gallyamov, M.; Turner, J.H.; Yeo, S.; Cardaci, G.; Lenzo, N.P. Efficacy and haematologic toxicity of palliative radioligand therapy of metastatic castrate-resistant prostate cancer with lutetium-177-labeled prostate-specific membrane antigen in heavily pre-treated patients. *Diagnostics* **2021**, *11*, 515. [CrossRef]
70. Devos, G.; Berghen, C.; Van Eecke, H.; Stichele, A.V.; Van Poppel, H.; Goffin, K.; Mai, C.; De Wever, L.; Albersen, M.; Everaerts, W.; et al. Oncological outcomes of metastasis-directed therapy in oligorecurrent prostate cancer patients following radical prostatectomy. *Cancers* **2020**, *12*, 2271. [CrossRef]
71. Steele, E.M.; Holmes, J.A. A review of salvage treatment options for disease progression after radiation therapy for localized prostate cancer. *Urol. Oncol.* **2019**, *37*, 582–598. [CrossRef]
72. Mazzola, R.; Francolini, G.; Triggiani, L.; Napoli, G.; Cuccia, F.; Nicosia, L.; Livi, L.; Magrini, S.M.; Salgarello, M.; Alongi, F. Metastasis-directed therapy (SBRT) guided by PET-CT 18F-CHOLINE versus PET-CT 68Ga-PSMA in castration-sensitive oligorecurrent prostate cancer: A comparative analysis of effectiveness. *Clin. Genitourin. Cancer* **2021**, *19*, 230–236. [CrossRef]
73. Tsumura, H.; Ishiyama, H.; Tabata, K.; Sekiguchi, A.; Kawakami, S.; Satoh, T.; Kitano, M.; Iwamura, M. Long-term outcomes of combining prostate brachytherapy and metastasis-directed radiotherapy in newly diagnosed oligometastatic prostate cancer: A retrospective cohort study. *Prostate* **2019**, *79*, 506–514. [CrossRef] [PubMed]
74. Perez-Lopez, R.; Tunariu, N.; Padhani, A.R.; Oyen, W.J.G.; Fanti, S.; Vargas, H.A.; Omlin, A.; Morris, M.J.; de Bono, J.; Koh, D.M. Imaging diagnosis and follow-up of advanced prostate cancer: Clinical perspectives and state of the art. *Radiology* **2019**, *292*, 273–286. [CrossRef] [PubMed]
75. Ng, C.K.C. Diagnostic performance of artificial intelligence-based computer-aided detection and diagnosis in pediatric radiology: A systematic review. *Children* **2023**, *10*, 525. [CrossRef] [PubMed]
76. Ng, C.K.C. Generative adversarial network (generative artificial intelligence) in pediatric radiology: A systematic review. *Children* **2023**, *10*, 1372. [CrossRef] [PubMed]
77. Sun, Z.; Ng, C.K.C. Artificial intelligence (enhanced super-resolution generative adversarial network) for calcium deblooming in coronary computed tomography angiography: A feasibility study. *Diagnostics* **2022**, *12*, 991. [CrossRef] [PubMed]
78. Sun, Z.; Ng, C.K.C. Finetuned super-resolution generative adversarial network (artificial intelligence) model for calcium deblooming in coronary computed tomography angiography. *J. Pers. Med.* **2022**, *12*, 1354. [CrossRef] [PubMed]

79. Ng, C.K.C. Artificial intelligence for radiation dose optimization in pediatric radiology: A systematic review. *Children* **2022**, *9*, 1044. [CrossRef]
80. Ng, C.K.C.; Leung, V.W.S.; Hung, R.H.M. Clinical evaluation of deep learning and atlas-based auto-contouring for head and neck radiation therapy. *Appl. Sci.* **2022**, *12*, 11681. [CrossRef]

Disclaimer/Publisher's Note: The statements, opinions and data contained in all publications are solely those of the individual author(s) and contributor(s) and not of MDPI and/or the editor(s). MDPI and/or the editor(s) disclaim responsibility for any injury to people or property resulting from any ideas, methods, instructions or products referred to in the content.

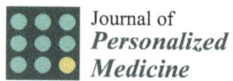

Article

Impact of the COVID-19 Pandemic on the Epidemiological Situation of Pulmonary Tuberculosis–Using Natural Language Processing

Diego Morena [1,2,*], Carolina Campos [1], María Castillo [1], Miguel Alonso [1], María Benavent [3] and José Luis Izquierdo [1,4]

1. Servicio de Neumología, Hospital Universitario de Guadalajara, 19002 Guadalajara, Spain; ccampos.bm@gmail.com (C.C.); mariacastillogarcia37@gmail.com (M.C.); alonsomiguel23@gmail.com (M.A.); jlizquierdoa@gmail.com (J.L.I.)
2. Programa de Doctorado en Ciencias de la Salud, Universidad de Alcalá, 28801 Madrid, Spain
3. SAVANA, Medsavana S.L., 28013 Madrid, Spain; mbenavent@savanamed.com
4. Departamento de Medicina y Especialidades Médicas, Universidad de Alcalá, 28801 Madrid, Spain
* Correspondence: diegomorenavalles6@gmail.com; Tel.: +346-2788-9489

Abstract: Background: We aimed to analyze the impact of the COVID-19 pandemic on pulmonary tuberculosis (TB) using artificial intelligence. To do so, we compared the real-life situation during the pandemic with the pre-2020 situation. Methods: This non-interventional, retrospective, observational study applied natural language processing to the electronic health records of the Castilla-La Mancha region of Spain. The analysis was conducted from January 2015 to December 2020. Results: A total of 2592 patients were diagnosed with pulmonary tuberculosis; 64.6% were males, and the mean age was 53.5 years (95%CI 53.0–54.0). In 2020, pulmonary tuberculosis diagnoses dropped by 28% compared to 2019. In total, 62 (14.2%) patients were diagnosed with COVID-19 and pulmonary tuberculosis coinfection in 2020, with a mean age of 52.3 years (95%CI 48.3–56.2). The main symptoms in these patients were dyspnea (27.4%) and cough (35.5%), although their comorbidities were no greater than patients with isolated TB. The female sex was more frequently affected, representing 53.4% of this patient subgroup. Conclusions: During the first year of the COVID-19 pandemic, a decrease was observed in the incidence of pulmonary tuberculosis. Women presented a significantly higher risk for pulmonary tuberculosis and COVID-19 coinfection, although the symptoms were not more severe than patients diagnosed with pulmonary tuberculosis alone.

Keywords: pulmonary tuberculosis; COVID-19; artificial intelligence

Citation: Morena, D.; Campos, C.; Castillo, M.; Alonso, M.; Benavent, M.; Izquierdo, J.L. Impact of the COVID-19 Pandemic on the Epidemiological Situation of Pulmonary Tuberculosis–Using Natural Language Processing. *J. Pers. Med.* **2023**, *13*, 1629. https://doi.org/10.3390/jpm13121629

Academic Editor: Daniele Giansanti

Received: 14 October 2023
Revised: 13 November 2023
Accepted: 17 November 2023
Published: 22 November 2023

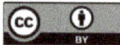

Copyright: © 2023 by the authors. Licensee MDPI, Basel, Switzerland. This article is an open access article distributed under the terms and conditions of the Creative Commons Attribution (CC BY) license (https://creativecommons.org/licenses/by/4.0/).

1. Introduction

Infections that cause respiratory tract diseases continue to be the cause of the greatest morbidity and mortality from infectious diseases in the world. In 2019, just three pathogens featured on the WHO Blueprint priority list for research and development. These were severe acute respiratory syndrome coronavirus (SARS-CoV), Middle East respiratory syndrome coronavirus (MERS-CoV), and Mycobacterium tuberculosis. In 2020, SARS-CoV2 was included [1].

Since then, COVID-19 has been the direct cause of hundreds of thousands of deaths worldwide over the last 3 years. During the first months of the COVID-19 pandemic, almost all countries in the world experienced a devastating impact. As the virus spread rapidly, health systems faced unprecedented pressure. Confinement measures were implemented in several countries to slow the spread, affecting the daily lives of the population. The situation generated international collaboration in search of solutions, evidencing the need for a coordinated global response to public health emergencies. The acute respiratory syndrome associated with the SARSCoV-2 virus has caused serious distortions in healthcare systems, surpassing the HIV situation of 40 years ago [1].

The pandemic has had countless economic, social, and healthcare-related effects, both direct and indirect. Spain was one of the first European countries to be affected by COVID-19 and, along with Italy, also one of the first to implement confinement as a control measure [1].

The impact of COVID-19 on hospital services was dramatic, causing personnel and financial resources to be diverted. Thus, the ability to correctly diagnose and control other pathologies was limited. In fact, the burden on health services caused by the COVID-19 emergency has led to several changes in the ordinary management of both communicable and non-communicable diseases, following the reduction in or suspension of non-urgent outpatient care [1,2].

The World Health Organization has reported that certain pathologies, such as pulmonary tuberculosis (TB), may have suffered a delay in diagnosis and the start of treatment [2].

Pulmonary TB is one of the leading causes of death and disease in many countries around the world. Mycobacterium tuberculosis is the second deadliest pathogen after the virus that causes COVID-19 [2]. Transmission of pulmonary tuberculosis occurs through the inhalation of saliva droplets or respiratory secretions from infected individuals. Once inhaled, the bacteria can establish themselves in the lungs and trigger an immune response, forming granulomas that encapsulate the bacteria. However, these structures can also act as reservoirs of infection, making it difficult to completely eradicate the bacteria. Symptoms of pulmonary tuberculosis include persistent fever, weight loss, and fatigue. Early diagnosis is crucial to prevent the spread of the disease. In 2018, countries attending the United Nations high-level meeting on tuberculosis committed to intensify their efforts to achieve the ambitious goals of treating an additional 40 million people with tuberculosis and providing prophylaxis to at least 30 million people who are at risk of contracting the disease until 2030 [3]. It is considered a true healthcare problem, reaching a prevalence of 10 million patients and 1.5 million deaths in 2020, the majority registered in Asia (55%) and Africa (30%) [2,3]. The number of deaths increased from 2019 to 2020, reversing the trend of previous years [3–6]. These data are far from reaching the goal of eradicating TB in 2030 [4].

Around the world, there have been reports that some 18% of patients with pulmonary TB were not diagnosed in 2020, as the number of notified cases dropped from 7.1 million subjects in 2019 to 5.8 million in 2020 [2–5,7–10]. Although 6.4 million cases were diagnosed in 2021, we are still far below pre-pandemic levels. In Europe, a total of 47 of 504 cases of tuberculosis were reported in 2019, which is equivalent to a rate of 9.2 cases per 100,000. In 2020, however, 33,000 cases were reported, most of whom were male [4] (54%), causing increased comorbidities and risk of mortality in this population [3–5]. In Spain, the impact of the pandemic represented a 50% drop in the inclusion of patients in 2020 compared to 2019 [4]. Pulmonary tuberculosis can be prevented and cured. About 85% of people who contract it progress satisfactorily with a therapeutic regimen of 4 to 6 months [11]. In addition, treatment reduces transmission. For this reason, it is important to make a quick and correct diagnosis of this pathology [12].

The public health and social measures implemented during the SARSCoV-2 pandemic, such as social distancing and respiratory isolation, may have had a beneficial effect on the transmission of certain infectious agents [13]. A significant decrease in transmission has been demonstrated in infections with short incubation periods, such as influenza or respiratory syncytial virus [14,15]. In pulmonary TB, the precise impact of these measures has still not been determined [16,17]. Furthermore, various studies have stated that the coinfection of SARSCoV-2 and tuberculosis disease could lead to an increase in the severity of COVID-19 and accelerate the progression of TB [15–17].

Our working hypothesis is that by leveraging artificial intelligence methodologies on large-scale patient datasets, we can attain a more nuanced understanding of these interrelationships within the context of real-world clinical practice. Big data applications in the health sector, and specifically the application of new technologies to manage and extract value from complex data generated in large volumes of electronic health records, are a reality. Most of the information contained in the medical electronic files is found in an unstructured way, as free text, its analysis being possible through analysis techniques, like artificial intelligence.

The aim of this real-life study is to analyze the epidemiological situation of pulmonary tuberculosis and SARS-CoV-2 coinfection during the first year of the pandemic and to compare the current situation to that existing before the appearance of COVID-19 using artificial intelligence techniques, specifically natural language processing with the Savana Manager 3.0 platform.

2. Materials and Methods

This study was conducted in the autonomous community of Castilla-La Mancha, Spain, from January 2015 to December 2020. It is a retrospective observational study designed to follow the guidelines of the Strengthening the Reporting of Observational Studies in Epidemiology (STROBE) Statement.

Data on pulmonary tuberculosis were collected from 2015 to 2020, while data for TB in association with COVID-19 were collected from January 2020 to December 2020. The total population was 2,866,188, and all information was collected from the electronic health records (EHRs) of patients diagnosed with pulmonary tuberculosis and COVID-19.

The data were analyzed using the Savana Manager 3.0 natural language processor, which uses artificial intelligence and big data techniques. This processor is able to analyze unstructured information in EHRs made available by the Castilla-La Mancha Health Service (SESCAM), and then the data are extracted for use in research. A detailed description of the system has been previously published [18–21]. In addition, through the use of computational linguistic techniques, comprehensive clinical content is scientifically detected and validated using the SNOMED CT tool [22]. This international database uses comprehensive, multilingual, and codified clinical terminology. This concept carries a clinical idea associated with a unique identifier, which is permanent and unalterable. In this way, it attempts to solve the problem of semantic interoperability presented by some classifications such as ICD 10–11, and at the same time, to create an agile mapping with these commonly used classifications. The terms proposed by the SNOMED coding will be used for both COVID-19 and pulmonary TB.

Using EHRead technology, the free text contained in the EHR was analyzed and processed with natural language processing (NLP) techniques. Medical concepts were detected by using computational linguistic techniques and comprehensive clinical content. These unstructured data were treated as big data. We have previously evaluated the performance of Savana to verify the accuracy of the system to identify records that contain mentions of TB, COVID-19, and related variables. The lack of coded clinical data in Spain requires the development of an annotated corpus known as the 'gold standard' to carry out this evaluation. This gold standard consists of a set of clinical documents where the appearance of entities/concepts related to pulmonary TB and COVID-19 are manually verified by experts. Specifically, the corpus used in this evaluation is a set of 450 documents reviewed by three experts to guarantee the reliability of the manual annotation and review. Subsequently, a judge external to the study confirms the correct verification of the reviewers. Savana's performance was automatically calculated using the expert-created 'gold standard' as an evaluation resource. This means that the precision of Savana to identify records, in which the presence of the pathology under study and the related variables have been detected, was measured compared to the 'gold standard'. The evaluation of the system was calculated in terms of the standard metrics of precision (P), recall (R), and its F-score.

Precision (P) = $tp/(tp + fp)$. This parameter offers an indicator of reliability with which the system retrieves the information.

Range (R) = $tp/(tp + fn)$. This parameter offers an indicator of the quantity of information that the system retrieves.

F-measure = $(2 \times precision \times recall)/(precision \times recall)$. This parameter offers an indicator of the overall data retrieval performance.

In all cases, a true positive (*tp*) was defined as a correctly identified record, a false positive (*fp*) as a wrongly identified record, and a false negative (*fn*) as a record that should have been identified.

Our results regarding Savana's performance for evaluating pulmonary TB and COVID-19 information are shown in Table 1.

Table 1. Performance of Savana in terms of precision, recall, and F-measure for IPF and COVID 19.

	Precision	Recall	F-Measure
PULMONARY TB	1.0	0.94	0.97
COVID-19	0.99	0.75	0.93

The data collection system complies with the General Data Protection Regulation (GDPR) of the European Union, and it is impossible to identify doctor or patient information when extracting data.

This study has followed all local regulations, procedures for the correct use of big data, Guidelines for Good Pharmacoepidemiology Practices, and the latest edition of the Declaration of Helsinki. The study was approved by the Research Ethics Committee of the Guadalajara healthcare administration (CEIm: 2022.28.EO; acceptance date 19 December 2022). As it is a retrospective observational study that uses patient data anonymously, patient informed consent was not required.

The statistical analysis that was carried out in this study was a descriptive analysis of all the variables evaluated. Absolute frequencies and percentages are expressed as qualitative variables, and means, 95%CI, and standard deviations are expressed as quantitative variables. Student's *t*-test of the independent samples was used for the analysis of numerical variables. The chi-squared test was used to measure the association and compare proportions between qualitative variables. Differences where the *p*-value was less than 0.05 were considered significant. OpenEpi (v3.0) and SSPS (v25; IBM Corporation, Armonk, NY, USA) were used for the statistical analysis.

3. Results

During the study period (January 2015–December 2020), a total of 2592 patients were diagnosed with pulmonary tuberculosis of a total population of 2,866,188 subjects. The flowchart for the study population is shown in Figure 1.

In total, 64.6% of patients diagnosed with pulmonary tuberculosis were men with a mean age of 53.5 years (95%CI 53.0–54.0), and 35.4% were women with a mean age of 52.3 years (95%CI 51.4–53.2).

From January 2020 to December 2020, a total of 210,164 (11.1%) patients were diagnosed with COVID-19. That same year, a total of 438 (0.02%) patients were diagnosed with pulmonary TB, 59.5% of which were male with a mean age of 55.0 years (95%CI 53.4–56.7), and 40.5% were female with a mean age of 53.9 years (95%CI 52.6–55.2). Figure 2 shows the evolution of TB diagnoses annually since 2015. Above the columns, the number of patients diagnosed with pulmonary TB per 100,000 inhabitants is shown. A higher incidence of pulmonary TB was not observed in the first year of the pandemic; instead, a 28% reduction was observed compared to 2019.

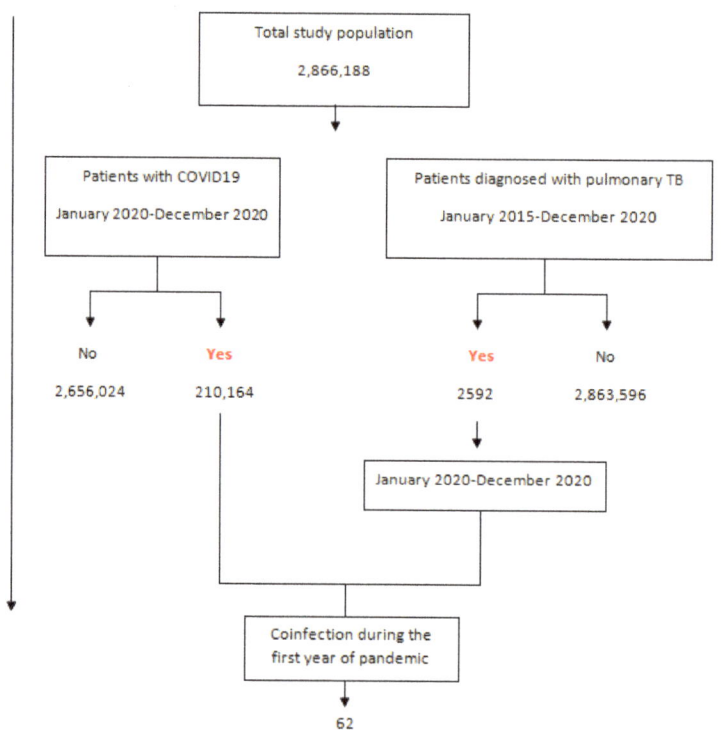

Figure 1. Flowchart showing the total study population, patients diagnosed with COVID-19, patients diagnosed with pulmonary TB, as well as patients with coinfection of these two diseases during the first year of the pandemic.

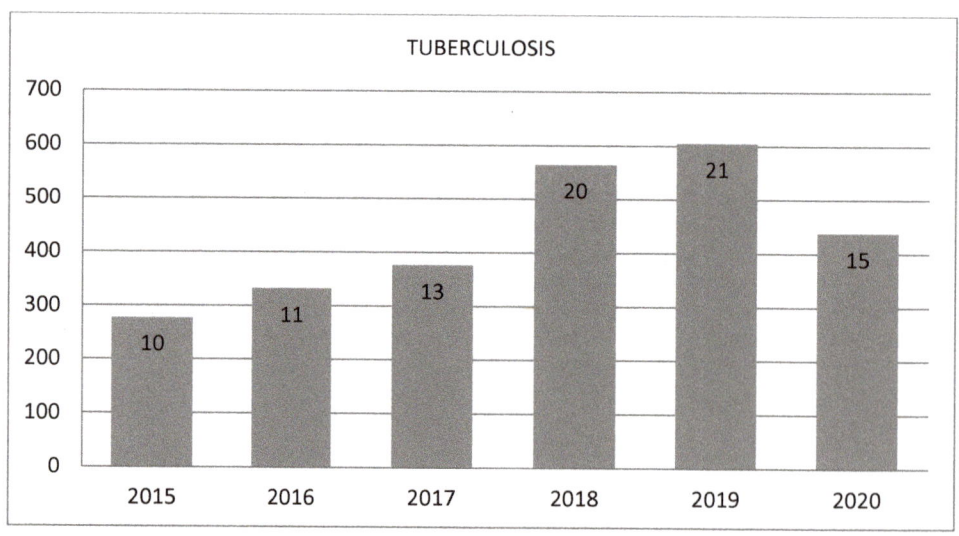

Figure 2. Annual prevalence of pulmonary TB from 2015 to 2020. Within the columns, TB pulmonary patients per 100,000 inhabitants are shown.

Table 2 compares the pulmonary TB diagnoses of 2019 versus 2020, as well as the percentage reduction in diagnoses from one year to the next. A comparative variability between the 2 years stands out (marked in the gray rows of the table), which is probably related to the first and second waves of the COVID-19 pandemic in our setting (March to May, and October to November).

Table 2. Comparison of pulmonary TB diagnosis in 2019 and 2020.

	Pulmonary Tuberculosis		
	2019	2020	Reduction
January	62	59	4.84%
February	50	40	20.00%
March	58	33	43.10%
April	60	10	83.33%
May	69	30	56.52%
June	43	41	4.65%
July	49	45	8.16%
August	23	21	8.70%
September	34	31	8.82%
October	70	45	35.71%
November	52	50	3.85%
December	35	33	5.71%

A total of 62 (14.2%) patients diagnosed with TB presented COVID-19 coinfection over the course of 2020, with a mean age of 52.3 years (95%CI 48.3–56.2). In this instance, women were more frequently affected (53.4%; OR 1.8, 95%CI 1.1–3.2). No statistically significant age differences were found between patients with coinfection versus those with a diagnosis of pulmonary TB alone ($p = 0.18$).

The main symptoms of patients with coinfection were dyspnea (27.4%), cough (35.5%), and fever (27.4%). The symptoms of patients diagnosed with TB alone were similar (32%, 36%, and 20%, respectively). Table 3 shows the main comorbidities of patients with coinfection versus patients with pulmonary TB alone. The only statistically significant difference found was for arterial hypertension ($p = 0.02$).

Table 3. Main comorbidities in patients with TB + COVID-19 coinfection versus patients with pulmonary TB alone.

	Pulmonary TB +COVID	%	Pulmonary TB	%	OR (IC 95%)
Arterial hypertension	21	33.9	200	45.7	0.6 (0.3–0.9)
Diabetes mellitus	15	24.2	136	31.1	0.7 (0.4–1.3)
Dyslipidemia	20	32.3	160	36.5	0.8 (0.5–1.4)
Obesity	6	9.7	45	10.3	0.9 (0.4–2.3)
COPD	5	8.1	58	13.2	0.5 (0.2–1.4)
Asthma	4	6.4	29	6.6	0.9 (0.3–2.8)
Ischemic cardiopathy	2	3.2	24	5.5	0.5 (0.1–2.3)
Human immunodeficiency virus (HIV)	3	4.8	44	10.0	0.4 (0.1–1.4)

Among patients diagnosed with TB and COVID-19 in 2020, no deaths were recorded from this cause during the study period.

4. Discussion

The integration of artificial intelligence (AI) systems plays a pivotal role in assessing the repercussions of the COVID-19 pandemic on the diagnosis and monitoring of various pathologies. In the realm of medicine, AI has emerged as a groundbreaking scientific frontier, orchestrating a paradigm shift in healthcare and biomedical research. Its presence in our everyday clinical practice holds the promise of enhancing the diagnosis, prognosis, and treatment of respiratory diseases. This transformative potential is particularly evident in the application of big data techniques, where AI in healthcare facilitates the management and extraction of valuable insights from the vast and intricate data archived in electronic health records. One of the notable strengths of AI lies in its capacity to handle extensive datasets and discern intricate patterns, fundamentally altering our approach to understanding and managing respiratory diseases. The integration of AI technologies allows for a comprehensive evaluation of the key indicators within specific clinical processes. Crucially, this approach mitigates selection biases, transcending the limitations imposed solely by the existence of a registry.

In the context of the COVID-19 pandemic, where the volume and complexity of medical data have surged, AI systems offer unparalleled advantages. These systems contribute significantly to the rapid and accurate diagnosis of respiratory conditions, enabling timely interventions and personalized treatment strategies. Moreover, AI's capabilities extend beyond diagnosis, encompassing prognosis and treatment planning. The technology's ability to sift through massive datasets facilitates the identification of subtle patterns and correlations, potentially unveiling new insights into the progression and management of respiratory diseases.

As we navigate the complexities of the modern healthcare landscape, the symbiosis of AI and medicine stands as a beacon of progress. It not only expedites processes but also ensures a more nuanced and individualized approach to patient care. The ongoing evolution of AI in the medical domain holds vast potential, fostering a future where technology augments our understanding and management of respiratory diseases, contributing to improved patient outcomes and shaping a more resilient healthcare ecosystem.

The aim of this study was to demonstrate this impact on the population diagnosed with pulmonary tuberculosis in 2020 using NLP. The prevalence of this pathology in our setting has been confirmed, which predominantly affected males from 2015 to 2020. This higher prevalence in men has already been described in recent previous studies [11,12].

In 2020, we observed a drop in the incidence of pulmonary TB compared to previous years (shown in Figure 2), including a marked decrease in patients diagnosed in the months of February to April and in October, which was probably due to the first and second waves of COVID-19 in Spain. These results are in line with previous studies from other regions of the Iberian Peninsula and other countries [3–5,23–28]. The majority of studies previously carried out are of the Italian population, since within Europe it was the country that most quickly suffered the direct causes of the pandemic. These studies present populations studied with a low number of patients, our study being the first to analyze with artificial intelligence the epidemiological situation of pulmonary TB during the pandemic and its possible co-infection with COVID-19.

Several possible explanations exist for this decrease in the incidence of pulmonary TB, which are not necessarily mutually exclusive. The reorganization of hospital services and community health centers due to the pressure of the COVID-19 pandemic could have indirectly affected the management and identification of patients with TB, while also reducing the diagnostic and treatment capabilities for this pathology. Second, it may have caused an underreporting of cases, increasing the number of patients with undiagnosed and untreated pulmonary tuberculosis. Also, the fear of COVID-19 infection or the presence of minor symptoms could have deterred patients from going to medical centers. The same reasons may justify the increase in the proportion of cases who are lost to follow-up.

Another cause of the lower incidence of pulmonary TB during the first year of the pandemic could be the public health and social measures that were implemented. Quarantine, the mandatory use of masks, and social distancing may have had a beneficial effect on certain diseases, resulting in the lower propagation of pathogens spread by airborne transmission, such as pulmonary tuberculosis. In this way, COVID-19 not only aggravates the disaster of this disease, as previously described, but also provides experience in the fight against tuberculosis. People from all social sectors have learned and practiced intervention programs related to respiratory infectious diseases, giving the opportunity for better management of these diseases in the future, raising awareness among the population about taking safety measures.

Coinfection with tuberculosis (TB) and COVID-19 presents a significant medical challenge due to the intersection of two respiratory pathologies with a great global impact. Coinfection can lead to a complex interaction between the two diseases, potentially exacerbating severity and complicating prognosis. The presence of TB can compromise the host's immune response, increasing the susceptibility and severity of COVID-19 [17]. At the same time, SARS-CoV-2 infection could influence the clinical course of TB, especially in individuals with compromised immune systems. The COVID-19 pandemic has impacted TB control programs, with disruptions to healthcare services and the reallocation of resources. These factors have contributed to delays in the diagnosis and treatment of TB, increasing the risks of transmission and drug resistance. Current research focuses on understanding the mechanisms of interaction between both infections [15–17], as well as evaluating the impact of coinfection on progression and clinical outcome. These studies have described a probable increased risk of disease severity in patients with COVID-19 and pulmonary tuberculosis coinfection [15–17], which would lead to accelerated progression and symptoms of the latter. With these data documented in the previous bibliography, it is reasonable to speculate that the hyperinflammatory environment induced by COVID-19 could accelerate the progression of TB disease and vice versa. A worrying importance of coinfection with active TB, in addition to the worst results of the treatment, is the possibility of missing a TB diagnosis due to overlapping clinical features.

Strategies are being explored to optimize clinical management and coordination between TB and COVID-19 programs, recognizing the importance of a comprehensive approach that addresses the complexities of these co-occurring respiratory diseases [25–27]. Preventing and effectively managing coinfection require close collaboration among health professionals, as well as continued efforts to ensure equitable access to appropriate health services and treatments. A deep understanding of TB-COVID-19 co-infection is essential to guide public health policies and clinical strategies that minimize the impact of this duality of respiratory diseases globally.

In our study population, a total of 62 patients presented coinfection. This study has one of the largest cohorts (both European and worldwide) of pulmonary TB and COVID-19. The female sex was most often affected, as opposed to males in the case of isolated pulmonary TB, and this difference was statistically significant. The increased risk of co-infection in women raises important questions about the interaction between tuberculosis and SARS-CoV-2, as well as potential gender disparities in immune response. Further research is needed to fully understand these findings and determine whether there are biological, sociodemographic, or other factors that explain this association. There were no major changes with respect to age when diagnosed with pulmonary TB alone, remaining at around 50 years of age. The symptoms presented by coinfected patients were similar to patients who presented TB alone, which were dyspnea, cough, and fever. The comorbidities of these patients were also studied, although patients with COVID-19 and TB did not present more comorbidities. This information could have important implications for clinical management and public health strategies, as it suggests that people with co-infection do not necessarily experience a more severe course of the disease. However, continued surveillance and more extensive research is needed to fully understand the clinical and epidemiological ramifications of this dual interaction between pulmonary tuberculosis and COVID-19. In this group, no related deaths were registered.

5. Conclusions

Despite the emergence of the COVID-19 pandemic, we have not observed a rebound in the incidence of pulmonary tuberculosis. This may be due to the delay in the diagnosis of the disease in the first wave or the public health and social measures adopted in that timeframe. In our setting, women presented an increased risk of pulmonary TB and SARS-CoV-2 coinfection. These patients did not present more comorbidities or worsened symptoms compared to patients with isolated TB diagnosis. This finding suggests a unique dynamic between tuberculosis and COVID-19, where specific factors, yet to be determined, could influence women's susceptibility to this co-infection.

Author Contributions: Conceptualization, D.M. and J.L.I.; methodology, D.M.; software, M.B.; validation, D.M., M.A., C.C. and M.C.; investigation, D.M.; writing—original draft preparation, D.M.; writing—review and editing, D.M. and J.L.I.; visualization, D.M.; supervision, J.L.I. All authors have read and agreed to the published version of the manuscript.

Funding: Supported by the Chair of inflamatory Diseases of Airways, University of Alcalá (Alcala de Henares, Spain).

Institutional Review Board Statement: The study was conducted in accordance with the Declaration of Helsinki, and approved by the Ethics Committee of Guadalajara's Hospital, for studies involving humans.

Informed Consent Statement: Informed consent was not required because the study is anonymous, observational, and retrospective.

Data Availability Statement: The data presented in this study are available upon request from the corresponding author. The data are not publicly available because they belong to the national health system of Castilla La Mancha.

Conflicts of Interest: Author Maria Benavent was employed by the company Savana. JL Izquierdo reports having received personal fees from ASTRA ZENECA, BAYER, BOEHRINGER INGELHEIM, CHIESI, GSK, GRIFOLS, MENARINI, NOVARTIS, ORION, PFIZER, SANDOZ, TEVA, Zambon, during the study pe-riod. The remaining authors declare that the research was conducted in the absence of any commercial or financial relationships that could be construed as a potential conflict of interest.

References

1. World Health Organization. Pulse Survey on Continuity of Essential Health Services During the Covid-19 Pandemic. 2020. Available online: https://www.who.int/teams/integrated-health-services/monitoring-health-services/global-pulse-survey-on-continuity-of-essential-health-services-during-the-covid-19-pandemic (accessed on 25 October 2023).
2. World Health Organization. Global Tuberculosis Report 2022. 2022. Available online: https://www.who.int/teams/global-tuberculosis-programme/tb-reports/global-tuberculosis-report-2022 (accessed on 25 October 2023).
3. Migliori, G.B.; Thong, P.M.; Akkerman, O.; Alffenaar, J.-W.; Álvarez-Navascués, F.; Assao-Neino, M.M.; Bernard, P.V.; Biala, J.S.; Blanc, F.-X.; Bogorodskaya, E.M.; et al. Worldwide Effects of Coronavirus Disease Pandemic on Tuberculosis Services January–April 2020. *Emerg. Infect. Dis.* **2020**, *26*, 2709–2712. [CrossRef] [PubMed]
4. World Health Organization. Impact of the COVID-19 Pandemic on TB Detection and Mortality in 2020. 2021. Available online: https://www.who.int/publications/m/item/impact-of-the-covid-19-pandemic-on-tb-detection-and-mortality-in-2020 (accessed on 25 October 2023).
5. Vázquez-Temprano, N.; Ursúa-Díaz, M.I.; Salgado-Barreira, Á.; Vázquez-Gallardo, R.; Bastida, V.T.; Anibarro, L. Decline of Tuberculosis Rates and COVID-19 Pandemic. Fact or Fiction? *Arch. Bronconeumol.* **2022**, *58*, 272–274. [CrossRef] [PubMed]
6. McQuaid, C.F.; McCreesh, N.; Read, J.M.; Sumner, T.; Houben, R.M.G.J.; White, R.G.; Harris, R.C. The potential impact of COVID-19-related disruption on tuberculosis burden. *Eur. Respir. J.* **2020**, *56*, 2001718. [CrossRef]
7. Cilloni, L.; Fu, H.; Vesga, J.F.; Dowdy, D.; Pretorius, C.; Ahmedov, S.; Nair, S.A.; Mosneaga, A.; Masini, E.; Sahu, S.; et al. The potential impact of the COVID-19 pandemic on the tuberculosis epidemic a modelling analysis. *EClinicalMedicine* **2020**, *28*, 100603. [CrossRef]

8. Barrett, J.; Painter, H.; Rajgopal, A.; Keane, D.; John, L.; Papineni, P.; Whittington, A. Increase in disseminated TB during the COVID-19 pandemic. *Int. J. Tuberc. Lung Dis.* **2021**, *25*, 160–166. [CrossRef] [PubMed]
9. Bhatia, V.; Mandal, P.P.; Satyanarayana, S.; Aditama, T.Y.; Sharma, M. Mitigating the impact of the COVID-19 pandemic on progress towards ending tuberculosis in the WHO South-East Asia Region WHO South East Asia. *J. Public Health* **2020**, *9*, 95–99. [CrossRef] [PubMed]
10. Berardi, C.; Antonini, M.; Genie, M.G.; Cotugno, G.; Lanteri, A.; Melia, A.; Paolucci, F. The COVID-19 pandemic in Italy: Policy and technology impact on health and non-health outcomes. *Health Policy Technol.* **2020**, *9*, 454–487. [CrossRef]
11. Sreeramareddy, C.T.; Qin, Z.Z.; Satyanarayana, S.; Subbaraman, R.; Pai, M. Delays in diagnosis and treatment of pulmonary tuberculosis in India: A systematic review. *Int. J. Tuberc. Lung Dis.* **2014**, *18*, 255–266. [CrossRef]
12. Ong, C.W.M.; Migliori, G.B.; Raviglione, M.; MacGregor-Skinner, G.; Sotgiu, G.; Alffenaar, J.W.; Tiberi, S.; Adlhoch, C.; Alonzi, T.; Archuleta, S.; et al. Epidemic and pandemic viral infections: Impact on tuberculosis and the lung: A consensus by the World Association for Infectious Diseases and Immunological Disorders (WAidid), Global Tuberculosis Network (GTN), and members of the European Society of Clinical Microbiology and Infectious Diseases Study Group for Mycobacterial Infections (ESGMYC). *Eur. Respir. J.* **2020**, *56*, 2001727.
13. Alfano, V.; Ercolano, S. The Efficacy of Lockdown Against COVID-19: A Cross-Country Panel Analysis. *Appl. Health Econ. Health Policy* **2020**, *18*, 509–517. [CrossRef]
14. Pang, Y.; Liu, Y.; Du, J.; Gao, J.; Li, L. Impact of COVID-19 on tuberculosis control in China. *Int. J. Tuberc. Lung Dis.* **2020**, *24*, 545–547. [CrossRef] [PubMed]
15. Stochino, C.; Villa, S.; Zucchi, P.; Parravicini, P.; Gori, A.; Raviglione, M.C. Clinical characteristics of COVID-19 and active tuberculosis co-infection in an Italian reference hospital. *Eur. Respir. J.* **2020**, *56*, 2001708. [CrossRef] [PubMed]
16. Tadolini, M.; Codecasa, L.R.; García-García, J.-M.; Blanc, F.-X.; Borisov, S.; Alffenaar, J.-W.; Andréjak, C.; Bachez, P.; Bart, P.-A.; Belilovski, E.; et al. Active tuberculosis, sequelae and COVID-19 co-infection: First cohort of 49 cases. *Eur. Respir. J.* **2020**, *56*, 2001398. [CrossRef] [PubMed]
17. Chen, H.; Zhang, K. Insight into the impact of the COVID-19 epidemic on tuberculosis burden in China. *Eur. Respir. J.* **2020**, *56*, 2002710. [CrossRef]
18. Izquierdo, J.L.; Morena, D.; González, Y.; Paredero, J.M.; Pérez, B.; Graziani, D.; Gutierrez, M.; Rodriguez, J.M. Manejo clínico de la EPOC en situación de vida real. Análisis a partir de big data. *Arch. Bronconeumol.* **2020**, *57*, 94–100. [CrossRef]
19. Izquierdo, J.L.; Ancochea, J.; Soriano, J.B. Savana COVID-19 Research Group; et al. Clinical characteristics and prognostic factors for intensive care unit admission of patients With COVID-19: Retrospective study using machine learning and natural language processing. *J. Med. Internet Res.* **2020**, *22*, e21801. [CrossRef]
20. Izquierdo, J.L.; Almonacid, C.; González, Y.; Del Rio-Bermudez, C.; Ancochea, J.; Cárdenas, R.; Lumbreras, S.; Soriano, J.B. The impact of COVID-19 on patients with asthma: A Big data analysis. *Eur. Respir. J.* **2021**, *57*, 2003142. [CrossRef]
21. Morena, D.; Fernández, J.; Campos, C.; Castillo, M.; López, G.; Benavent, M.; Izquierdo, J.L. Clinical Profile of Patients with Idiopathic Pulmonary Fibrosis in Real Life. *J. Clin. Med.* **2023**, *12*, 1669. [CrossRef]
22. Benson, T. *Principles of Health Interoperability HL7 and SNOMED*; Springer: London, UK, 2012.
23. Di Gennaro, F.; Gualano, G.; Timelli, L.; Vittozzi, P.; Di Bari, V.; Libertone, R.; Cerva, C.; Pinnarelli, L.; Nisii, C.; Ianniello, S.; et al. Increase in tuberculosis diagnostic delay during first wave of the COVID-19 Pandemic: Data from an Italian infectious disease referral hospital. *Antibiotics* **2021**, *10*, 272. [CrossRef]
24. Cronin, A.M.; Railey, S.; Fortune, D.; Wegener, D.H.; Davis, J.B. Notes from the Field: Effects of the COVID-19 Response on Tuberculosis Prevention and Control Efforts—United States March-April 2020. *Morb. Mortal. Wkly. Rep.* **2020**, *69*, 971. [CrossRef]
25. Magro, P.; Formenti, B.; Marchese, V.; Gulletta, M.; Tomasoni, L.R.; Caligaris, S.; Castelli, F.; Matteelli, A. Impact of the SARS-CoV-2 epidemic on tuberculosis treatment outcome in Northern Italy. *Eur. Respir. J.* **2020**, *56*, 2002665. [CrossRef] [PubMed]
26. Zumla, A.; McHugh, B.; Maeurer, M.; Zumla, A.; Kapata, N. COVID-19 and tuberculosis—Threats and opportunities. *Int. J. Tuberc. Lung Dis.* **2020**, *24*, 18–25. [CrossRef] [PubMed]
27. Louie, J.K.; Reid, M.; Stella, J.; Agraz-Lara, R.; Graves, S.; Chen, L.; Hopewell, P. A decrease in tuberculosis evaluations and diagnoses during the COVID-19 pandemic. *Int. J. Tuberc. Lung Dis.* **2020**, *24*, 860–862. [CrossRef] [PubMed]
28. Datiko, D.G.; Jerene, D.; Suarez, P. Patient and health system delay among TB patients in Ethiopia: Nationwide mixed method cross-sectional study. *BMC Public Health* **2020**, *20*, 1126. [CrossRef] [PubMed]

Disclaimer/Publisher's Note: The statements, opinions and data contained in all publications are solely those of the individual author(s) and contributor(s) and not of MDPI and/or the editor(s). MDPI and/or the editor(s) disclaim responsibility for any injury to people or property resulting from any ideas, methods, instructions or products referred to in the content.

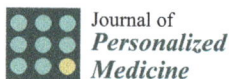

Systematic Review

The Use of Artificial Intelligence Algorithms in the Prognosis and Detection of Lymph Node Involvement in Head and Neck Cancer and Possible Impact in the Development of Personalized Therapeutic Strategy: A Systematic Review

Luca Michelutti [1,†], Alessandro Tel [1,†], Marco Zeppieri [2,*], Tamara Ius [3], Salvatore Sembronio [1] and Massimo Robiony [1]

1. Clinic of Maxillofacial Surgery, Head-Neck and NeuroScience Department, University Hospital of Udine, p.le S. Maria della Misericordia 15, 33100 Udine, Italy; alessandro.tel@asufc.sanita.fvg.it (A.T.)
2. Department of Ophthalmology, University Hospital of Udine, Piazzale S. Maria della Misericordia 15, 33100 Udine, Italy
3. Neurosurgery Unit, Head-Neck and NeuroScience Department, University Hospital of Udine, p.le S. Maria della Misericordia 15, 33100 Udine, Italy
* Correspondence: markzeppieri@hotmail.com
† These authors contributed equally to this work, shared first authorship.

Abstract: Given the increasingly important role that the use of artificial intelligence algorithms is taking on in the medical field today (especially in oncology), the purpose of this systematic review is to analyze the main reports on such algorithms applied for the prognostic evaluation of patients with head and neck malignancies. The objective of this paper is to examine the currently available literature in the field of artificial intelligence applied to head and neck oncology, particularly in the prognostic evaluation of the patient with this kind of tumor, by means of a systematic review. The paper exposes an overview of the applications of artificial intelligence in deriving prognostic information related to the prediction of survival and recurrence and how these data may have a potential impact on the choice of therapeutic strategy, making it increasingly personalized. This systematic review was written following the PRISMA 2020 guidelines.

Keywords: machine learning; deep learning; artificial intelligence; oral cancer; head and neck cancer; prognosis; therapy; follow-up; recurrence; maxillofacial surgery

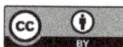

1. Introduction

Artificial intelligence in recent years has spread to all fields, from socio-economic to health care. The purpose of this systematic review is to propose an overview of the applications of artificial intelligence algorithms in oncology in head and neck cancer patients and to focus on the assessment of lymph node status through these new technological tools.

Head and neck cancer represents the sixth most common cancer in the world, with about 630,000 new patients diagnosed each year and more than 350,000 deaths each year. They are lethal cancers that have a high rate of metastasis and recurrence [1,2]. The application of artificial intelligence algorithms can potentially be one of many new tools at our disposal to better manage this disease [3,4]. There are already several recent studies that have investigated the application of artificial intelligence in the assessment of oncological outcomes, such as the study conducted by Chinnery et al. (2021) that evaluated different prognostic prediction models through the application of artificial intelligence and radiomics, demonstrating how these tools may have potential application in the clinical setting (although further studies are needed regarding the creation of standardized protocols) [5].

When we talk about artificial intelligence, we refer to a branch of computer science that deals with creating algorithms tasked with performing tasks traditionally performed by human intelligence. Machine learning (ML) is within this branch; it is a subset of artificial intelligence that allows computers to learn through data input. In addition to ML, there is also deep learning (DL), which is a subset of artificial neural networks that fall into the group of artificial intelligence and function by mimicking the functioning of the neural networks in our brains [3].

The use of artificial intelligence algorithms (in the analysis of clinical, epidemiologic, radiomic, histologic, and genomic data) in the field of oncology is proving to be a potential tool for the study of pathogenetic mechanisms, diagnosis, prediction of malignant transformation of precancerous lesions, and prognostic evaluation, both through the study of known prognostic and predictive factors and through the identification of new ones. Therefore, these computational strategies would enable improved research and prognosis of head and neck cancer [3,6–8].

There have been several studies in the literature that evaluate the clinical applications of these algorithms for the management of head and neck cancer. ML and AI have shown to be useful tools for grading, staging, prognostic evaluation, predicting response to therapy, and deriving information on prognostic endpoints, such as overall survival (OS), through the analysis of radiomic data. A significant and conspicuous source of data being analyzed by these machine learning and deep learning algorithms is imaging (e.g., CT, MRI, and PET images) [4,9].

Given that imaging data are an important source of information, the use of machine learning in the analysis of radiomic data can have the goal of creating models that reflect the genesis and evolution of head and neck cancer. Thanks to radiomics, quantitative features can be extracted from conventional medical images and combined with other data, such as molecular biomarkers or clinical data, to assess tumor status more accurately with positive repercussions on diagnosis and therapy, with the latter being increasingly personalized [10].

Prognostic evaluation is critical, as this has a significant impact on the choice of therapeutic strategy. The aim of this systematic review is to provide an overview of the applications of artificial intelligence algorithms in the prognostic evaluation of head and neck cancer patients; in particular, the creation of prognostic models and their impact on the therapeutic strategy. Considering that more than 65% of patients with squamous cell head and neck cancer have recurrent or metastatic disease [11], we understand how crucial it is to have at our disposal innovative tools that can best predict the patient's prognosis and to identify those patients who present greater risk of recurrence and thus would benefit from a particular treatment compared with the standard treatment.

We also decided to focus on the evaluation and prediction of lymph node status as a prognostic factor. Lymph node metastasis is the main way of dissemination of head and neck carcinoma, and its presence has a substantial impact on the prognosis and consequent therapy [12].

2. Materials and Methods

This study was conducted according to the preferred reporting items for systematic review and meta-analyses (PRISMA) statement [13]. The PRISMA checklist is reported in the Supplementary Materials.

The research question of this systematic review was built according to the PICOS framework (participant, interventions, comparators, outcomes, and study design) (Table 1) and can be summarized as follows: "Does artificial intelligence algorithm-mediated prognostic evaluation of head and neck cancer patients provide useful data to improve and personalize therapeutic strategy?".

Table 1. PICOS framework.

Participant	Patients with head and neck cancer that have already been diagnosed.
Interventions	Evaluation of prognostic factors using artificial intelligence algorithms.
Comparators	Comparison to other artificial intelligence algorithms or the same algorithm but with different types of data processing or prognostic models based on clinical pathological data (e.g., TNM staging).
Outcomes	Recurrence-free survival, distant metastasis-free survival, loco-regional failure, overall survival, tumor-related death, and disease-free survival.
Study design	Clinical trials, randomized clinical trials, cohort studies, research articles, and original articles

This review was registered in the PROSPERO database (International Prospective Register of Systematic Reviews; ID number 474750).

2.1. Literature Search

The literature search was performed in accordance with the PICOS framework (Table 1); specifically, the items "participants" and "outcome" were used to compose the query. The query used was: ((artificial intelligence) OR (machine learning) OR (deep learning)) AND ((oral cancer) OR (head and neck cancer) OR (OSCC) OR (mouth neoplasm)). Using combinations of keywords, the literature search was conducted until 29 September 2023 by consulting the following medical literature databases: MEDLINE, Cochrane Central Register of Controlled Trials (CENTRAL), ClinicalTrials.gov, ScienceDirect, Embase, Scopus, and CINAHL.

For database searching, filters were applied to select English-only articles conducted on human species with publication dates between 2013 and 2023. The selected articles were clinical trials, randomized clinical trials, cohort studies, original articles, and research articles.

After a primary search, the articles were imported into EndNote21 (Clarivate, Analytics, Philadelphia, PA, USA), and all saved articles were screened by two independent investigators (L.M. and A.T.) through an evaluation of the title and abstract, as reported in the PRISMA flowchart (Figure 1). In case of doubts or disagreements between the two investigators, a third independent investigator (M.R.) was involved.

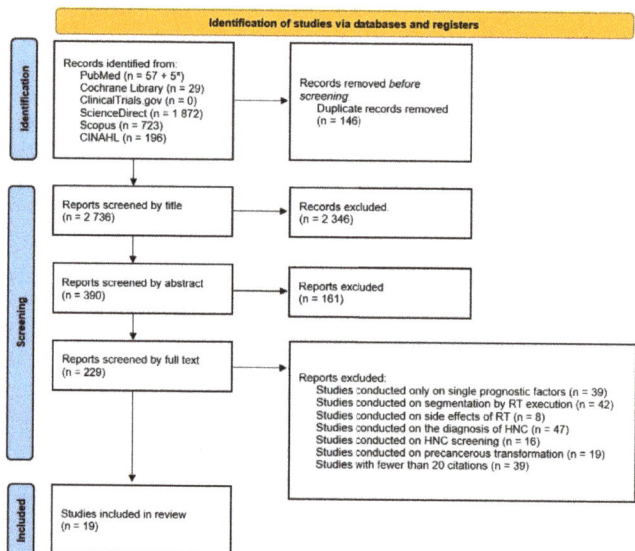

Figure 1. PRISMA flowchart of the systematic review process. * The first number indicates the results obtained via the keywords, while the second number refers to results identified via MeSH.

2.2. Inclusion and Exclusion Criteria

The two independent investigators (L.M.) and (A.T.) applied the following inclusion and exclusion criteria by first evaluating the title of the collected studies, then the abstract, and finally, for the remaining studies, by reading the full text. Non-randomized and randomized clinical trials, cohort studies, original articles, and research articles published from 2013 to 2023 in English only and performed on humans were included. From the results obtained from the database search, all studies dealing with artificial intelligence applied for head and neck cancer diagnosis and screening, detection and prediction of transformation of potentially malignant lesions, and segmentation used for radiotherapy planning were not considered. In addition, review articles and meta-analyses were not considered. Studies for which an abstract was not available were also excluded. Studies conducted on single prognostic factors were removed, except for those that evaluated the application of artificial intelligence for the assessment and prediction of lymph node status. Studies with fewer than 20 citations were removed.

To summarize the studies included in this review, they were grouped into two categories based on the type of topic (Table 2):

1. Prognostic models (n = 11).
2. Diagnosis and prediction of lymph node status (n = 8).

The first group included studies evaluating the efficacy of prognostic models based on artificial intelligence algorithms and studies demonstrating how these prognostic models can have a significant impact on patients' treatment strategy, while the second group included studies evaluating the efficacy of artificial intelligence algorithms in assessing lymph node metastasis, diagnosing and predicting extracapsular lymph node extent, and predicting lymph node metastasis.

Table 2. Breakdown of selected articles by topic.

Main Groups	Topics
1. Prognostic models (n = 11)	a. Creation of prognostic models (n = 9);
	b. Example of prognostic models with the ability to guide therapeutic choice (n = 2).
2. Diagnosis and prediction of lymph node status (n = 8)	a. Diagnosis of lymph node metastasis (n = 1);
	b. Diagnosis and prediction of extracapsular lymph node extension (n = 3);
	c. Prediction of lymph node metastasis (n = 4).

2.3. Data Collection

From the selected studies, the following data were extracted: study topic, study objective, endpoints examined, number of patients examined, treatment of patients examined, type of tumor examined (oral squamous cell carcinoma, oropharyngeal carcinoma, hypopharyngeal carcinoma, nasopharyngeal carcinoma, or laryngeal carcinoma), data analyzed to create the algorithm (clinical, pathological, imaging, or genetic/molecular data), the algorithm used (ML or DL), comparison (to other artificial intelligence algorithms or prognostic models based on clinical/histologic data such as TNM staging), and the summary of results obtained.

Data were manually extracted by the two independent researchers (L.M. and A.T.) and collected in a Microsoft Excel spreadsheet. This information was then displayed in Table 3; Table 4 in the Section 3.

2.4. Bias Assessment

The risk of bias was assessed by the two independent investigators (L.M.) and (A.T.) using the Robvis tool [14]. Five types of bias were assessed: bias arising from the randomization process, bias due to deviations from the intended interventions, bias due to missing outcome data, bias in outcome measurement, and bias in reported outcome selection (Figures 2 and 3).

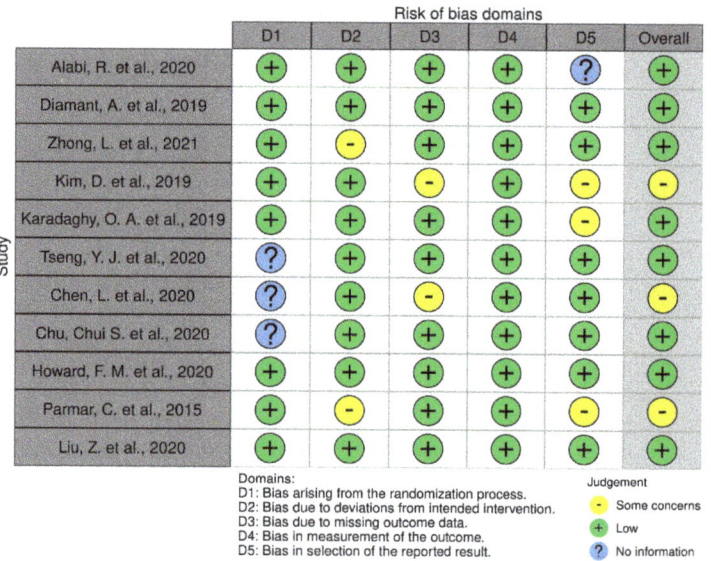

Figure 2. Robvis tool for assessing the risk of bias in studies concerning prognostic models.

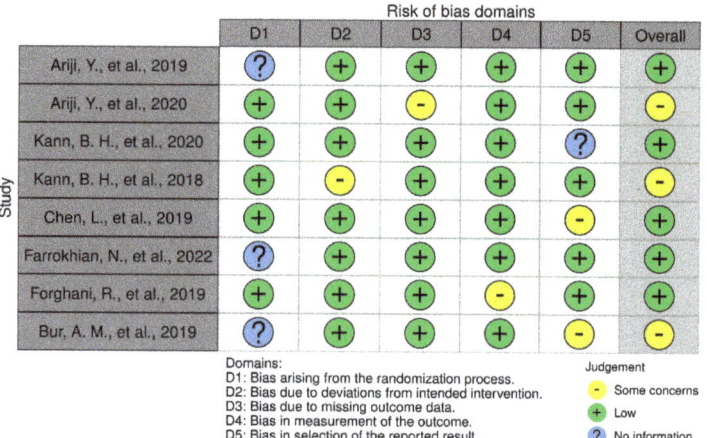

Figure 3. Robvis tool for assessing the risk of bias in studies concerning evaluation and prediction of lymph node status.

3. Results

Figure 2 shows the PRISMA flowchart describing the study selection process. Using a combination of keywords, the investigators retrieved 2882 studies. All articles were imported into EndNote. After identifying duplicates, 146 studies were removed. The remaining 2736 were screened by title, with the removal of 2346 papers. Subsequent screening by abstract led to the exclusion of an additional 161 reports. The full texts of 229 studies were read and, following the application of the inclusion and exclusion criteria, 19 studies were included in this systematic review.

Of the 19 selected studies, we assessed the risk of bias using the Robvis tool [14]; 11 articles concerning prognostic models are shown in Figure 2, and 8 articles concerning lymph node status assessment are shown in Figure 3.

The included studies were grouped into two groups based on the type of topic addressed (Table 2): "prognostic models" and "evaluation and prediction of lymph node status". The following data were collected for prognostic models (as summarized in Table 3) and for lymph node status assessment (as summarized in Table 4): study topic, study objective, endpoints examined, number of patients examined, treatment of patients examined, type of tumor examined (oral squamous cell carcinoma, oropharyngeal carcinoma, hypopharyngeal carcinoma, nasopharyngeal carcinoma, or laryngeal carcinoma), data analyzed to create the algorithm (clinical, pathological, imaging, or genetic/molecular data), algorithm used (machine learning or deep learning), comparison (to other artificial intelligence algorithms or prognostic models based on clinical/histologic data such as TNM staging), and summary of results obtained.

3.1. Prognostic Models (Table 3)

Several studies demonstrated that they succeeded in developing prognostic models capable of assessing parameters, such as overall survival (OS) and disease-free survival (DFS), by processing clinical, imaging, histopathological, and/or genomic data.

3.1.1. Endpoint

Analyzing the data collected and summarized in Table 3, the following endpoints were evaluated from these studies: recurrence-free survival, distant metastasis-free survival, loco-regional failure, overall survival, tumor-related death, and disease-free survival. This demonstrates the broad ability of these algorithms to evaluate multiple prognostic endpoints.

3.1.2. Data Analyzed

The data processed by the different artificial intelligence algorithms to obtain these prognostic results are also varied: about 73% of the studies analyze clinical data, 64% clinical/pathological data (age, sex, grading, depth of invasion, perineural invasion, lymph/vascular invasion, tumor budding, bone marrow invasion, persistence of tumor at resection margin, extranodal extension, tumor site), 36% analyze treatments already performed on the patient (radiotherapy, chemotherapy, adjuvant CT-RT, concomitant CT-RT, cervical dissection, surgical resection of primary tumor), 45% analyze imaging data with radiomic processing and patterns (CT images, CT with contrast medium, MRI, PET, PET-TC), 18% analyze socio-demographic data, and 9% analyze genetic data. All this information is not simply processed as individual data but is integrated because of the ability of artificial intelligence algorithms to do so. In fact, as the study conducted by Tseng, Y.J. et al. (2020) [15] shows, the integration of genetic data together with clinical/pathological data goes a long way toward improving the performance of the prognostic model in assessing recurrence-free survival (endpoint examined by this study).

3.1.3. Types of Head and Neck Tumors Studied

The tumors analyzed are oral squamous cell carcinoma (addressed in 64% of the selected studies), oropharyngeal carcinoma (in 36%), hypopharyngeal carcinoma (in 27%), nasopharyngeal carcinoma (in 18%), and laryngeal carcinoma (in 45%).

3.1.4. Artificial Intelligence Algorithms

The algorithms employed in the different studies are various, from ML models to DL models to convolutional neural networks. These models once developed are trained with data from the training cohort (training set) and then validated (analyzing the processing by these models of data from the validation cohort (testing set). They are then compared either to other artificial intelligence algorithms or to prognostic models based on clinical/pathological data (such as TNM staging or DOI (depth of invasion)). For instance, in the Alabi study (R. et al. (2020) [16]), a first comparison is made between several different types of artificial intelligibility algorithms to assess which one has better performance and to compare the most accurate model to that obtained from the DOI (depth of invasion) study.

A total of 64% of the studies reported in Table 3 evaluate the application of ML algorithms for prognostic modeling, while 36% analyze applications of DL.

The algorithms used in the selected studies are: support vector machine (SVM), naïve Bayes (NB), boosted decision tree (BDT), decision forest (DF), convolutional neural network (CNN), random forest (RF), random survival forest (RSF), linear regression (LR), decision tree (DT), support vector machine (SVM), k-nearest neighbors (KNN), bagging (BAG), Bayesian (BY), boosting (BST), decision Tree (DT), generalized linear models (GLM), multiple adaptive regression splines (MARS), nearest neighbors, neural network (Nnet), and partial least square and principle component regression (PLSR).

3.1.5. Comparison

About 27% of the studies reported in Table 3 compare artificial intelligence algorithms to prognostic models based solely on the study of staging or other clinical/histologic parameters such as DOI (depth of invasion). About 36% of the reported studies compare the performance of different types of prognostic algorithms in processing the same data, while 18% of the studies compare the same algorithm in processing different data. There are several studies in the current literature that analyze the use of certain artificial intelligence algorithms but without performing a comparison, evaluating only their performance in deriving prognostic data (about 27% of the reported studies).

Table 3. Studies evaluating the effectiveness of prognostic models based on artificial intelligence algorithms.

	Endpoint Analyzed	Objective of the Study	Tumor Type Examined	Data Analyzed	Algorithm Used	Results
Alabi et al., 2020 [16]	Risk of recurrences in early stage	Evaluation of 4 ML algorithms in the prediction of loco-regional recurrence risk	OTSCC	Clinical/pathological data and treatment given.	ML: 4 ML algorithms (SVM, NB, BDT, DF)	BDT proved to be the best among the 4 algorithms and was then compared to a DOI-based prognostic model. Using the DOI model, only 49.5% of the examinees were correctly identified as having recidivism, while the BDT correctly recognized 78.9% as having recidivism.
Diamant et al., 2019 [17]	Risk of distant metastasis, loco-regional failure, overall survival (OS)	Compare traditional radiomic framework to CNN algorithm for predicting treatment outcomes	OPC, HPC, NPC, and LC	CT images pre-treatment	DL: CNN	The use of a single end-to-end CNN trained de novo (without secondary automatic learning algorithms) predicts oncology outcomes better than "traditional radiomics", i.e., an approach in which an automatic learning algorithm such as random forest is used.
Kim et al., 2019 [18]	Risk of loco-regional recurrence and tumor-related death	Comparison of CPH model, RSF and DeepSurv	OSCC	Clinical/pathological data and treatment (postoperative radiation therapy, postoperative CCRT)	DL: DeepSurv	DeepSurv (DL) shows better performance among the three models (CPH, RSF, and DeepSurv) in prognostic evaluation and derivation of the following endpoints: risk of loco-regional recurrence and tumor-related death.
Karadaghy et al., 2019 [19]	Overall survival (OS)	Develop a prediction model using ML and compare it to a prediction model created by the TNM stage	OSCC	Clinical/pathological and socio-demographic data	ML: 2-class DF architecture	ML algorithm proves to have greater accuracy and precision than TNM-based model for 5-year OS assessment.
Tseng et al., 2020 [15]	Cancer-specific survival, loco-regional recurrence-free survival, distant metastasis-free survival	Develop a risk stratification model and compare the performance of the same ML algorithm but with different data processing.	OSCC	Clinical, pathological, and genetics data	ML: EN (model based on both clinical/pathological and genetic data)	In postoperative patients treated with adjuvant CCRT, the model that also included genetic data improved the prediction of loco-regional recurrence-free survival compared with the model that did not include genetic data.

Table 3. Cont.

	Endpoint Analyzed	Objective of the Study	Tumor Type Examined	Data Analyzed	Algorithm Used	Results
Chen et al., 2020 [20]	Overall survival (OS)	Assess the prognostic value of radiomic signature and nomogram based on CT with contrast	LC	CT with contrast enhancement, clinical/pathological data	ML: Radiomic nomogram	Radiomic nomogram manages to discriminate better than cancer staging in the training cohort and validation cohort
Chu et al., 2020 [21]	Risk of loco-regional recurrence and distant metastasis	Evaluation of ML algorithms to improve prediction of clinical outcomes	OSCC	Clinical/pathological data, cervical lymph node dissection, and/or adjuvant CT-RT regimens	ML: LR, DT, SVM, KNN	The DT model was better in identifying progressive disease by analyzing the risk of local recurrence and distant metastasis.
Parmar et al., 2015 [22]	OS	Evaluation, in terms of OS prediction and ML classification methods	OPC and LC	CT images	ML: BAG, BY, BST, DT, GLM, MARS, NN, Nnet, PLSR, RF, SVM	Through AUC, the prognostic performance of different ML methods and the feasibility of these algorithms in deriving the patient's overall survival (OS) by processing imaging data (CT images) was evaluated.
Liu et al., 2020 [23]	OS and DFS	Assessing the prediction of OS and DFS through the use of models based on radiomic signatures	OPC, LC, HPC, and OSCC	18F-PET/CT pre- and posttreatment	ML: Model with clinicopathological + radiomic data	Combining clinicopathologic and radiologic data substantially improves the prediction of OS and DFS compared with models that analyze only clinicopathologic data.
Zhong et al., 2021 [24]	Predicting the prognosis of patients with NPC with different optimal treatment regimens with DFS as the primary endpoint	Development of a DL-based model for treatment decision making by comparing CPTDN to 3 clinical models (the first based on all patients, the second only on those who received CCRT, and the third on those who received ICT + CCRT.	NPC	MR images pretreatment and clinical factors	CPTDN based on a shared backbone Nnet and two subnetworks to simultaneously predict prognosis and treatment response	Excellent prognostic ability for DFS in both the group receiving CCRT and the group receiving ICT + CCRT. Based on the prognostic difference between the two types of treatments, patients were divided into two groups: preferential ICT and preferential CCRT. In the first group, patients who received ICT + CCRT had better DFS than those who received CCRT. In the second group, however, the opposite trend occurred.

Table 3. Cont.

Endpoint Analyzed	Objective of the Study	Tumor Type Examined	Data Analyzed	Algorithm Used	Results
Howard et al., 2020 [25] OS associated with treatment according to model recommendations	Identify patients with intermediate risk head and neck cancer who would benefit from adjuvant chemotherapy	OSCC, OPC, HPC, and LC	Demographic, clinical/pathological data, treatment (chemotherapy performance, radiation dose)	DL: DS, NMLR, and SF models	The 3 DL models recommended CT-RT in 44–52% of the cases examined. It was shown to have the potential for stratifying patients and selecting those who would need trimodal therapy (and excluding those who would not need this treatment approach, avoiding possible complications related to chemotherapy and RT).

Shown in blue are the two studies that represent an example of how these prognostic models may impact the choice of therapeutic strategy. Legends: AUC—area under the curve; BAG—bagging; BY—Bayesian; BDT—boosted decision tree; BST—boosting; CCRT—concurrent chemoradiotherapy; CNN: convolutional neural networks; CPH: Cox proportional hazards model; CPTDN: combined prognosis and treatment decision nomogram; CT: computed tomography; CT-RT—chemotherapy–radiotherapy; DOI—depth of invasion; DL—deep learning; DF—decision forest; DFS—disease free survival; DS—DeepSurv; DT—decision tree; EN—elastic net; GLM—generalized linear models; HPC—hypopharyngeal cancer; ICT—induction chemotherapy; KNN—k-nearest neighbors; LC—laryngeal cancer; LR—linear regression; ML: machine learning; MARS: Multiple adaptive regression splines; NB: Naïve Bayes; NMLR: neural multitasking logistic regression; NN: Nearest neighbors; Nnet—neural networks; NPC—nasopharyngeal carcinoma; OPC—oropharyngeal cancer; OS—overall survival; OSCC—oral squamous cell carcinoma; OTSCC—oral tongue squamous cell carcinoma; PET—positron emission tomography; PLSR—partial least square and principle component regression; RF—random forest; RSF—random survival forest; RT—radiotherapy; MR—magnetic resonance; SF—survival forest; SVM—support vector machine.

3.1.6. Evaluation of Prognostic Endpoint

The application of ML and DL algorithms have proven to be very useful in evaluating different types of endpoints, including recurrence-free survival, distant metastasis-free survival, loco-regional failure, overall survival, tumor-related death, and disease-free survival.

The study conducted by Alabi et al. (2020) [16] compared the performance of four different types of ML algorithms (support vector machine, naïve Bayes, boosted decision tree, and decision forest) in deriving the risk of recurrence in patients with oral tongue squamous cell carcinoma by processing clinical/pathological data. The algorithm that proved best among the four, namely the boosted decision tree (BDT), was then compared to a prognostic model based solely on DOI (depth of invasion). This study showed how the DOI model correctly identified only 49.5 percent of patients with recurrence, while the ML model (the BDT) recognized 78.9 percent, demonstrating greater accuracy. Another study demonstrated how artificial intelligence algorithms were more effective in assessing the overall survival of five patients with oral squamous cell carcinoma (OSCC), namely the study conducted by Karadaghy et al. (2019) [19]. This study compared an ML algorithm to a prognostic model obtained through TNM staging, demonstrating how the former had greater accuracy and precision than the latter in calculating overall survival.

As mentioned earlier, studies comparing the same type of diagnostic algorithm but with different data processing were included. The study conducted by Liu et al. (2020) [23] showed that processing by the same ML algorithm of both clinical/pathological data together with radiomic data obtained from PET/CT scans was better in predicting overall survival (OS) and disease-free survival (DFS) than processing clinical data alone in a patient with oropharyngeal, laryngeal, hypopharyngeal, and oral cavity cancer. The study conducted by Tseng et al. (2020) [15] showed that processing both clinical data and genetic data, again performed by the same ML algorithm, was better in predicting cancer-specific survival, loco-regional recurrence-free survival, and distant metastasis-free survival than processing only clinical/pathological data in patients with oral squamous cell carcinoma.

In contrast, the study conducted by Diamant et al. (2019) [17], which examined patients with oropharyngeal, hypopharyngeal, nasopharyngeal, and laryngeal cancer, showed how the DL algorithm (the convolutional neural network) performed better than the ML (random forest) algorithm in calculating the risk of distant metastasis (DM), loco-regional failure (LRF), and overall survival (OS) by analysis of CT images performed during presurgical treatment.

3.2. Diagnosis and Prediction of Lymph Node Status (Table 4)

Knowing the lymph node status is crucial in the management of a patient with a head/neck tumor. The following studies have been divided into three parts:
1. Studies on the "Assessment of cervical lymph node metastasis";
2. Studies on the "Diagnosis and prediction of ENE (extranodal extension)";
3. Studies on "Prediction of lymph node metastasis".

3.2.1. Topics

The topics of these studies are to develop models based on artificial intelligence in order to perform more precise diagnoses and evaluation of lymph node metastasis, to diagnose and predict the occurrence of extranodal extension (ENE), and to predict the occurrence of lymph node metastasis.

3.2.2. Data Analyzed

The data analyzed for the evaluation of these prognostic models are mostly radiomic in nature: 75% of the selected studies present imaging data for the creation and validation of machine learning and deep learning algorithms, while the remaining 25% exploit clinical/pathological data. Particularly, of that 75%, data come from CT scans (66%), PET-CT (17%), and DECT dual-energy CT (17%).

3.2.3. Type of Head and Neck Tumors Studied

The tumors analyzed are oral squamous cell carcinoma (addressed in 87% of the selected studies), oropharyngeal carcinoma (50%), hypopharyngeal carcinoma (37%), nasopharyngeal carcinoma (25%), and laryngeal carcinoma (50%).

3.2.4. Comparison

A total of 37.5% of the studies reported in Table 4 compare the performance of artificial intelligence algorithms to the analytical ability of professional radiologists (in studies in which the data to be analyzed are CT images), 37.5% of the studies compare these algorithms to models based on the study of clinical/pathological factors (such as DOI), 12.5% of the studies compare different types of algorithms to the same types of data processed, and another 12.5% of the studies reported compare the performance of the same algorithms but with different data processing.

Table 4. Studies evaluating assessment and prediction of lymph node status.

	Topics	Objective of the Study	Tumor Type Examined	Data Analyzed	Algorithm Used	Results
Ariji et al., 2019 [26]	Assessment of cervical lymph node metastasis	Evaluation of DL performance for diagnosis of lymph node metastasis	OSCC	CT images	DL	The results obtained by DL models are similar to those obtained by experienced radiologists in terms of accuracy, sensitivity, specificity, and positive and negative predictive value. This indicates the reliability of these algorithms in the diagnosis of lymph node metastasis and their potential use as an aid tool for radiologists.
Ariji et al., 2020 [27]	Diagnosis and prediction of ENE	Clarifying the diagnostic performance of CT in ENE by applying DL algorithms	OSCC	CT images	DL	The diagnostic performance of the DL is superior to that obtained by radiologists.
Kann et al., 2020 [28]	Diagnosis and prediction of ENE	Evaluation of the application of DL algorithms in the pretreatment identification of ENEs	OPC, LC, HPC, NPC, OSCC	Contrast-enhanced CT scans	DL	The DL algorithm achieved higher AUC values than those obtained by the two radiologists. Implementation of these DL algorithms in a radiologist's work would provide increased AUC and sensitivity.
Kann et al., 2018 [29]	Diagnosis and prediction of ENE	Evaluation of the application of DL algorithms in the prediction of lymph node metastasis and ENE	OPC, LC, HPC, NPC, OSCC	CT images	DL	In the testing set, DL predicted ENE and lymph node metastasis with an AUC of 0.91, while the logistic regression model (based on clinical risk factors and lymph node ROI diameter) obtained an AUC of 0.81.
Chen et al., 2019 [30]	Prediction of lymph node metastasis	Evaluation of an automatic prediction model for lymph node metastasis	OPC and LC	CT-PET images pretreatment	"Hybrid" predictive model based on radiomics and DL strategies (fusion of MaO-radiomics and 3D-CNN)	Hybrid model achieved higher accuracy than XmasNet and radiomics models.
Farrokhian et al., 2022 [31]	Prediction of lymph node metastasis	Evaluation of an ML model for prediction of occult early-stage lymph node metastasis	OSCC	Clinical/pathological data (obtained after surgical resection of the primary tumor)	ML	The ML predictive model outperformed the DOI-based model in terms of AUC, sensitivity, specificity, and positive and negative predictive value.

Table 4. *Cont.*

Topics	Objective of the Study	Tumor Type Examined	Data Analyzed	Algorithm Used	Results
Forghani et al., 2019 [32]	Prediction of lymph node metastasis	Development and evaluation of risk stratification model by dual-energy texture analysis (DECT) by ML to predict lymphadenopathy	OPC, HPC, LC, OSCC	Dual-energy by texture analysis (DECT)	ML (RF patterns)	The application of an ML algorithm in the analysis of multi-energy DECT textures has been shown to be superior in predicting lymph node metastasis compared with models based solely on single-energy CT.
Bur et al. 2019 [33]	Prediction of lymph node metastasis	Development and evaluation of an ML algorithm to predict lymph node metastasis	OSCC	Clinical/pathological data	ML (DF algorithm)	The decision forest algorithm outperformed the performance achieved by the DOI model in the external test.

Studies dealing with the diagnosis of lymph node metastasis are shown in yellow, those dealing with the prediction of lymph node metastasis are shown in blue, and those dealing with the prediction of extranodal extension (ENE) are shown in green. Legends: AUC—area under the curve; CT—computed tomography; CNN—convolutional neural net; DECT—dual-energy computed tomography; DF—decision forest; DL—depth learning; DOI—deep of invasion; ENE—extranodal extension; HPC—hypopharyngeal cancer; LC—laryngeal cancer; ML—machine learning; NPC—nasopharyngeal cancer; OPC—oropharyngeal cancer; OSCC—oral squamous cell carcinoma; RF—random forest.

3.2.5. Lymph Node Status Assessment

Artificial intelligence algorithms have proven to be especially useful in diagnosing and predicting lymph node metastasis and predicting extranodal extension (a very important prognostic factor that severely impacts a patient's prognosis). The study conducted by Ariji et al. (2019) [26] investigated the ability of DL to diagnose lymph node metastasis in patients with oral squamous cell carcinoma through CT image processing. The results obtained were then compared to those of two experienced radiologists. It was shown that the results obtained by the DL models were similar to those obtained by the two radiologists in terms of accuracy, sensitivity, and specificity, emphasizing how these algorithms can be useful tools to be used in the work of radiologists.

On the subject of extranodal extension, the study conducted by Ariji et al. (2020) [27] instead examined the ability of DL algorithms to diagnose the presence of ENE in patients with oral squamous cell carcinoma. The performance of these algorithms was shown to be superior to that of three radiologists who were tasked with reviewing the same CT images. In contrast, the study conducted by Kann et al. (2018) [29] focused on evaluating the ability of DL algorithms in predicting ENE in patients with oropharyngeal, laryngeal, hypopharyngeal, nasopharyngeal, and oral cavity cancer. The DL model was compared to a regression model of clinical risk factors and diagnostic controls performed by radiologists, showing that the application of the DL algorithm achieved superior performance in predicting both ENE and lymph node metastasis.

Regarding the prediction of lymph node metastasis, another study also demonstrated interesting results. The study by Farrokhian et al. (2022) [31] compared the performance of an ML algorithm to that of a model that relied solely on DOI (depth of invasion) assessment, showing how the predictive ML model was better in terms of AUC (area under the curve), sensitivity, and specificity.

4. Discussion

As stated in the introduction, the purpose of this paper is to provide an overview of the potential performance of artificial intelligence as applied in the prognostic evaluation of head and neck cancer patients, particularly in prognostic modeling, clinical endpoint assessment, and lymph node status assessment.

When the clinician assesses the prognosis of the cancer patient, several prognostic factors are assessed through the study of the clinical, imaging, and histologic report and the possible presence of certain molecular alterations that, in addition to having prognostic significance, may add predictive value to the use of certain treatments. We understand how precisely knowing the patient's prognosis allows for the best management of the disease with proper therapy and follow-up.

The application of artificial intelligence algorithms is proving useful for this purpose because of their ability to process information in a way that the human mind alone cannot. Studies demonstrating the validity of ML for predicting treatment outcomes in cancers such as prostate and breast cancer have been published for some time now [34].

There are recent studies demonstrating how the application of artificial intelligence algorithms can be a useful tool for outcome prediction in patients with head and neck cancer, such as the study conducted by Chinnery et al. (2021) [5] that demonstrated how the use of these algorithms can be applied in prognostic evaluation through the analysis of imaging data, the study conducted by Adeoye et al. (2021) [35] that demonstrated how these tools have excellent accuracy in predicting both lymph node metastasis and prognosis in the patient with oral cavity cancer, or the study conducted by Zhang et al. (2023) [36] that showed how radiomics can be a means to the clinician's advantage in assessing clinical endpoints.

From the studies we have collected in our review, it can be understood how ML and DL algorithms provide excellent performance in assessing different types of prognostic endpoints (such as, for example, overall survival) and in predicting posttreatment outcomes, demonstrating how they can be an essential tool to better personalize therapy. The application of these algorithms has demonstrated greater accuracy both in terms of AUC (area under the curve) and in terms of specificity and sensitivity than models commonly used in clinical practice for prognostic evaluation, such as prognostic models based on TNM staging or DOI (depth of invasion). Moreover, by being able to process multiple types of information (clinical, radiological, histological, and molecular data), together these tools have demonstrated a greater ability to stratify patients according to their prognosis by even being able to identify which subgroups of patients with the same tumor and stage would benefit from specific treatments and which would not. In this regard, the study conducted by Howard et al. (2020) [25] (that we include in our review) demonstrated how different DL algorithms (DeepSurv, neural multitasking logistic regression, and survival forest) were able, through the analysis of demographics and clinical/pathological data and according to the type of treatment received, to stratify patients with early-stage head and neck cancer into different subgroups, identifying those who would receive a benefit from adding adjuvant chemotherapy to surgical treatment. This has a major impact on the lives of patients, as it means more aggressive treatments against early-stage cancer in those who have a higher risk of recurrence and metastasis, while sparing those who would not benefit from such treatments from the side effects of chemotherapy and radiotherapy (mucositis, osteonecrosis, dermatitis, dysphagia, and many others) [37–39].

Studies conducted on lymph node metastasis prediction also prove to be useful for patient stratification and therapy personalization, such as the study conducted by Farrokhian et al. (2022) [31] that examined the application of ML in lymph node metastasis prediction and demonstrated how it is superior to the DOI (depth of invasion)-based prognostic model, succeeding in selecting which patients with early-stage head and neck cancer would benefit from cervical lymph node dissection. Thus, artificial intelligence algorithms prove to be much more accurate in predicting lymph node metastasis and extranodal extension (ENE) than assessments conducted by DOI (depth of invasion)-based models. For the diagnosis of lymph node metastasis, through the study of radiologic images, we have observed how these algorithms perform the same if not in some cases even better than those of experienced radiologists. This shows, in our opinion, how these algorithms can be considered reliable and how they can be used as an auxiliary tool for the clinician in tumor assessment.

However, we must emphasize some aspects that we consider limiting. Although these algorithms show excellent performance in prognostic evaluation, further studies are needed to have a significant impact on clinical practice, especially through the implementation of standardized protocols. Ther are numerous studies addressing the issue of head and neck cancer prognosis, but not all of them analyze the same algorithms and the same types of data (clinical, radiological, histological, and molecular), not to mention the type of treatment received by the patient. Moreover, the fact that there are studies analyzing the same types of prognostic factors for different types of head and neck cancer that could represent a risk, they would neglect the study of prognostic factors that are peculiar only to certain types of cancer, such as HPV positivity. In oropharyngeal cancer, the presence of HPV has a recognized prognostic role, while, for oral squamous cell carcinoma, they recognize this role during prognosis [40,41]. It must also be borne in mind that certain types of data, such as molecular data, cannot be obtained in all hospitals, as not all centers have the required facilities and laboratories.

5. Conclusions

Although more studies and standardized protocols are needed for them to have a significant impact on clinical practice, artificial intelligence algorithms demonstrate excellent performances in predicting outcomes after treatment, evaluating clinical endpoints, and predicting metastasis and recurrence in head and neck cancer patients. These algorithms exhibit better accuracy than commonly used prognostic models such as those that rely on TNM staging or DOI (depth of invasion). The application of ML and DL algorithms in prognostic evaluation has also shown how it is possible to stratify cancer patients with the same tumor and at the same stage into multiple subgroups, identifying which patients would benefit from more aggressive treatments toward the tumor (such as, for example, the trimodal approach of surgery, chemotherapy, and radiotherapy) and who would not, with the aim of avoiding the patient side effects that would result from such an approach. AI is showing great promise. However, prospective clinical trials comparing AI to standard prognostic algorithms are required to evaluate AI as a tool for disease management. We believe that the application of artificial intelligence in the management of oncology patients can play an important role in the medicine of the future.

Supplementary Materials: The following supporting information can be downloaded at: https://www.mdpi.com/article/10.3390/jpm13121626/s1.

Author Contributions: Conceptualization, L.M., A.T. and M.Z.; methodology, L.M., A.T., M.Z., T.I., S.S. and M.R.; software, L.M., and A.T. validation, L.M., A.T., M.Z., T.I., S.S. and M.R.; formal analysis, L.M. and A.T.; investigation, L.M. and A.T.; resources, M.R.; data curation, L.M. and A.T.; writing—original draft preparation, L.M. and A.T.; writing—review and editing, L.M., A.T. and M.Z.; visualization, L.M., A.T., M.Z., T.I., S.S. and M.R.; supervision, M.R.; project administration, M.R.; funding acquisition, M.R. All authors have read and agreed to the published version of the manuscript.

Funding: This research received no external funding.

Conflicts of Interest: The authors declare no conflict of interest.

References

1. Vigneswaran, N.; Williams, M.D. Epidemiologic Trends in Head and Neck Cancer and Aids in Diagnosis. *Oral Maxillofac. Surg. Clin. N. Am.* **2014**, *26*, 123–141. [CrossRef]
2. Bray, F.; Ferlay, J.; Soerjomataram, I.; Siegel, R.L.; Torre, L.A.; Jemal, A. Global Cancer Statistics 2018: GLOBOCAN Estimates of Incidence and Mortality Worldwide for 36 Cancers in 185 Countries. *CA Cancer J. Clin.* **2018**, *68*, 394–424. [CrossRef]
3. Chen, M.M.; Terzic, A.; Becker, A.S.; Johnson, J.M.; Wu, C.C.; Wintermark, M.; Wald, C.; Wu, J. Artificial Intelligence in Oncologic Imaging. *Eur. J. Radiol. Open* **2022**, *9*, 100441. [CrossRef]
4. Abdel Razek, A.A.K.; Khaled, R.; Helmy, E.; Naglah, A.; AbdelKhalek, A.; El-Baz, A. Artificial Intelligence and Deep Learning of Head and Neck Cancer. *Magn. Reson. Imaging Clin. N. Am.* **2022**, *30*, 81–94. [CrossRef]
5. Chinnery, T.; Arifin, A.; Tay, K.Y.; Leung, A.; Nichols, A.C.; Palma, D.A.; Mattonen, S.A.; Lang, P. Utilizing Artificial Intelligence for Head and Neck Cancer Outcomes Prediction From Imaging. *Can. Assoc. Radiol. J.* **2021**, *72*, 73–85. [CrossRef]
6. Mahmood, H.; Shaban, M.; Indave, B.I.; Santos-Silva, A.R.; Rajpoot, N.; Khurram, S.A. Use of Artificial Intelligence in Diagnosis of Head and Neck Precancerous and Cancerous Lesions: A Systematic Review. *Oral Oncol.* **2020**, *110*, 104885. [CrossRef]
7. Resteghini, C.; Trama, A.; Borgonovi, E.; Hosni, H.; Corrao, G.; Orlandi, E.; Calareso, G.; De Cecco, L.; Piazza, C.; Mainardi, L.; et al. Big Data in Head and Neck Cancer. *Curr. Treat. Options Oncol.* **2018**, *19*, 62. [CrossRef]
8. Mäkitie, A.A.; Alabi, R.O.; Ng, S.P.; Takes, R.P.; Robbins, K.T.; Ronen, O.; Shaha, A.R.; Bradley, P.J.; Saba, N.F.; Nuyts, S.; et al. Artificial Intelligence in Head and Neck Cancer: A Systematic Review of Systematic Reviews. *Adv. Ther.* **2023**, *40*, 3360–3380. [CrossRef]
9. Gharavi, S.M.H.; Faghihimehr, A. Clinical Application of Artificial Intelligence in PET Imaging of Head and Neck Cancer. *PET Clin.* **2022**, *17*, 65–76. [CrossRef]
10. Peng, Z.; Wang, Y.; Wang, Y.; Jiang, S.; Fan, R.; Zhang, H.; Jiang, W. Application of Radiomics and Machine Learning in Head and Neck Cancers. *Int. J. Biol. Sci.* **2021**, *17*, 475–486. [CrossRef]
11. Chow, L.Q.M. Head and Neck Cancer. *N. Engl. J. Med.* **2020**, *382*, 60–72. [CrossRef]
12. Karatzanis, A.D.; Koudounarakis, E.; Papadakis, I.; Velegrakis, G. Molecular Pathways of Lymphangiogenesis and Lymph Node Metastasis in Head and Neck Cancer. *Eur. Arch. Otorhinolaryngol.* **2012**, *269*, 731–737. [CrossRef]
13. Page, M.J.; McKenzie, J.E.; Bossuyt, P.M.; Boutron, I.; Hoffmann, T.C.; Mulrow, C.D.; Shamseer, L.; Tetzlaff, J.M.; Akl, E.A.; Brennan, S.E.; et al. The PRISMA 2020 Statement: An Updated Guideline for Reporting Systematic Reviews. *BMJ* **2021**, *372*, n160. [CrossRef]
14. McGuinness, L.A.; Higgins, J.P.T. Risk-of-bias VISualization (Robvis): An R Package and Shiny Web App for Visualizing Risk-of-bias Assessments. *Res. Synth. Methods* **2021**, *12*, 55–61. [CrossRef]
15. Tseng, Y.-J.; Wang, H.-Y.; Lin, T.-W.; Lu, J.-J.; Hsieh, C.-H.; Liao, C.-T. Development of a Machine Learning Model for Survival Risk Stratification of Patients with Advanced Oral Cancer. *JAMA Netw. Open* **2020**, *3*, e2011768. [CrossRef]
16. Alabi, R.O.; Elmusrati, M.; Sawazaki-Calone, I.; Kowalski, L.P.; Haglund, C.; Coletta, R.D.; Mäkitie, A.A.; Salo, T.; Almangush, A.; Leivo, I. Comparison of Supervised Machine Learning Classification Techniques in Prediction of Locoregional Recurrences in Early Oral Tongue Cancer. *Int. J. Med. Inform.* **2020**, *136*, 104068. [CrossRef]

17. Diamant, A.; Chatterjee, A.; Vallières, M.; Shenouda, G.; Seuntjens, J. Deep Learning in Head & Neck Cancer Outcome Prediction. *Sci. Rep.* **2019**, *9*, 2764. [CrossRef]
18. Kim, D.W.; Lee, S.; Kwon, S.; Nam, W.; Cha, I.-H.; Kim, H.J. Deep Learning-Based Survival Prediction of Oral Cancer Patients. *Sci. Rep.* **2019**, *9*, 6994. [CrossRef]
19. Karadaghy, O.A.; Shew, M.; New, J.; Bur, A.M. Development and Assessment of a Machine Learning Model to Help Predict Survival Among Patients with Oral Squamous Cell Carcinoma. *JAMA Otolaryngol. Head Neck Surg.* **2019**, *145*, 1115. [CrossRef]
20. Chen, L.; Wang, H.; Zeng, H.; Zhang, Y.; Ma, X. Evaluation of CT-Based Radiomics Signature and Nomogram as Prognostic Markers in Patients with Laryngeal Squamous Cell Carcinoma. *Cancer Imaging* **2020**, *20*, 28. [CrossRef]
21. Chu, C.S.; Lee, N.P.; Adeoye, J.; Thomson, P.; Choi, S. Machine Learning and Treatment Outcome Prediction for Oral Cancer. *J. Oral. Pathol. Med.* **2020**, *49*, 977–985. [CrossRef]
22. Parmar, C.; Grossmann, P.; Rietveld, D.; Rietbergen, M.M.; Lambin, P.; Aerts, H.J.W.L. Radiomic Machine-Learning Classifiers for Prognostic Biomarkers of Head and Neck Cancer. *Front. Oncol.* **2015**, *5*, 272. [CrossRef]
23. Liu, Z.; Cao, Y.; Diao, W.; Cheng, Y.; Jia, Z.; Peng, X. Radiomics-Based Prediction of Survival in Patients with Head and Neck Squamous Cell Carcinoma Based on Pre- and Post-Treatment 18F-PET/CT. *Aging* **2020**, *12*, 14593–14619. [CrossRef]
24. Zhong, L.; Dong, D.; Fang, X.; Zhang, F.; Zhang, N.; Zhang, L.; Fang, M.; Jiang, W.; Liang, S.; Li, C.; et al. A Deep Learning-Based Radiomic Nomogram for Prognosis and Treatment Decision in Advanced Nasopharyngeal Carcinoma: A Multicentre Study. *EBioMedicine* **2021**, *70*, 103522. [CrossRef]
25. Howard, F.M.; Kochanny, S.; Koshy, M.; Spiotto, M.; Pearson, A.T. Machine Learning—Guided Adjuvant Treatment of Head and Neck Cancer. *JAMA Netw. Open* **2020**, *3*, e2025881. [CrossRef]
26. Ariji, Y.; Fukuda, M.; Kise, Y.; Nozawa, M.; Yanashita, Y.; Fujita, H.; Katsumata, A.; Ariji, E. Contrast-Enhanced Computed Tomography Image Assessment of Cervical Lymph Node Metastasis in Patients with Oral Cancer by Using a Deep Learning System of Artificial Intelligence. *Oral Surg. Oral Med. Oral Pathol. Oral Radiol.* **2019**, *127*, 458–463. [CrossRef]
27. Ariji, Y.; Sugita, Y.; Nagao, T.; Nakayama, A.; Fukuda, M.; Kise, Y.; Nozawa, M.; Nishiyama, M.; Katumata, A.; Ariji, E. CT Evaluation of Extranodal Extension of Cervical Lymph Node Metastases in Patients with Oral Squamous Cell Carcinoma Using Deep Learning Classification. *Oral Radiol.* **2020**, *36*, 148–155. [CrossRef]
28. Kann, B.H.; Hicks, D.F.; Payabvash, S.; Mahajan, A.; Du, J.; Gupta, V.; Park, H.S.; Yu, J.B.; Yarbrough, W.G.; Burtness, B.A.; et al. Multi-Institutional Validation of Deep Learning for Pretreatment Identification of Extranodal Extension in Head and Neck Squamous Cell Carcinoma. *J. Clin. Oncol.* **2020**, *38*, 1304–1311. [CrossRef]
29. Kann, B.H.; Aneja, S.; Loganadane, G.V.; Kelly, J.R.; Smith, S.M.; Decker, R.H.; Yu, J.B.; Park, H.S.; Yarbrough, W.G.; Malhotra, A.; et al. Pretreatment Identification of Head and Neck Cancer Nodal Metastasis and Extranodal Extension Using Deep Learning Neural Networks. *Sci. Rep.* **2018**, *8*, 14036. [CrossRef]
30. Chen, L.; Zhou, Z.; Sher, D.; Zhang, Q.; Shah, J.; Pham, N.-L.; Jiang, S.; Wang, J. Combining Many-Objective Radiomics and 3D Convolutional Neural Network through Evidential Reasoning to Predict Lymph Node Metastasis in Head and Neck Cancer. *Phys. Med. Biol.* **2019**, *64*, 075011. [CrossRef]
31. Farrokhian, N.; Holcomb, A.J.; Dimon, E.; Karadaghy, O.; Ward, C.; Whiteford, E.; Tolan, C.; Hanly, E.K.; Buchakjian, M.R.; Harding, B.; et al. Development and Validation of Machine Learning Models for Predicting Occult Nodal Metastasis in Early-Stage Oral Cavity Squamous Cell Carcinoma. *JAMA Netw. Open* **2022**, *5*, e227226. [CrossRef]
32. Forghani, R.; Chatterjee, A.; Reinhold, C.; Pérez-Lara, A.; Romero-Sanchez, G.; Ueno, Y.; Bayat, M.; Alexander, J.W.M.; Kadi, L.; Chankowsky, J.; et al. Head and Neck Squamous Cell Carcinoma: Prediction of Cervical Lymph Node Metastasis by Dual-Energy CT Texture Analysis with Machine Learning. *Eur. Radiol.* **2019**, *29*, 6172–6181. [CrossRef]
33. Bur, A.M.; Holcomb, A.; Goodwin, S.; Woodroof, J.; Karadaghy, O.; Shnayder, Y.; Kakarala, K.; Brant, J.; Shew, M. Machine Learning to Predict Occult Nodal Metastasis in Early Oral Squamous Cell Carcinoma. *Oral Oncol.* **2019**, *92*, 20–25. [CrossRef]
34. Kourou, K.; Exarchos, T.P.; Exarchos, K.P.; Karamouzis, M.V.; Fotiadis, D.I. Machine Learning Applications in Cancer Prognosis and Prediction. *Comput. Struct. Biotechnol. J.* **2015**, *13*, 8–17. [CrossRef]
35. Adeoye, J.; Tan, J.Y.; Choi, S.-W.; Thomson, P. Prediction Models Applying Machine Learning to Oral Cavity Cancer Outcomes: A Systematic Review. *Int. J. Med. Inform.* **2021**, *154*, 104557. [CrossRef]
36. Zhang, Y.-P.; Zhang, X.-Y.; Cheng, Y.-T.; Li, B.; Teng, X.-Z.; Zhang, J.; Lam, S.; Zhou, T.; Ma, Z.-R.; Sheng, J.-B.; et al. Artificial Intelligence-Driven Radiomics Study in Cancer: The Role of Feature Engineering and Modeling. *Mil. Med. Res.* **2023**, *10*, 22. [CrossRef]
37. Alfouzan, A.F. Radiation Therapy in Head and Neck Cancer. *Saudi Med. J.* **2021**, *42*, 247–254. [CrossRef]
38. Gau, M.; Karabajakian, A.; Reverdy, T.; Neidhardt, E.-M.; Fayette, J. Induction Chemotherapy in Head and Neck Cancers: Results and Controversies. *Oral Oncol.* **2019**, *95*, 164–169. [CrossRef]
39. Dreno, B. Mucocutaneous Side Effects of Chemotherapy. *Biomed. Pharmacother.* **1990**, *44*, 163–167. [CrossRef]
40. Huang, S.H.; O'Sullivan, B. Overview of the 8th Edition TNM Classification for Head and Neck Cancer. *Curr. Treat. Options Oncol.* **2017**, *18*, 40. [CrossRef]
41. Hübbers, C.U.; Akgül, B. HPV and Cancer of the Oral Cavity. *Virulence* **2015**, *6*, 244–248. [CrossRef]

Disclaimer/Publisher's Note: The statements, opinions and data contained in all publications are solely those of the individual author(s) and contributor(s) and not of MDPI and/or the editor(s). MDPI and/or the editor(s) disclaim responsibility for any injury to people or property resulting from any ideas, methods, instructions or products referred to in the content.

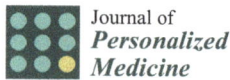

Perspective

Anterior Open Bite Malocclusion: From Clinical Treatment Strategies towards the Dissection of the Genetic Bases of the Disease Using Human and Collaborative Cross Mice Cohorts

Iqbal M. Lone [1], Osayd Zohud [1], Kareem Midlej [1], Eva Paddenberg [2], Sebastian Krohn [2], Christian Kirschneck [3], Peter Proff [2], Nezar Watted [4,5,6] and Fuad A. Iraqi [1,2,6,*]

1. Department of Clinical Microbiology and Immunology, Sackler Faculty of Medicine, Tel-Aviv University, Tel-Aviv 69978, Israel; iqbalzoo84@gmail.com (I.M.L.); osaydzohud@mail.tau.ac.il (O.Z.); kareemmidlej@mail.tau.ac.il (K.M.)
2. Department of Orthodontics, University Hospital of Regensburg, D-93053 Regensburg, Germany; eva.paddenberg@ukr.de (E.P.); sebastian.krohn@klinik.uni-regensburg.de (S.K.); peter.proff@klinik.uni-regensburg.de (P.P.)
3. Department of Orthodontics, University of Bonn, D-53111 Bonn, Germany; christian.kirschneck@uni-bonn.de
4. Center for Dentistry Research and Aesthetics, Jatt 45911, Israel; nezar.watted@gmx.net
5. Department of Orthodontics, Faculty of Dentistry, Arab America University, Jenin 919000, Palestine
6. Gathering for Prosperity Initiative, Jatt 45911, Israel
* Correspondence: fuadi@tauex.tau.ac.il

Abstract: Anterior open bite malocclusion is a complex dental condition characterized by a lack of contact or overlap between the upper and lower front teeth. It can lead to difficulties with speech, chewing, and biting. Its etiology is multifactorial, involving a combination of genetic, environmental, and developmental factors. Genetic studies have identified specific genes and signaling pathways involved in jaw growth, tooth eruption, and dental occlusion that may contribute to open bite development. Understanding the genetic and epigenetic factors contributing to skeletal open bite is crucial for developing effective prevention and treatment strategies. A thorough manual search was undertaken along with searches on PubMed, Scopus, Science Direct, and Web of Science for relevant studies published before June 2022. RCTs (clinical trials) and subsequent observational studies comprised the included studies. Orthodontic treatment is the primary approach for managing open bites, often involving braces, clear aligners, or other orthodontic appliances. In addition to orthodontic interventions, adjuvant therapies such as speech therapy and/or physiotherapy may be necessary. In some cases, surgical interventions may be necessary to correct underlying skeletal issues. Advancements in technology, such as 3D printing and computer-assisted design and manufacturing, have improved treatment precision and efficiency. Genetic research using animal models, such as the Collaborative Cross mouse population, offers insights into the genetic components of open bite and potential therapeutic targets. Identifying the underlying genetic factors and understanding their mechanisms can lead to the development of more precise treatments and preventive strategies for open bite. Here, we propose to perform human research using mouse models to generate debatable results. We anticipate that a genome-wide association study (GWAS) search for significant genes and their modifiers, an epigenetics-wide association study (EWAS), RNA-seq analysis, the integration of GWAS and expression-quantitative trait loci (eQTL), and micro-, small-, and long noncoding RNA analysis in tissues associated with open bite in humans and mice will uncover novel genes and genetic factors influencing this phenotype.

Keywords: malocclusion; open bite; etiology; treatment; Collaborative Cross mice

Citation: Lone, I.M.; Zohud, O.; Midlej, K.; Paddenberg, E.; Krohn, S.; Kirschneck, C.; Proff, P.; Watted, N.; Iraqi, F.A. Anterior Open Bite Malocclusion: From Clinical Treatment Strategies towards the Dissection of the Genetic Bases of the Disease Using Human and Collaborative Cross Mice Cohorts. *J. Pers. Med.* **2023**, *13*, 1617. https://doi.org/10.3390/jpm13111617

Academic Editor: Daniele Giansanti

Received: 17 October 2023
Revised: 7 November 2023
Accepted: 15 November 2023
Published: 17 November 2023

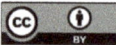

Copyright: © 2023 by the authors. Licensee MDPI, Basel, Switzerland. This article is an open access article distributed under the terms and conditions of the Creative Commons Attribution (CC BY) license (https://creativecommons.org/licenses/by/4.0/).

1. Introduction

Malocclusion, a common dental condition impacting many individuals worldwide, refers to the misalignment of the teeth and jaws. This condition can adversely affect oral health, impairing eating, speaking, and the maintenance of good oral hygiene. Moreover, malocclusion can influence appearance, diminishing self-confidence and self-esteem [1]. The causes of malocclusion are multifactorial and intricate, involving genetic, environmental, and developmental factors [1]. Dental research has made significant progress in understanding the molecular mechanisms underlying malocclusion, particularly through exploring genetics and genomics. These studies have revealed specific genes and signaling pathways that influence jaw formation, tooth emergence, and tooth closure. However, fully comprehending the intricate interplay between hereditary and environmental variables which leads to malocclusion remains a challenging task [2].

Anterior open bite is a type of malocclusion that occurs when there is no contact or overlap between the upper and lower front teeth. It can also occur with all forms of skeletal Dysgnathy (Figure 1A–E). Prolonged use of a pacifier may contribute to its development. It is a complex dental problem that can be triggered by a number of circumstances, such as genetics, environmental factors, and habits such as thumb-sucking or tongue-thrusting [3]. An open bite can be classified as either functional, skeletal, or dentoalveolar, or as a combination of all three, depending on the underlying cause (Figure 2). Skeletal open bite is caused by excessive vertical growth of the dentoalveolar complex, especially in the posterior molar region. In this patient category, there is an increased lower face height compared to the upper face height (long face syndrome). Cephalometric open bite is a hyperdevirgence of the InterBase angles (angles between the upper and lower jaw base). This long face can be seen extra-orally (Figure 3A,B). At the same time, dental open bite is generally found in the anterior region within the area of the cuspids and incisors and is associated with a normal craniofacial pattern, proclined and undererupted anterior teeth, and thumb- or finger-sucking habits. In this patient category, there is a harmony between the upper and lower facial height. Nothing is noticeable extra-orally, as shown in Figure 4A,B [3]. The third category consists of the combination of skeletal and dentoalveolar open bite, in which the intraoral and the extra-oral symptoms can be seen (Figure 5A,B). An open bite can cause difficulties with speech, chewing, and biting and can also lead to temporomandibular joint (TMJ) disorders [4]. Treatment of an open bite can be challenging and may require a combination of orthodontic and surgical interventions (Figure 6). This article reviews the etiologies, dentofacial morphology, treatment modalities, retention, and stability of anterior open bite [3].

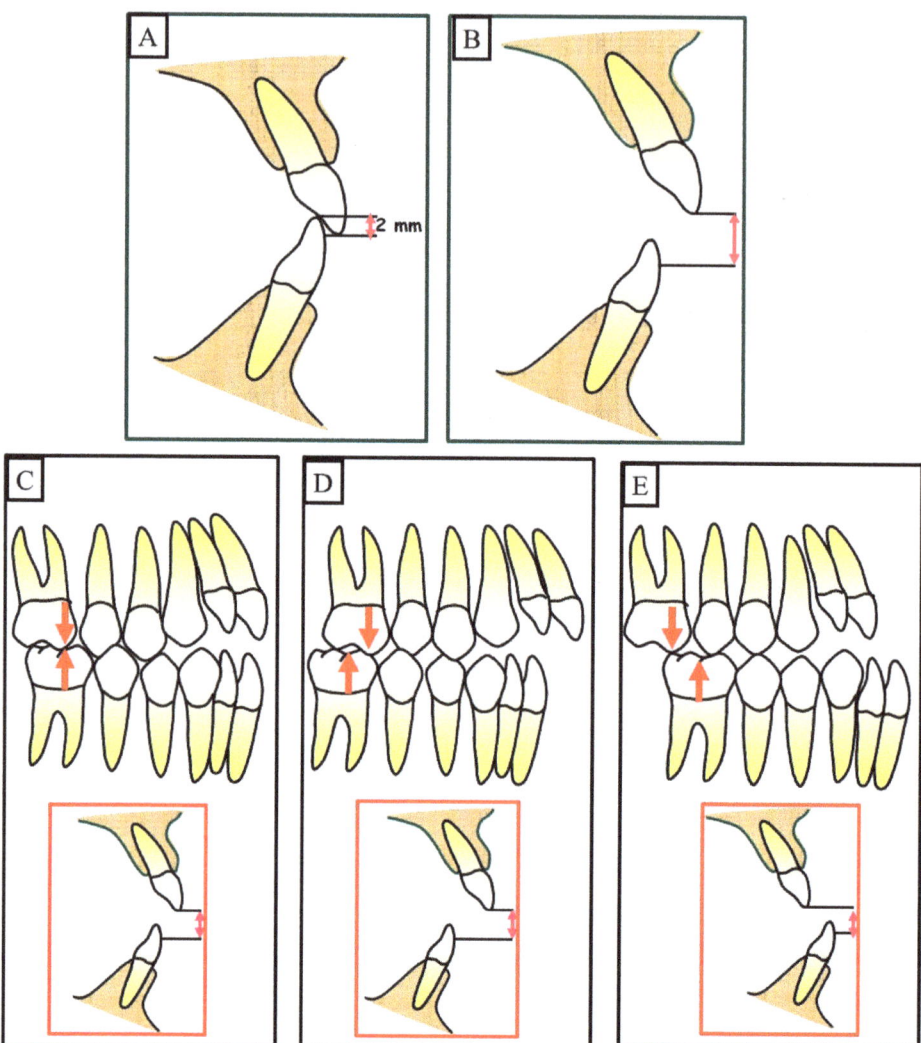

Figure 1. Overbite denotes the vertical alignment or the space between the upper central incisor of the maxilla and the corresponding central incisor of the mandible. (**A**) A normal or physiological overbite typically measures about 2–3 mm. (**B**) An open bite refers to a reduced overbite, usually measuring less than 0 mm. (**C**) Open bite combined with a Class I dental relationship. (**D**) Open bite in association with a Class II dental relationship. (**E**) Open bite in connection with a Class III dental relationship.

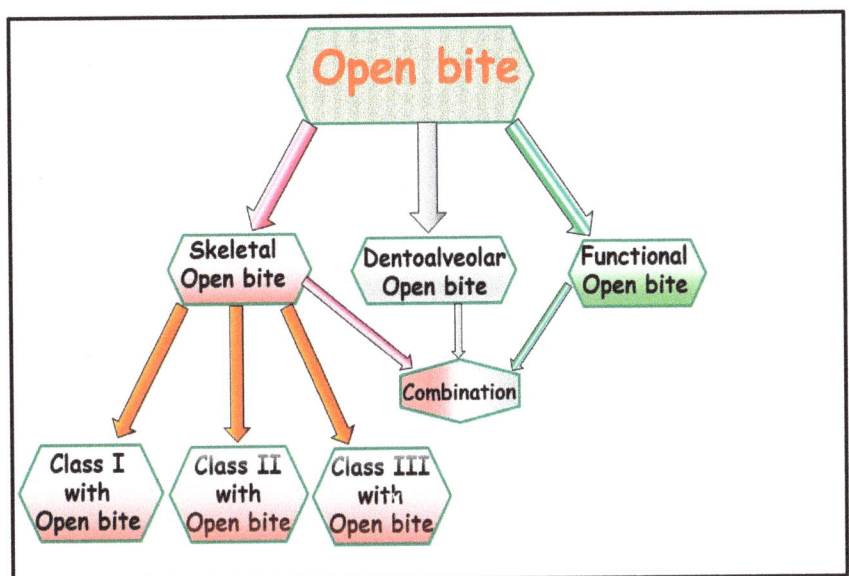

Figure 2. Various categories of open bites exist, and a visual representation in the form of a diagram can help elucidate these distinctions.

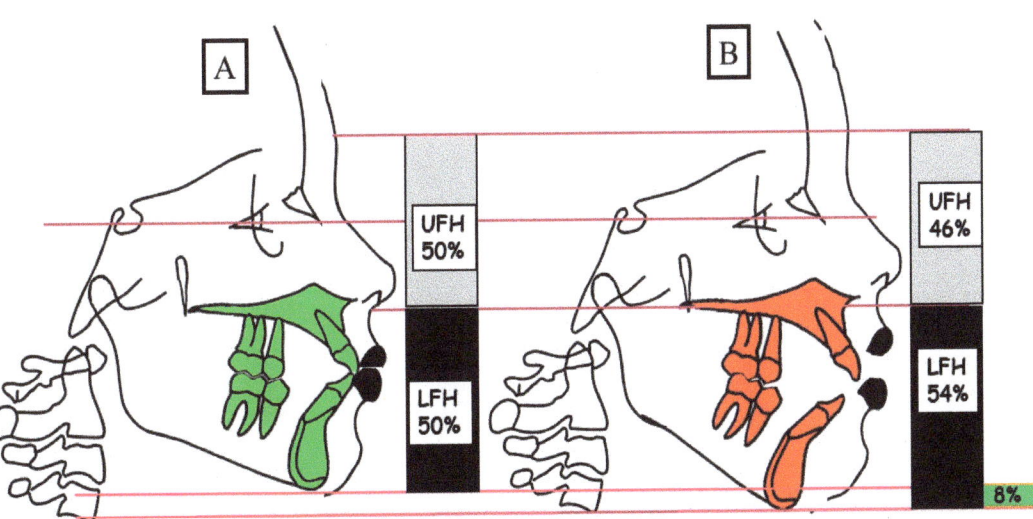

Figure 3. A schematic depiction of the vertical dimension illustrates a physiological overbite (**A**) and a skeletal open bite (**B**). (**A**) In a physiological vertical dimension, there is a balanced relationship between the upper facial height (UFH 50%) and lower facial height (LFH 50%). (**B**) A skeletal open bite is characterized by an elevated lower facial height (LFH 54%) in comparison to the upper facial height (UFH 46%).

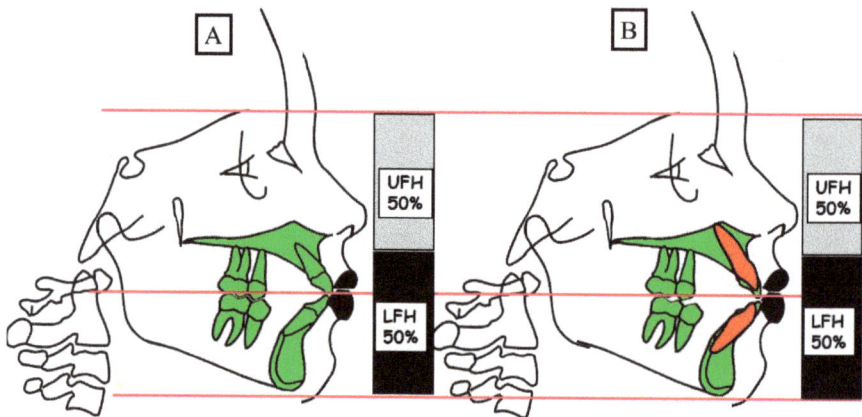

Figure 4. A schematic illustration of the vertical dimension showcases a physiological overbite (**A**) and a dentoalveolar open bite (**B**). (**A**) In a physiological vertical dimension, there exists a harmonious relationship between the upper facial height (UFH 50%) and lower facial height (LFH 50%). (**B**) A dentoalveolar open bite occurs due to the infraocclusion or protrusion of the front teeth, maintaining a balanced relation between the upper facial height (UFH 50%) and lower facial height (LFH 50%).

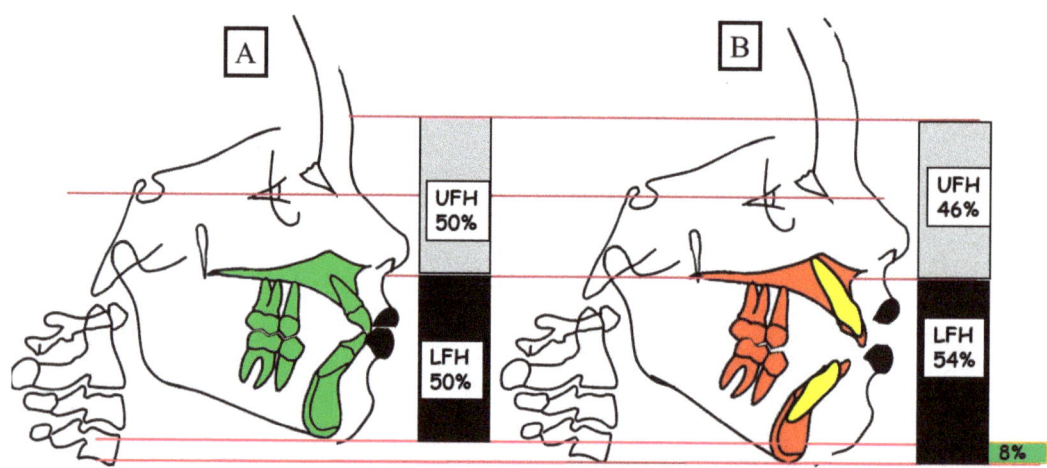

Figure 5. A schematic portrayal of the vertical dimension demonstrates a physiological overbite (**A**) and the coexistence of a skeletal and dentoalveolar open bite (**B**). (**A**) In a physiological vertical dimension, there is an equilibrium between the upper facial height (UFH 50%) and lower facial height (LFH 50%). (**B**) A combined skeletal and dentoalveolar open bite results from the posterior rotation of the mandible and the infraocclusion of the front teeth, leading to an elevated lower facial height (LFH 54%) in contrast to the upper facial height (UFH 46%).

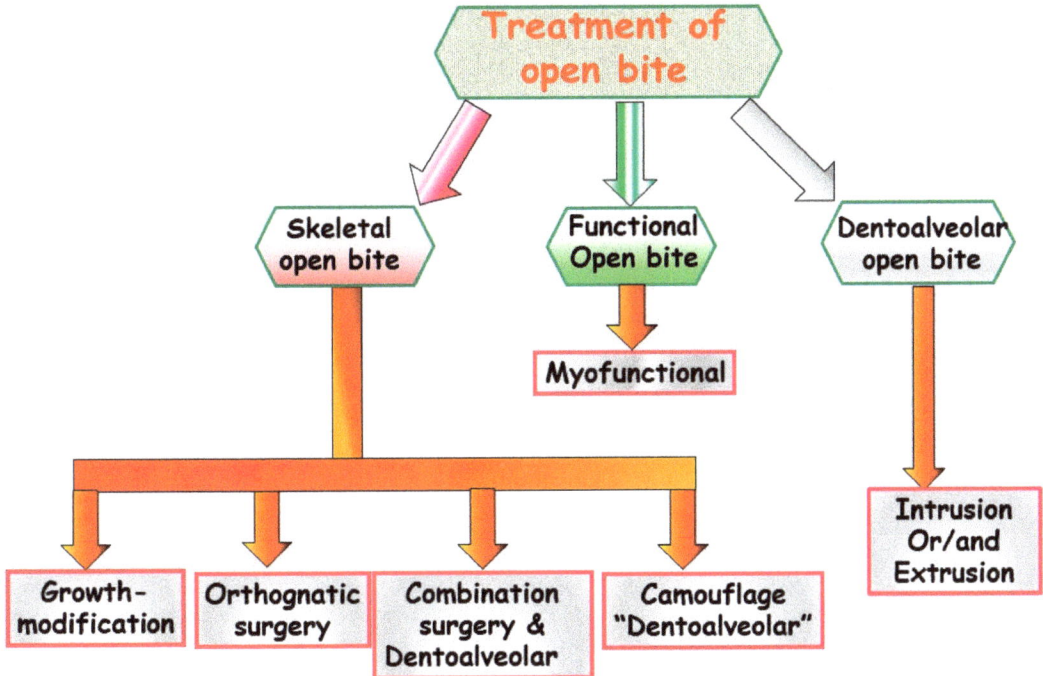

Figure 6. A diagram depicting various treatment approaches for open bite, which can be categorized based on factors such as age, growth stage, causative factors, functional considerations, and aesthetic concerns.

2. Top of Form

Open bite malocclusion can be classified into different types based on its location and etiology. According to Moyer, simple open bite is limited to the teeth and their surrounding alveolar process, whereas a complex open bite is primarily the result of vertical dysplasia and is often linked to Class I, Class II, and Class III malocclusions (Figure 1A–E and Figure 2). False or dental open bite is characterized by proclined teeth without alteration of the osseous bases, while true or skeletal open bite involves deformed alveolar processes and dolichofacial characteristics. Posterior open bite is defined as the failure of contact between the posterior teeth when the teeth occlude in centric occlusion. Open bites can also be classified based on their location, such as anterior open bite, which can be dental or skeletal, and posterior open bite. The classification of open bite includes simple open bite, compound open bite, and infantile open bite. Understanding the different types and classifications of open bite is crucial in diagnosing and planning treatment for such cases [5].

Strong pieces of evidence suggest that genetics and heredity can play a significant role in the development of open bite malocclusion. Evolution has led to genetically determined smaller jaws and more vertical facial structures, which can increase the risk of open bite. Height may also be a hereditary factor, and was shown to be a coounder involved in affecting understanding of the genetic and environmental variables that contribute to open bite, which are critical for precise diagnosis and therapy [6].

The utilization of animal models has greatly contributed to the advancement of molecular analysis in the field of malocclusion research. By leveraging these models, researchers are able to delve into the intricate interplay between environmental and genetic variables that possess a role in the formation of tooth misalignment, as well as to explore and evaluate diverse preventive and therapeutic strategies. Among the various animal models available, mice have emerged as a particularly advantageous choice due to their small physical stature, ease of breeding, and remarkable genetic resemblance to humans [7].

An animal model that has proven to be highly effective in investigating complex genetic traits like malocclusion is the Collaborative Cross (CC) mouse. Through meticulous breeding techniques, CC mice can give rise to a genetically diverse population, which considerably expands the range of genetic variations available for comprehensive examination. This particular mouse population serves as an exceptional model for the thorough investigation of the intricate genetic underpinnings associated with malocclusion, owing to its possession of a distinct and heterogeneous assortment of genetic variants [7]. Notably, CC mice have been successfully harnessed in previous studies to unravel the complexities underlying a wide array of genetic traits, including but not limited to body mass index and metabolic diseases [8]. Consequently, the inherent genetic diversity present within the CC mouse population offers an invaluable resource for gaining a comprehensive understanding of the multifaceted genetic components implicated in malocclusion, thereby facilitating the targeted identification of specific genetic variants that contribute to the manifestation of complex traits [9]. The role of genetic factors in the emergence of open bite will be addressed in this paper, and the potential of the CC mouse population in identifying genetic variants that contribute to open bite will be highlighted. We also suggest that the implications of this proposed research will lead to the development of precise treatments and preventive strategies for open bite. The use of the CC mice cohort is pivotal in our research. This unique mouse model, created through meticulous breeding, replicates the genetic diversity encountered in human populations. CC mice have proven effective in unraveling the complexities of diverse genetic traits, offering a dynamic platform for genetic studies. By harnessing the CC mice, we aim to simulate and understand the genetic components of open bite and identify specific genetic variants which contribute to its manifestation.

3. Etiology

The etiology of open bite is complex and multifactorial, involving a combination of genetic, environmental, and developmental factors. Interaction between genetic and environmental factors can influence open bite development. For example, a genetic predisposition to malocclusion combined with oral habits such as thumb-sucking can lead to more severe malocclusion. Understanding these factors and their interactions is critical for developing effective prevention and treatment strategies for open bite [10]. Genetic factors are believed to play a significant role in the development of open bite. Studies have identified specific genes and signaling pathways implicated in the growth of the jaw and the eruption of teeth, and variations in these genes may contribute to open bite development.

Genetic factors do not solely influence the development of malocclusion, as epigenetic mechanisms also contribute to its manifestation. Epigenetic processes, encompassing DNA methylation, histone modification, and microRNA regulation, have been identified as influential elements in the intricate web of malocclusion development. These epigenetic changes possess the ability to modify patterns of gene expression, thereby impacting the growth and development of teeth and jaws. Research has demonstrated that patients with malocclusion exhibit altered DNA methylation patterns, which, in turn, can disrupt transcriptome profiles that are crucial for the development of the jaw and the emergence of the teeth [11]. Furthermore, it is important to note that environmental factors, including diet, stress, and exposure to toxins, can influence epigenetic modifications. For instance, research has revealed that maternal stress experienced by mothers throughout gestation can cause changes in DNA methylation patterns in children, eventually leading to craniofacial deformities and malocclusion [12].

To summarize, the bases for malocclusion development extend beyond genetic differences alone. They also involve intricate interactions between genes, signaling pathways, and epigenetic factors. The genetic factors encompass variations in genes responsible for mandibular development, the eruption of teeth, and oral occlusion. However, epigenetic mechanisms, including DNA methylation and microRNA control of microRNA activity, exert their influence on malocclusion development as well. By comprehensively gaining insights into the genetic and epigenetic elements that play a role in the development of malocclusion, researchers can provide the foundation for the creation of innovative preventative and therapeutic solutions aimed at addressing this prevalent dental condition.

4. Classification of Open Bite

4.1. Anterior Open Bite

A malocclusion, in this context, refers to an anterior portion of the dental arches without any contact, and the posterior teeth in occlusion are shown in Figure 1A–E and Figure 7A,B. When a malocclusion affects the posterior segment, it is referred to as a combined open bite [13]. Anterior open bite is one of the most widespread and challenging to treat of the malocclusions that are most frequently encountered in clinic practice. When the etiology is multifactorial, the pathology results in aesthetic changes, harm to the articulation of some phonemes, and unfavorable psychological states [14,15]. Functional, dentoalveolar, skeletal, or a combination of other factors may be the cause of the open bite. Using fixed appliances for orthodontic treatments makes treating dental open bite simple. For the treatment of skeletal open bite, which may necessitate orthognathic surgery, a more thorough strategy is needed. Myofunctional appliances can be used to repair dental open bite in growing patients, and afterward, orthodontic removable appliances can be used to fix it during the retention phase [16]. The prepubertal and pubertal growth should be evaluated for nasal obstruction [17]. The axial inclinations of the incisors might change as a result of excessive activity of the tongue while swallowing or even when it is at rest, which may cause an open bite [18].

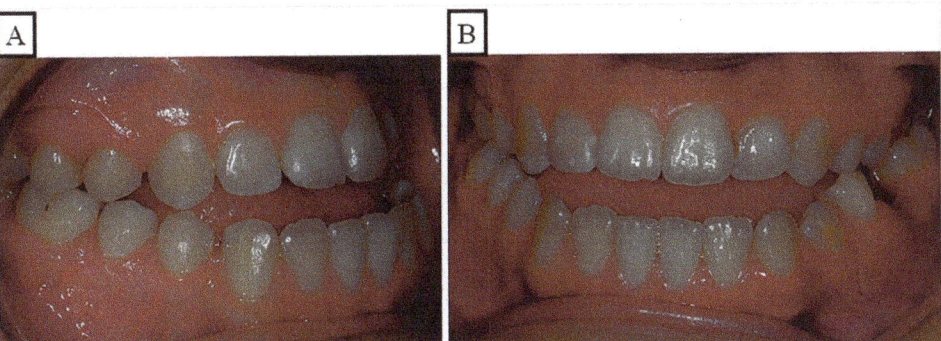

Figure 7. An anterior portion of the dental arches without contact is meant by a malocclusion in this context (**A**); (**B**) the posterior teeth in occlusion.

4.2. Posterior Open Bite

When the teeth occlude in centric occlusion, posterior open bite is the loss of contact between the posterior teeth, as shown in Figure 8A,B. The maxillary and mandibular premolars are not occluded, as seen in the figures. Insignificant contact exists between the mandibular and maxillary molars in a typical anterior overjet and overbite.

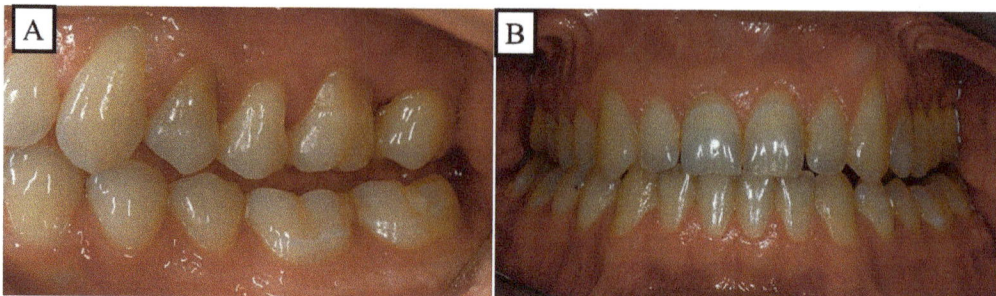

Figure 8. Posterior open bite is the loss of contact between the posterior teeth. Subfigure (**A**) shows the posterior open bite from first premolar to the second molar, and (**B**) the same patient shows contact in anterior area, while open in the posterior area.

4.3. Types of Open Bite

4.3.1. False or Dental Open Bite

The osseous roots of the teeth in this bite are unaltered, and the procline does not reach past the canine. This individual displays a pseudo-bite, a dentoalveolar issue, normal facial morphology, and proper bone relationships, all of which are shown in Figure 9A–F and fully discussed by Meyer-Marcotty et al. and Rodriguez and Casasa [19,20].

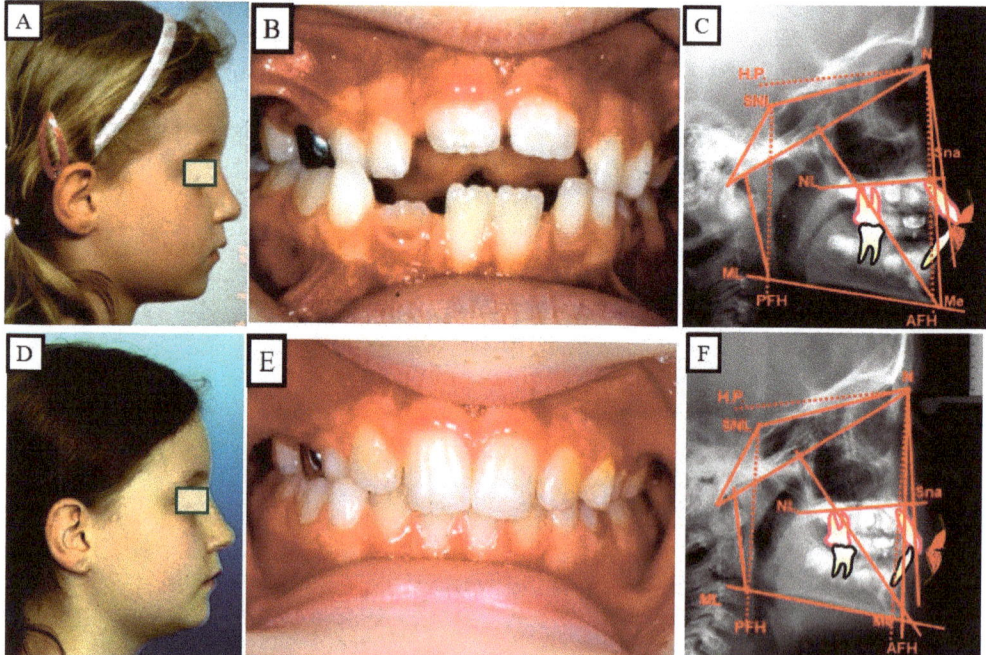

Figure 9. False (**A**) or dental (**B**) open bite. (**A–C**) During tooth development and tooth eruption. (**D–F**) After tooth development and complete tooth eruption.

4.3.2. True or Skeletal Open Bite

Alveolar processes that are implicated or malformed as well as dolichofacial characteristics are found in this kind of open bite. The lower third and vertical dimensions of this patient's face are increased, and they have hyper-divergency in their maxilla, as shown in Figure 3A,B and Figure 5A,B and discussed by Chang and Moon [21].

Open bites are classified into anterior and posterior open bites based on the region in which they occur. From an etiological standpoint, these two divisions correspond to dental and skeletal open bites. A dental eruption obstruction causes the dental anterior open bite, while posterior facial development causes the skeletal open bite. The posterior open bite is defined by the inability of a significant number of teeth in either or both of the opposing buccal segments to achieve occlusion despite incisor contact. It occurs seldom and may be brought on by the tongue interposing, eruptional disturbances (such as ankylosis), a basic lack of eruption, or a fully open bite, as presented in Figure 5A,B and Figure 7A,B and discussed by Greenlee et al. [22].

4.4. Andrew Richardson Classification

4.4.1. Transitional Open Bite

When the permanent teeth start erupting, this kind of open bite happens. An anterior open bite is the outcome of the dentoalveolar region's inadequate development. Alveolar growth that continues and the typical growth increase in the lower anterior face height cause spontaneous adjustments.

4.4.2. Digit-Sucking Open Bite

An anterior open bite results from digit sucking, which prevents the incisor teeth from erupting fully. By stopping the habit, such open bites can be avoided (Figure 10A–C). Rarely do these open bites last throughout adulthood, despite being uncommon during pubertal growth stages. Anterior open bites often spontaneously close due to the growth of the dentoalveolar process and the incisor uprighting. Cysts, dilacerations, and ankylosis are a few of the local pathological diseases that can cause an anterior open bite. A proper surgical procedure to remove the local disease facilitates dentoalveolar development. In contrast, an open bite brought on by the skeletal pathology or abnormalities becomes visible near the conclusion of the growing phase. These illnesses include cleft palate, craniofacial dysostosis, cleidocranial dysostosis, and achondroplasia. The nonpathological skeletal group is divided into three subgroups.

Open bite during the early tooth development phase which closes throughout growth periods before and during puberty is caused by dentoalveolar growth compensation. As a result, the frequency of open bites tends to decline with age. The second subgroup is noticeable in the pre-pubertal period, but it disappears throughout adolescence and reemerges during the post-pubertal stage. This is a result of the interaction between the vertical facial growth and compensatory dentoalveolar growth, which is enough to seal the open bite. However, vertical facial growth takes over in the post-pubertal period and results in an open bite. The third category poses the most challenging clinical orthodontic issue, as facial development predominates and causes a gross anterior open bite as people mature [23].

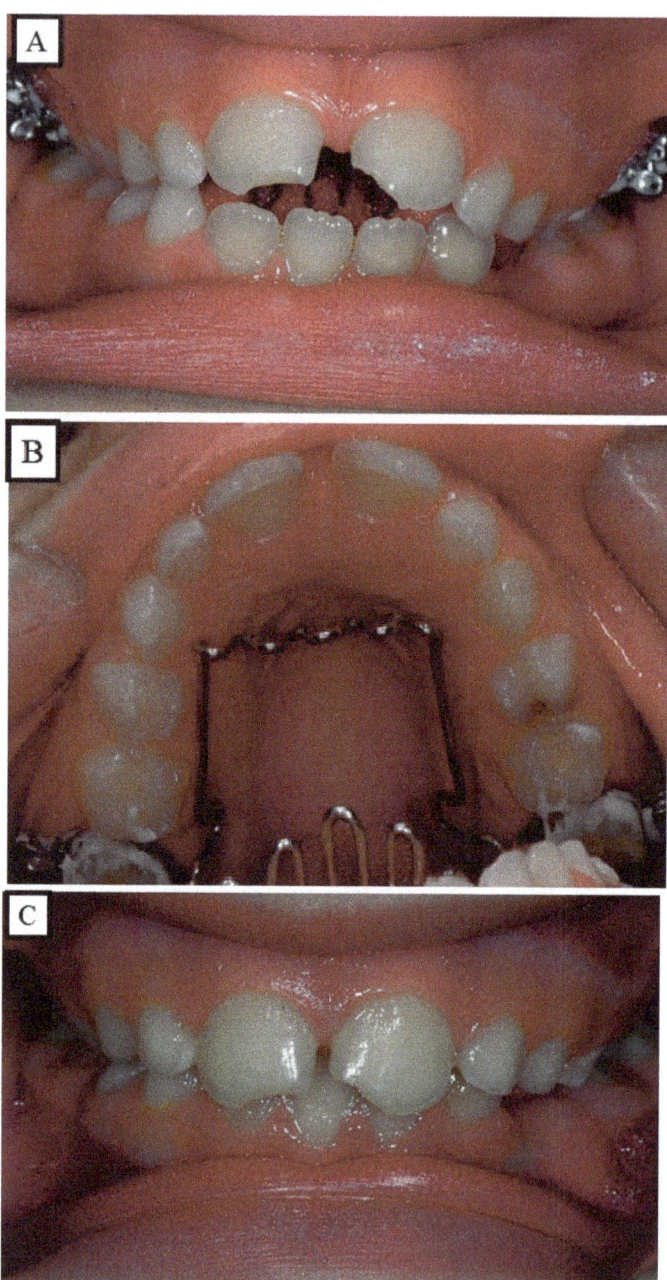

Figure 10. An anterior open bite results from digit sucking. After preventing finger sucking by using a special device, spontaneous closure of the anterior open bite occurred (**A–C**).

4.5. Factors and Characteristics of Open Bite

One of the most challenging orthodontic issues is open bite malocclusion, which is regarded as a problem. Multiple variables, including genetic and environmental influences, can contribute to open bites. Two general categories—skeletal and dental—can be used to classify open bites. A real skeletal open bite might require dental surgery in addition to orthodontic therapy, while a dental open bite can be corrected with braces. An open bite can cause people to experience problems with their appearance, oral function, and mental health. Children's development is hampered by functional issues, which include speech, mastication, and deglutition defects. The open bite frequency might reach up to 17% in mixed dentition [24]. Recurrent adenoid infections can result in a malpositioned tongue, a chronic infantile swallow, and bad oral habits that can be observed as the incisors are partially erupting. Dento-alveolar anterior open bite is caused by bad oral practices such as finger or lip sucking, breathing through the mouth, and tongue pushing. This is easily remedied with just orthodontic care. This is true if the patient receives a diagnosis early and the related practices can be changed. Mouth breathing is frequently accompanied by difficulty in speaking, particularly spitting consonants, and dry nasal passages. There is a propensity for vertical dentofacial dysplasia to recur. Both open bite and deep bite malocclusions result in this [25]. Anterior open bite found in vertical dysplasia is multifactorial [26,27].

4.6. Hereditary Factors

Most frequently, inherited facial expansion is connected to the open bite abnormality. Dysplasias in the vertical plane may be inherited since horizontal skeletal dysplasias appear to be inherited [28]. Research on the causes of craniofacial growth have focused on three significant ideas in the last few years [29]. Similar to other tissues, bone determines its own growth to a large extent [30]. Cartilage controls skeletal development, with the bone acting incidentally and passively [31].

4.7. Non-Hereditary Factors

Maciel and Leite [32] and Arat et al. [33] have emphasized aberrant functioning patterns and harmful oral habits of the tongue, as well as atypical swallowing habits (Figure 10A–C) and speech issues, as contributing to and being part of the open bite phenomena. An irregular swallowing pattern may be the root cause or the outcome of a tongue problem.

The location of the open bite defect varies depending on the pressures present and the teeth and supporting structures' capacity to resist change, according to Wajid et al. [5]. There may be a propensity toward an anterior open bite, for instance, if the swallowing pattern is incorrect and the tongue is propelled forward strongly. Additionally, the existence of harmful thumb, finger, or lip suckling, as well as poor oral breathing practices and weak labial muscles, have a significant impact on the severity of the anterior open bite.

5. Sucking Habits

The duration, frequency, severity, and location of the sucking practices all play a role in the extent of the harm done to the teeth and underlying tissues. When a child is between the ages of four and five, thumb- or finger-sucking habits might be observed. This is regarded as a typical habit that does not cause a malocclusion to become permanent. An anterior open bite, however, may well occur if thumb sucking continues unabated up until the age groups of mixed and permanent dentition [34]. Some youngsters actively suck their thumbs or fingers, while others just let their thumbs passively lie in their mouths. The malocclusions will have varied degrees of severity depending on the intensity and consistency of the habit. The anterior aspect of the maxillary complex may be subjected to upward and forward stress as a result of frequent thumb sucking (Figure 11A,B).

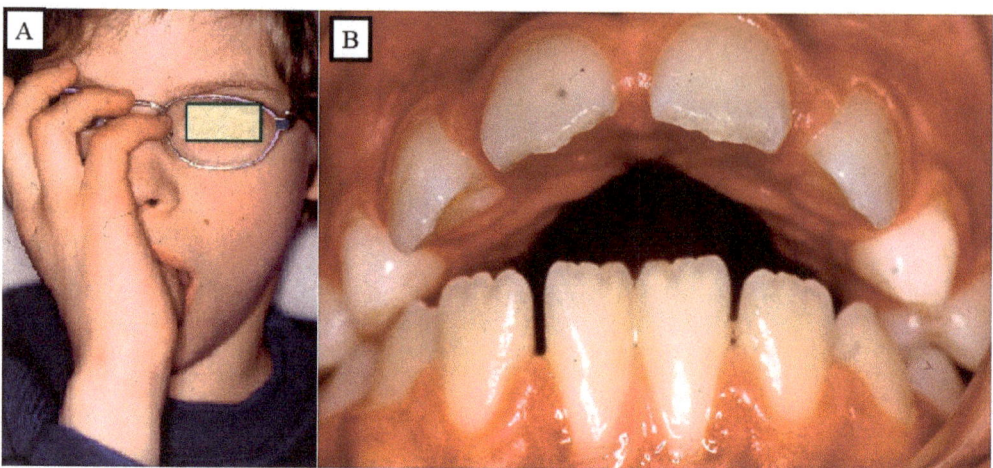

Figure 11. An anterior open bite (**A**), the upper jaw shape results from thumb sucking during growth (**B**).

6. Adaptability

According to Reichert et al. [35], an open bite with ineffective lips may occur from an excessive rearward rotation of the mandible. For the purpose of forming an oral seal during deglutition, hyperactive mentalis and tongue muscles may be needed [36].

7. Environmental Factors

Habits, neurological impairments, trauma, and illnesses are examples of environmental variables. According to Park et al. [37], macroglossia is frequently accompanied by harmful oral behaviors such as tongue thrusting and mouth breathing. According to Togawa et al. [38], the neuromuscular inadequacies classify the open bite's skeletal component. Leptoprosopic patients with muscular dystrophy exhibit supra eruption of the posterior buccal segment, precipitating as an anterior open bite. Skeleto-facial or dentoalveolar trauma are two possible types. Ankylosis of the condyle, which manifests as abnormal vertical growth of the mandible, or the stoppage of condyle growth, which causes a clearly defined anterior open bite, are the most common causes of this condition (Figure 12A–D). An anterior open bite is a sign of dental trauma, especially to the incisors. Prior to the patient's full growth, damaged teeth begin to ankylose [39]. Condylar resorption frequently coexists with degenerative conditions such as idiopathic condylar resorption and juvenile rheumatoid arthritis [40].

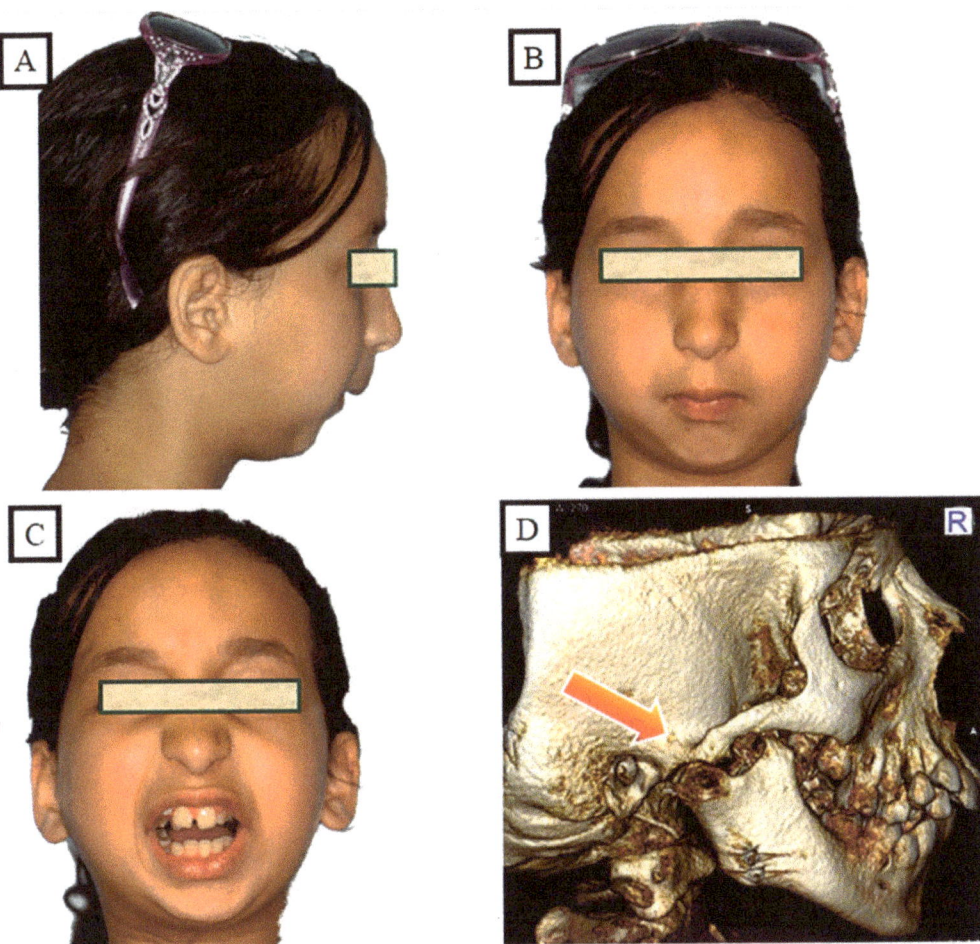

Figure 12. Patient with a temporomandibular joint fracture in the growth phase, the result was ankylosis and growth disorders in the ramus mandible, an open bite developed (**A–D**).

8. Genetics

The genetic make-up of the body controls innate growth potentials. For instance, control over the sagittal, transverse, and vertical dimensions is typically passed on in families, like the Hapsburg jaw. The patient's genetic makeup is also responsible for growth and growth rotations that take place in the late maturation stage. Molars can erupt vertically in facial types like the hyper and leptoprosopic types, which results in an excessively vertical skeletal architecture [41].

9. Findings of Literature Search

Although the etiology of posterior open bite (POB) is poorly understood, a possible genetic cause has been suggested in an investigation of a non-syndromic family collection of cases with strong POB penetrance over two generations [42]. The intricate interaction of environmental and genetic variables contributes to the root cause of POB, a complex issue to understand and comprehend. However, the possibility of a genetic cause for POB exists [42]. The majority of genetic investigations on the genesis of malocclusion have been on syndromic disorders. Many single-gene correlated diseases, such as Apert's syndrome,

Treacher Collins syndrome, and cleidocranial dysplasia, are characterized by craniofacial and oral symptoms and are triggered by alterations in fibroblast growth factor receptor 2 (FGFR2), treacle ribosome biogenesis factor 1 (TCOF1), and Runt-related transcription factor 2 (RUNX2), correspondingly [42]. Malocclusions in these illnesses tend to be components of and subsequent to a complicated pattern of several dentofacial abnormalities. Although there has been no evidence in the literature of any genetic etiology of POB (excluding those indirectly induced by primary failure of eruption (PFE)), the potential remains [42]. There is an unusual pedigree of POB patients with strong penetrance spanning two generations in the orthodontic clinic at Rutgers School of Dental Medicine, but no syndromic disorders have been recorded. Patients MM1, MM2, and MM3 are three Caucasian siblings who all have POB. They all have straight to somewhat concave profiles, perioral muscular tension, and several missing teeth. The study implies that identifying the implicated gene(s) and their roles will assist scientists in comprehending the etiology and processes of POB, as well as in building the groundwork for improved therapies and results [42]. This article highlights the importance of identifying the fundamental genetic component of POB by genetic linkage analysis or whole genome sequencing to better understand its mechanisms. Further investigations into the gene(s) and mechanism(s) implicated cannot just offer an exceptional chance to better comprehend POB and the complex muscular–occlusal interaction, it can also provide strong insight into the most successful treatments.

Several studies have investigated the genetic factors contributing to this malocclusion [43]. One of the main findings of these studies is that open bite is a polygenic characteristic, indicating that it is caused by the simultaneous segregation of many genes [43]. The specific genes leading to a particular skeletal variability are not yet fully understood, but studies have demonstrated that vertical characteristics are more genetically regulated than anteroposterior parameters, and heredity is displayed anteriorly rather than posteriorly [43]. The mandibular shape also seems to be determined more genetically than mandibular size. Different inheritance models have been suggested for mandibular prognathism, which is sometimes associated with open bite, including the simple recessive or autosomal dominant with incomplete penetrance models. However, the polygenic nature of craniofacial features makes determining the precise genes responsible for skeletal variations difficult [43]. In addition to genetic factors, environmental factors such as thumb sucking, tongue thrusting, and mouth breathing can also lead to the formation of open bite. However, the relative contribution of genetic and environmental factors to open bite development is not yet fully understood [43]. A genetic syndrome might accompany some malocclusions with severe skeletal discrepancies, and mutations in specific genes can cause these syndromes. For example, mutations in the Fibrillin (FBN) 1 gene are the major cause of Marfan syndrome, which can lead to maxillary/mandibular retrognathia, a long face, a highly arched palate, and other craniofacial abnormalities. In conclusion, the genetic basis of open bite is complex and not fully understood. Open bite is a polygenic trait, and the specific genes leading to particular skeletal variabilities are not yet fully understood. Further genetic investigations are needed to identify all of the individual genes that contribute to certain skeletal variations, which could pave the way to the genetic repair of genetically regulated dentofacial malformations and malocclusions in the future [43].

Another research article explores the relationship between amelogenesis imperfecta, which is a genetic disorder that affects the development of tooth enamel, which is the hard, outer layer of the teeth. This condition can cause teeth to be discolored, to be pitted, or to have an abnormal shape. In some cases, the enamel may be so thin that the teeth are more prone to damage or decay. Amelogenesis imperfecta can be inherited in an autosomal dominant, autosomal recessive, or X-linked pattern, and there are several different types of the condition with varying degrees of severity, including anterior open bite, a dental condition where the front teeth do not touch. The study found that an anterior open bite was always associated with a severe discrepancy in the vertical relationship of the jaws and that this vertical dysgnathia was the primary etiological factor predisposing patients to an anterior open bite. The article suggests that the frequent association of anterior open bite and amelogenesis imperfecta is caused by a genetically determined anomaly of craniofacial development, rather than by local factors influencing alveolar growth. The article highlights the importance of cephalometric analyses in identifying other derangements within the cranial base and facial skeleton [44].

Other studies have investigated genetic factors that contribute to the development of open bite, and have found that genes involved in the growth and development of bones, teeth, and soft tissues may be associated with this malocclusion [45]. Several genes have been identified, including CYP19A1, GHR, TNF-α, RANKL/RANK, OPG, MYO1H, MMP, TIMPs, α-actin, and PTHR1 [46]. However, environmental factors are also important, and the occurrence of open bite is multifactorial, resulting from the interaction of genetic and environmental factors. Habits such as pacifier sucking and digital sucking are among the most prominent environmental variables involved in the establishment of open bite.

According to Nishio and Huynh [47], there is evidence to suggest that genetics play a role in the development of open bite. One study mentioned in the document found that two candidate genes, PAX5 and ABCA4-ARHGAP29, have been associated with vertical discrepancies ranging from skeletal deep to open bite. Additionally, another study found that patients with deep bite and the hypodivergent phenotype had a significant occurrence of palatally displaced maxillary canines, which suggests a genetic component to the etiology of this dental anomaly. However, further studies are necessary to clarify the frequency of occurrence of these dental disturbances in patients with vertical skeletal malocclusions and whether there is a genetically aetiological association between these disorders. A cross-sectional study aimed to evaluate whether polymorphisms of four genes (TNF-α, MTR, MTRR, and TGFβ1) could be biomarkers for oral health-related quality of life (OHRQoL) in preschoolers with anterior open bite (AOB). Overall, the study provides valuable insights into the genetic background of AOB and its impact on OHRQoL in preschool children [48].

In our research, we will employ a variety of advanced genetic analysis techniques to unravel the complex etiology of open bite. Genome-Wide Association Studies (GWAS) will allow for a comprehensive exploration of the entire genome, revealing specific genetic loci associated with open bite malocclusion and offering crucial insights into the genetic basis of this condition. Epigenome-Wide Association Studies (EWAS) will provide an in-depth analysis of epigenetic modifications, such as DNA methylation and histone modifications, which significantly influence open bite development by shaping gene expression patterns. Furthermore, through RNA sequencing (RNA-seq) analysis, we will seek to identify genes that exhibit differential expressions in tissues related to open bite, providing valuable insights into the molecular mechanisms underlying this condition and uncovering potential therapeutic targets. The integration of GWAS data with Expression Quantitative Trait Loci (eQTL) analysis will offer a comprehensive approach to understanding the intricate relationship between genetics and the manifestation of this dental condition. These genetic analysis methods will be pivotal in advancing our knowledge of open bite etiology and will hold promise for innovative prevention and treatment strategies.

10. Treatment

The degree and form of malocclusion, the dysfunction, the age of the patient, and the general well-being, along with other individualized variables, all influence open bite therapy. Orthodontic therapy is generally considered the first line of treatment for open bite, and may involve the use of braces, clear aligners, or other orthodontic devices to reposition the teeth correctly and close the open space. In some cases, a surgical approach may be essential to address the fundamental skeletal problem responsible for the open bite.

There are different treatment strategies depending on the type of dysgnathy or dentoalveolar malformation, age, and desired treatment goals in terms of function, aesthetics, and stability:

10.1. Myofunctional Therapy

The aim of this treatment is to normalize function. The most common example is unphysiological breathing due to the position of the tongue in the oral cavity. This disorder leads to a narrowing of the airways, which causes an unphysiological tongue position. This malposition of the tongue can cause growth and tooth eruption disorders. With this treatment strategy, the function changes as well as the occlusion and the profile (Figure 13A–H).

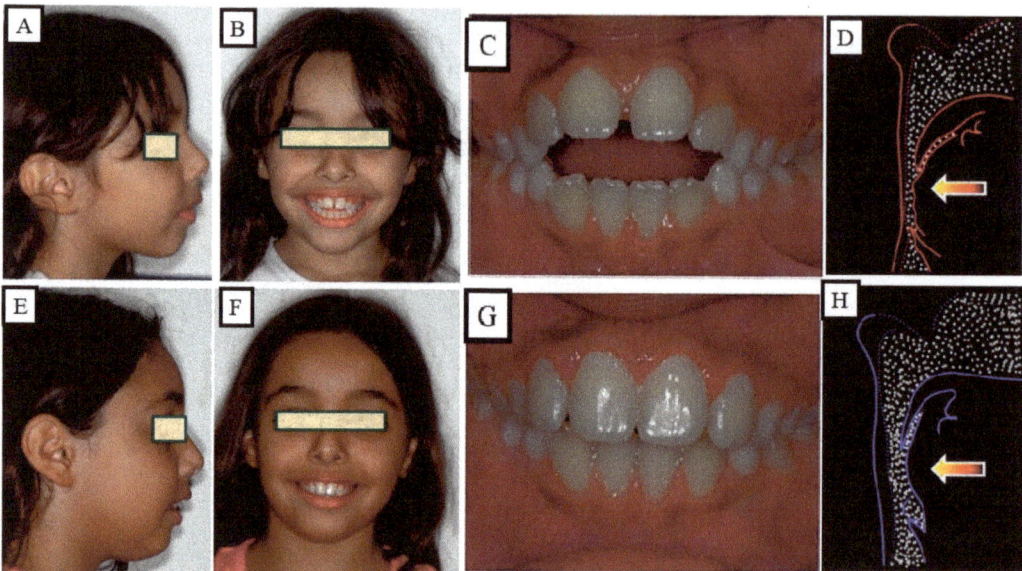

Figure 13. Patient with an anterior open bite. Due to the narrowed tongue space in the upper jaw and, thus, narrowed airways, there was a developmental disorder of the alveolar bone and the teeth. (**A–D**) Situation before treatment, (**D**) shows the narrowed airway. (**E–H**) The extra-oral and intraoral images after treatment, there was spontaneous bite closure after maxillary expansion. The physiological tongue position led to an expansion of the airways.

10.2. Skeletal Treatment by Influencing Growth

The existence of sufficient growth is a prerequisite for this treatment strategy. The growth of the maxilla can be reduced by vertical forces so that the mandible autorotates when the mandibular growth is undisturbed. This autorotation changes the position of the mandible in the vertical and sagittal dimensions. This leads to a reduction in the lower facial height and closure of the open bite. With this treatment strategy, the function changes as well as the occlusion and the profile (Figure 14A–I).

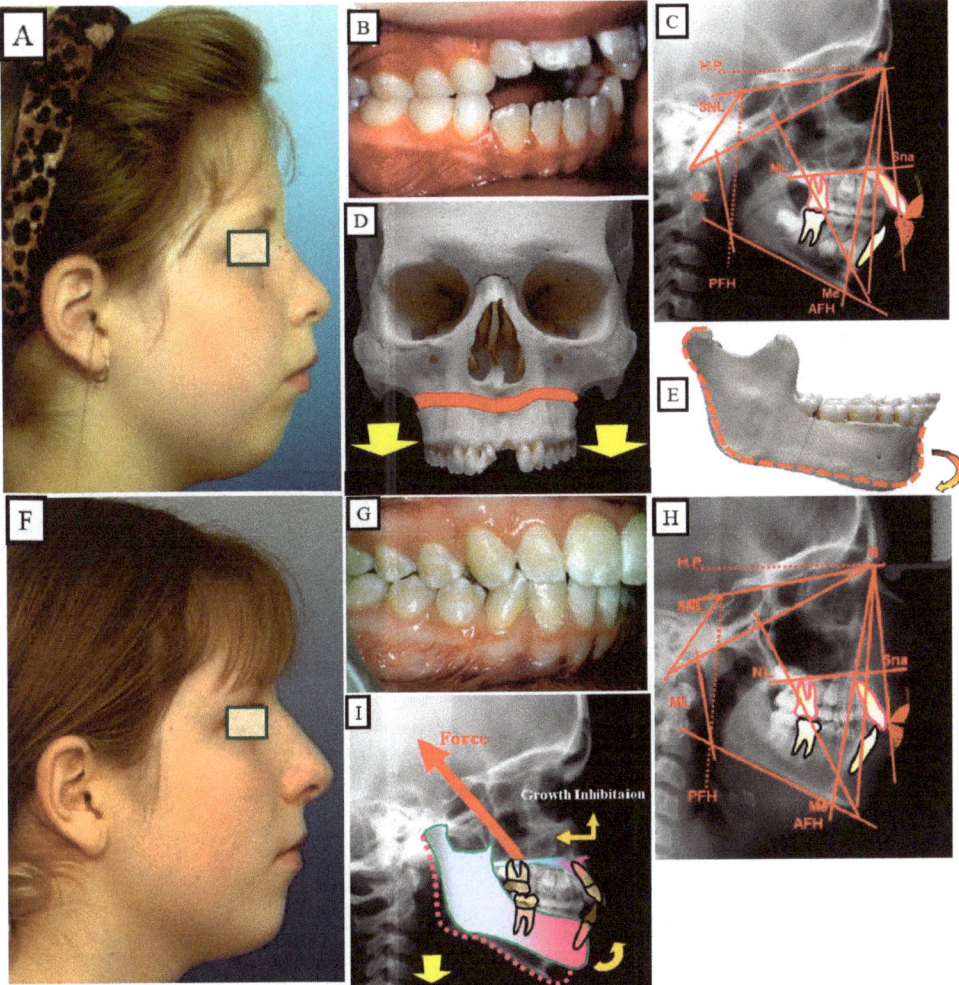

Figure 14. Skeletal open bite in a 10-year-old female patient, treated with growth-influencing measures. (**A–C**) Profile photo shows a long face with a skeletal open bite, which is confirmed intraorally and skeletal or cephalometrically. (**D,E**) Overdevelopment of the maxilla and alveolar bone resulted in posterior rotation of the mandible and thus posterior displacement of the mandible, resulting in the lower face lengthening. (**F–H**) treatment results of influencing the growth of the upper jaw in the vertical dimension, a harmonization of function and form, and, thus, a change in aesthetics. (**I**) Representation of the growth inhibition of the maxilla in the vertical direction, the autorotation of the mandible, and the alteration in position of the mandible.

10.3. Skeletal Treatment through Orthognathic Surgery

A prerequisite for this treatment strategy is completed growth. The skeletal open bite is corrected by surgically changing the vertical emission (upper jaw impaction), thus shortening the height of the lower face. A precisely planned maxillary impaction results in vertical and ventral autorotation of the mandible (Figure 15A–L).

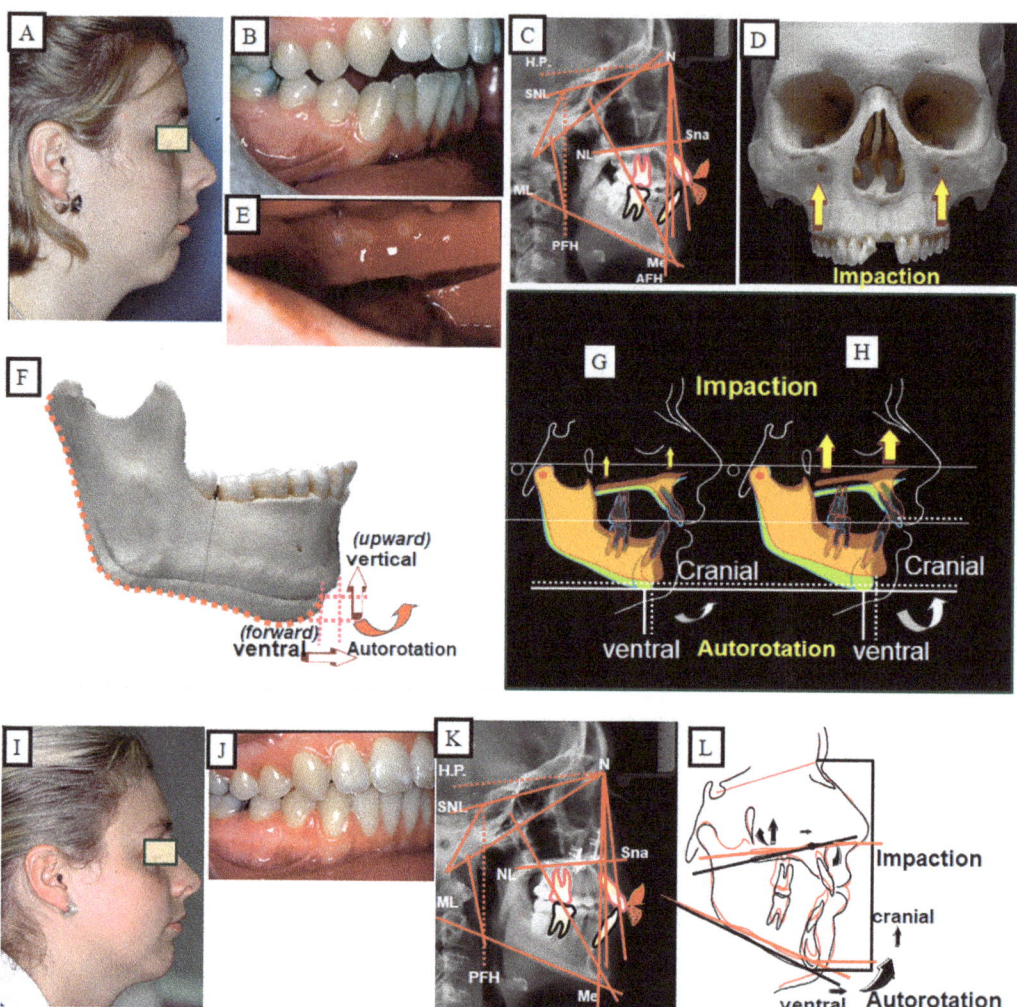

Figure 15. Skeletal open bite of a 25-year-old patient treated by orthognathic surgery. (**A–C**) The photograph shows a long face with a skeletal open bite, which is confirmed intraorally and is skeletal or cephalometric. (**D,E**) To correct the vertical relation, impaction of the maxilla was performed, and the excess bone of the maxilla was reduced. (**F**) A result of the maxillary action, the mandible autorotates with a change in sagittal and vertical position. (**G,H**) Simulation of the surgical impaction of the maxilla and the reaction of the mandible as described with cranial and simultaneous ventral autorotation. The greater the impact, the greater the autorotation of the mandible. (**I–K**) Situation after the treatment. (**L**) Superposition of the cephalograms pretreatment (black) and posttreatment (red).

Presurgical preparation sometimes requires dentoalveolar corrections by extrusion of the anterior teeth for a stable and perfect treatment result (Figure 16A–M). With this treatment strategy, the occlusion and the profile change, in addition to the function, are improved.

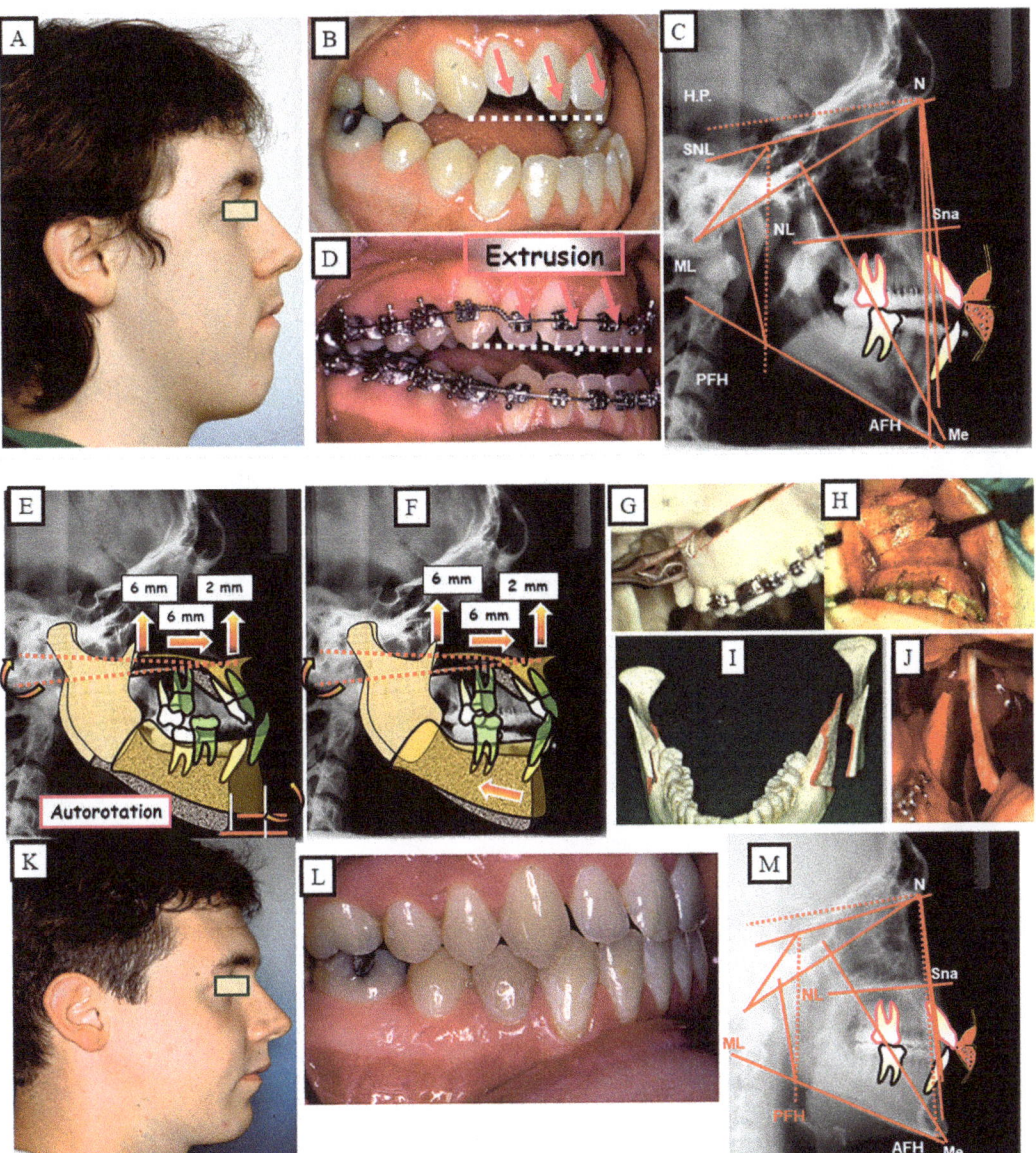

Figure 16. Skeletal and dental open bite in a 23-year-old man treated by orthognathic surgery. (**A–C**) Situation before the treatment, extended lower face due to the skeletal structure. The open bite has additionally strengthened the infra occlusion of the front teeth. (**D**) During the pre-surgical preparation, part of the open bite was corrected by extruding the front teeth. (**E,F**) Simulation of the surgical procedure. After impaction of the maxilla, the mandible autorotated with a change in position in the vertical and sagittal planes (**E**); for the final correction of the skeletal disgnathia, a dorsal displacement of the mandible (**F**) was carried out. (**G,H**) Description of maxillary impaction. (**I,J**) Representation of the surgical adjustment of the mandible for the correction of the position of the mandible. (**K–M**) Situation after the treatment.

10.4. Dentoalveolar Compensation Therapy (Camouflage Therapy) of Skeletal Dysgnathia

Some of the prerequisites for this therapy are that there are no functional disorders (such as difficult lip and mouth closure) and no serious extra-oral impairments (aesthetic disorders). This therapy uses intrusive biomechanics of the posterior teeth and extrusion biomechanics of the anterior teeth (Figure 17A–G). With this treatment strategy, the occlusion and the dental aesthetics change in addition to the function.

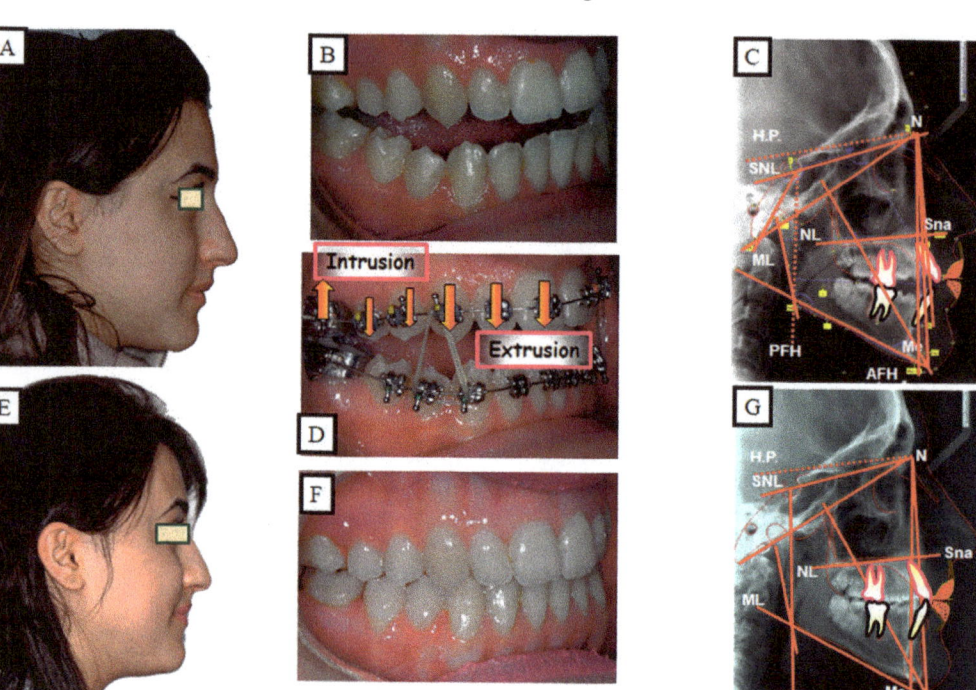

Figure 17. The Skeletal and dental open bite in a 25-year-old patient, treatment is dentoalveolar. It is crucial that the patient does not have any functional or aesthetic disorders extra-orally. (**A–C**) Situation before the treatment. (**D**) Presentation of the biomechanics used for ventoalveolar closure of the open bite; extrusion of the front and intrusion of the molars. (**E–G**) Situation after the treatment.

10.5. Dentoalveolar Treatment Strategy of the Dental Open Bite

No abnormalities can be seen extra-orally because the harmony is in the bones and in the soft tissue structures. Therefore, the treatment focuses on the dental malformations. The most common dental malformation is infraocclusion of the front teeth. When smiling, these patients show an inverted smile compared to an ideal smile. With this treatment strategy, the occlusion and the dental aesthetics change in addition to the function (Figure 18A–J).

In addition to the aforementioned factors, significant advancements in technology have brought about promising prospects in the realm of malocclusion treatment. Innovations including technologies like 3D printing and computer-assisted design and manufacturing (CAD/CAM) have revolutionized the field by enabling the production of personalized orthodontic appliances and surgical guides. This breakthrough facilitates the attainment of enhanced treatment precision and efficiency, as the appliances can be tailored to meet the specific requirements of each patient. The utilization of these cutting-edge technologies holds great potential in optimizing treatment outcomes for individuals with malocclusion.

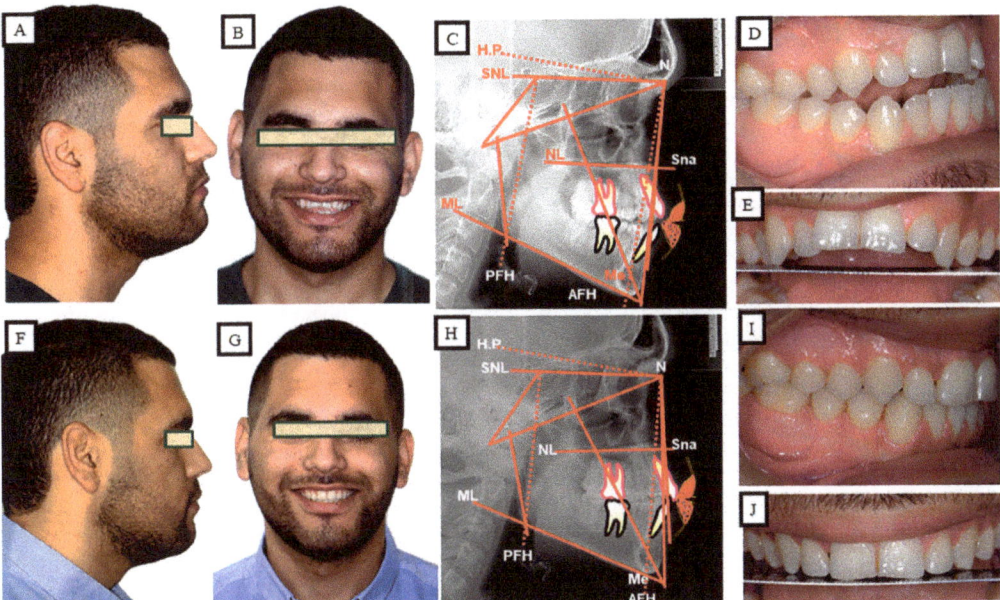

Figure 18. Dentoalveolar open bite in a 27-year-old patient, the treatment is dentoalveolar. The patient has no extra-oral functional or aesthetic disorders. There were intraoral dental functional and aesthetic disorders. (**A–E**) Before treatment, the infraocclusion of the front teeth in the upper jaw is clearly visible (**E**). (**F–J**) After treatment, to close the open bite, the maxillary front was extruded (**J**).

However, it is important to recognize that achieving the best possible results in malocclusion treatment necessitates the development of a personalized treatment plan under the guidance of a qualified orthodontic specialist. Several crucial factors must be taken into account, including the age and general well-being of the patient, as well as the degree and form of the malocclusion. By carefully considering these aspects, orthodontists can tailor treatment approaches to suit the unique needs and expectations of each patient. Therefore, fostering open and effective patient–orthodontist communication is essential, as it ensures the establishment of a comprehensive treatment plan that aligns with the individual's specific circumstances, leading to optimal outcomes.

11. Exploring the Etiology of the Open Bite through A Collaborative Cross Mouse Model

Dental conditions like open bite have significant implications for dental and overall wellness. To develop effective treatment strategies, it is imperative to comprehend the fundamental genetic and environmental variables that contribute to these conditions. In recent years, the utilization of mouse models, including the Collaborative Cross population, has emerged as a powerful method for investigating complex features and deciphering the underlying causes of dental problems. This section delves into how such creative methodologies can provide insights into the phenotypes of open bite, shedding light on underlying causes as well as prospective treatment methods [49].

12. Unveiling the Genetic Basis

Animal models provide an excellent platform for studying the genetic variables that contribute to deep bite and open bite. Scientists can develop mice with oral characteristics similar to these disorders by altering certain genes or causing mutations. This enables the study of potential genes implicated in the formation and preservation of dental occlusion. Scientists can investigate the impacts of specific genes and their connections on dental morphology and occlusal relations using knockout or knock-in mice models. Such investigations provide valuable insights into the genetic basis of deep bite and open bite, expanding our understanding of the complex genetic networks underlying these conditions [50].

The Collaborative Cross (CC) mouse population offers an exceptional chance to explore the multidimensional character of the open bite. The CC population is made up of genetically varied recombinant inbred mouse strains descended from many founder strains. This genetic diversity allows scientists to examine the effects of variation in genetic backgrounds on phenotypic variability. By thoroughly phenotyping the dental occlusion of CC mice, researchers can identify genetic loci associated with deep bite or open bite traits. Subsequent mapping studies help pinpoint specific genomic regions and candidate genes contributing to the observed phenotypes, enabling a more comprehensive understanding of the underlying biological mechanisms [51–56].

13. Discussion

Open bite malocclusion is a complex dental condition that can have genetic, environmental, and developmental causes. Genetic factors have an important impact on the development of open bite, involving certain genes and signaling pathways that play a part in jaw development, the eruption of teeth, and dental occlusion. Epigenetic mechanisms like DNA methylation and microRNA regulation may additionally impact malocclusion progression. Recognizing the genetic and epigenetic elements involved in open bite can lead to the development of better prevention and treatment strategies.

The treatment of open bite depends on various factors, and orthodontic treatment is generally the first line of approach. This may involve the use of braces, clear aligners, or other orthodontic appliances to move the teeth into the correct position and close the open space. In some cases, surgical intervention may be necessary to address the underlying skeletal issue causing the open bite. Advancements in technology, such as 3D printing and CAD/CAM, have improved treatment precision and efficiency.

Research using animal models, particularly the Collaborative Cross mouse population, has provided valuable insights into the genetic components of malocclusion. The genetic diversity of the CC mouse population allows researchers to study the genetic variants that contribute to open bite and understand its underlying mechanisms. Identifying the genetic factors involved in open bite can lead to the development of more targeted and effective treatment approaches.

Beyond genetic factors, environmental influences play a pivotal role in the development of dental occlusion abnormalities. The Collaborative Cross mouse approach provides researchers with the means to study the interactions between genes and the environment by exposing CC mice to various environmental conditions. Scientists can test how external variables interact with genetic predispositions to alter dental occlusion by altering factors such as food, mechanical loading, or hormone effects. This holistic approach allows for a deeper exploration of the intricate interaction between genetic and environmental variables in the formation of open bite [49].

The findings from mice models and CC populations hold immense potential for improving diagnostic and therapeutic strategies in human dentistry. Understanding the genetic and environmental variables that contribute to deep bite and open bite in mouse models can enable scientists to find possible biomarkers and genetic susceptibility factors in humans. These results can help to guide the creation of focused therapies and tailored treatment plans. Moreover, mouse models facilitate the preclinical testing of novel therapeutic interventions, including gene therapies and pharmacological treatments, before advancing them to clinical trials. This translational approach ensures a more comprehensive and evidence-based approach to addressing the challenges posed by deep bite and open bite [49]. Figure 19 demonstrates the procedure for creating system genetic databases using cellular, molecular, and clinical trait data in order to investigate associations between malocclusion and open bite phenotypes [57]. The regulatory genomic regions linked in phenotypic variance monitoring characteristics may be discovered using QTL mapping in the CC mouse model and humans by merging SNP genotype data and RNA expression. Combining existing data with future potential gene association studies in people offers the potential to find vulnerability genes linked to the development of open bite malocclusion in humans.

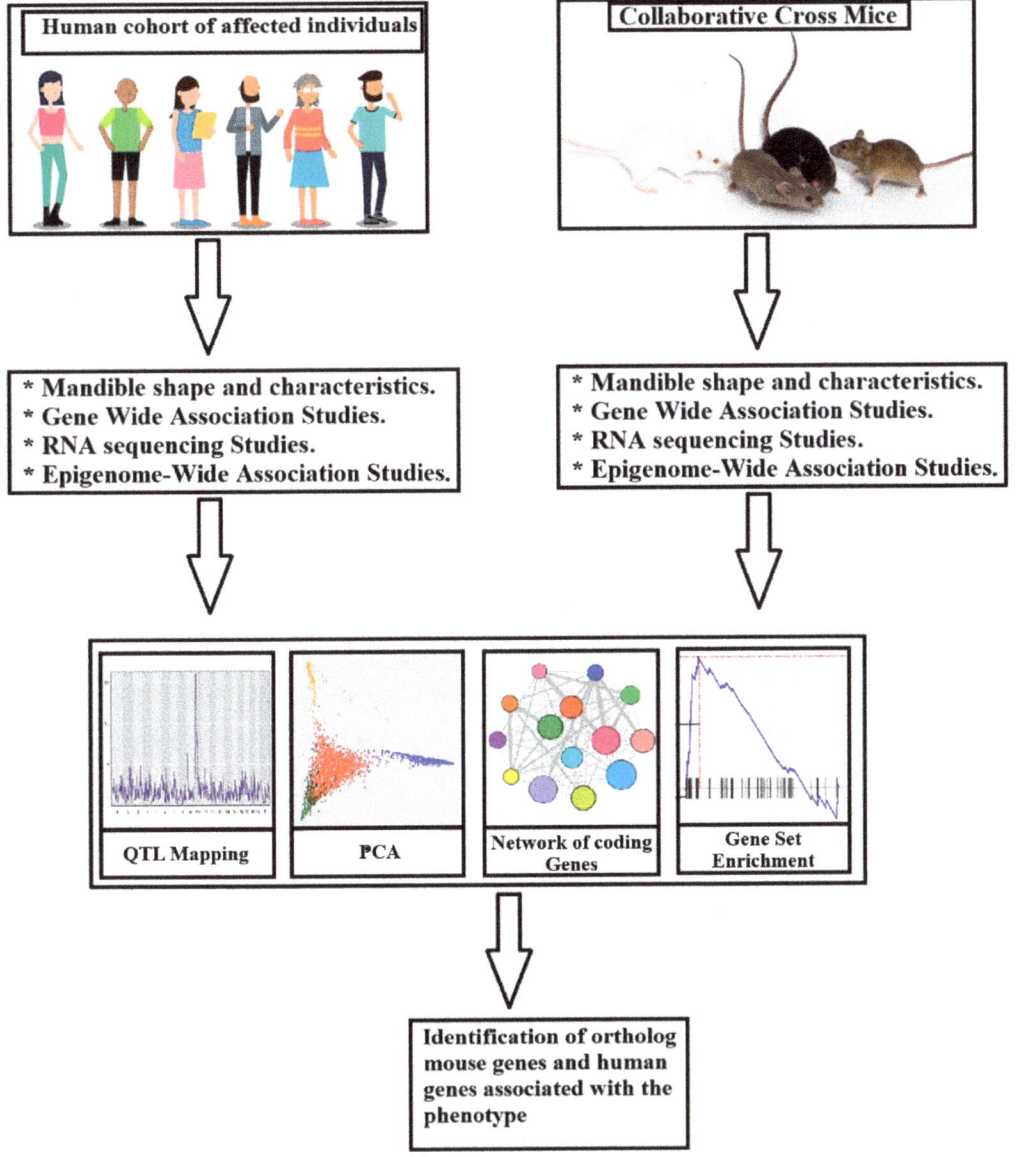

Figure 19. Process for creating system genetic datasets using cellular, molecular, and clinical trait data in order to investigate relationships between malocclusion and open bite phenotypes. Using QTL mapping in the CC mouse model and humans, regulatory genomic areas associated in phenotypic variance monitoring characteristics may be discovered by integrating SNP genotype data and RNA expression. The combination of existing data with future candidate gene association studies in people has the potential to find susceptibility genes linked to the development of open bite malocclusion in humans.

14. Conclusions

Orthodontists find it challenging to correct open bite malocclusion. Functional appliances and adult surgery are two common treatment techniques for growing children. Fixed orthodontics and other habit-breaking appliances are effective treatments for minor cases. With this kind of malocclusion, relapse rates are higher. The stomatognathic system's ability to function effectively is compromised in such circumstances. Since any mistake in determining the etiology could have negative consequences, more care should be given when diagnosing and arranging therapy for situations like this. As we delve into the intricate genetic underpinnings of open bite malocclusion, emerging tools and models like Collaborative Cross (CC) mice offer a promising avenue for research. The utilization of genetic insights and CC mice can lead to a deeper understanding of the genetic components governing this condition. By elucidating these genetic factors and their interactions, we pave the way for more precise diagnostic methods and targeted therapies. In this evolving landscape of malocclusion research, a paramount consideration is careful and meticulous diagnosis and treatment planning. Given the potential repercussions of errors in determining etiology, practitioners should exercise the utmost diligence. With genetics and CC mice at the forefront of exploration, the path toward innovative preventive and therapeutic strategies for open bite malocclusion is being illuminated, heralding a new era of dental care.

Author Contributions: Conceptualization, F.A.I., P.P. and N.W.; Methodology, I.M.L., O.Z., E.P., S.K., C.K. and K.M.; Validation, F.A.I.; Investigation, I.M.L., O.Z., K.M., E.P., S.K., C.K. and N.W.; Resources, F.A.I., P.P. and N.W.; Data Curation, I.M.L., O.Z. and K.M.; Writing—Original Draft Preparation, O.Z. and I.M.L.; Writing—Review and Editing, P.P., N.W. and F.A.I.; Supervision, F.A.I., P.P. and N.W.; Project Administration, F.A.I.; Funding Acquisition, F.A.I., P.P. and N.W. All authors have read and agreed to the published version of the manuscript.

Funding: This study was supported by core funds from Tel Aviv University, Arab American University in Jenin, and the University Hospital of Regensburg.

Institutional Review Board Statement: Ethical review and approval were waived for this study since there was no intervention procedure involved with patients or biological sample collection. However, we used ICS from patients for using their cephalometric images.

Informed Consent Statement: Informed consent was obtained from all subjects involved in the study.

Data Availability Statement: This study did not report any data.

Conflicts of Interest: The authors declare no conflict of interest.

References

1. Neela, P.K.; Atteeri, A.; Mamillapalli, P.K.; Sesham, V.M.; Keesara, S.; Chandra, J.; Monica, U.; Mohan, V. Genetics of dentofacial and orthodontic abnormalities. *Glob. Med. Genet.* **2020**, *7*, 95–100. [CrossRef] [PubMed]
2. Moreno Uribe, L.M.; Miller, S.F. Genetics of the dentofacial variation in human malocclusion. *Orthod. Craniofac. Res.* **2015**, *18* (Suppl. S1), 91–99. [CrossRef] [PubMed]
3. Lin, L.-H.; Huang, G.-W.; Chen, C.-S. Etiology and treatment modalities of anterior open bite malocclusion. *J. Exp. Clin. Med.* **2013**, *5*, 1–4. [CrossRef]
4. Watted, N.; Wieber, M.; Reuther, J. Treatment of a Class II Deformity with Skeletal Open Bite and Lateroocclusion. *Clin. Orthod. Res.* **2001**, *4*, 50–59. [CrossRef]
5. Kulshrestha, R.; Wajid, M.A.; Chandra, P.; Singh, K.; Rastogi, R.; Umale, V. Open bite malocclusion: An overview. *J. Oral Health Craniofacial Sci.* **2018**, *3*, 011–020.
6. Rijpstra, C.; Lisson, J.A. Etiology of anterior open bite: A review. *J. Orofac. Orthop.* **2016**, *77*, 281–286. [CrossRef]
7. Lone, I.M.; Midlej, K.; Nun, N.B.; Iraqi, F.A. Intestinal cancer development in response to oral infection with high-fat diet-induced Type 2 diabetes (T2D) in collaborative cross mice under different host genetic background effects. *Mamm. Genome* **2023**, *34*, 56–75. [CrossRef]
8. Lone, I.M.; Iraqi, F.A. Genetics of murine type 2 diabetes and comorbidities. *Mamm. Genome* **2022**, *33*, 421–436. [CrossRef]
9. Iraqi, F.A.; Churchill, G.; Mott, R. The Collaborative Cross, developing a resource for mammalian systems genetics: A status report of the Wellcome Trust cohort. *Mamm. Genome* **2008**, *19*, 379–381. [CrossRef]

10. Achmad, H.; Armedina, R.N.; Timokhina, T. Literature review: Problems of dental and oral health primary school children. *Indian J. Forensic Med. Toxicol.* **2021**, *15*, 2.
11. Huh, A.; Horton, M.J.; Cuenco, K.T.; Raoul, G.; Rowlerson, A.M.; Ferri, J.; Sciote, J.J. Epigenetic influence of KAT6B and HDAC4 in the development of skeletal malocclusion. *Am. J. Orthod. Dentofac. Orthop.* **2013**, *144*, 568–576. [CrossRef] [PubMed]
12. Kundakovic, M.; Jaric, I. The Epigenetic Link between Prenatal Adverse Environments and Neurodevelopmental Disorders. *Genes* **2017**, *8*, 104. [CrossRef]
13. Moyers, R.E. *Ortodontia*, 4th ed.; Trad. Coord. Por Aloysio Cariello. Rio de Janeiro; Guanabara Koogan: Chicago, IL, USA, 1991.
14. Teittinen, M.; Tuovinen, V.; Tammela, L.; Schätzle, M.; Peltomäki, T. Long-term stability of anterior open bite closure corrected by surgical-orthodontic treatment. *Eur. J. Orthod.* **2012**, *34*, 238–243. [CrossRef]
15. Farret, M.M.B.; Tomé, M.C.; Jurach, E.M.; Pires, R.T.T. Efeitos na mordida aberta anterior a partir do reposicionamento postural da língua. *Ortodon. Gaúch* **1999**, *3*, 118–124.
16. Kim, Y.H.; Han, U.K.; Lim, D.D.; Serraon, M.L. Stability of anterior openbite correction with multiloop edgewise archwire therapy: A cephalometric follow-up study. *Am. J. Orthod. Dentofac. Orthop.* **2000**, *118*, 43–54. [CrossRef] [PubMed]
17. Sodré, A.S.; Franco, E.A.; Monteiro, D.F. Mordida aberta anterior. *J. Bras. Ortodon. Ortop. Facial* **1998**, *3*, 80–94.
18. Pedrazzi, M.E. Treating the open bite. *J. Gen. Orthod.* **1997**, *8*, 5–16.
19. Meyer-Marcotty, P.; Hartmann, J.; Stellzig-Eisenhauer, A. Dentoalveolar open bite treatment with spur appliances. *J. Orofac. Orthop.* **2007**, *68*, 510–521. [CrossRef]
20. Esequiel, E.; Casasa, R. *Ortodoncia Contemporánea–Diagnóstico y Tratamiento*. In *Cap. Xv. Reabsorción Radicular Y Ortodoncia*, 1st ed.; Editorial Amolca. México DF: Ciudad de México, Mexico, 2005.
21. Chang, Y.I.; Moon, S.C. Cephalometric evaluation of the anterior open bite treatment. *Am. J. Orthod. Dentofac. Orthop.* **1999**, *115*, 29–38. [CrossRef]
22. Greenlee, G.M.; Huang, G.J.; Chen, S.S.-H.; Chen, J.; Koepsell, T.; Hujoel, P. Stability of treatment for anterior open-bite malocclusion: A meta-analysis. *Am. J. Orthod. Dentofac. Orthop.* **2011**, *139*, 154–169. [CrossRef]
23. Lawry, D.M.; Heggie, A.A.; Crawford, E.C.; Ruljancich, M.K. A review of the management of anterior open bite malocclusion. *Aust. Orthod. J.* **1990**, *11*, 147–160.
24. Stahl, F.; Grabowski, R. Malocclusion and caries prevalence: Is there a connection in the primary and mixed dentitions? *Clin. Oral Investig.* **2004**, *8*, 86–90. [CrossRef] [PubMed]
25. Cozza, P.; Mucedero, M.; Baccetti, T.; Franchi, L. Early orthodontic treatment of skeletal open-bite malocclusion: A systematic review. *Angle Orthod.* **2005**, *75*, 707–713. [CrossRef] [PubMed]
26. Shapiro, P.A. Stability of open bite treatment. *Am. J. Orthod. Dentofac. Orthop.* **2002**, *121*, 566–568. [CrossRef] [PubMed]
27. Bilodeau, J.E. Nonsurgical treatment of a Class III patient with a lateral open-bite malocclusion. *Am. J. Orthod. Dentofac. Orthop.* **2011**, *140*, 861–868. [CrossRef] [PubMed]
28. Justus, R. Correction of Anterior Open Bite with Spurs: Long-Term Stability. *World J. Orthod.* **2001**, *2*, 219–231.
29. Carlson, D.S. Theories of craniofacial growth in the postgenomic era. *Semin. Orthod.* **2005**, *11*, 172–183. [CrossRef]
30. Thilander, B. Basic mechanisms in craniofacial growth. *Acta Odontol. Scand.* **1995**, *53*, 144–151. [CrossRef]
31. Proffit, W.R.; Fields, H.W.; Larson, B.; Sarver, D.M. *Contemporary Orthodontics-E-Book*; Elsevier Health Sciences: Amsterdam, The Netherlands, 2018.
32. Maciel, C.T.V.; Leite, I.C.G. Etiological aspects of anterior open bite and its implications to the oral functions. *Pro Fono Rev. Atualizacao Cient.* **2005**, *17*, 293–302. [CrossRef]
33. Arat, Z.M.; Akcam, M.O.; Esenlik, E.; Arat, F.E. Inconsistencies in the differential diagnosis of open bite. *Angle Orthod.* **2008**, *78*, 415–420. [CrossRef]
34. Sandler, P.J.; Madahar, A.K.; Murray, A. Anterior open bite: Aetiology and management. *Dent Update* **2011**, *38*, 522–524, 527. [CrossRef] [PubMed]
35. Reichert, I.; Figel, P.; Winchester, L. Orthodontic treatment of anterior open bite: A review article--is surgery always necessary? *Oral Maxillofac. Surg.* **2014**, *18*, 271–277. [CrossRef]
36. Dixit, U.B.; Shetty, R.M. Comparison of soft-tissue, dental, and skeletal characteristics in children with and without tongue thrusting habit. *Contemp. Clin. Dent.* **2013**, *4*, 2–6. [CrossRef] [PubMed]
37. Park, Y.-C.; Lee, H.-A.; Choi, N.-C.; Kim, D.-H. Open Bite Correction by Intrusion of Posterior Teeth with Miniscrews. *Angle Orthod.* **2008**, *78*, 699–710. [CrossRef]
38. Togawa, R.; Iino, S.; Miyawaki, S. Skeletal Class III and open bite treated with bilateral sagittal split osteotomy and molar intrusion using titanium screws. *Angle Orthod.* **2010**, *80*, 1176–1184. [CrossRef] [PubMed]
39. Proffit, W.R.; Bailey, L.T.J.; Phillips, C. Long-term stability of surgical open-bite correction by Le Fort I osteotomy. *Angle Orthod.* **2000**, *70*, 112–117.
40. Nielsen, I. Vertical malocclusion: Etiology, development, diagnosis and some aspects of treatment. *Angle Orthod.* **1991**, *61*, 247–260.
41. Torres, F.C.; de Almeida, R.R.; de Almeida-Pedrin, R.R.; Pedrin, F.; Paranhos, L.R. Dentoalveolar comparative study between removable and fixed cribs, associated to chincup, in anterior open bite treatment. *J. Appl. Oral Sci.* **2012**, *20*, 531–537. [CrossRef]
42. Huang, W.; Shan, B.; Ang, B.S.; Ko, J.; Bloomstein, R.D.; Cangialosi, T.J. Review of etiology of posterior open bite: Is there a possible genetic cause? *Clin. Cosmet. Investig. Dent.* **2020**, *12*, 233–240. [CrossRef]

43. Cakan, D.G.; Ulkur, F.; Taner, T.U. The genetic basis of facial skeletal characteristics and its relation with orthodontics. *Eur. J. Dent.* **2012**, *6*, 340–345. [CrossRef]
44. Rowley, R.; Hill, F.J.; Winter, G.B. An investigation of the association between anterior open-bite and amelogenesis imperfecta. *Am. J. Orthod.* **1982**, *81*, 229–235. [CrossRef] [PubMed]
45. Küchler, E.C.; Barreiros, D.; da Silva, R.O.; de Abreu, J.G.B.; Teixeira, E.C.; da Silva, R.A.B.; da Silva, L.A.B.; Nelson Filho, P.; Romano, F.L.; Granjeiro, J.M.; et al. Genetic polymorphism in MMP9 may be associated with anterior open bite in children. *Braz. Dent. J.* **2017**, *28*, 277–280. [CrossRef] [PubMed]
46. Leal, M.F.C.; Lemos, A.; Costa, G.F.; Lopes Cardoso, I. Genetic and Environmental Factors Involved in The Development of Oral Malformations Such As Cleft Lip/Palate In Non-Syndromic Patients And Open Bite Malocclusion. *EJMED* **2020**, *2*, 1–11. [CrossRef]
47. Nishio, C.; Huynh, N. Skeletal Malocclusion and Genetic Expression: An Evidence-Based Review. *JDSM* **2016**, *3*, 57–63. [CrossRef]
48. Teixeira, E.C.; das Neves, B.M.; Castilho, T.; Silva Ramos, T.; Flaviana, A.; Carelli, J.; Kuchler, E.C.; Germano, F.N.; Alves Antunes, L.A.; Antunes, L.S. Evidence of Association between MTRR and TNF-α Gene Polymorphisms and Oral Health-Related Quality of Life in Children with Anterior Open Bite. *J. Clin. Pediatr. Dent.* **2022**, *46*, 249–258. [CrossRef] [PubMed]
49. Lone, I.M.; Zohud, O.; Nashef, A.; Kirschneck, C.; Proff, P.; Watted, N.; Iraqi, F.A. Dissecting the Complexity of Skeletal-Malocclusion-Associated Phenotypes: Mouse for the Rescue. *Int. J. Mol. Sci.* **2023**, *24*, 2570. [CrossRef]
50. Carver, E.A.; Oram, K.F.; Gridley, T. Craniosynostosis in Twist heterozygous mice: A model for Saethre-Chotzen syndrome. *Anat. Rec. Off. Publ. Am. Assoc. Anat.* **2002**, *268*, 90–92. [CrossRef]
51. Collaborative Cross Consortium. The genome architecture of the Collaborative Cross mouse genetic reference population. *Genetics* **2012**, *190*, 389–401. [CrossRef]
52. Yehia, R.; Lone, I.M.; Yehia, I.; Iraqi, F.A. Studying the Pharmagenomic effect of Portulaca oleracea extract on anti-diabetic therapy using the Collaborative Cross mice. *Phytomed. Plus* **2023**, *3*, 100394. [CrossRef]
53. Lone, I.M.; Zohud, O.; Midlej, K.; Proff, P.; Watted, N.; Iraqi, F.A. Skeletal Class II Malocclusion: From Clinical Treatment Strategies to the Roadmap in Identifying the Genetic Bases of Development in Humans with the Support of the Collaborative Cross Mouse Population. *J. Clin. Med.* **2023**, *12*, 5148. [CrossRef]
54. Lone, I.M.; Nun, N.B.; Ghnaim, A.; Schaefer, A.S.; Houri-Haddad, Y.; Iraqi, F.A. High-fat diet and oral infection induced type 2 diabetes and obesity development under different genetic backgrounds. *Anim. Models Exp. Med.* **2023**, *6*, 131–145. [CrossRef]
55. Ghnaim, A.; Lone, I.M.; Ben Nun, N.; Iraqi, F.A. Unraveling the Host Genetic Background Effect on Internal Organ Weight Influenced by Obesity and Diabetes Using Collaborative Cross Mice. *Int. J. Mol. Sci.* **2023**, *24*, 8201. [CrossRef] [PubMed]
56. Lone, I.M.; Zohud, O.; Midlej, K.; Awadi, O.; Masarwa, S.; Krohn, S.; Kirschneck, C.; Proff, P.; Watted, N.; Iraqi, F.A. Narrating the Genetic Landscape of Human Class I Occlusion: A Perspective-Infused Review. *J. Pers. Med.* **2023**, *13*, 1465. [CrossRef] [PubMed]
57. Watted, N.; Lone, I.M.; Osayd Zohud, O.; Midlej, K.; Proff, P.; Iraqi, F.A. Comprehensive Deciphering the Complexity of the Deep Bite: Insight from Animal Model to Human Subjects. *J. Pers. Med.* **2023**, *13*, 1472. [CrossRef] [PubMed]

Disclaimer/Publisher's Note: The statements, opinions and data contained in all publications are solely those of the individual author(s) and contributor(s) and not of MDPI and/or the editor(s). MDPI and/or the editor(s) disclaim responsibility for any injury to people or property resulting from any ideas, methods, instructions or products referred to in the content.

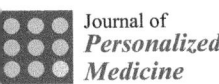

Review

Systems Biology in Cancer Diagnosis Integrating Omics Technologies and Artificial Intelligence to Support Physician Decision Making

Alaa Fawaz, Alessandra Ferraresi and Ciro Isidoro *

Laboratory of Molecular Pathology, Department of Health Sciences, Università del Piemonte Orientale, 28100 Novara, Italy; 20041632@studenti.uniupo.it (A.F.); alessandra.ferraresi@med.uniupo.it (A.F.)
* Correspondence: ciro.isidoro@med.uniupo.it; Tel.: +39-0321-660507; Fax: +39-0321-620421

Abstract: Cancer is the second major cause of disease-related death worldwide, and its accurate early diagnosis and therapeutic intervention are fundamental for saving the patient's life. Cancer, as a complex and heterogeneous disorder, results from the disruption and alteration of a wide variety of biological entities, including genes, proteins, mRNAs, miRNAs, and metabolites, that eventually emerge as clinical symptoms. Traditionally, diagnosis is based on clinical examination, blood tests for biomarkers, the histopathology of a biopsy, and imaging (MRI, CT, PET, and US). Additionally, omics biotechnologies help to further characterize the genome, metabolome, microbiome traits of the patient that could have an impact on the prognosis and patient's response to the therapy. The integration of all these data relies on gathering of several experts and may require considerable time, and, unfortunately, it is not without the risk of error in the interpretation and therefore in the decision. Systems biology algorithms exploit Artificial Intelligence (AI) combined with omics technologies to perform a rapid and accurate analysis and integration of patient's big data, and support the physician in making diagnosis and tailoring the most appropriate therapeutic intervention. However, AI is not free from possible diagnostic and prognostic errors in the interpretation of images or biochemical–clinical data. Here, we first describe the methods used by systems biology for combining AI with omics and then discuss the potential, challenges, limitations, and critical issues in using AI in cancer research.

Keywords: artificial intelligence; medical technology; smart health; digital health; omics technologies; imaging; diagnosis; personalized medicine

Citation: Fawaz, A.; Ferraresi, A.; Isidoro, C. Systems Biology in Cancer Diagnosis Integrating Omics Technologies and Artificial Intelligence to Support Physician Decision Making. *J. Pers. Med.* **2023**, *13*, 1590. https://doi.org/10.3390/jpm13111590

Academic Editor: Daniele Giansanti

Received: 17 October 2023
Revised: 7 November 2023
Accepted: 8 November 2023
Published: 10 November 2023

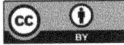

Copyright: © 2023 by the authors. Licensee MDPI, Basel, Switzerland. This article is an open access article distributed under the terms and conditions of the Creative Commons Attribution (CC BY) license (https://creativecommons.org/licenses/by/4.0/).

1. Introduction

Delayed diagnoses, misdiagnoses, and missed diagnoses impact patient health and safety, and have great societal consequences. Mistakes in diagnosis may account for up to 60% of all medical errors and are accountable for up to 80,000 deaths in U.S. medical centers each year [1]. Typically, clinicians have limited time to make decisions based on the interpretation of huge amounts of laboratory, imaging, and clinical data, and this increases the risk of underestimating (or sometimes overestimating) some data. Furthermore, subjective factors, such as personal experience and medical specialty, are potential bias factors that influence the accuracy of diagnosis [2].

Artificial Intelligence (AI), a field of computer science used for prediction and automation, has emerged as a potential solution to promote a precision approach in healthcare and is expected to reduce errors caused by human judgment in various medical domains [3].

Cancer is the leading cause of death in people, accounting for an estimated 10 million deaths by 2020 [4]. It is a complex disease resulting from anomalies in physiological processes involving genes, coding and non-coding RNAs, proteins, metabolites, and other biomolecules [5,6]. To understand such a complex disease from its onset to its progression, multi-omics analysis of these numerous bio-entities is required. Modern biotechnologies allow for the high throughput analysis of the sequence and expression of many genes (genomics and epigenomics), proteins and their post-translational modifications (proteomics, phospho-proteomics and glycol-proteomics), RNAs (RNA transcriptomics), non-coding RNAs (including miRNAs and long-non-coding RNAs), and metabolites (metabolomics) from the same organism [7]. However, a platform where all these big data are integrated to uncover correlations and synergisms among the biological pathways and processes is required. Systems biology combines the power of AI and of multi-omics technologies for modeling the signaling and metabolic signature of a given cancer. This is instrumental for designing effective diagnostic and prognostic markers and novel and patient-tailored therapeutic interventions.

Despite difficulties in providing individualized and data-driven care, advancements in screening, diagnosis, treatment, and survival rate in cancer patients have been remarkable in recent decades [8]. Early detection and prognosis prediction represent two crucial clinical needs for limiting cancer progression. Body and organ computed scan methodologies, the histopathology imaging of biopsies, and a range of blood tests for detecting biomarkers are instrumental in the initial diagnosis process and for determining cancer staging, the grade of malignancy, and prognosis. These approaches do not provide information on the molecular alterations that precede and follow the onset of cancer. Molecular and omics technologies can provide a genetic, epigenetic, and metabolic profile of the tumor that can better define such alterations thus helping to determine the most appropriate treatment as well as predict the response to therapy [9,10].

The development and extensive use of high-throughput technologies has ushered in the era of biological and medical big data. This has led to the accumulation of data sets on a large scale, thereby opening a wide range of potential applications for data-driven methods in cancer treatment, spanning from basic research to clinical practice: molecular tumor characterization, tumor heterogeneity, drug discovery and potential therapeutic strategies. As a result, the data-driven research field of bioinformatics adapts data mining techniques, such as systems biology, machine learning, and deep learning, which are discussed in this review paper. Systems biology uses a data-driven approach to identify important signaling pathways. The pathway-oriented analysis is extremely important in cancer research because it helps researchers comprehend the molecular features and heterogeneity of tumors and tumor subtypes [11]. In this context, the proper clinical care for cancer patients can be improved by the introduction of AI in cancer detection, diagnosis, and treatment [12–15].

AI-based technologies applied to oncology aim at improving clinical practice, including but not limited to the early and accurate diagnosis and prediction of personalized outcomes (i.e., prognosis and therapy response), by acquiring a profound perception of tumor molecular biology through the association of multiple biological parameters [16].

Artificial Intelligence in Medicine at Glance

AI is meant to mimic human cognitive abilities in elaborating the information but at a much higher speed and with no emotional interference. The main types of AI that apply to cancer-patient healthcare include machine learning (ML) and its evolved subtype deep learning (DL), which can assist in making a rapid and more accurate diagnosis (based on biochemical, clinical data, and medical imaging), in discovering and developing new drugs, in designing personalized therapy, in predicting the therapy response, and in guiding the robotic surgery [17,18] (Figure 1).

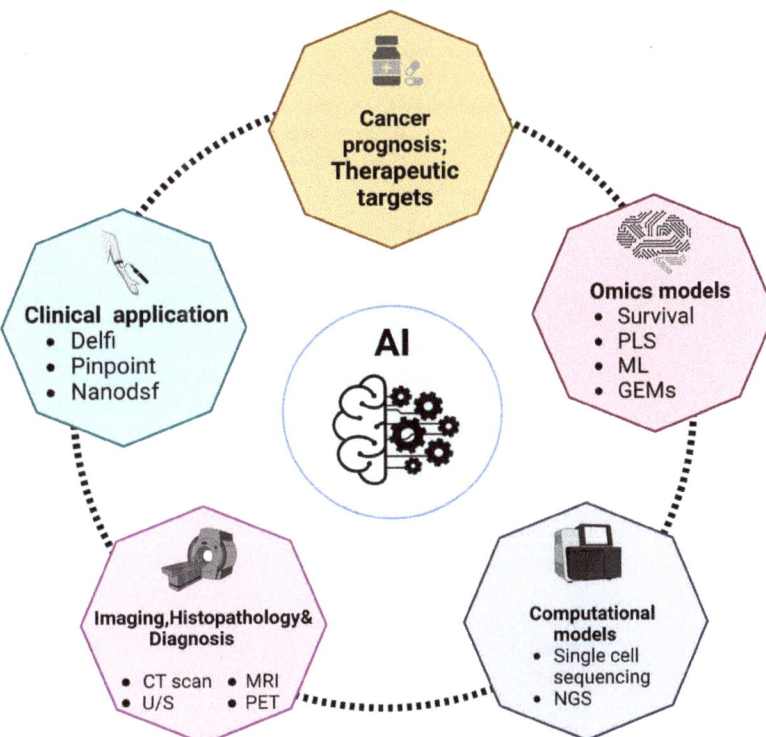

Figure 1. Overview of the applications of AI to cancer diagnosis and oncology research field. The scheme depicts the main fields of application of AI discussed in this review. Abbreviations: computed tomography, CT; gene expression models, GEMs; machine learning, ML; magnetic resonance imaging, MRI; nano differential scanning fluorimetry, Nanodsf; next-generation sequencing, NGS; positron emission tomography, PET; partial least squares analysis, PLS; ultrasound imaging, U/S.

Current AI systems have been involved to be used in a variety of clinical settings, including (i) image-based computer-aided discovery and diagnosis in various medical specialties, (ii) the translation of genomic information for recognizing genetic variants using high-throughput sequencing technologies, and (iii) the prediction and tracking of patient's prognosis [19,20]. Moreover, they have been implemented as well in (iv) the discovery of new biomarkers by combining omics and phenotype data, (v) the detection of health status using biological signals (e.g., enzyme activity and protein concentration) obtained from wearable devices, and (vi) the production and implementation of autonomous robots in medical procedures [19,20].

The creation of AI models that predict the properties of vast and interconnected networks found in living organisms would allow for a thorough examination of how signaling molecules generate functional cellular reactions. Machine learning (ML) algorithms, a subset of AI, are capable of making decisive interpretations of large, complex data sets, making them an effective tool for analyzing and comprehending multi-omics data for patient-specific observations [20]. We can anticipate the remarkable growth of AI in the medical field in light of the digital acquisition of high-dimensional and annotated medical data, the progress of ML methods, open ML data science, and advancements in computational power and storage services [20]. AI is expected to make it easier to diagnose specific illnesses in patients. Commonly, deep learning (DL) architectures are analogous to artificial neural networks of multiple non-linear tiers. Over the past decade, a large variety of DL designs have been developed depending on the input data type and the purpose of the research. Moreover, the assessment of the model's efficiency has revealed that DL application on cancer prognosis surpasses other traditional ML techniques. DL frameworks have also been used in cancer diagnosis, classification, and treatment by utilizing genomic profiles and phenotype information. Systems biology has been an effective method to comprehend the complex molecular profile of cancers, interpret the mechanisms of tumor progression, and allow for the amalgamation of omics data as well as the characterization of diverse tumors [21,22].

2. Omics Data for Identifying Cancer Metabolic Biomarkers

Omics technologies allow for the in depth analysis of the molecular characteristics of cancer at both bulk and single-cell level, providing a wealth of multi-omics data that challenge the capability of scientists and medical doctor to combine for drawing a consistent picture of the multilayer complexity of cancer biology. Genomic, epigenomic, transcriptomic, proteomic, and metabolomic data can be elaborated using appropriate models for making predictions about prognosis and treatment response in a patient-tailored (personalized) manner [13,15,22].

2.1. Survival Models

To find cancer metabolic biomarkers, survival models have been used more frequently than partial least squares (PLS) models, ML models, and gene expression modeling (GEM) [23] (Figure 2). The Kaplan–Meier method, the log-rank test, and/or the Cox regression model are representative survival models used in cancer studies. These models are used to describe the likelihood of survival (or survival curve) for a group of patients after treatment, compare the survival curves of two or more treatment groups, and describe the effects of multiple explanatory (independent) variables, profiles of gene expression, and metabolite concentration) on survival curves, respectively. In contrast to Kaplan–Meier models, which must discretize their data, the Cox regression model has the advantage of processing continuous values directly, minimizing data loss [24]. In their study, based on GEM of seven major metabolic pathways, Peng and colleagues identified 30 tumor subtypes in 33 different cancer types (such as breast invasive carcinoma, cholangiocarcinoma, colorectal cancer, glioblastoma multiforme, gastrointestinal tumors, lung cancer, pancreatic cancer, and ovarian serous cystadenocarcinoma, among others) and evaluated the clinical utility of so-called metabolic expression subtypes. For this, correlations between metabolic expression subtypes and their corresponding prognosis were investigated using the Kaplan–Meier method, log-rank test, and Cox regression model. Consequently, subtypes with upregulated lipid metabolism appeared to have a better prognosis than subtypes with upregulated glycemic, nucleotide, vitamin, and cofactor metabolism. The association of various somatic mutations in cancer driver genes with metabolic expression subtypes has also been discovered. Two transcription factors, SNAI1 and RUNX1, were identified from knockdown studies as potential therapeutic targets for a subtype of cancer with upregulated carbohydrate metabolism that consistently had a poor prognosis across cancer types [23].

2.2. PLS Models

Partial least squares regression (PLS) was initially created as a regression model that processes numerous independent variables that are correlated and produce numerous dependent variables, which many statistical and ML techniques cannot directly handle. PLS models and their variations, particularly PLS-discriminant analysis (PLS-DA) are frequently used for the analysis of omics data with a focus on metabolomics [25]. PLS-DA has been primarily used to extract insights from large datasets of omics data, such as identifying metabolites from metabolome data that differentiate between cancer cells in their various statuses. PLS-DA might have an overfitting issue too, like other data mining techniques, so it needs thorough validation, frequently performed through cross-validation [26].

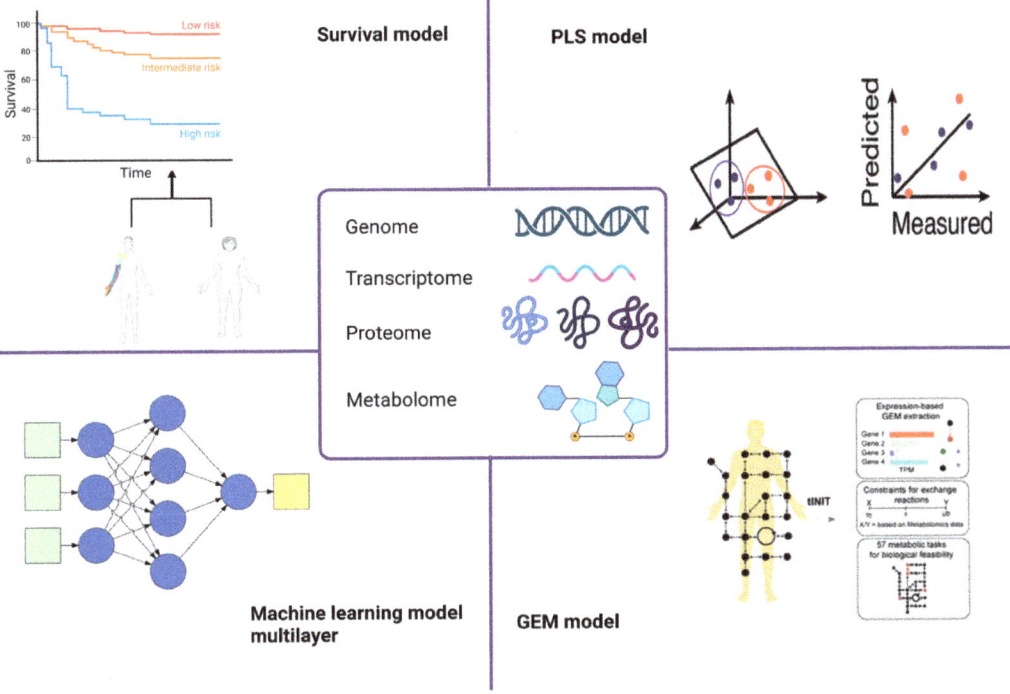

Figure 2. Overview of the omics technologies exploited in cancer diagnosis/prognosis. The scheme depicts the main omics models currently used in biomarker identification. Abbreviations: gene expression modeling, GEM; partial least squares analysis, PLS.

PLS-DA and its variants have been used to analyze metabolome data to identify a variety of cancers, including breast cancer, glioma, non-small cell lung cancer, oral precancerous cells, cervical precancerous lesions, and prostate cancer [27,28]. Among its advantages, PLS-DA allows for the analysis of highly collinear and noisy data. Moreover, the calibration model provides a subset of useful statistics, including prediction accuracy, scores and loading plots. However, a potential limitation has emerged when this method was applied to metabolomics; the use of this model by non-experts may produce inaccurate results, owing to a lack of appropriate statistical validation [29] (Table 1).

Table 1. Summary of the main advantages and limitations of PLS models.

Advantages	Limitations
Ability to robustly handle more descriptor variables	Higher risk of overlooking 'real' correlations
Provide more predictive accuracy	Sensitivity to the relative scaling of the descriptor variables
Low risk of chance correlation	

2.3. Genome-Scale Metabolic Models

Gene expression modeling (GEM) is a computational model based on the law of mass conservation of metabolites and allows for the prediction of metabolic fluxes for entire biochemical reactions taking place inside a cell by using numerical optimization [30,31]. Technically, GEM describes the participation of each metabolite for an entire set of biochemical reactions in the form of a stoichiometric matrix and is simulated using varied forms of objective functions and constraints that reflect genetic and environmental conditions of interest. As a result, GEM allows for the efficient simulation of a target cell's metabolic phenotypes under a wide range of genetic and environmental conditions. GEM can also be integrated with omics data, such as RNA-seq, for building a cell-specific model and thereafter modeling multicellular organisms. In comparison with ML models, GEMs generate more interpretable prediction outcomes that grasp a cell-specific metabolic phenotype. GEM simulations, however, demand consideration. Due to the possibility of biologically incorrect objective functions or constraints, it is advised to proceed with the analysis of the predicted intracellular metabolic flux distributions from GEMs with caution. A representative issue is the use of constraints that do not accurately reflect a culture medium. Finally, GEMs do not directly produce additional data for regulatory and signaling networks, which are also crucial for understanding the physiology of a cell [32,33] (Table 2).

Table 2. Summary of the main advantages and limitations of GEM models.

Advantages	Limitations
Explore metabolism in multiple cell types	Uncertainties in the estimated parameters regarding quantitative flux predictions
Validating or discovering biomarkers for screening, diagnostics, prognostics, and/or patient stratification	Ambiguous normalization of experimentally quantified fluxes
Identify cancer-specific metabolic features that constitute generic potential drug targets for cancer treatment	

2.4. Machine Learning Models

The classification task of disease prediction has been thoroughly studied in medical oncology and cancer research, based on well-established machine learning algorithms for dealing with binary or multi-class learning problems. Patient categorization would allow for the development of ML-based predictive models capable of assessing risk stratification with generalizable performance. Based on images and genetic data, DL models were trained to classify and detect disease subtypes. These data-driven approaches demonstrated the superiority of ML-based frameworks for leveraging heterogeneous datasets for improved diagnosis and treatment [34].

2.5. Deep Neural Networks (DNNs)

Deep neural network (DNN) models are rapidly evolving and becoming more sophisticated. They have been widely used in biomedical research across the board. Initially, large-scale imaging and video data aided its development. While most biomedical data sets are not considered big data, the rapid data accumulation enabled by NGS made it suitable for the application of DNN models that require a large amount of training data [35]. In 2019, for example, Samiei et al. used TCGA-based large-scale cancer data as benchmark datasets for bioinformatics machine learning research, such as Image-Net in computer vision [36]. Following that, large-scale public cancer data sets like the TCGA encouraged the widespread use of DNNs in cancer research [37] (Table 3).

Table 3. Summary of the main advantages and limitations of DNN models.

Advantages	Limitations
Ability to handle complex data and relationships	Massive data requirement
Effective at producing high-quality results	High processing and computational power
Extremely scalable because of its capacity to analyze large volumes of data	Black box problem making them hard to debug and understand how they make decisions

2.6. Graph Neural Networks (GNNs)

Graph neural networks (GNNs) have achieved great results and are being progressively employed in a node classification task. It offers a strategy to acquire novel representations of nodes by combining the features of its local neighborhood and connectivity. Recently, some GNN-based approaches have been proposed to forecast the molecular subtyping of cancer. Rhee et al. created a graph convolutional network (GCN)-based model to investigate the gene–gene alliance and information transmission for cancer subtyping [38]. Lee et al. developed a GCN model with a focus on the mechanisms to learn pathway-level representations of cancer samples for their subtype classification [39]. Even though GNNs are strong, it is reported that they are susceptible when the structure of the graph and nodes' features are polluted with noise [40]. Thus, a robust GNN model is required for the precise and stable prediction of cancer subtypes [41] (Table 4).

Table 4. Summary of the main advantages and limitations of GNN models.

Advantages	Limitations
Rapid processing of massive data	Limited to a fixed number of points
Reliable performance in mining deep-level topological information	Time and space complexity are higher
Extracting text relationship and reasoning the structure of graphics and images	Less handling of edges of graphs based on their types and relations

3. Computational Models for the Prediction of Cancer Metabolic Biomarkers

Single-cell sequencing allows for the study of the molecular changes occurring in individual cells within the tumor mass. Nonetheless, attributing a specific cellular annotation (in terms of cell type or metabolic state) is challenging, in particular to distinguish cancer cells in single-cell or spatial sequencing experiments. The information provided by high-throughput single-cell sequencing provides not only the description of distinct cellular annotations but also the functional annotation of single cells, for example the estimation of the differentiation potential, vulnerability to metabolic changes, and a prediction of cellular crosstalk [42]. However, the use of this technology also raises computational difficulties [43]. One of the major challenges in single-cell data analysis is to attribute a cell annotation to each cell analyzed [44]. The magnitude of the generated datasets renders the manual annotation processes unfeasible, whereas the peculiarities of data generation have stimulated the spread of novel and creative classification methods [45]. This limitation is particularly found in datasets coming from cancer tissues, in which the variability in the transcriptomic states does not conform to traditionally defined cell types [46,47].

In addition to the genome data, the transcriptome, proteome, and metabolome data offer snapshots of a cell's phenotype space. As shown by PCAWG58 and TCGA59, which also provide transcriptome data in addition to genome data, the transcriptome, particularly RNA sequencing (RNA-seq), is the most frequently generated omics data among these. To perform more complex transcriptomic analyses, bulk RNA-seq has evolved into single-cell RNA-seq (scRNA-seq) and spatial RNA-seq. To enable a greater understanding of cell phenotypes, massive amounts of proteome and metabolome data are being generated for various human cells [48,49]. The Human Metabolome Database (HMDB) and Human Protein Atlas (HPA) are representative databases for the human proteome and metabolome, respectively. Integrative omics analysis has gained importance since these omics data are complementary to one another, and multiple omics data are frequently generated for a target cell [50,51].

Several studies have combined NGS data with ML to propose a novel data-driven methodology in systems biology [52]. Several network-based ML models have been implemented to analyze cancer data and aid in the understanding of novel mechanisms in cancer development [53,54]. Furthermore, the use of DNN models for large-scale data analysis enhanced the accuracy of computational models for the prediction of the mutational landscape, molecular subtyping and drug repurposing [55–58]. A growing number of DNN-based applications have recently integrated multi-omics and systems biology data into the learned models. Such approaches aim to apply the DNN model to well-established biomedical knowledge, thereby improving our understanding of diseases and therapeutic effects in novel ways [59,60].

A common aim of NGS data analysis in cancer research is the identification of potential biomarkers that are predictive of specific cancer types or subtypes. A variety of bioinformatics tools and ML models, for example, aim to identify a molecular signature that is significantly altered in cancer cells on a genomic, transcriptomic, or epigenomic level. Statistical and ML methods are typically used to identify the best set of biomarkers, such as single nucleotide polymorphisms (SNPs), mutations, or differentially expressed genes that are important in cancer progression. Previously, those markers had to be discovered or validated using time-consuming in vitro analysis. As a result, systems biology provides in silico solutions to validate such findings by utilizing biological pathways or gene ontology data [61].

4. AI in Cancer Prognosis

Detecting and predicting the course of the disease are key components to controlling tumor enlargement and providing adequate treatment to cancer patients. With the understanding that cancer can affect individuals differently, AI has been utilized to isolate subgroups within the patient population based on prognosis and survival data. Aside from segmentation, AI has pinpointed biomarkers that can indicate the recurrence of the disease. AI has been implemented to prognosticate high-risk neuroblastoma patients. Utilizing combined gene expression and copy number variations, an unsupervised learning algorithm called auto encoder determined significant features, which were then used for division into two clusters [62]. In a separate study, Francescatto et al. employed the integrative network fusion framework together with an ML classifier to distinguish features that could differentiate between distinct outcomes of patients [63].

DL-based neural networks have also been applied to breast cancer survival prognosis. To prevent overfitting effects due to the vast size of omics data, the SALMON survival analysis algorithm operates on eigengene matrices of co-expression network modules. To enhance robustness, it brings together traditional cancer biomarkers and multi-omics information and pinpoints key feature genes and cytobands [64]. The use of a DL-based algorithm allows for the combination of the information from the same gene across different types of omics data, thus resulting in a successful and insightful analysis [65].

5. AI in the Identification of Therapeutic Targets

A subset of alternative network approaches to identifying cancer targets are provided by network-based biology analysis algorithms. More importantly, because different algorithms can look at network data from different angles, they can compensate for each other to provide accurate biological explanations [66].

Interactome data can be organized and represented in the form of network structures to explain the molecular mechanisms underlying carcinogenesis, where the nodes are biological entities (genes, proteins, mRNAs, and metabolites) while the edges represent the associations–interactions between them (gene co-expression, signaling transduction, gene regulation, and physical interaction between proteins) [67,68]. AI algorithms could efficiently process biological network data by implementing classification, clustering, and prediction tasks in biological networks using machines or programs that enhance human intelligence [69]. As a result, AI algorithms will be able to elucidate the complexity of cancer behavior that rely on the interactions between genes and their products in biological network structures [70], allowing us to better understand carcinogenesis and identify novel anti-cancer targets [71].

One of the fundamental needs of precision oncology is anticipating therapy response for a patient population. The advantages of ML strategies have been tried for treatment response displaying and expectation following both center-based and component choice-based strategies [72]. The profound neural system-based examination has been used to predict therapy response. MOLI, a multi-omics late mix strategy in light of a profound neural system, consolidates somatic transformation, and duplicates number variation and quality articulation information to anticipate medication reaction conduct. MOLI is additionally utilized for board medication information, and information on medications with a similar target [73].

The Support Vector Machine (SVM) and the Leave-One-Out Cross-Validation (LOOCV) models have been employed to detect significant changes in RNA and miRNA transcriptomics data between from pancreatic ductal adenocarcinoma specimens and normal tissues. These features (selected RNAs and miRNAs) in combination with miRNA target expression data were further exploited to identify efficient diagnostic markers that were validated in other distinct datasets and biologically interpreted by pathway analysis of the corresponding target genes [74]. Moreover, ML-based analysis has been utilized to discover specific anticancer drug targets for breast tumors [75]. The characteristic genes extracted from multi-omics data of breast cancer with the aid of capsule network-based modeling were compared with well-known oncogenes, and novel genes were identified [76].

Recently, a comprehensive examination of nine cancers has demonstrated that proteomics data combined with gene expression, miRNAs expression and genomics is more effective in predicting the responsiveness of drugs and molecules specifically designed to target them. This research was conducted across 58 cell lines over nine cancers with Bayesian Efficient Multiple Kernel Learning (BEMKL) models [72]. This confirms the robustness of multi-omics data analysis across cancer types.

6. AI Clinical Application

The DELFI technology, which uses a blood test to indirectly evaluate the packing of DNA in the nucleus of a cell by assessing the bulk and amount of cell-free DNA present in the flow from various regions of the genome, is one example of AI in clinical practice. Cancer cells release DNA into the bloodstream when they die. DELFI uses ML to investigate millions of cell-free DNA pieces for unusual design in order to distinguish the occurrence of cancer. The strategy provides a perspective on cell-free DNA known as the "fragmentome" and only requires low-coverage genome sequencing, allowing the technology to be economically affordable in a screening setting [77].

The DELFI methodology finds that patients who were later diagnosed positive for cancer had a wide fluctuation in their fragmentome profiles, while those who had a negative cancer diagnosis had predictable fragmentome profiles. Overall, the technique was able to distinguish more than 90 percent of patients with lung cancer (including those with early stages) and displaying different subtypes [78].

Another study focused on glioblastoma, whose diagnosis is based on resection or biopsy which can be especially arduous and perilous in the case that the tumor mass is located in a deep position. Moreover, tracking cancer progression also necessitates repeated biopsies that are often impracticable. Consequently, there is an urgent requirement to identify biomarkers to diagnose and follow-up glioblastoma evolution by limiting the invasive approaches. Recently, an innovative cancer detection method has been developed based on plasma denaturation profiles obtained by a novel use of differential scanning fluorimetry. By comparing the denaturation profiles of blood samples collected from glioma patients and from healthy subjects, the researchers demonstrated that ML-based algorithms can automatically distinguish the cancer patients from the healthy individuals (with a precision around 92%). Additionally, this high-throughput workflow can be applied to any type of cancer and may represent a potent pan-cancer diagnostic and monitoring tool that requires only a plain blood test [79].

Among the limitations of the current approaches, tissue biopsy presents a fixed overview of the tumor that fails to record the intratumor distinguishment and dynamic changes occurring during carcinogenesis, also determined by clonal pressure caused by the applied medication [80]. On top of that, it is an invasive procedure, which usually cannot be performed multiple times on request, making this system unfeasible to be conducted as a regular practice for cancer patients' long-term supervision and treatment adjustment. The emergence of liquid biopsy has been a revolutionary development for the current clinical practice, offering great potential to improve the management of ongoing cancer patients for the diagnosis, prognosis, and tailoring of treatment. This approach presents the advantage of being a minimally invasive procedure that utilizes tumor-derived materials obtained from several body fluids, such as peripheral blood, urine, pleural liquid, saliva, or ascites [81]. This solution is not limited by space or time, and it supplies clinically meaningful information related to both primary and metastatic malignant lesions. Among the components of tumor-derived materials that can be analyzed by liquid biopsy, circulating tumor cells, cell-free circulating nucleic acids, and extracellular vesicles are the most extensively studied and characterized cancer markers and are used for various objectives, for instance, the early detection of cancer, staging, prognosis, drug resistance, and minimal residual disease [82].

Another AI approach is the PinPoint test, a cost-effective AI-driven blood test for cancer that is meant to upgrade rapid cancer referral paths. The test is found on an algorithm that uses ML to investigate regular constituents, as well as the patient's age and sex. It can calibrate and combine these individual variables into one solid and highly precise result, such as the likelihood that a patient has cancer [83]. The PinPoint test has been crafted as a decision support tool to give medical professionals the data they need to better sort patients when they initially present with symptoms. Those with high risk can be given precedence for speedy examination in secondary care, while those with the lowest risk can be securely excluded from the "2 week wait" pathway for further discussion with their physicians [84]. This strategy of pinpointing those at the greatest risk for prioritization will promote early detection, contribute to a more dependable pathway, and assist in decreasing post-pandemic delays [85].

7. AI imaging in Cancer Diagnosis

In the field of cancer imaging, AI displays a great utility in three main clinical tasks: tumor detection, characterization, and monitoring [86]. The localization of objects of interest in radiographs is referred to as detection, and it is a subset of computer-aided detection (CADe). AI-based detection tools can be used to reduce observational errors and serve as a first line of defense against omission errors [87].

Characterization in general includes tumor segmentation, diagnosis, and staging. It can also include a disease-specific prognosis as well as outcome prediction based on specific treatment modalities. Segmentation determines the extent of abnormalities and can range from simple 2D measurements of the maximum in plane tumor diameter to more involved volumetric segmentations that assess the entire tumor as well as any surrounding tissues. This information could be exploited for future diagnostic purposes as well as for calculating the appropriate dose administration during radiation planning. AI has the capability to significantly improve the efficiency, reproducibility, and reliability of tumor measurements through automated segmentation. In computer-aided diagnosis (CADx) systems, systematic processing of quantitative tumor features is used, allowing for more reproducible descriptors. In the case of inconsistencies in interpretation by different human readers, CADx systems have been used to diagnose lung nodules in thin-section CT and prostate lesions in multiparametric MRI [88].

Staging is another aspect of tumor characterization in which tumors are classified into predefined groups based on the size and spread of the tumor mass, thus providing information regarding the expected clinical course and for the decision of the most appropriate treatment strategies [89]. The application of AI-based methods to cancer imaging allows for the estimation of tumor size, shape, morphology, texture, and kinetics. Additionally, the use of dynamic assessment of contrast uptake on MRI enables physicians to characterize the tumor mass in terms of heterogeneity, phenotypes of spatial features and dynamic characteristics [90]. Another variable taken in consideration from AI-based tools is entropy, a mathematical descriptor of randomness that provides information on how heterogeneous the pattern is within the tumor, thereby describing the heterogeneous pattern of vascular system uptake (contrast uptake) within tumors imaged on contrast-enhanced breast MRI. As demonstrated by the NCI's The Cancer Genome Atlas (TCGA) breast cancer dataset, such analyses could reflect the heterogeneous nature of angiogenesis and treatment susceptibility [91].

DL systems have been used to simultaneously detect and classify prostate lesions. For training convolutional neural networks (CNNs) for prostate cancer diagnosis by MRI, both de novo training [92] and the transfer learning of pre-trained models [93] have been successful. The implementation of CNNs models with anatomically aware features has been shown to improve their performance [94,95]. In addition to MRI, AI techniques for prostate cancer classification have shown promising results by integrating ultrasound data, specifically radiofrequency. Again, both traditional ML and DL approaches were used to train classifiers to estimate the grading of prostate cancer by exploiting temporal ultrasound data [96].

8. Critical Issues, Challenges, and Limitations

The accuracy and consistency of AI systems are frequently restricted by their training data and the hardware used. We must keep in mind that AI can make mistakes in some situations because its decision-making ability is predictive and probabilistic. As a result, there are no clear regulations or guidelines in place to determine who is legally liable when AI malfunctions occur or causes issues while providing a service. Another factor to take in consideration is that most of the places where the potential of AI in healthcare has been evaluated are basically high-income and resource-driven areas. When used in low-income countries with a shortage of well-trained physicians and oncological specialists, AI-based prediction tools are expected to have a greater impact and increment the success of cancer treatment.

The improvement in the AI interpretation is a crucial step toward mitigating this risk and providing a decision-making rationale. One limitation is represented by the lack of a human verification step in the process unless a physician supervises the AI system. As a result, no one expects AI to entirely replace medical professionals. AI-based precision medicine will be critical for cancer treatment in the future. Living databases will exploit extremely complex models capable of making a personalized therapy selection, estimation of the drug dose, follow-up schedule, and so on. However, the transition from artificial narrow intelligence to artificial general intelligence will result in the automation of all the steps involved in cancer prediction, diagnosis, and treatment.

Despite its numerous benefits, AI presents several challenges and constraints that hinder it from fully functioning in cancer research. Particularly, three layers of complexity must be considered: (i) cancer is a highly heterogeneous organoid-like structure that, at the time of diagnosis, is made up of many different cancer subclones embedded in a stroma (the tumor microenvironment) that itself contributes to cancer progression; (ii) as cancer progresses, tumor evolution leads to increased intratumor heterogeneity so that by the time therapy is started, the targeted cancer may not respond; (iii) cancers with the same molecular and histological signatures behave differently in each single patient because of individual epigenetic and immunological modulations [97–99]. Thus, the final clinical outcome will depend on the complex interplay between the cancer (with its multiple subclones) and the tumor microenvironment (which includes the stroma composition and the inflammatory and immune response), and, finally, the general pathophysiological condition of the patient (e.g., the body mass, the adipose tissue mass, the nutrition status, the psychological status, the immune status, etc.). This poses an important limit to the capability of AI in predicting the therapy efficacy and the prognosis, which once again stresses the fundamental role of the clinician that cannot be substituted by an algorithm.

The new era of innovation brings with it many challenges that should be overcome to drastically improve oncology procedures at several levels. The lack of inclusive and different datasets for training represents a significant obstacle to the widespread adoption of AI algorithms and decision-support systems in cancer care. Most of the powerful AI models require a large sample size to efficiently train the tool. Although there are dimensionality reduction and feature selection methods for addressing these aspects, proper implementation is critical for achieving better and reliable results. The number and type of data annotated influences the constructions of algorithms, and an imbalance in data from patients differing for gender, age, race, nutritional state, lifestyle, and environment will affect AI and ML training. Thus, the lack of sensible data may increase the risk of missed diagnosis. Therefore, experts are fundamental in data curation and data annotation to provide reliable datasets to be used for training AI classifier and predictors models.

In medical data sets, particularly in the case of cancer data, classes are typically distributed unequally. The continuous use of AI- and ML-based tools for diagnosis and treatment decisions can be risky due to distributional shifts, which means that target data may not match the ongoing patient data employed to train the model, resulting in incorrect outputs. Predictions made by AI at the time of diagnosis likely changes during the course of the therapy and the evolution of the disease along with changes in patient's habit (style of life, diet, medications, etc.).

Changes in technology, healthcare, and population, such as the gene pool, are likely to have an impact on the relationship between the data items. The actual application of AI models in clinics is not being actively considered. The predictions achieved with these models frequently require validation in the clinical practice to assist medical experts in confirming diagnosis decisions.

Significant issues regarding data availability and interpretability caused by AI's "black box" process, in parallel with the emergence of an inherent bias toward limited cohorts that reduces the reproducibility of AI models and perpetuates disparities in the healthcare, collectively prevent the widespread application of AI in clinics. Additionally, the distribution of AI-based technologies in many developing countries may be hampered by a lack of knowledge in computing algorithms and technologies of the physicians.

Taken together, the clinically relevant achievements discussed in the present review need to become more solid to be translated into the right treatment for the right patient. Hence, the rapidly ongoing evolution of AI-based medical data analysis will significantly improve the treatments in cancer.

9. Conclusions and Perspectives

In this paper, we present an overview of the models applied in diagnosing and identifying therapeutic targets, and we discussed the challenges and future perspectives of AI in cancer research (Figure 3). As the power and potential of AI are increasingly demonstrated, in the coming future several other biomedical fields may exploit the use of AI in their routine clinical practice. AI methodologies' accuracy and predictive power must be significantly improved, as well as demonstrated efficacy comparable to, or better than, human experts in controlled studies [100]. Up to now, AI shows early promising results in the management of several disease conditions, but more efforts in prospective trials and in the education of physicians, technologists, and physicists are needed before it can be widely used. Although there will always be a "black box" for human experts to view AI-generated results, data visualization tools are becoming more widely available to provide some visual understanding of how algorithms make decisions [101]. It is to be stressed that AI is meant to complement the medical doctor facilitating his work, but it will not replace the medical doctor.

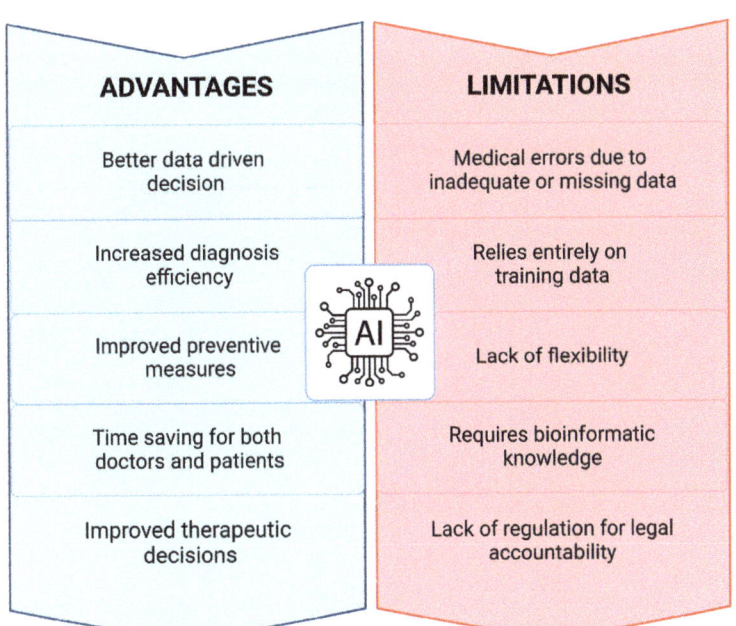

Figure 3. Advantages and limitations of AI. The scheme summarizes the main benefits along with the current concerns related to the use of AI in the clinical practice.

Author Contributions: Conceptualization, A.F. (Alaa Fawaz) and C.I.; writing—original draft preparation, A.F. (Alaa Fawaz) and A.F. (Alessandra Ferraresi); writing—review and editing, C.I.; visualization, A.F. (Alaa Fawaz) and A.F. (Alessandra Ferraresi). All authors have read and agreed to the published version of the manuscript.

Funding: This research received no external funding.

Institutional Review Board Statement: Not applicable.

Informed Consent Statement: Not applicable.

Data Availability Statement: No new data were created or analyzed in this study. Data sharing is not applicable to this article.

Acknowledgments: A.F. (Alessandra Ferraresi) is the recipient of a post-doctoral fellowship from Fondazione Umberto Veronesi (FUV 2023).

Conflicts of Interest: The authors declare no conflict of interest.

Abbreviations

Artificial Intelligence, AI; Bayesian Efficient Multiple Kernel Learning, BEMKL; computed tomography, CT; computer-aided detection, CADe; computer-aided diagnosis, CADx; convolutional neural networks, CNNs; deep learning, DL; deep neural network, DNN; gene expression modeling, GEM; graph convolutional network, GCN; graph neural networks, GNNs; Human Metabolome Database, HMDB; Human Protein Atlas, (HPA); Leave-One-Out Cross-Validation, LOOCV; machine learning, ML; magnetic resonance imaging, MRI; nano differential scanning fluorimetry, Nanodsf; next-generation sequencing, NGS; positron emission tomography, PET; partial least squares-discriminant analysis, PLS-DA; single nucleotide polymorphisms, SNPs; single-cell RNA sequencing, scRNA-seq; Support Vector Machine, SVM; The Cancer Genome Atlas, TCGA; ultrasound imaging, US.

References

1. Committee on Diagnostic Error in Health Care; Board on Health Care Services; Institute of Medicine; The National Academies of Sciences, Engineering, and Medicine. *Improving Diagnosis in Health Care*; Balogh, E.P., Miller, B.T., Ball, J.R., Eds.; National Academies Press: Washington, DC, USA, 2015. Available online: http://www.ncbi.nlm.nih.gov/books/NBK338596/ (accessed on 3 May 2023).
2. Rodziewicz, T.L.; Houseman, B.; Hipskind, J.E. Medical Error Reduction and Prevention. In *StatPearls*; StatPearls Publishing: St. Petersburg, FL, USA, 2023. Available online: http://www.ncbi.nlm.nih.gov/books/NBK499956/ (accessed on 3 May 2023).
3. Taylor, N. Duke Report Identifies Barriers to Adoption of AI Healthcare Systems. MedTech Dive. Available online: https://www.medtechdive.com/news/duke-report-identifies-barriers-to-adoption-of-ai-healthcare-systems/546739/ (accessed on 3 May 2023).
4. Bray, F.; Laversanne, M.; Weiderpass, E.; Soerjomataram, I. The Ever-Increasing Importance of Cancer as a Leading Cause of Premature Death Worldwide. *Cancer* 2021, *127*, 3029–3030. [CrossRef]
5. Ponomarenko, E.A.; Poverennaya, E.V.; Ilgisonis, E.V.; Pyatnitskiy, M.A.; Kopylov, A.T.; Zgoda, V.G.; Lisitsa, A.V.; Archakov, A.I. The Size of the Human Proteome: The Width and Depth. *Int. J. Anal. Chem.* 2016, *2016*, 7436849. [CrossRef]
6. Nadhan, R.; Kashyap, S.; Ha, J.H.; Jayaraman, M.; Song, Y.S.; Isidoro, C.; Dhanasekaran, D.N. Targeting Oncometabolites in Peritoneal Cancers: Preclinical Insights and Therapeutic Strategies. *Metabolites* 2023, *13*, 618. [CrossRef] [PubMed]
7. Hasin, Y.; Seldin, M.; Lusis, A. Multi-Omics Approaches to Disease. *Genome Biol.* 2017, *18*, 83. [CrossRef] [PubMed]
8. Perkins, D.O.; Jeffries, C.; Sullivan, P. Expanding the 'Central Dogma': The Regulatory Role of Nonprotein Coding Genes and Implications for the Genetic Liability to Schizophrenia. *Mol. Psychiatry* 2005, *10*, 69–78. [CrossRef] [PubMed]
9. Tsakiroglou, M.; Evans, A.; Pirmohamed, M. Leveraging Transcriptomics for Precision Diagnosis: Lessons Learned from Cancer and Sepsis. *Front. Genet.* 2023, *14*, 1100352. [CrossRef] [PubMed]
10. Haga, Y.; Minegishi, Y.; Ueda, K. Frontiers in Mass Spectrometry–Based Clinical Proteomics for Cancer Diagnosis and Treatment. *Cancer Sci.* 2023, *114*, 1783–1791. [CrossRef]
11. Janes, K.A.; Yaffe, M.B. Data-Driven Modelling of Signal-Transduction Networks. *Nat. Rev. Mol. Cell Biol.* 2006, *7*, 820–828. [CrossRef]
12. Luo, J.; Pan, M.; Mo, K.; Mao, Y.; Zou, D. Emerging Role of Artificial Intelligence in Diagnosis, Classification and Clinical Management of Glioma. *Semin. Cancer Biol.* 2023, *91*, 110–123. [CrossRef]
13. Wang, S.; Wang, S.; Wang, Z. A Survey on Multi-Omics-Based Cancer Diagnosis Using Machine Learning with the Potential Application in Gastrointestinal Cancer. *Front. Med.* 2023, *9*, 1109365. [CrossRef]
14. Liao, J.; Li, X.; Gan, Y.; Han, S.; Rong, P.; Wang, W.; Li, W.; Zhou, L. Artificial Intelligence Assists Precision Medicine in Cancer Treatment. *Front. Oncol.* 2023, *12*, 998222. [CrossRef] [PubMed]
15. He, X.; Liu, X.; Zuo, F.; Shi, H.; Jing, J. Artificial Intelligence-Based Multi-Omics Analysis Fuels Cancer Precision Medicine. *Semin. Cancer Biol.* 2023, *88*, 187–200. [CrossRef] [PubMed]
16. Dembrower, K.; Wåhlin, E.; Liu, Y.; Salim, M.; Smith, K.; Lindholm, P.; Eklund, M.; Strand, F. Effect of Artificial Intelligence-Based Triaging of Breast Cancer Screening Mammograms on Cancer Detection and Radiologist Workload: A Retrospective Simulation Study. *Lancet Digit. Health* 2020, *2*, e468–e474. [CrossRef] [PubMed]
17. Davenport, T.; Kalakota, R. The potential for artificial intelligence in healthcare. *Future Healthc. J.* 2019, *6*, 94–98. [CrossRef] [PubMed]
18. Bohr, A.; Memarzadeh, K. The rise of artificial intelligence in healthcare applications. In *Artificial Intelligence in Healthcare*; Elsevier: Amsterdam, The Netherlands, 2020; pp. 25–60. [CrossRef]
19. Venkatesan, D.; Elangovan, A.; Winster, H.; Pasha, M.Y.; Abraham, K.S.; Satheeshkumar, J.; Sivaprakash, P.; Niraikulam, A.; Gopalakrishnan, A.V.; Narayanasamy, A.; et al. Diagnostic and therapeutic approach of artificial intelligence in neuro-oncological diseases. *Biosens. Bioelectron. X* 2022, *11*, 100188. [CrossRef]
20. Swanson, K.; Wu, E.; Zhang, A.; Alizadeh, A.A.; Zou, J. From patterns to patients: Advances in clinical machine learning for cancer diagnosis, prognosis, and treatment. *Cell* 2023, *186*, 1772–1791. [CrossRef]
21. Mohammed, M.; Biegert, G.; Adamec, J.; Helikar, T. Identification of Potential Tissue-Specific Cancer Biomarkers and Development of Cancer versus Normal Genomic Classifiers. *Oncotarget* 2017, *8*, 85692–85715. [CrossRef]
22. Zhang, Y.; Xiong, S.; Wang, Z.; Liu, Y.; Luo, H.; Li, B.; Zou, Q. Local Augmented Graph Neural Network for Multi-Omics Cancer Prognosis Prediction and Analysis. *Methods* 2023, *213*, 1–9. [CrossRef]
23. Peng, X.; Chen, Z.; Farshidfar, F.; Xu, X.; Lorenzi, P.L.; Wang, Y.; Cheng, F.; Tan, L.; Mojumdar, K.; Du, D.; et al. Molecular Characterization and Clinical Relevance of Metabolic Expression Subtypes in Human Cancers. *Cell Rep.* 2018, *23*, 255–269.e4. [CrossRef]
24. Yokota, K.; Uchida, H.; Sakairi, M.; Abe, M.; Tanaka, Y.; Tainaka, T.; Shirota, C.; Sumida, W.; Oshima, K.; Makita, S.; et al. Identification of Novel Neuroblastoma Biomarkers in Urine Samples. *Sci. Rep.* 2021, *11*, 4055. [CrossRef]
25. Barker, M.; Rayens, W. Partial Least Squares for Discrimination. *J. Chemom.* 2003, *17*, 166–173. [CrossRef]
26. Rohart, F.; Gautier, B.; Singh, A.; Lê Cao, K.-A. MixOmics: An R Package for 'omics Feature Selection and Multiple Data Integration. *PLoS Comput. Biol.* 2017, *13*, e1005752. [CrossRef] [PubMed]
27. Westerhuis, J.A.; Hoefsloot, H.C.J.; Smit, S.; Vis, D.J.; Smilde, A.K.; van Velzen, E.J.J.; van Duijnhoven, J.P.M.; van Dorsten, F.A. Assessment of PLSDA Cross Validation. *Metabolomics* 2008, *4*, 81–89. [CrossRef]

28. Brereton, R.G.; Lloyd, G.R. Partial Least Squares Discriminant Analysis: Taking the Magic Away: PLS-DA: Taking the Magic Away. *J. Chemom.* **2014**, *28*, 213–225. [CrossRef]
29. Gromski, P.S.; Muhamadali, H.; Ellis, D.I.; Xu, Y.; Correa, E.; Turner, M.L.; Goodacre, R. A Tutorial Review: Metabolomics and Partial Least Squares-Discriminant Analysis—A Marriage of Convenience or a Shotgun Wedding. *Anal. Chim. Acta* **2015**, *879*, 10–23. [CrossRef]
30. Gu, C.; Kim, G.B.; Kim, W.J.; Kim, H.U.; Lee, S.Y. Current Status and Applications of Genome-Scale Metabolic Models. *Genome Biol.* **2019**, *20*, 121. [CrossRef]
31. Fang, X.; Lloyd, C.J.; Palsson, B.O. Reconstructing Organisms in Silico: Genome-Scale Models and Their Emerging Applications. *Nat. Rev. Microbiol.* **2020**, *18*, 731–743. [CrossRef]
32. Thiele, I.; Palsson, B.O. A Protocol for Generating a High-Quality Genome-Scale Metabolic Reconstruction. *Nat. Protoc.* **2010**, *5*, 93–121. [CrossRef]
33. O'Brien, J.E.; Monk, J.M.; Palsson, B.O. Using Genome-Scale Models to Predict Biological Capabilities. *Cell* **2015**, *161*, 971–987. [CrossRef]
34. Chand, S. A comparative study of breast cancer tumor classification by classical machine learning methods and deep learning method. *Mach. Vis. Appl.* **2020**, *31*, e270.
35. Angermueller, C.; Pärnamaa, T.; Parts, L.; Stegle, O. Deep Learning for Computational Biology. *Mol. Syst. Biol.* **2016**, *12*, 878. [CrossRef]
36. Samiei, M.; Würfl, T.; Deleu, T.; Weiss, M.; Dutil, F.; Fevens, T.; Boucher, G.; Lemieux, S.; Cohen, J.P. The TCGA Meta-Dataset Clinical Benchmark. *arXiv* **2019**, arXiv:1910.08636.
37. Jin, S.; Zeng, X.; Xia, F.; Huang, W.; Liu, X. Application of Deep Learning Methods in Biological Networks. *Brief. Bioinform.* **2021**, *22*, 1902–1917. [CrossRef] [PubMed]
38. Rhee, S.; Seo, S.; Kim, S. Hybrid Approach of Relation Network and Localized Graph Convolutional Filtering for Breast Cancer Subtype Classification. *arXiv* **2018**, arXiv:1711.05859.
39. Lee, S.; Lim, S.; Lee, T.; Sung, I.; Kim, S. Cancer Subtype Classification and Modeling by Pathway Attention and Propagation. *Bioinformatics* **2020**, *36*, 3818–3824. [CrossRef]
40. Dai, H.; Li, H.; Tian, T.; Huang, X.; Wang, L.; Zhu, J.; Song, L. Adversarial Attack on Graph Structured Data. In Proceedings of the 35th International Conference on Machine Learning (ICML 2018), Stockholm, Sweden, 10–15 July 2018. Available online: https://proceedings.mlr.press/v80/dai18b.html (accessed on 3 May 2023).
41. Zhang, X.; Zitnik, M. GNNGuard: Defending Graph Neural Networks against Adversarial Attacks. In *Advances in Neural Information Processing Systems*; Curran Associates, Inc.: New York, NY, USA, 2020; Volume 33, pp. 9263–9275. Available online: https://papers.nips.cc/paper/2020/hash/690d83983a63aa1818423fd6edd3bfdb-Abstract.html (accessed on 3 May 2023).
42. Abdelaal, T.; Michielsen, L.; Cats, D.; Hoogduin, D.; Mei, H.; Reinders, M.J.T.; Mahfouz, A. A Comparison of Automatic Cell Identification Methods for Single-Cell RNA Sequencing Data. *Genome Biol.* **2019**, *20*, 194. [CrossRef]
43. Tan, Y.; Cahan, P. SingleCellNet: A Computational Tool to Classify Single Cell RNA-Seq Data Across Platforms and Across Species. *Cell Syst.* **2019**, *9*, 207–213.e2. [CrossRef]
44. Hu, J.; Li, X.; Hu, G.; Lyu, Y.; Susztak, K.; Li, M. Iterative Transfer Learning with Neural Network for Clustering and Cell Type Classification in Single-Cell RNA-Seq Analysis. *Nat. Mach. Intell.* **2020**, *2*, 607–618. [CrossRef]
45. Andreatta, M.; Corria-Osorio, J.; Müller, S.; Cubas, R.; Coukos, G.; Carmona, S.J. Interpretation of T Cell States from Single-Cell Transcriptomics Data Using Reference Atlases. *Nat. Commun.* **2021**, *12*, 2965. [CrossRef]
46. Michielsen, L.; Reinders, M.J.T.; Mahfouz, A. Hierarchical Progressive Learning of Cell Identities in Single-Cell Data. *Nat. Commun.* **2021**, *12*, 2799. [CrossRef]
47. Ranjan, B.; Schmidt, F.; Sun, W.; Park, J.; Honardoost, M.A.; Tan, J.; Rayan, N.A.; Prabhakar, S. ScConsensus: Combining Supervised and Unsupervised Clustering for Cell Type Identification in Single-Cell RNA Sequencing Data. *BMC Bioinform.* **2021**, *22*, 186. [CrossRef]
48. Gao, J.; Aksoy, B.A.; Dogrusoz, U.; Dresdner, G.; Gross, B.E.; Sumer, S.O.; Sun, Y.; Jacobsen, A.; Sinha, R.; Larsson, E.; et al. Integrative Analysis of Complex Cancer Genomics and Clinical Profiles Using the CBioPortal. *Sci. Signal.* **2013**, *6*, pl1. [CrossRef]
49. Grossman, R.L.; Heath, A.P.; Ferretti, V.; Varmus, H.E.; Lowy, D.R.; Kibbe, W.A.; Staudt, L.M. Toward a Shared Vision for Cancer Genomic Data. *N. Engl. J. Med.* **2016**, *375*, 1109–1112. [CrossRef]
50. Goldman, M.J.; Craft, B.; Hastie, M.; Repečka, K.; McDade, F.; Kamath, A.; Banerjee, A.; Luo, Y.; Rogers, D.; Brooks, A.N.; et al. Visualizing and Interpreting Cancer Genomics Data via the Xena Platform. *Nat. Biotechnol.* **2020**, *38*, 675–678. [CrossRef]
51. Manzoni, C.; Kia, D.A.; Vandrovcova, J.; Hardy, J.; Wood, N.W.; Lewis, P.A.; Ferrari, R. Genome, Transcriptome and Proteome: The Rise of Omics Data and Their Integration in Biomedical Sciences. *Brief. Bioinform.* **2018**, *19*, 286–302. [CrossRef] [PubMed]
52. Creixell, P.; Reimand, J.; Haider, S.; Wu, G.; Shibata, T.; Vazquez, M.; Mustonen, V.; Gonzalez-Perez, A.; Pearson, J.; Sander, C.; et al. Pathway and Network Analysis of Cancer Genomes. *Nat. Methods* **2015**, *12*, 615–621. [PubMed]
53. Ngiam, K.Y.; Khor, I.W. Big Data and Machine Learning Algorithms for Health-Care Delivery. *Lancet Oncol.* **2019**, *20*, e262–e273. [CrossRef] [PubMed]
54. Reyna, M.A.; Haan, D.; Paczkowska, M.; Verbeke, L.P.C.; Vazquez, M.; Kahraman, A.; Pulido-Tamayo, S.; Barenboim, J.; Wadi, L.; Dhingra, P.; et al. Pathway and Network Analysis of More than 2500 Whole Cancer Genomes. *Nat. Commun.* **2020**, *11*, 729. [CrossRef]

55. Luo, P.; Ding, Y.; Lei, X.; Wu, F.-X. DeepDriver: Predicting Cancer Driver Genes Based on Somatic Mutations Using Deep Convolutional Neural Networks. *Front. Genet.* **2019**, *10*, 13. [CrossRef]
56. Jiao, W.; Atwal, G.; Polak, P.; Karlic, R.; Cuppen, E.; PCAWG Tumor Subtypes and Clinical Translation Working Group; Danyi, A.; de Ridder, J.; van Herpen, C.; Lolkema, M.P.; et al. A Deep Learning System Accurately Classifies Primary and Metastatic Cancers Using Passenger Mutation Patterns. *Nat. Commun.* **2020**, *11*, 728. [CrossRef]
57. Chaudhary, K.; Poirion, O.B.; Lu, L.; Garmire, L.X. Deep Learning-Based Multi-Omics Integration Robustly Predicts Survival in Liver Cancer. *Clin. Cancer Res. Off. J. Am. Assoc. Cancer Res.* **2018**, *24*, 1248–1259. [CrossRef]
58. Gao, F.; Wang, W.; Tan, M.; Zhu, L.; Zhang, Y.; Fessler, E.; Vermeulen, L.; Wang, X. DeepCC: A Novel Deep Learning-Based Framework for Cancer Molecular Subtype Classification. *Oncogenesis* **2019**, *8*, 44. [CrossRef] [PubMed]
59. Zeng, X.; Zhu, S.; Liu, X.; Zhou, Y.; Nussinov, R.; Cheng, F. DeepDR: A Network-Based Deep Learning Approach to in Silico Drug Repositioning. *Bioinformatics* **2019**, *35*, 5191–5198. [CrossRef] [PubMed]
60. Issa, N.T.; Stathias, V.; Schürer, S.; Dakshanamurthy, S. Machine and Deep Learning Approaches for Cancer Drug Repurposing. *Semin. Cancer Biol.* **2021**, *68*, 132–142. [CrossRef] [PubMed]
61. Park, Y.; Heider, D.; Hauschild, A.-C. Integrative Analysis of Next-Generation Sequencing for Next-Generation Cancer Research toward Artificial Intelligence. *Cancers* **2021**, *13*, 3148. [CrossRef]
62. Zhang, L.; Lv, C.; Jin, Y.; Cheng, G.; Fu, Y.; Yuan, D.; Tao, Y.; Guo, Y.; Ni, X.; Shi, T. Deep Learning-Based Multi-Omics Data Integration Reveals Two Prognostic Subtypes in High-Risk Neuroblastoma. *Front. Genet.* **2018**, *9*, 477. [CrossRef]
63. Francescatto, M.; Chierici, M.; Dezfooli, S.R.; Zandonà, A.; Jurman, G.; Furlanello, C. Multi-Omics Integration for Neuroblastoma Clinical Endpoint Prediction. *Biol. Direct* **2018**, *13*, 5. [CrossRef] [PubMed]
64. Huang, Z.; Zhan, X.; Xiang, S.; Johnson, T.S.; Helm, B.; Yu, C.Y.; Zhang, J.; Salama, P.; Rizkalla, M.; Han, Z.; et al. SALMON: Survival Analysis Learning with Multi-Omics Neural Networks on Breast Cancer. *Front. Genet.* **2019**, *10*, 166. [CrossRef]
65. Xie, G.; Dong, C.; Kong, Y.; Zhong, J.F.; Li, M.; Wang, K. Group Lasso Regularized Deep Learning for Cancer Prognosis from Multi-Omics and Clinical Features. *Genes* **2019**, *10*, 240. [CrossRef]
66. Chen, L.; Wu, J. Bio-Network Medicine. *J. Mol. Cell Biol.* **2015**, *7*, 185–186. [CrossRef]
67. Song, H.; Chen, L.; Cui, Y.; Li, Q.; Wang, Q.; Fan, J.; Yang, J.; Zhang, L. Denoising of MR and CT Images Using Cascaded Multi-Supervision Convolutional Neural Networks with Progressive Training. *Neurocomputing* **2022**, *469*, 354–365. [CrossRef]
68. Zhang, Z.; Zhang, L.; Guo, Y.; Xiao, M.; Feng, L.; Yang, C.; Wang, G.; Ouyang, L. MCDB: A Comprehensive Curated Mitotic Catastrophe Database for Retrieval, Protein Sequence Alignment, and Target Prediction. *Acta Pharm. Sin. B* **2021**, *11*, 3092–3104. [CrossRef] [PubMed]
69. Zhou, Y.; Wang, F.; Tang, J.; Nussinov, R.; Cheng, F. Artificial Intelligence in COVID-19 Drug Repurposing. *Lancet Digit. Health* **2020**, *2*, e667–e676. [CrossRef] [PubMed]
70. Suhail, Y.; Cain, M.P.; Vanaja, K.; Kurywchak, P.A.; Levchenko, A.; Kalluri, R.; Kshitiz. Systems Biology of Cancer Metastasis. *Cell Syst.* **2019**, *9*, 109–127. [CrossRef]
71. Barabási, A.-L.; Oltvai, Z.N. Network Biology: Understanding the Cell's Functional Organization. *Nat. Rev. Genet.* **2004**, *5*, 101–113. [CrossRef]
72. Ali, M.; Khan, S.A.; Wennerberg, K.; Aittokallio, T. Global Proteomics Profiling Improves Drug Sensitivity Prediction: Results from a Multi-Omics, Pan-Cancer Modeling Approach. *Bioinformatics* **2018**, *34*, 1353–1362. [CrossRef]
73. Sharifi-Noghabi, H.; Zolotareva, O.; Collins, C.C.; Ester, M. MOLI: Multi-Omics Late Integration with Deep Neural Networks for Drug Response Prediction. *Bioinformatics* **2019**, *35*, i501–i509. [CrossRef]
74. Kwon, M.-S.; Kim, Y.; Lee, S.; Namkung, J.; Yun, T.; Yi, S.G.; Han, S.; Kang, M.; Kim, S.W.; Jang, J.-Y.; et al. Integrative Analysis of Multi-Omics Data for Identifying Multi-Markers for Diagnosing Pancreatic Cancer. *BMC Genom.* **2015**, *16*, S4. [CrossRef]
75. Gautam, P.; Jaiswal, A.; Aittokallio, T.; Al-Ali, H.; Wennerberg, K. Phenotypic Screening Combined with Machine Learning for Efficient Identification of Breast Cancer-Selective Therapeutic Targets. *Cell Chem. Biol.* **2019**, *26*, 970–979.e4. [CrossRef]
76. Peng, C.; Zheng, Y.; Huang, D.-S. Capsule Network Based Modeling of Multi-Omics Data for Discovery of Breast Cancer-Related Genes. *IEEE/ACM Trans. Comput. Biol. Bioinform.* **2020**, *17*, 1605–1612. [CrossRef]
77. Mazzone, P.J.; Sears, C.R.; Arenberg, D.A.; Gaga, M.; Gould, M.K.; Massion, P.P.; Nair, V.S.; Powell, C.A.; Silvestri, G.A.; Vachani, A.; et al. Evaluating Molecular Biomarkers for the Early Detection of Lung Cancer: When Is a Biomarker Ready for Clinical Use? An Official American Thoracic Society Policy Statement. *Am. J. Respir. Crit. Care Med.* **2017**, *196*, e15–e29. [CrossRef] [PubMed]
78. Seijo, L.M.; Peled, N.; Ajona, D.; Boeri, M.; Field, J.K.; Sozzi, G.; Pio, R.; Zulueta, J.J.; Spira, A.; Massion, P.P.; et al. Biomarkers in Lung Cancer Screening: Achievements, Promises, and Challenges. *J. Thorac. Oncol. Off. Publ. Int. Assoc. Study Lung Cancer* **2019**, *14*, 343–357. [CrossRef] [PubMed]
79. Tsvetkov, P.O.; Eyraud, R.; Ayache, S.; Bougaev, A.A.; Malesinski, S.; Benazha, H.; Gorokhova, S.; Buffat, C.; Dehais, C.; Sanson, M.; et al. An AI-Powered Blood Test to Detect Cancer Using NanoDSF. *Cancers* **2021**, *13*, 1294. [CrossRef] [PubMed]
80. Parikh, A.R.; Leshchiner, I.; Elagina, L.; Goyal, L.; Levovitz, C.; Siravegna, G.; Livitz, D.; Rhrissorrakrai, K.; Martin, E.E.; Van Seventer, E.E.; et al. Liquid versus Tissue Biopsy for Detecting Acquired Resistance and Tumor Heterogeneity in Gastrointestinal Cancers. *Nat. Med.* **2019**, *25*, 1415–1421. [CrossRef]
81. Lu, T.; Li, J. Clinical Applications of Urinary Cell-Free DNA in Cancer: Current Insights and Promising Future. *Am. J. Cancer Res.* **2017**, *7*, 2318–2332. [PubMed]

82. Heitzer, E.; Haque, I.S.; Roberts, C.E.S.; Speicher, M.R. Current and Future Perspectives of Liquid Biopsies in Genomics-Driven Oncology. *Nat. Rev. Genet.* **2019**, *20*, 71–88. [CrossRef]
83. Savage, R.; Messenger, M.; Neal, R.D.; Ferguson, R.; Johnston, C.; Lloyd, K.L.; Neal, M.D.; Sansom, N.; Selby, P.; Sharma, N.; et al. Development and Validation of Multivariable Machine Learning Algorithms to Predict Risk of Cancer in Symptomatic Patients Referred Urgently from Primary Care: A Diagnostic Accuracy Study. *BMJ Open* **2022**, *12*, e053590. [CrossRef]
84. Cohen, J.D.; Li, L.; Wang, Y.; Thoburn, C.; Afsari, B.; Danilova, L.; Douville, C.; Javed, A.A.; Wong, F.; Mattox, A.; et al. Detection and Localization of Surgically Resectable Cancers with a Multi-Analyte Blood Test. *Science* **2018**, *359*, 926–930. [CrossRef]
85. Cree, I.A.; Uttley, L.; Woods, H.B.; Kikuchi, H.; Reiman, A.; Harnan, S.; Whiteman, B.L.; Philips, S.T.; Messenger, M.; Cox, A.; et al. The Evidence Base for Circulating Tumour DNA Blood-Based Biomarkers for the Early Detection of Cancer: A Systematic Mapping Review. *BMC Cancer* **2017**, *17*, 697. [CrossRef]
86. Aerts, H.J.W.L.; Velazquez, E.R.; Leijenaar, R.T.H.; Parmar, C.; Grossmann, P.; Carvalho, S.; Bussink, J.; Monshouwer, R.; Haibe-Kains, B.; Rietveld, D.; et al. Decoding Tumour Phenotype by Noninvasive Imaging Using a Quantitative Radiomics Approach. *Nat. Commun.* **2014**, *5*, 4006. [CrossRef]
87. Hosny, A.; Parmar, C.; Quackenbush, J.; Schwartz, L.H.; Aerts, H.J.W.L. Artificial Intelligence in Radiology. *Nat. Rev. Cancer* **2018**, *18*, 500–510. [CrossRef]
88. Chan, H.-P.; Hadjiiski, L.; Zhou, C.; Sahiner, B. Computer-aided diagnosis of lung cancer and pulmonary embolism in computed tomography-a review. *Acad. Radiol.* **2008**, *15*, 535–555. [CrossRef] [PubMed]
89. Rasch, C.; Barillot, I.; Remeijer, P.; Touw, A.; van Herk, M.; Lebesque, J.V. Definition of the Prostate in CT and MRI: A Multi-Observer Study. *Int. J. Radiat. Oncol. Biol. Phys.* **1999**, *43*, 57–66. [CrossRef]
90. Chen, W.; Giger, M.L.; Li, H.; Bick, U.; Newstead, G.M. Volumetric Texture Analysis of Breast Lesions on Contrast-Enhanced Magnetic Resonance Images. *Magn. Reson. Med.* **2007**, *58*, 562–571. [CrossRef] [PubMed]
91. Zhu, B.; Song, N.; Shen, R.; Arora, A.; Machiela, M.J.; Song, L.; Landi, M.T.; Ghosh, D.; Chatterjee, N.; Baladandayuthapani, V.; et al. Integrating Clinical and Multiple Omics Data for Prognostic Assessment across Human Cancers. *Sci. Rep.* **2017**, *7*, 16954. [CrossRef] [PubMed]
92. Liu, S.; Zheng, H.; Feng, Y.; Li, W. Prostate Cancer Diagnosis Using Deep Learning with 3D Multiparametric MRI. *arXiv* **2017**, arXiv:1703.04078.
93. Chen, Q.; Xu, X.; Hu, S.; Li, X.; Zou, Q.; Li, Y. A Transfer Learning Approach for Classification of Clinical Significant Prostate Cancers from MpMRI Scans. *Proc. SPIE* **2017**, *10134*, 101344F.
94. Seah, J.C.Y.; Tang, J.S.N.; Kitchen, A. Detection of Prostate Cancer on Multiparametric MRI. In *Medical Imaging 2017: Computer-Aided Diagnosis*; Armato, S.G., Petrick, N.A., Eds.; SPIE: Orlando, FL, USA, 2017; Volume 10134, p. 1013429.
95. Mehrtash, A.; Sedghi, A.; Ghafoorian, M.; Taghipour, M.; Tempany, C.M.; Wells, W.M.; Kapur, T.; Mousavi, P.; Abolmaesumi, P.; Fedorov, A. Classification of Clinical Significance of MRI Prostate Findings Using 3D Convolutional Neural Networks. *Proc. SPIE Int. Soc. Opt. Eng.* **2017**, *10134*, 101342A.
96. Azizi, S.; Bayat, S.; Yan, P.; Tahmasebi, A.; Nir, G.; Kwak, J.T.; Xu, S.; Wilson, S.; Iczkowski, K.A.; Lucia, M.S.; et al. Detection and Grading of Prostate Cancer Using Temporal Enhanced Ultrasound: Combining Deep Neural Networks and Tissue Mimicking Simulations. *Int. J. Comput. Assist. Radiol. Surg.* **2017**, *12*, 1293–1305. [CrossRef]
97. Al Bakir, M.; Huebner, A.; Martínez-Ruiz, C.; Grigoriadis, K.; Watkins, T.B.K.; Pich, O.; Moore, D.A.; Veeriah, S.; Ward, S.; Laycock, J.; et al. The Evolution of Non-Small Cell Lung Cancer Metastases in TRACERx. *Nature* **2023**, *616*, 534–542. [CrossRef]
98. Martínez-Ruiz, C.; Black, J.R.M.; Puttick, J.; Hill, M.S.; Demeulemeester, J.; Cadieux, E.L.; Thol, K.; Jones, T.P.; Veeriah, S.; Naceur-Lombardelli, C.; et al. Genomic–Transcriptomic Evolution in Lung Cancer and Metastasis. *Nature* **2023**, *616*, 543–552. [CrossRef] [PubMed]
99. Chen, C.; Wang, Z.; Ding, Y.; Wang, L.; Wang, S.; Wang, H.; Qin, Y. DNA Methylation: From Cancer Biology to Clinical Perspectives. *Front. Biosci. Landmark* **2022**, *27*, 326. [CrossRef] [PubMed]
100. Olaronke, I.; Oluwaseun, O. Big Data in Healthcare: Prospects, Challenges and Resolutions. In Proceedings of the 2016 Future Technologies Conference (FTC), San Francisco, CA, USA, 6–7 December 2016; pp. 1152–1157.
101. Esteva, A.; Kuprel, B.; Novoa, R.A.; Ko, J.; Swetter, S.M.; Blau, H.M.; Thrun, S. Dermatologist-Level Classification of Skin Cancer with Deep Neural Networks. *Nature* **2017**, *542*, 115–118. [CrossRef] [PubMed]

Disclaimer/Publisher's Note: The statements, opinions and data contained in all publications are solely those of the individual author(s) and contributor(s) and not of MDPI and/or the editor(s). MDPI and/or the editor(s) disclaim responsibility for any injury to people or property resulting from any ideas, methods, instructions or products referred to in the content.

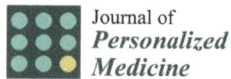

Perspective

The Next Frontier in Sarcoma Care: Digital Health, AI, and the Quest for Precision Medicine

Bruno Fuchs [1,2,*], Gabriela Studer [1], Beata Bode-Lesniewska [3], Philip Heesen [4] and on behalf of the Swiss Sarcoma Network [†]

1 Sarcoma Service, University Teaching Hospital LUKS, University of Lucerne, 6000 Lucerne, Switzerland
2 Sarcoma Service, Kantonsspital Winterthur, 8400 Winterthur, Switzerland
3 Patho Enge, SSN Reference Sarcoma Pathology, University of Zurich, 8000 Zurich, Switzerland
4 University Hospital USZ, University of Zurich, 8000 Zurich, Switzerland
* Correspondence: fuchs@sarcoma.surgery
† Additional collaborators of the Swiss Sarcoma Network are indicated in the Acknowledgement.

Abstract: The landscape of sarcoma care is on the cusp of a transformative era, spurred by the convergence of digital health and artificial intelligence (AI). This perspectives article explores the multifaceted opportunities and challenges in leveraging these technologies for value-based, precision sarcoma care. We delineate the current state-of-the-art methodologies and technologies in sarcoma care and outline their practical implications for healthcare providers, administrators, and policymakers. The article also addresses the limitations of AI and digital health platforms, emphasizing the need for high-quality data and ethical considerations. We delineate the promise held by the synergy of digital health platforms and AI algorithms in enhancing data-driven decision-making, outcome analytics, and personalized treatment planning. The concept of a sarcoma digital twin serves as an illustrative paradigm for this integration, offering a comprehensive, patient-centric view of the healthcare journey. The paper concludes with proposals for future research aimed at advancing the field, including the need for randomized controlled trials or target trial emulations and studies focusing on ethical and economic aspects. While the road to this transformative care is laden with ethical, regulatory, and practical challenges, we believe that the potential benefits far outweigh the obstacles. We conclude with a call to action for multidisciplinary collaboration and systemic adoption of these technologies, underscoring the urgency to act now for the future betterment of sarcoma care and healthcare at large.

Keywords: digital health; artificial intelligence; value-based healthcare; sarcoma; precision medicine; benchmarking; interoperable platforms; quality indicators

Citation: Fuchs, B.; Studer, G.; Bode-Lesniewska, B.; Heesen, P.; on behalf of the Swiss Sarcoma Network. The Next Frontier in Sarcoma Care: Digital Health, AI, and the Quest for Precision Medicine. *J. Pers. Med.* **2023**, *13*, 1530. https://doi.org/10.3390/jpm13111530

Academic Editor: Daniele Giansanti

Received: 17 September 2023
Revised: 16 October 2023
Accepted: 23 October 2023
Published: 25 October 2023

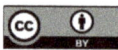

Copyright: © 2023 by the authors. Licensee MDPI, Basel, Switzerland. This article is an open access article distributed under the terms and conditions of the Creative Commons Attribution (CC BY) license (https://creativecommons.org/licenses/by/4.0/).

1. Introduction

Sarcoma, a rare and heterogenous group of malignant tumors originating from mesenchymal tissues, poses unique challenges for healthcare providers and patients alike. With over 100 subtypes and often complex clinical presentations, treating sarcoma requires a multidisciplinary, data-driven approach—an approach that modern healthcare is progressively leaning towards but has not yet fully realized [1–5]. In terms of the state of the art, recent advancements in genomics, targeted therapies, and immunotherapy have begun to reshape the landscape of sarcoma treatment. However, these advancements are often isolated in their impact, lacking a cohesive, data-driven strategy for implementation across healthcare systems. The integration of artificial intelligence (AI) and digital health platforms represents the next frontier in this context. These technologies have the potential to synthesize large and complex datasets, from genomic information to real-world-time patient outcomes, thereby enabling more precise and personalized care. This is particularly crucial for sarcoma, given its heterogeneity and the consequent need for highly individualized treatment plans. The dawn of precision medicine has ushered in an era where treatment is personalized, not just to the disease but to the individual [6]. Yet, while the promise of precision medicine is substantial, its full realization is intricately tied to the evolution of healthcare systems towards value-based models, especially for complex conditions like sarcoma [7,8].

The notion of value-based healthcare (VBHC) emphasizes patient-centricity, focusing on metrics that matter most to the patient's well-being. This patient-centricity must be supported by robust, real-world-time data analytics that not only gauge the quality of care but also its cost-effectiveness [9,10]. Recent advancements in digital health technologies and AI have demonstrated unprecedented potential to empower this transition, offering an innovative toolkit for data collection, management, and predictive analytics [11–13].

However, the intersection of digital health and AI remains an underexplored terrain, especially in the context of sarcoma care [14]. This article aims to go beyond a mere review of existing technologies and methodologies. Instead, it seeks to offer a forward-looking perspective on how the confluence of these technologies could redefine the very essence of sarcoma care, contributing to a future where diagnosis is precise, treatment is personalized, and outcomes are continually optimized [15] (Figure 1).

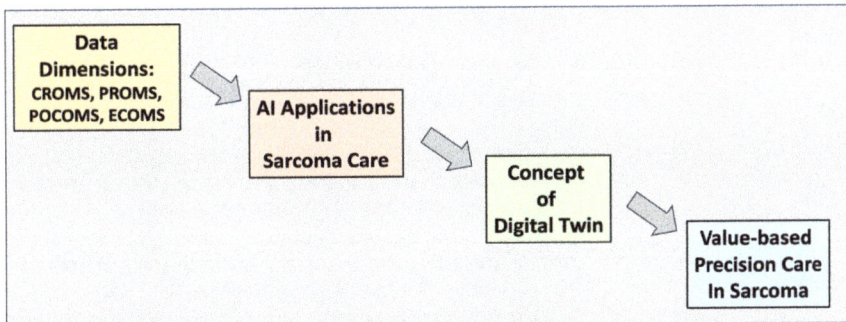

Figure 1. The figure depicts the evolution of sarcoma care, emphasizing patient-centricity and a data-driven approach. Digital health technologies, like Sarconector, form the foundation, streamlining patient data integration. Building on this, AI employs advanced algorithms to precisely characterize sarcoma subtypes and predict treatment outcomes. The pinnacle is the 'digital twin', a virtual patient profile that harnesses AI for predictive modeling and treatment optimization. CROMS = clinician-reported outcome measures; PROMS = patient-reported outcomes measures; POCOMS = patient-omics-centric outcome measures; ECOMS = economic measures.

In doing so, this article embarks on a visionary journey to explore the untapped potential of digital health and AI. It aims to serve as a catalyst for multidisciplinary dialogue and research, encouraging healthcare professionals, policymakers, and technologists to collaborate in transforming the future of sarcoma care—making it more precise, sustainable, and, above all, value-based.

2. The Vision for Value-Based Precision Care in Sarcoma

The pursuit of value-based healthcare is not merely a trend but a paradigm shift—one that brings the patient to the center of the healthcare universe [16]. In the context of sarcoma, a complex and rare malignancy, this transformation is not just aspirational but essential [15]. The heterogeneity of sarcoma, spanning multiple subtypes and clinical complexities, demands an individualized, outcomes-focused approach [17,18]. Traditional healthcare systems, largely built on a volume-based model, often fall short in providing the comprehensive, personalized care that sarcoma patients require. Value-based care in sarcoma envisions a healthcare ecosystem where every stakeholder, from surgeons and oncologists to data scientists and policymakers, collaborates to enhance the patient experience—from diagnosis to treatment and follow-up. It is an approach that goes beyond the immediate clinical outcomes to consider the patient's quality of life, long-term wellbeing, and the economic sustainability of the care provided. In this envisioned ecosystem, treatment protocols are not rigid pathways but dynamic algorithms, constantly updated with real-world-time data and adapted to each patient's unique medical history, genomic profile, and even psychosocial needs [19–21].

This vision is not utopian; it is attainable. Emerging technologies in digital health, coupled with advances in artificial intelligence and machine learning, offer the tools needed to actualize this vision. Imagine a future where an interoperable digital platform integrates multi-dimensional data, from medical imaging to genomic sequencing and patient-reported outcomes. These data are then processed by sophisticated AI algorithms to provide actionable insights, ranging from predicting treatment responses to estimating healthcare costs [19,22]. Moreover, the continuous benchmarking against quality indicators ensures that the care provided is not just effective but continually optimized [22].

However, the transition from vision to reality entails overcoming significant barriers—technological, ethical, and institutional. The subsequent sections of this article delve into these challenges, offering a multi-faceted perspective on how the confluence of digital health and AI can serve as the linchpin in materializing the vision for value-based care in sarcoma.

3. Potential of Digital Health

Digital health stands as a cornerstone in the realization of value-based care, especially in the intricate landscape of sarcoma [23,24]. The advent of technologies such as interoperable Electronic Health Records (EHRs), telemedicine, and real-world-time data platforms has enabled healthcare systems to move beyond the siloed structures of the past [19,22]. These technologies permit the seamless integration of multi-dimensional patient data—from diagnostic imaging and laboratory results to patient-reported outcomes and follow-up care metrics [25]. The role of digital health in sarcoma care is not merely auxiliary; it is transformative. For instance, telemedicine has proven to be invaluable in providing specialized sarcoma care to patients in remote locations, breaking down geographical barriers to quality healthcare. This is particularly crucial for a rare and complex disease like sarcoma, where specialized expertise may not be readily available in all regions. Interoperable EHRs, on the other hand, facilitate multi-disciplinary collaboration by allowing seamless data sharing between oncologists, radiologists, pathologists, and even primary care physicians. This is vital in sarcoma care, which often requires a multi-disciplinary approach for optimal outcomes. The EHRs can also be integrated with AI algorithms to flag potential issues or suggest alternative treatment pathways based on historical data and predictive analytics. Moreover, real-world-time data platforms can serve as a tool for continuous quality improvement. By tracking key performance indicators in real-time, healthcare providers can identify areas for improvement almost instantaneously, allowing for rapid intervention and adaptation of care protocols [19].

But the potential of digital health is not just in data collection; it is in data utilization. Advanced digital platforms can streamline the diagnostic journey, enhance treatment personalization, and even predict clinical outcomes, thereby offering a more holistic, patient-centric model of care. For example, digital platforms can automate the pre-diagnostic phase by gathering and analyzing patient history, symptoms, and preliminary test results, thereby aiding clinicians in making more accurate initial assessments. These platforms can also integrate with wearable devices that monitor patient vitals and other health metrics, providing a continuous stream of data that can be invaluable for ongoing care and monitoring. Furthermore, digital health technologies can facilitate patient engagement by providing platforms for virtual consultations, remote monitoring, and even digital therapeutics. These technologies empower patients to take an active role in their healthcare journey, thereby aligning with the principles of value-based care.

In essence, digital health technologies serve as the scaffolding upon which value-based care in sarcoma can be constructed, offering the dual advantages of operational efficiency and clinical efficacy.

4. Future Applications of AI in Sarcoma Care

As we look toward the horizon of sarcoma care, artificial intelligence (AI) emerges as a highly promising tool for advancing the field [26,27]. While current applications have been instrumental in diagnosis and treatment planning, the future holds even greater promise. Advanced machine learning algorithms are poised to delve into multi-omics data, offering unprecedented levels of precision in characterizing sarcoma subtypes and predicting treatment responses. The application of machine learning in sarcoma research extends beyond clinical data and can incorporate environmental, genetic, and lifestyle factors. By creating more comprehensive models that consider these variables, AI has the potential to identify new risk factors and even suggest preventative measures for at-risk populations. Deep learning techniques, a subset of machine learning, could be particularly impactful in image analysis. These algorithms can analyze complex patterns in radiological images that may be too subtle for the human eye, thereby aiding in early diagnosis and more accurate staging of the disease. This is crucial for sarcoma, where early diagnosis can significantly improve prognosis.

These algorithms could also integrate radiomic features with pathological and clinical data, refining prognostic accuracy [28]. Moreover, AI has the potential to support real-time decision making during surgeries through augmented reality interfaces, allowing for more precise surgical interventions. The introduction of natural language processing (NLP) can further enhance patient engagement by automating the analysis of patient-reported outcomes, thereby incorporating the patient's voice directly into the care continuum. NLP's real strength lies in its ability to convert unstructured data, such as patient narratives or free-text clinical notes, into structured data that can be easily analyzed. This is particularly valuable in sarcoma care, where patient experiences and symptoms can be highly variable and complex. By applying NLP algorithms to these unstructured data sources, healthcare providers can gain insights into patient well-being, treatment side effects, and even early indicators of complications that may not be readily apparent through traditional structured data. These structured data can then be integrated into machine learning models to improve predictive accuracy, thereby contributing to more personalized and effective treatment plans.

In a value-based healthcare framework, AI can enable more personalized, efficient, and outcome-oriented care, serving as a catalyst for transforming the ideal of precision sarcoma care into a tangible reality.

5. The Concept of Sarcoma Digital Twin

The notion of a "Digital Twin" in sarcoma care is a groundbreaking concept that aligns closely with the goals of precision medicine and value-based healthcare [29]. Drawing inspiration from the Swiss Sarcoma Network's robust digital platform, the Sarconector, a sarcoma digital twin serves as a virtual replica of an individual patient's medical profile, integrating real-world-time data including Clinical-Reported Outcome Measures (CROMS), Patient-Reported Outcome Measures (PROMS), POCOMS (patient-omics-centric outcome measures), ECOMS (economic measures), and other metrics from multiple sources like Electronic Health Records (EHR), surveys, and interviews [22,30].

The concept of a digital twin goes beyond merely storing or aggregating data; it serves as a dynamic, interactive model that evolves in real-world-time. As new clinical data become available, whether they are from imaging studies, laboratory tests, or patient-reported symptoms, the digital twin updates accordingly. This dynamic nature allows for a more nuanced understanding of the patient's condition, thereby facilitating more informed clinical decisions. Moreover, the digital twin concept is not limited to the individual patient level. When aggregated across a population of sarcoma patients, these digital twins can serve as a rich data repository for observational studies, clinical trials, and even epidemiological research. This collective data pool can be invaluable for identifying patterns or trends in sarcoma treatment and outcomes, thereby contributing to evidence-based medicine.

By leveraging AI-driven analytical tools, the digital twin can assist in predictive modeling, optimizing treatment plans, and even simulating potential outcomes of various therapeutic strategies. This creates an innovative ecosystem for quality-centric, value-based sarcoma care, enabling iterative improvement based on ongoing assessments and benchmarking. The utility of AI in this context is multifold. For instance, machine learning algorithms can analyze the digital twin data to predict patient responses to different treatment modalities, thereby aiding in personalized treatment planning. Furthermore, natural language processing (NLP) algorithms can sift through clinical notes and patient interviews to extract valuable insights that may not be readily apparent through quantitative data alone. These AI-driven analyses can be integrated into the digital twin, providing a comprehensive, 360-degree view of the patient's health status and treatment options. The concept of a sarcoma digital twin also has implications for healthcare economics. By providing a more accurate and personalized treatment plan, it has the potential to reduce unnecessary tests and treatments, thereby contributing to cost-effectiveness and sustainability in healthcare systems. In doing so, the concept of a sarcoma digital twin pushes the frontier of what is possible in delivering personalized, effective, and efficient care to sarcoma patients.

6. Roadmap to the Future

The Swiss Sarcoma Network's comprehensive roadmap to sarcoma care offers a visionary blueprint for the future, highlighting the synergy between AI and digital health in achieving a sustainable healthcare system. From a practical standpoint, this roadmap serves as a guide for healthcare providers, administrators and policymakers. It outlines actionable steps such as the adoption of interoperable digital platforms, the integration of AI in diagnostic and treatment protocols, and the establishment of quality indicators for continuous improvement. These practical measures aim to facilitate the transition from traditional, volume-based healthcare models to a more dynamic, value-based approach. The roadmap also suggests the use of real-world-time data to validate and refine AI algorithms, thereby ensuring that technological advancements are rooted in tangible clinical benefits. The roadmap outlines a multi-faceted approach that includes real-world-time data collection, interoperable digital platforms for data management, automated analysis employing AI algorithms, and benchmarking against quality indicators specific to sarcoma care [19,26]. These elements come together to assess various dimensions of care, including clinical outcomes and patient experiences. The ultimate aim is to continuously refine sarcoma care through iterative improvements, bringing the healthcare system closer to realizing value-based precision care. Adding another layer of innovation, the roadmap aims to incorporate the concept of a sarcoma digital twin, a virtual replica of an individual patient's medical condition that integrates seamlessly with AI-driven predictive modeling. As the roadmap evolves, there will be an increasing focus on aligning costs with value, thereby contributing to a more sustainable, efficient, and patient-centric healthcare system. Thus, the roadmap represents not just a pathway for sarcoma care but also serves as a model for the broader application of precision medicine and value-based healthcare.

While the Swiss Sarcoma Network provides a innovative model, its potential is not confined to Switzerland alone. By fostering international collaborations and partnerships, this roadmap can be scaled globally, adapted to diverse healthcare infrastructures and socio-cultural contexts. Key to this expansion is the network's emphasis on interoperability and standardization, facilitating seamless data exchange across borders. The establishment of international sarcoma care consortiums, working cohesively within the potential of such platform, can harmonize methodologies, share best practices, and collectively advance the vision of precision medicine. As more regions adopt this model, there is an opportunity for global real-world-time data aggregation, enhancing AI's predictive capabilities and refining treatment strategies. Thus, the roadmap represents not just a pathway for sarcoma care but also serves as a model for the broader application of precision medicine and value-based healthcare on a global scale.

7. Ethical and Regulatory Forethought

As we advance toward a new paradigm of value-based precision care in sarcoma, underpinned by digital health and AI, ethical and regulatory considerations must be addressed with the same vigor as technological innovations [31,32]. The collection, storage, and analysis of patient data pose questions about data security, privacy, and informed consent. Ensuring equitable access to advanced sarcoma treatments catalyzed by AI and digital tools is paramount to preventing disparities in care. However, it is important to acknowledge the limitations of our approach. While AI and digital health platforms offer transformative potential, they are no without their drawbacks. The quality of AI algorithms is highly dependent on the quality and quantity of the data fed into them. Incomplete or biased data can lead to inaccurate or even harmful clinical decisions. Additionally, the ethical implications of AI decision making in healthcare are still not fully understood and require further study. There is also the risk of over-reliance on technology, which could potentially undermine the role of medical professionals in patient care. Furthermore, the cost of implementing advanced digital solutions may be prohibitive for smaller healthcare facilities, potentially widening the gap in the quality of care. Regulatory bodies and ethical committees must work in concert with healthcare providers, technology developers, and policymakers to standardize protocols, ensuring that they are universally applicable and ethically sound. These protocols must also be flexible enough to adapt to rapid technological advancements without compromising patient safety or data integrity. As real-world data platforms become more integrated into the healthcare system, legal frameworks will play a critical role in shaping the ethical landscape of digital health and AI in sarcoma care. Thus, ethical and regulatory forethought is not a mere afterthought but an integral component of the roadmap to value-based precision care.

8. Challenges and Barriers: A Call to Action

While the horizon is bright with the promise of digital health and AI ushering in a new era of value-based precision care in sarcoma, the path is fraught with challenges that require immediate attention. Practically speaking, the implementation of this roadmap will necessitate substantial investments in technology and human resources. Hospitals and healthcare providers will need to upgrade their existing infrastructures to support data-intensive AI algorithms. Training programs will be essential for clinicians to effectively interpret and act upon AI-generated insights. Moreover, the roadmap calls for a collaborative effort involving not just the medical community but also regulatory bodies and insurance providers. This multi-stakeholder approach is crucial for overcoming the financial, ethical, and logistical barriers to implementing a value-based healthcare model in sarcoma care. Resource constraints, a lack of standardized data protocols, and resistance to change within medical institutions all pose significant barriers. The dearth of expertise in data science within the medical community adds another layer of complexity. Furthermore, data privacy concerns and regulatory hurdles can slow down the pace of innovation. However, these challenges should not deter us; rather, they should serve as a clarion call to action. This involves not only healthcare professionals and technologists but also policymakers, patient advocacy groups, and regulatory bodies. A collective, multidisciplinary effort is crucial to overcome these barriers. Funding must be allocated for research and development, educational initiatives must be put in place, and policy frameworks need to be developed to encourage data sharing and interoperability. By acknowledging and addressing these challenges head-on, we can accelerate the journey toward realizing the full potential of digital health and AI in transforming sarcoma care.

9. Conclusions and Proposals for Future Research

In the evolving landscape of sarcoma care, the convergence of digital health and artificial intelligence offers a beacon of hope for personalized, efficient, and value-based treatment options. We have explored the promise this union holds—from the integration of real-world-time data and interoperable digital platforms to the application of AI for predictive analytics, all the way to the conceptualization of the sarcoma digital twin, thereby enabling predictive and value-based precision sarcoma care. As we look to the future, several avenues for research emerge. First, there is a need for randomized controlled trials (or, alternatively, target trial emulations) to validate the efficacy of AI algorithms in sarcoma diagnosis and treatment planning. Second, research should focus on the ethical implications of AI in healthcare, particularly in the context of data privacy and informed consent. Third, the economic aspects of implementing digital health platforms and AI in sarcoma care warrant in-depth study, including cost–benefit analyses and long-term sustainability assessments. Lastly, future work could explore the integration of other emerging technologies, such as blockchain for secure data sharing or augmented reality for enhanced surgical planning, into the existing digital health ecosystem. These research proposals aim to fill the existing gaps in our understanding and provide a comprehensive framework for the adoption of digital health and AI in sarcoma care. While the challenges are significant, they are not insurmountable. We stand at the cusp of a transformative era in healthcare, one where the systematic adoption of these technologies could revolutionize the way we approach not just sarcoma, but complex diseases at large. However, to realize this vision, a coordinated, multidisciplinary effort is essential. The time for action is now; let us seize this moment to propel sarcoma care into a future replete with the benefits of digital health and AI, ultimately improving outcomes and quality of life for patients around the globe.

Author Contributions: Conceptualization, B.F. and P.H.; methodology, B.F.; writing—original draft preparation, B.F. and P.H.; writing—review and editing, G.S. and B.B.-L.; project administration, B.F., G.S., B.B.-L. and P.H.; funding acquisition, B.F., G.S., B.B.-L. and P.H. All authors have read and agreed to the published version of the manuscript.

Funding: This research received no external funding.

Institutional Review Board Statement: Not applicable.

Informed Consent Statement: Not applicable.

Data Availability Statement: Not applicable.

Acknowledgments: The Swiss Sarcoma Network (SSN; www.swiss-sarcoma.net; URL accessed on 30 August 2023) is organized as a non-profit association with the goal of defining and improving the quality of sarcoma care. Its members are institutions that are committed to transparently sharing information of all their consecutive patients with suspicion/confirmation of sarcoma at the weekly MDT/SB and to prospectively register the patients in a common real-world-time database. This database is designed for predictive modelling and the creation of the sarcoma digital twin to realize predictive and value-based precision sarcoma care. We would like to thank all representatives and members of the SSN: Silke Gillessen-Sommer, Barbara Kopf, Glauco Martinetti (Ente Ospedaliero Cantonale, Bellinzona, Locarno, Lugano), Markus Furrer, Christian Michelitsch, Hugo Keune (Kantonsspitäler Graubünden KSGR), Paul Magnus Schneider, Marco Gugolz (Hirslanden Zürich); Markus Weber, Marc Widmer (Stadtspital Zürich); Beata Bode, Marianne Tinguely (Patho Enge, Zurich), Stefan Breitenstein, Hansjörg Lehmann (Kantonsspital Winterthur), Gabriela Studer, Benno Fuchs (LUKS Teaching University Hospital Luzern), and the Faculty of Medicine and Health Sciences, University of Lucerne, Switzerland (Reto Babst, Stefan Boes).

Conflicts of Interest: The authors declare no conflict of interest.

References

1. Kubicek, P.; Cesne, A.L.; Lervat, C.; Toulmonde, M.; Chevreau, C.; Duffaud, F.; Le Nail, L.-R.; Morelle, M.; Gaspar, N.; Vérité, C.; et al. Management and outcomes of adolescent and young adult sarcoma patients: Results from the French nationwide database NETSARC. *BMC Cancer* **2023**, *23*, 69. [CrossRef] [PubMed]
2. Blay, J.-Y.; Penel, N.; Gouin, F.; Le Cesne, A.; Toulmonde, M. Improving at a nationwide level the management of patients with sarcomas with an expert network. *Ann. Oncol.* **2022**, *33*, 659–661. [CrossRef] [PubMed]
3. Blay, J.-Y.; Casali, P.; Bouvier, C.; Dehais, C.; Galloway, I.; Gietema, J.; Halámková, J.; Hindi, N.; Idbaih, A.; Kinloch, E.; et al. European Reference Network for rare adult solid cancers, statement and integration to health care systems of member states: A position paper of the ERN EURACAN. *ESMO Open Cancer Horizons* **2021**, *6*, 100174. [CrossRef] [PubMed]
4. Blay, J.Y.; Bonvalot, S.; Gouin, F.; Le Cesne, A.; Penel, N. Criteria for reference centers for sarcomas: Volume but also long-term multidisciplinary organisation. *Ann. Oncol.* **2019**, *30*, 2008–2009. [CrossRef] [PubMed]
5. Blay, J.Y.; Soibinet, P.; Penel, N.; Bompas, E.; Duffaud, F.; Stoeckle, E.; Mir, O.; Adam, J.; Chevreau, C.; Bonvalot, S.; et al. Improved survival using specialized multidisciplinary board in sarcoma patients. *Ann. Oncol.* **2017**, *28*, 2852–2859. [CrossRef]
6. Hoeben, A.; Joosten, E.A.J.; van den Beuken-van Everdingen, M.H.J. Personalized Medicine: Recent Progress in Cancer Therapy. *Cancers* **2021**, *13*, 242. [CrossRef]
7. Jameson, J.L.; Longo, D.L. Precision medicine—Personalized, problematic, and promising. *N. Engl. J. Med.* **2015**, *372*, 2229–2234. [CrossRef]
8. Denny, J.C.; Collins, F.S. Precision medicine in 2030-seven ways to transform healthcare. *Cell* **2021**, *184*, 1415–1419. [CrossRef]
9. Porter, M.E. A strategy for health care reform—Toward a value-based system. *N. Engl. J. Med.* **2009**, *361*, 109–112. [CrossRef]
10. Porter, M.E.; Pabo, E.A.; Lee, T.H. Redesigning primary care: A strategic vision to improve value by organizing around patients' needs. *Health Aff.* **2013**, *32*, 516–525. [CrossRef]
11. Obermeyer, Z.; Emanuel, E.J. Predicting the Future—Big Data, Machine Learning, and Clinical Medicine. *N. Engl. J. Med.* **2016**, *375*, 1216–1219. [CrossRef] [PubMed]
12. Obermeyer, Z.; Topol, E.J. Artificial intelligence, bias, and patients' perspectives. *Lancet* **2021**, *397*, 2038. [CrossRef] [PubMed]
13. Chen, J.H.; Asch, S.M. Machine Learning and Prediction in Medicine—Beyond the Peak of Inflated Expectations. *N. Engl. J. Med.* **2017**, *376*, 2507–2509. [CrossRef] [PubMed]
14. Zilchman, E.; Nicklin, W.; Aggarwal, R.; Bates, D. Health Care 2030: The coming transformatrion. *NEJM Catalyst* **2021**, *1*, 1–11.
15. Fuchs, B.; Studer, G.; Bode, B.; Wellauer, H.; Frei, A.; Theus, C.; Schupfer, G.; Plock, J.; Windegger, H.; Breitenstein, S.; et al. Development of a value-based healthcare delivery model for sarcoma patients. *Swiss Med. Wkly.* **2021**, *151*, w30047. [CrossRef]
16. Kaplan, R.S.; Porter, M.E. How to solve the cost crisis in health care. *Harv. Bus. Rev.* **2011**, *89*, 46–52.
17. Blay, J.Y.; Hindi, N.; Bollard, J.; Aguiar, S.; Angel, M.; Araya, B.; Badilla, R.; Bernabeu, D.; Campos, F.; Caro-Sánchez, C.H.S.; et al. SELNET clinical practice guidelines for soft tissue sarcoma and GIST. *Cancer Treat. Rev.* **2022**, *102*, 102312. [CrossRef]
18. Blay, J.Y.; Palmerini, E.; Bollard, J.; Aguiar, S.; Angel, M.; Araya, B.; Badilla, R.; Bernabeu, D.; Campos, F.; Chs, C.S.; et al. SELNET Clinical practice guidelines for bone sarcoma. *Crit. Rev. Oncol. Hematol.* **2022**, *174*, 103685. [CrossRef]
19. Fuchs, B.; Schelling, G.; Elyes, M.; Studer, G.; Bode-Lesniewska, B.; Scaglioni, M.F.; Giovanoli, P.; Heesen, P. Unlocking the Power of Benchmarking: Real-World-Time Data Analysis for Enhanced Sarcoma Patient Outcomes. *Cancers* **2023**, *15*, 4395. [CrossRef]
20. Bates, D.W. How to regulate evolving AI health algorithms. *Nat. Med.* **2023**, *29*, 26. [CrossRef]
21. Haug, C.J.; Drazen, J.M. Artificial Intelligence and Machine Learning in Clinical Medicine, 2023. *N. Engl. J. Med.* **2023**, *388*, 1201–1208. [CrossRef] [PubMed]
22. Heesen, P.; Studer, G.; Bode, B.; Windegger, H.; Staeheli, B.; Aliu, P.; Martin-Broto, J.; Gronchi, A.; Blay, J.Y.; Le Cesne, A.; et al. Quality of Sarcoma Care: Longitudinal Real-Time Assessment and Evidence Analytics of Quality Indicators. *Cancers* **2022**, *15*, 47. [CrossRef] [PubMed]
23. Topol, E.J. High-performance medicine: The convergence of human and artificial intelligence. *Nat. Med.* **2019**, *25*, 44–56. [CrossRef] [PubMed]
24. Rajpurkar, P.; Chen, E.; Banerjee, O.; Topol, E.J. AI in health and medicine. *Nat. Med.* **2022**, *28*, 31–38. [CrossRef]
25. Steinhubl, S.R.; Muse, E.D.; Topol, E.J. Can mobile health technologies transform health care? *JAMA* **2013**, *310*, 2395–2396. [CrossRef]
26. Esteva, A.; Robicquet, A.; Ramsundar, B.; Kuleshov, V.; DePristo, M.; Chou, K.; Cui, C.; Corrado, G.; Thrun, S.; Dean, J. A guide to deep learning in healthcare. *Nat. Med.* **2019**, *25*, 24–29. [CrossRef]
27. Jiang, F.; Jiang, Y.; Zhi, H.; Dong, Y.; Li, H.; Ma, S.; Wang, Y.; Dong, Q.; Shen, H.; Wang, Y. Artificial intelligence in healthcare: Past, present and future. *Stroke Vasc. Neurol.* **2017**, *2*, 230–243. [CrossRef]
28. Bera, K.; Braman, N.; Gupta, A.; Velcheti, V.; Madabhushi, A. Predicting cancer outcomes with radiomics and artificial intelligence in radiology. *Nat. Rev. Clin. Oncol.* **2021**, *19*, 132–146. [CrossRef]
29. Hernandez-Boussard, T.; Macklin, P.; Greenspan, E.J.; Gryshuk, A.L.; Stahlberg, E.; Syeda-Mahmood, T.; Shmulevich, I. Digital twins for predictive oncology will be a paradigm shift for precision cancer care. *Nat. Med.* **2021**, *27*, 2065–2066. [CrossRef]
30. Mosku, N.; Heesen, P.; Christen, S.; Scaglioni, M.F.; Bode, B.; Studer, G.; Fuchs, B. The Sarcoma-Specific Instrument to Longitudinally Assess Health-Related Outcomes of the Routine Care Cycle. *Diagnostics* **2023**, *13*, 1206. [CrossRef]

31. Char, D.S.; Shah, N.H.; Magnus, D. Implementing Machine Learning in Health Care—Addressing Ethical Challenges. *N. Engl. J. Med.* **2018**, *378*, 981–983. [CrossRef] [PubMed]
32. Price, W.N., 2nd; Cohen, I.G. Privacy in the age of medical big data. *Nat. Med.* **2019**, *25*, 37–43. [CrossRef] [PubMed]

Disclaimer/Publisher's Note: The statements, opinions and data contained in all publications are solely those of the individual author(s) and contributor(s) and not of MDPI and/or the editor(s). MDPI and/or the editor(s) disclaim responsibility for any injury to people or property resulting from any ideas, methods, instructions or products referred to in the content.

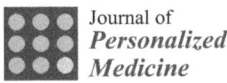

Review

Digital Twins in Healthcare: Methodological Challenges and Opportunities

Charles Meijer, Hae-Won Uh and Said el Bouhaddani *

Department Data Science & Biostatistics, Julius Center, UMC Utrecht, 3584 CX Utrecht, The Netherlands; h.w.uh@umcutrecht.nl (H.-W.U.)
* Correspondence: s.elbouhaddani@umcutrecht.nl

Abstract: One of the most promising advancements in healthcare is the application of digital twin technology, offering valuable applications in monitoring, diagnosis, and development of treatment strategies tailored to individual patients. Furthermore, digital twins could also be helpful in finding novel treatment targets and predicting the effects of drugs and other chemical substances in development. In this review article, we consider digital twins as virtual counterparts of real human patients. The primary aim of this narrative review is to give an in-depth look into the various data sources and methodologies that contribute to the construction of digital twins across several healthcare domains. Each data source, including blood glucose levels, heart MRI and CT scans, cardiac electrophysiology, written reports, and multi-omics data, comes with different challenges regarding standardization, integration, and interpretation. We showcase how various datasets and methods are used to overcome these obstacles and generate a digital twin. While digital twin technology has seen significant progress, there are still hurdles in the way to achieving a fully comprehensive patient digital twin. Developments in non-invasive and high-throughput data collection, as well as advancements in modeling and computational power will be crucial to improve digital twin systems. We discuss a few critical developments in light of the current state of digital twin technology. Despite challenges, digital twin research holds great promise for personalized patient care and has the potential to shape the future of healthcare innovation.

Keywords: virtual twins; personalized medicine; precision medicine; digital twin methodology; multi-modal data sources; AI; data integration

Citation: Meijer, C.; Uh, H.-W.; el Bouhaddani, S. Digital Twins in Healthcare: Methodological Challenges and Opportunities. *J. Pers. Med.* **2023**, *13*, 1522. https://doi.org/10.3390/jpm13101522

Academic Editor: Daniele Giansanti

Received: 16 August 2023
Revised: 14 October 2023
Accepted: 15 October 2023
Published: 23 October 2023

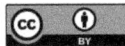

Copyright: © 2023 by the authors. Licensee MDPI, Basel, Switzerland. This article is an open access article distributed under the terms and conditions of the Creative Commons Attribution (CC BY) license (https://creativecommons.org/licenses/by/4.0/).

1. Introduction

Digital twin technologies have seen a rise in popularity in various industries, including manufacturing, engineering, and rocketry, from where the term originated [1]. This rise can be attributed to the developments in rapidly collecting, storing, and sharing data, together with computers being able to apply complex models and algorithms in a short amount of time [2]. In several fields of healthcare, such as precision medicine, clinical trials, and public health, the application of digital twins has become more and more apparent as they may serve as a tool to understand and simulate complex physiological processes. Moreover, digital twins may also reduce the need for animal experimentation, which takes an estimated 200 million animals per year [3], as it allows a direct translation of in vitro measurements into what could be expected in vivo either in digital animal models or humans [4].

General definitions of a digital twin have been given in the literature [5–9]. In this narrative review, we work with the general definition of healthcare digital twins [10] as virtual replicas of real human patients, through which clinicians can gain valuable insights, optimize treatment strategies, and deliver personalized care [5,11,12]. For specific healthcare domains, the operationalization of this definition depends very much on the underlying methodology and data used to construct the digital twin. Though the general aim is expected to align with the definition above, a *'cardiac'* digital twin (e.g., Section 2.2 below) differs considerably from a *'drug response'* digital twin (e.g., Section 2.6 below) in methodology, data types, and implementation. One of our goals is to take a deeper look into the methodological aspects underlying digital twins across several healthcare domains where this technology is being applied. By gaining an understanding of the methods and data used, the potential value and important pitfalls of digital twins in future studies can be more easily identified.

Healthcare digital twins require large amounts of data and often multiple data types. These include measurements that can be made using a smartphone or -watch, like heart rate, temperature, and location [13], and data that can otherwise be gathered at home, such as blood pressure and blood oxygen saturation, but also medical imaging data recorded during CT or MRI scans, electrophysiology, and various types of -omics data, which can be collected through a wide range of techniques including sequencing, immunoprecipitation and mass-spectrometry [14]. After generating the digital twin, a variety of methods can be applied to make simulations and predictions. These range from fitting regression lines to the data to designing deep neural networks [15] and can be used for many different purposes. Apart from their clinical use, digital twin technologies may also be applied to identify novel drug targets, simulate the effectiveness and safety of new treatments, or predict patient traffic during a pandemic [5].

The aim of this narrative review is twofold. We aim to review the methodological development of digital twin systems across several healthcare domains. Second, we aim to identify the types of data required to construct the respective digital twins. Secondary to these aims, we further discuss how to overcome the challenges introduced by handling large amounts of data and standardization, integration, and interpretation of many different types of data. The research questions we desire to answer are: (1) which data types and sources are important for the development of healthcare digital twins? (2) What are the prevailing methods and techniques employed in healthcare digital twin systems, and how do they vary in their applications? (3) How can the challenges related to healthcare digital twin methods and data be transformed into opportunities? Addressing these aims and questions will be crucial to harnessing the full potential of digital twins, ensuring that this promising idea can be integrated successfully into clinical practice.

2. Case Studies

Digital twins of complex systems require vast amounts of data to accurately represent their physical counterparts. Different types of data can be gathered via different methods, and integrated into one model, to simulate pathways, organs, or entire organisms. However, gathering all that data may be especially challenging in medical care, compared to the original DT application in rocketry, for example. While a lot of environmental data can be continuously captured using body-worn sensors like a smartphone or -watch, more complicated and intrusive methods may be necessary to gain -omics or imaging information [5]. We present several key case studies in different healthcare fields where we review the data sources used and the methodology applied to construct digital twins. To aid in quickly searching the relevant literature regarding digital twin methodology, an annotated overview of the significant literature is presented in a searchable spreadsheet as Supplementary Material. Together with this supplementary overview, the case studies reviewed below provide an overview of the methodological cornerstones of digital twins across different healthcare domains.

2.1. Artificial Pancreas

One of the first digital twin-like systems is the artificial pancreas. It consists of two essential parts: a system capable of continuously measuring blood glucose levels, and a device containing a syringe used for insulin infusion when needed. Blood glucose levels used to be measured by having the user collect a drop of blood from their finger, but less invasive methods have been developed during the late 20th century and beyond. Instead of measuring true blood glucose levels, these values could be inferred by monitoring the glucose concentration in extracellular space. However, as the relation between the new interstitial glucose data and blood glucose levels is not one-to-one, the devices had to be calibrated with true blood glucose readings. Furthermore, even after successful calibration, this method was prone to loss of sensitivity and random noise. Addressing these issues is essential in order to be usable as a 'near-future' digital twin: for example, if glucose levels are predicted to be too high or too low in the near future, the system can generate preventive alerts, prompting the patient to take appropriate actions, such as adjusting insulin dosage or dietary choices.

To combat these issues, a collection of signal processing algorithms has been applied to ensure accurate prediction of blood glucose levels based on minimally invasive, interstitial readings [16]. The 'smart continuous glucose monitoring sensor' combines the existing glucose monitoring sensor with several software modules designed to reduce noise, improve accuracy, and predict future glucose concentration (Figure 1) [17].

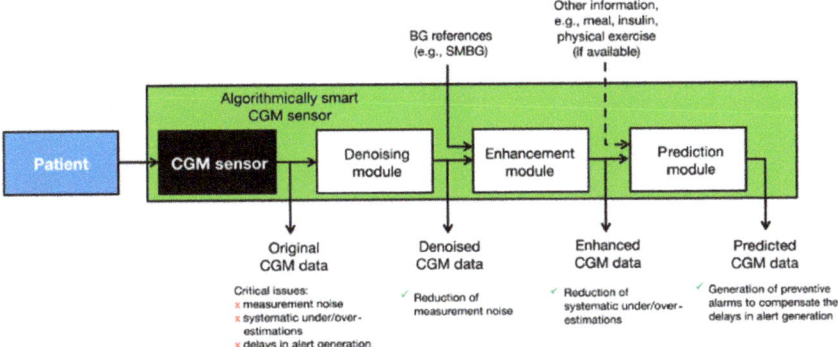

Figure 1. Schematic of the smart continuous glucose monitoring sensor which allows for subcutaneous glucose reading, signal processing, and future reading prediction to reduce measurement noise and under- and overestimations of blood glucose values. It also contains a prediction module to generate timelier alerts. Figure taken from [17].

Denoising is used to improve the subcutaneous glucose concentration readings from the sensor by reducing the impact of noise in the data. To estimate the true interstitial blood glucose concentration, the denoising algorithm uses a Bayesian interference algorithm that takes into account general information on signal-to-noise ratios, as well as the data it has collected previously from the specific individual, to determine which parts of the signal are noise. The algorithm also does not require user intervention and is designed to be adaptive to the signal-to-noise ratio of every individual user. Further, to combat under- and overestimations of blood glucose levels based on subcutaneous glucose readings, the data is enhanced using a least squares linear regression model. Briefly put, blood glucose measurements are fit against blood glucose estimations made based on the interstitial readings taken at the same time. Then, the regression parameters are used to enhance future data collected by the subcutaneous sensor to more accurately estimate the corresponding blood glucose values. This linear regression can be updated in real-time, and it takes into account the influence of blood-to-interstitium glucose transport and its delay on the individual user. The addition of these two data processing steps resulted in a greatly improved blood glucose estimation accuracy, which is essential for devices using subcutaneous readings (Figure 2). Lastly, the smart sensor is capable of predicting future glucose concentrations to enable the device to generate timelier alerts. Glucose level prediction is achieved by reading all the past data generated by the sensor and assigning every measurement a different weight, based on an autoregressive model. The future values are subsequently calculated by multiplying each past data point by its weight in real-time, and a preventive alert can be generated when the predicted value is either too low or too high [17].

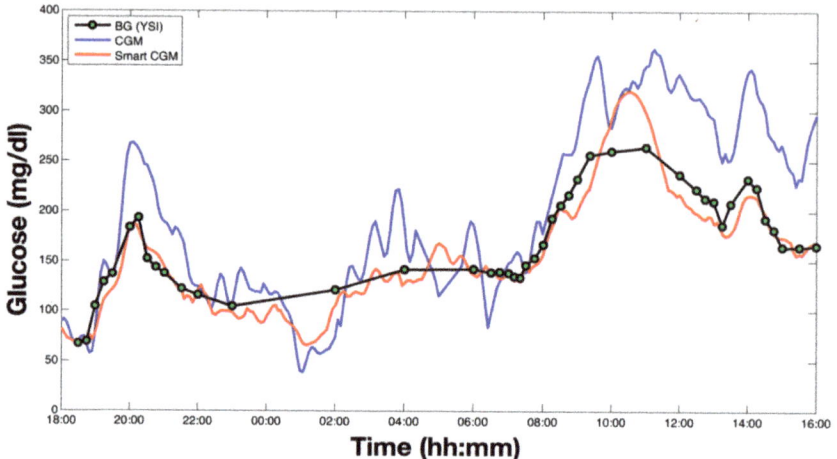

Figure 2. Results of application of the smart continuous glucose measuring system on a human subject. Original reading data are in blue, denoised and enhanced values are in red, and reference blood glucose measurements are shown as green dots. Figure taken from [17].

In the last few years, glucose monitors using these algorithms have been approved for use by the FDA without the need for calibration by capillary blood readings. These devices are capable of measuring patient data, applying data processing, and predicting future values in real-time [16]. However, many more variables other than blood glucose are needed to create a complex pancreas digital twin. In 1979, the rate of glucose processing was described in a nonlinear function [18] and that model has evolved into one describing a glucose–insulin network using many functions and parameters to take into account the glucose kinetics, insulin kinetics, rate of glucose appearance, endogenous glucose production, utilization, secretion and excretion [19]. Furthermore, models that describe the effect of external influences like physical activity and the delays associated with subcutaneous, rather than intravenous, insulin delivery were designed. These models make it possible to test the effect of any meal or insulin injection, as well as any extreme scenarios digitally, before use in clinical trials. Currently, an increasing number of variables are being added to the artificial pancreas systems. Heart rate monitoring, motion sensing, additional hormones, and glucagon have all been analyzed for their use in mitigating hypoglycemia during physical exercise. Technical developments, like the prevalence of smartphones capable of running algorithms and a wireless connection, may offer patients better monitoring of their glucose levels using a device that is already integrated into daily life as the controller [16].

2.2. Cardiac Digital Twins

In healthcare, generating digital twins to mimic a human organ has seen much popularity in cardiovascular research. Multiple types of data are combined to create a cardiac digital twin (CDT), which can be used to test patient-specific monitoring and treatment strategies (Figure 3). The process of creating a CDT can be split into two distinct stages; the anatomical and functional twinning stages. The anatomical twinning stage consists of creating a very detailed 3D copy of the physical twin, based on CT or MRI scans of the patient [20]. This cardiac 3D mesh is based on Universal Ventricular Coordinates. This model essentially describes the location of specific cardiac regions such as the apex or septum and can be automatically computed with relatively little input data. It requires an epicardial apex surface point, a left ventricular endocardial surface point, a right ventricular septal surface point, and surface points of the ventricular base, to compute the ventricular coordinates of the heart base, epicardium, left ventricular endocardium, and right ventricular endocardium and septum. The UVC algorithm is also capable of computing coordinates for trabeculae and certain heart valve openings [21]. A similar approach can be used to map Universal Torso Coordinates.

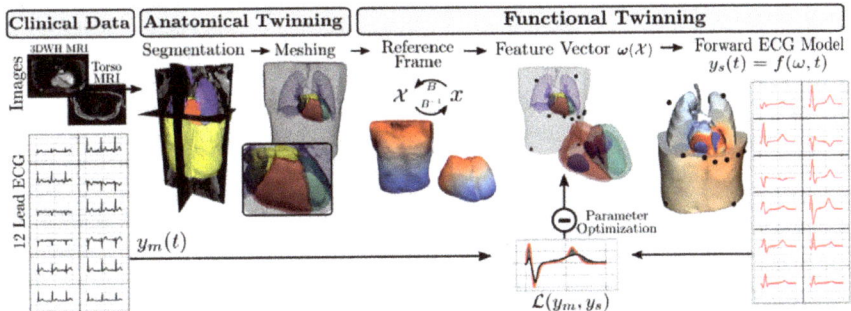

Figure 3. Schematic of workflow for CDT generation. MRI data is segmented and used to create anatomical meshes. A reference frame (X) is computed based on UVC and UTC. ECG waveforms generated with a forward ECG model are compared to clinically measured 12-lead ECG data for optimization of the model parameters contained in w(X). Figure taken from [20].

The input data is recorded during the MRI study of the patient. The 3D whole-heart MRI scans are segmented automatically by a convolutional neural network, and corrected manually. Automatic UVC computations are then run to create the cardiac mesh for the specific heart [20].

The second stage in creating the CDT, functional twinning, covers the electrophysiology of the heart. Four factors responsible for the ECG waveforms during activation and repolarization were defined mathematically: depolarization caused by the His–Purkinje system and distribution to the subendocardium, the conduction velocity within the ventricles, spatially varying action potential duration, and the conductivity of the torso surrounding the heart. Electrophysical activity of the anatomical reference frame was simulated using a fast-forward ECG model, and compared to clinical measurements of 12-lead ECGs (Figure 4). These comparisons show that with this two-stage twinning method, cardiac electrophysiology can be simulated automatically and in near real-time.

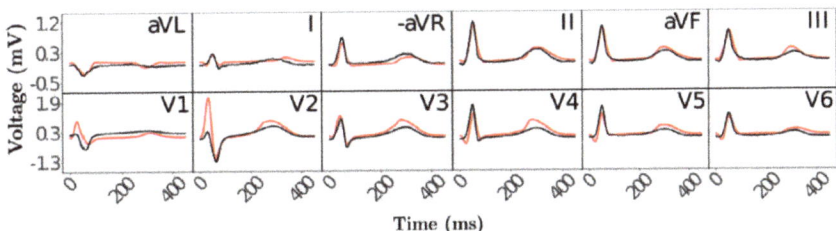

Figure 4. Simulated ECGs (red) compared to measured reference ECGs (black) after obtaining optimal parameter values. Electrodes were placed and simulated according to the 12-lead ECG setup. Figure taken from [20].

2.3. Single-Cell Flux Analysis

Apart from organ-specific measurements like heart electrophysiology and blood glucose levels, the vast amounts of data generated in omics research may also be used in generating digital twins. In cancer research, single-cell digital twins based on metabolomics and fluxomics, the analysis of production and consumption of metabolites, have been proposed as a tool to better discriminate between cancer phenotypes. The model used to create the single-cell digital twin integrates single-cell RNA (scRNA) sequencing data and extracellular metabolite fluxes to obtain a view of the single-cell metabolic phenotype at any given time [22].

The single-cell Flux Balance Analysis (scFBA) model requires three types of input (Figure 5). Firstly, it needs a template metabolic network, describing the different metabolites, their biochemical reactions, and their consumption or secretion [22]. The complete human metabolic network has been reconstructed by integrating pharmacogenomic associations, large-scale phenotypic data, and structural data for proteins and metabolites. The metabolic fluxes in this network have been predicted by models that have also been fed data from other omics analyses, describing the pathways that are expressed in any given cell or tissue [23]. Secondly, the scFBA model is given an scRNA-seq dataset that contains the normalized read count of each gene in each cell in the analysis. Lastly, extracellular fluxes in the patients' cell population are approximated from the measurement of metabolite concentrations in the cell culture medium of the patient-derived organoid or xenograft, for example.

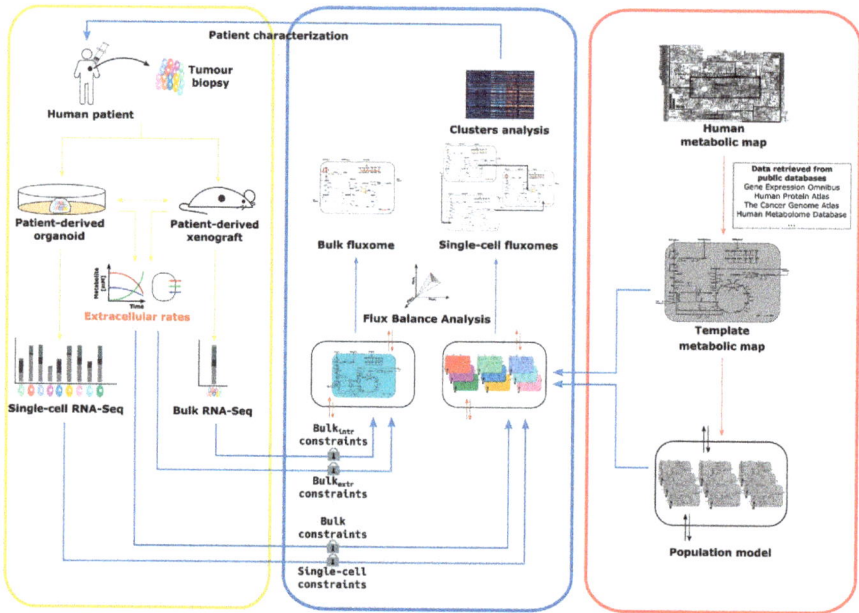

Figure 5. Schematic overview of the scFBA workflow. Single-cell RNA-seq and bulk RNA-seq are performed on patient-derived organoids or xenografts. Extracellular metabolite exchange rates are also measured. A template metabolic network is imported from a public database. The bulk RNA and flux data are integrated to form a population model. Single-cell networks can be computed by incorporating bulk constraints based on bulk data, and single-cell constraints based on the single-cell RNA-seq data. Figure taken from [22].

The scFBA pipeline starts with pre-processing, by removing genes with zero read count from the template metabolic network. Then, a population model is generated. This model is created by integrating all the RNA data of all the available cells in the template metabolite network. The resulting network corresponds to the scRNA of the average cell in the sample and is copied to produce a population model consisting of replicas of the single metabolic network. All the cells in the population now have the same set of metabolites as the template network. Each single-cell network can be reconstructed by introducing cooperation reactions, which allow metabolite exchange among cells and with the environment. These reactions are then linked to the scRNA data via logistically expressed rules. The 'AND' operator is used to describe genes that encode for different subunits of the same enzyme, while the 'OR' operator describes genes that encode for isoforms of the same enzyme. These logical operators are then used to calculate the reaction activity scores for each reaction. These scores represent the expression of the genes in transcripts per kilobase million. For the reactions that are caused by genes that are linked only through the AND operator, all the genes are necessary. This means that the reaction activity score can be defined as the expression of the least-expressed gene that is necessary for that reaction to occur. If the genes involved in the reaction are only linked through the OR operator, the activity score is calculated as the sum of the expression values.

After the population model and the reaction activity scores for each cell are computed, bulk and single-cell constraints are imposed. These represent boundaries on the metabolite exchanges with the environment and within the cells based on their reaction activity scores, respectively. The model, now describing the metabolite exchange between single cells and the environment, constrained by the reaction activity scores for each cell, as well as by boundaries set through measurements of the entire sample, can be used to simulate the effect of single gene deletions. The reactions that are associated with that gene which is only linked to other genes by the AND operator should be disabled by the deletion. These reactions are removed from the network, and the population model is reoptimized for total biomass production. This allows analysis of the effect of single genes on tumor growth in a patient-specific cell system, which may lead to identifying genes or clusters of cells that can be exploited to deregulate cancer metabolism [22].

2.4. Protein and DNA Interactions

Networks like the ones generated with scFBA may be created and applied in digital twin computations for other -omics data, as well. Protein interactions may be studied through multiple techniques. The yeast two-hybrid and LUMIER methods can both be applied to check for interaction between two specific proteins [24,25]. A high-throughput platform combining immunoprecipitation and high-throughput mass spectrometry (IP-HTMS) is capable of rapidly identifying novel protein interactions for a protein of interest (Figure 6).

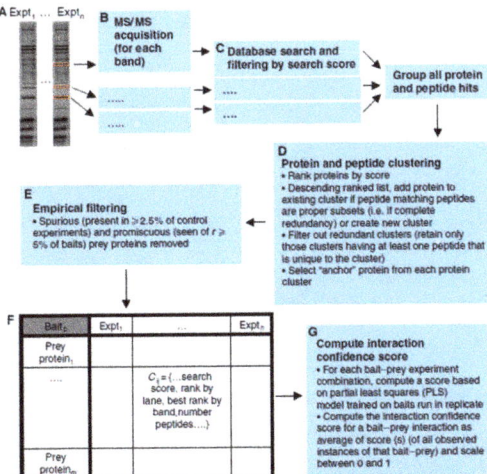

Figure 6. Schematic of the IP-HTMS pipeline. Bait proteins were isolated with their prey partners through immunoprecipitation and identified after SDS-PAGE and mass spectrometry. The proteins and peptides are clustered based on a scoring system and filtered. Finally, a confidence score is calculated for each bait–prey interaction. Figure taken from [26].

To demonstrate the IP-HTMS workflow, 407 'bait' proteins of interest were flag-tagged and isolated, together with any interacting 'prey' partners, via immunoprecipitation. The proteins were then subjected to SDS-PAGE and mass spectrometry for identification. All proteins and peptides that were associated with the same bait protein were clustered and an 'anchor' protein was selected for each cluster by ranking the proteins within the cluster based on the number of peptides. Interactions that were non-specific, bait–bait interactions, and interactions with contaminant proteins were removed from the interaction network. Several metrics were used to generate a measure of confidence in the bait–prey interactions, and high-scoring pairs were further analyzed by integrating other types of genomic information, such as gene expression, sub-cellular location, and function. With this pipeline, many protein interactions may be studied rapidly to create complex protein–protein interaction networks [26]. Networks like these can provide critical information to human digital twins, as they enable in-depth analysis of the effects of the absence or abundance of specific proteins on their pathways, which can lead to understanding why certain diseases occur, as well as pinpointing potential targets for treatment.

Protein–DNA interactions can also be analyzed, although the regulatory networks are more incomplete in comparison with protein–protein interaction networks, metabolic networks, and RNA networks [27]. Chromatin immunoprecipitation (ChIP), combined with next-generation sequencing can be used to identify DNA-bound proteins, as well as the DNA sequence they are bound to. This information may explain the effect of an altered DNA sequence if it results in a transcription factor not being able to interact with the DNA, for example. Protein–DNA interactions uncovered via ChIP-sequencing have been reported in databases like UniPROBE and JASPAR [28,29], but the technique is limited by the cost as well as the availability of the high-quality antibodies needed to retrieve the DNA–protein complexes [27].

2.5. Clinical Reports in Oncology

Advancements in machine learning and specifically natural language processing (NLP) have enabled the use of written records in creating digital twins. In cancer research, structured, written reports containing 'findings' and 'impressions' from CT-scan analysis of multiple organs were annotated for the presence or absence of metastases by five radiologists (Figure 7). Individual reports from each patient were concatenated in chronological order to enable multi-report analysis. This allows the model to access every previous report when it predicts the presence of metastases during the time of a patient's third report, for example. This is especially important in the event of no change compared to the last analysis being reported for a particular organ. The multi-report analysis enables the algorithm to decide whether 'no change' means an analysis based on the previous information.

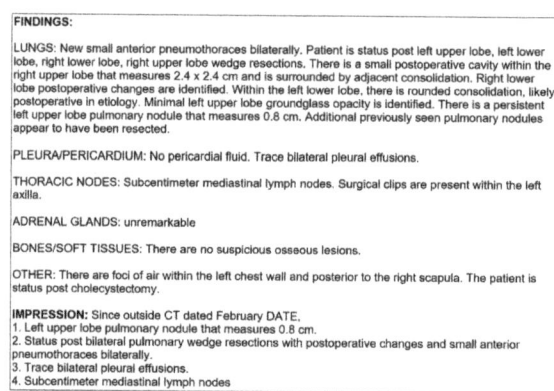

Figure 7. Example report of a chest CT containing organ site-specific 'findings', and 'impressions', with information about any organ. Figure taken from [30].

The structured reports are first converted into numeric vector representations to be used as inputs for the three machine learning models developed to predict metastasis presence over time. This can be achieved by removing the punctuation and unknown words in the report and assigning each word an index value. The strings of index values representing the written text are fed as input to the convolutional neural network (CNN), capable of learning which combinations of words mean the presence and which mean the absence of metastasis in each analyzed organ. An augmented CNN with an attention layer is used to better capture important information in the reports by assigning higher weights to the indices that represent more important words. Thirdly, to take the context into account, a bi-directional long short-term memory (LSTM) network was developed. This variant of a recurrent neural network is capable of processing the data both forward and backward. This allows the network model to account for both past and future contexts when learning the meaning of different word combinations. The LSTM network is designed to deal with long sequences, and it can determine what information needs to be remembered and what can be forgotten [30]. The three models were tested on over fourteen thousand radiology reports on the lung, liver, and adrenal glands. Prediction accuracies exceeded 96% across all combinations of models and organs. This shows that with the use of NLP algorithms, written report data could contribute to developing a cancer digital twin, as these texts still contain much of the information in the medical record [30].

2.6. Predicting Drug Effectiveness

Once available, healthcare digital twins may be used to predict treatment outcomes, simulate various events, or digitally test the effects of the absence of a certain protein, for example. Different goals require different statistical methods and, just like during the creation of the twins, speed, and accuracy are key in creating viable digital twin applications.

During clinical trials of a new treatment, the efficacy of the new treatment is usually tested against a standard treatment or a placebo when given to a random sample of the population. However, the new treatment could only be more beneficial to a select subgroup of patients in the sample. It is worth trying to analyze what characteristics define this subgroup, to understand why the treatment is especially effective for them [31]. Although selecting a couple of features to create subgroups is known to be prone to finding false positives, various statistical methods have shown to be capable of this task [32].

The classical method consists of fitting a regression model based on the interactions between treatments and patient data. One drawback of this model is that it is not suitable for use with datasets containing many different variables, as it would need to consider many different possible interactions [33]. Multiple new algorithms for defining the boundaries of a certain subgroup have been tested.

One method relies on the use of random forests and regression or classification trees to prioritize covariates that predict which patients will benefit most from a treatment. First, random forests are applied to the data which take the variable values, including the treatment group, as input, and give the probability of a certain outcome as output. The estimated treatment effect is subsequently calculated by subtracting the probability of a positive outcome under control from the positive outcome after treatment. So, a high estimated treatment-effect value means that the treatment greatly affected the patients' chances of a positive outcome. Then, the variables that have a strong effect on the estimated treatment-effect value are selected through either regression or classification trees. With the regression tree method, a regression tree is created with the estimated treatment effect as the response and the variables as the other input data. This tree is used to again predict the treatment-effect value for each patient, and patients with a high estimated value are grouped. The variable values that result in an increased effect can be found by analyzing the tree and finding the paths that lead to terminal nodes with high predicted-effect values [31]. With the classification method, the estimated treatment-effect value is dichotomized by splitting the outcomes using a threshold value. This binary estimated treatment-effect value is used to generate the classification tree that is used to classify the patients into either the 'low effect' or 'high effect' groups. This means that every variable used by the tree to classify a patient in the 'high effect' group can also be used to define a digital twin [31].

The random forest and regression tree approaches, as well as the classical model, have been tested on data from a clinical trial in 1019 patients, 517 of whom received the experimental treatment, while the others received a placebo. The patient's condition was possibly fatal, so the positive outcome was defined as survival 28 days after receiving the treatment or placebo. Both the regression and classification methods resulted in the identification of variables that could be used to define the subgroup of patients to whom the experimental treatment was especially beneficial. The models identified four variables that affected the estimated treatment effect the most, three of which were related to the severity of the patient's condition [31]. In this case, the differences in treatment effectiveness between patients in the subgroup and the average patient were not convincing enough to definitively prove that patients in the subgroup have a significantly better outcome. However, it shows that these digital twin-centric methods are an improvement on the classic logistic regression method when it comes to identifying and defining a subgroup of patients during clinical trials. The methods are more suited to bigger datasets, easier to interpret, and better at defining subgroup boundaries. Developments like these are essential for the application of digital twins in healthcare research.

2.7. Drug Repurposing for SARS-CoV-2

When the SARS-CoV-2 (or COVID-19) pandemic began, a lot of research was carried out to find agents that could either prevent or cure a COVID infection in a relatively short time. One quick way of obtaining suitable drugs on the market was to find drugs that had already been approved for use in another healthcare application and repurpose them for COVID treatment. One study started by searching for drugs that were approved for diseases with a similar molecular effect as COVID-19 [34]. To find these drugs, 332 host protein targets of the coronavirus were mapped to the human interactome. Of these targets, 208 turned out to be connected within the interactome network.

Three methods were used to identify potentially repurposable drugs for COVID-19 treatment (Figure 8). Firstly, an AI-based algorithm was used to map drug–protein targets and disease–protein targets. Secondly, a diffusion algorithm ranked the available drugs based on their ability to affect the pathways that contained the SARS-CoV-2 protein targets in the network. Lastly, a proximity algorithm was applied to calculate the distance between the host protein targets of SARS-CoV-2 and the closest proteins that were targeted by the drugs.

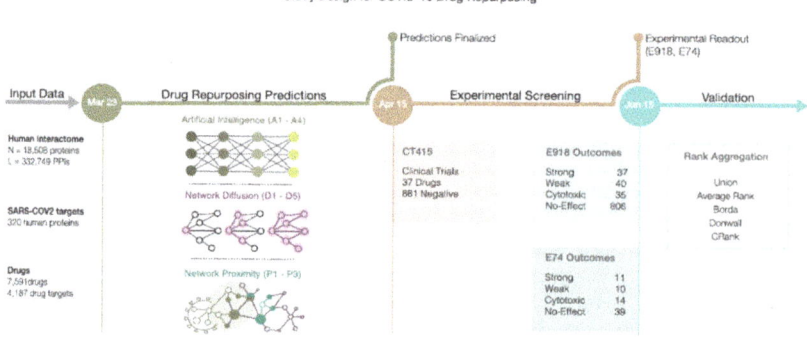

Figure 8. Schematic of the workflow for identifying drugs that could be repurposed for COVID-19 treatment. An AI-based method, network diffusion, and network proximity were used to identify possibly repurposable drugs, which were then validated through comparison with various clinical trials. Various rank aggregation algorithms were used to rank the drugs, based on their results in the different pipelines. Figure taken from [34].

The predictions made using the three methods were compared to compounds that had been experimentally screened for their efficacy in SARS-CoV-2 in monkey kidney cells. Of the 918 tested drugs, 77 had a positive effect, 806 showed no effect, and 35 turned out to be toxic to the cells. The drugs were subsequently compared to another dataset containing outcomes of clinical trials, as well [34]. Lastly, the drugs were given a rank based on their scores in the different pipelines described above. Multiple rank aggregation algorithms were tested for this purpose. CRank, capable of extracting the predictive power of the individual methods, consistently showed a strong predictive performance among datasets [34]. Of the 200 drugs ranked by this algorithm, 13 had positive outcomes in the monkey cells. Two drugs were already tested repeatedly, and of the remaining eleven, six showed potential for treating SARS-CoV-2 infection when tested on human cells. Of these drugs, three were highly ranked by CRank and had strong outcomes in the experimental tests, but were not yet used in clinical trials [34].

Studies like these show how digital twins containing protein–protein interaction networks may be used to estimate the effect of new treatments. In this case, a general interactome network was used to find drugs that may be potent in the treatment of COVID-19 infection in a population. However, these methods may also prove useful for a personal digital twin-based approach to evaluate treatment options for specific individuals.

3. Discussion

Recent developments in digital twin research in healthcare show great promise in understanding complex physiological processes, and may be applicable in several medical fields. To fully grasp the possibilities and pitfalls of these digital twins, we provide an in-depth look into the methodology and data types used in constructing digital twins. Though unified by their common goal, digital twins from different fields vary considerably in methods and data used. The main findings are summarized in Table 1.

Table 1. Summarizing overview of the various methodologies and data types used to construct digital twins across several healthcare fields.

Case Study	Aim of Digital Twin	Input Data	Methodology
Artificial Pancreas	Enhance blood glucose level monitoring and insulin delivery for individuals with diabetes, ensuring accurate predictions, noise reduction, and timely alerts without the need for frequent calibration.	Blood glucose data collected non-invasively via continuous monitoring. Calibration data for accurate glucose level predictions. Data related to glucose–insulin networks, external factors (e.g., physical activity), and additional hormones.	Signal processing algorithms for denoising and data enhancement. Bayesian inference for denoising. Least squares linear regression for data enhancement. Autoregressive modeling for future glucose concentration prediction.
Cardiac Digital Twin	Create detailed replicas of the heart (anatomical twinning) and simulate cardiac electrophysiology (functional twinning) for personalized testing and treatment strategies.	Three-dimensional heart scans from MRI. Clinical ECG measurements.	Universal Ventricular Coordinates for anatomical twinning. Mathematical models for cardiac electrophysiology. Fast-forward ECG modeling. Near real-time simulation of cardiac electrophysiology.
Single-cell Flux analysis	Integrate single-cell RNA sequencing data and metabolite fluxes to understand single-cell metabolic phenotypes, particularly in cancer research, aiding in phenotype discrimination.	Template metabolic networks. scRNA-seq datasets. Extracellular flux measurements.	scFBA model for metabolic analysis. Logical operators to calculate reaction activity scores. Constraints for metabolite exchanges.

Table 1. Cont.

Case Study	Aim of Digital Twin	Input Data	Methodology
Protein and DNA interactions	Construct protein–protein interaction networks for studying protein interactions and regulatory networks for protein–DNA interactions, enabling a deeper understanding of various biological processes and disease mechanisms.	Protein interaction data from techniques like IP-HTMS. Protein–DNA interaction data from ChIP-sequencing.	Bioinformatic analysis to identify and prioritize interactions. Integration with other genomic information for comprehensive analysis.
Clinical reports in oncology	Utilize natural language processing (NLP) to extract valuable information from clinical reports, particularly in cancer diagnosis, enabling better analysis and prediction of metastases presence over time.	Structured clinical reports from CT scans. Concatenated reports for multi-report analysis.	NLP for text processing. Machine learning models, including CNN and LSTM, for prediction. Multi-report analysis to improve accuracy.
Drug effectiveness	Identify subgroups of patients who may benefit from specific treatments during clinical trials, providing a more personalized and efficient approach to treatment evaluation.	Patient data and treatment outcomes. Variables describing patient characteristics.	Random forests, regression trees, and classification trees. Identification of variables affecting treatment effectiveness. Subgroup definition based on variables.
Drug repurposing for SARS-Cov-2	Identify existing drugs that can be repurposed for COVID-19 treatment by analyzing their interactions with the virus's protein targets and predicting their efficacy, thereby accelerating drug discovery for the pandemic.	A total of 332 host protein targets mapped to the human interactome. Experimental and clinical trial outcomes.	AI-based algorithms for drug mapping. Diffusion algorithms for pathway analysis. Proximity algorithms for target prediction. Rank aggregation for drug prioritization.

There exist several opportunities and challenges in the methodology and data types underlying digital twins. In diabetes management, the artificial pancreas is a prime example of a digital twin-like system that can greatly improve the ability to monitor and predict blood glucose levels and administer insulin based on non-invasive glucose monitoring methods. The data and methodology employed in the 'smart sensor' represent a multifaceted and data-driven approach, namely continuous glucose monitoring, signal processing algorithms, Bayesian interference, least squares linear regression, and autoregressive models. While this 'smart sensor' system can already offer great benefits to diabetes patients, there is still much room for improvement. The denoising and data enhancement methods could be combined and performed at the same time to reduce the complexity of the pipeline. Furthermore, the prediction module could be expanded to account for information such as meals, sleep, or physical activity. Even with these challenges that still need to be addressed, the reliability and effectiveness of these systems are demonstrated by the fact that the FDA has already approved them for personal use in their current state.

In cardiovascular research, a field that has seen many new ideas and improvements in digital twin systems recently, multiple types of data, including MRI and CT scans and electrophysiology measurements, can be integrated to compile a digital heart model through which ECG patterns can be simulated and predicted in any location and in real-time. This ability allows for the testing of patient-specific monitoring and treatment strategies and has the potential to significantly improve patient outcomes in cardiovascular diseases. The approach here consists of two distinct stages: anatomical twinning and functional twinning. In the anatomical twinning stage, detailed 3D representations of the heart are generated based on patient-specific CT or MRI scans. The second stage focuses on the electrophysiology of the heart, where mathematical models are used to describe and simulate electrophysiological activity of the heart. One important limitation of this method is that it requires accurate, multi-label segmentation to create anatomical CDTs. This is the largest computational time sink in the whole pipeline. While some studies have shown neural networks trained for this purpose, a fully automated method for segmentation of the cardiac chambers is not available at this time. The same is true for the segmentation of the torso. Models capable of fully automatically threshold-based segmentation that account for patient-specific anatomy will have to be achieved in the future. Additionally, the representation of the His–Purkinje System in the CDT may be too simplistic, as its workings are not yet fully understood. However, it was noted that once an activation profile has been identified, an automated workflow for integrating a topological representation of the HPS can be readily implemented [20].

Ultimately, a fully comprehensive healthcare digital twin would also require the integration of different types of omics data. The scFBA model can be used to incorporate single-cell RNA sequencing data and extracellular metabolite fluxes into digital twins that can provide insights into the metabolic phenotypes of cancer cells and allow for the analysis of the effect of genetic alterations. In the scFBA model, three main types of input are required: a template metabolic network, a single-cell RNA sequencing dataset, and approximated extracellular fluxes from the patient's cell population. Using these data, gene-to-metabolic reaction links are calculated and used to simulate the effect of single gene deletions. This approach offers a powerful tool to study cancer phenotypes and identify potential novel targets for therapeutic intervention.

Furthermore, the developments in machine learning and AI-based statistical methods allow for the prediction of drug effectiveness in patients (regression and random forests), identification of already approved drugs that may be repurposed for another cause (drug- and disease-protein mappings and rank aggregations), and the ability to extract data from clinical reports (natural language processing and neural networks), for example.

However, several challenges need to be addressed. Firstly, while the metabolic network maps are very comprehensive, protein–protein and regulatory networks are still considered incomplete. Gathering and integrating large amounts of data from diverse sources remains a significant hurdle and the continuous development of non-invasive and high-throughput data collection methods will be crucial to improve the accuracy and effectiveness of digital twin-based approaches. This is especially important for strategies that rely on digital twin systems to monitor health in real-time, to be able to predict a drop in blood glucose levels or to generate alerts based on simulated EEG patterns, for example. Additionally, a wide range of variables and parameters in digital twin models is necessary to accurately mimic complex physiological systems. Integration of these variables requires ongoing advancements in computational power and modeling techniques. Lastly, it is paramount to the practical application of digital twin systems that the privacy of the patient can be guaranteed, while large amounts of data are collected and ideally shared, to enable researchers to collaborate all over the world.

A lot of research is already being carried out to overcome these obstacles, and access to an ever-increasing amount of computational power allows for the use of more and more data, as well as complex models and algorithms. An increasing number of publicly available template models describing protein interactions, single-cell metabolomics, and thoracic cell coordinates, for example, will also be paramount in creating patient-specific digital twin systems in a short time. Additionally, modern systems and standards for data management will enable secure and efficient ways to store personal data and share them with others all over the world.

In conclusion, the development of digital twins in healthcare has the potential to revolutionize medical care and personalized treatments. The examples discussed in this review demonstrate the effectiveness of digital twin technology in artificial pancreas systems, cardiac digital twins, and single-cell digital twins for cancer research. By integrating diverse data sources and advanced modeling techniques, digital twins offer a powerful tool to simulate and understand complex physiological processes. Continued research and development in this field will pave the way for improved patient care and precision medicine.

4. Conclusions

Recent developments in digital twin research in healthcare hold great promise for understanding complex physiological processes and their potential applications in various medical fields. The examples discussed include digital twins in diabetes management, such as the artificial pancreas, which improves blood glucose monitoring and insulin administration. Challenges exist in denoising data and expanding prediction modules. In cardiovascular research, digital heart models enable real-time prediction of ECG patterns, allowing for patient-specific monitoring and treatment strategies, yet segmentation and representation challenges persist. Integrating omics data and AI-based methods in comprehensive healthcare digital twins provides insights into cancer phenotypes and drug effectiveness prediction. Addressing challenges in data integration, computational power, and privacy, is crucial for advancing digital twin-based approaches. Overall, digital twins have the potential to revolutionize medical care and precision medicine, offering personalized solutions for patients.

Supplementary Materials: The following supporting information can be downloaded at: https://www.mdpi.com/article/10.3390/jpm13101522/s1. Spreadsheet S1: Annotated overview of Digital Twin literature. An annotated overview of some of the literature covering digital twins is given in the form of a (searchable) Excel spreadsheet. Besides the complete citation, a brief summary, definition of a digital twin, and statement of value is given where needed.

Author Contributions: Conceptualization, C.M., H.-W.U. and S.e.B.; investigation, C.M. and S.e.B.; writing—original draft preparation, C.M. and S.e.B.; writing—review and editing, C.M., H.-W.U. and S.e.B.; visualization, C.M.; supervision, S.e.B and H.-W.U. All authors have read and agreed to the published version of the manuscript.

Funding: This research received no external funding.

Institutional Review Board Statement: Not applicable.

Informed Consent Statement: Not applicable.

Data Availability Statement: Not applicable.

Conflicts of Interest: The authors declare no conflict of interest.

References

1. Singh, M.; Fuenmayor, E.; Hinchy, E.; Qiao, Y.; Murray, N.; Devine, D. Digital Twin: Origin to Future. *Appl. Syst. Innov.* **2021**, *4*, 36. [CrossRef]
2. Yin, Y.; Zeng, Y.; Chen, X.; Fan, Y. The internet of things in healthcare: An overview. *J. Ind. Inf. Integr.* **2016**, *1*, 3–13. [CrossRef]
3. Taylor, K.; Alvarez, L.R. An Estimate of the Number of Animals Used for Scientific Purposes Worldwide in 2015. *Altern. Lab. Anim.* **2019**, *47*, 196–213. [CrossRef] [PubMed]
4. Subramanian, K. Digital Twin for Drug Discovery and Development—The Virtual Liver. *J. Indian Inst. Sci.* **2020**, *100*, 653–662. [CrossRef]
5. Barricelli, B.R.; Casiraghi, E.; Fogli, D. A Survey on Digital Twin: Definitions, Characteristics, Applications, and Design Implications. *IEEE Access* **2019**, *7*, 167653–167671. [CrossRef]
6. Björnsson, B.; Borrebaeck, C.; Elander, N.; Gasslander, T.; Gawel, D.R.; Gustafsson, M.; Jörnsten, R.; Lee, E.J.; Li, X.; Lilja, S.; et al. Digital twins to personalize medicine. *Genome Med.* **2019**, *12*, 4. [CrossRef] [PubMed]
7. Grieves, M.; Vickers, J. Digital Twin: Mitigating Unpredictable, Undesirable Emergent Behavior in Complex Systems. In *Transdisciplinary Perspectives on Complex Systems: New Findings and Approaches*; Kahlen, F.-J., Flumerfelt, S., Alves, A., Eds.; Springer International Publishing: Cham, Switzerland, 2017; pp. 85–113.
8. Chen, Y.; Yang, O.; Sampat, C.; Bhalode, P.; Ramachandran, R.; Ierapetritou, M. Digital Twins in Pharmaceutical and Biopharmaceutical Manufacturing: A Literature Review. *Processes* **2020**, *8*, 1088. [CrossRef]
9. Glaessgen, E.H.; Stargel, D.S. The Digital Twin Paradigm for Future NASA and US Air Force Vehicles. In Proceedings of the 53rd AIAA/ASME/ASCE/AHS/ASC Structures, Structural Dynamics and Materials Conference, Honolulu, HI, USA, 16 April 2012.
10. Venkatesh, K.P.; Raza, M.M.; Kvedar, J.C. Health digital twins as tools for precision medicine: Considerations for computation, implementation, and regulation. *Npj Digit. Med.* **2022**, *5*, 150. [CrossRef]

11. Kamel Boulos, M.N.; Zhang, P. Digital Twins: From Personalised Medicine to Precision Public Health. *J. Pers. Med.* **2021**, *11*, 745. [CrossRef]
12. Giansanti, D. Precision Medicine 2.0: How Digital Health and AI Are Changing the Game. *J. Pers. Med.* **2023**, *13*, 1057. [CrossRef]
13. Majumder, S.; Deen, M.J. Smartphone Sensors for Health Monitoring and Diagnosis. *Sensors* **2019**, *19*, 2164. [CrossRef]
14. Cozzolino, F.; Iacobucci, I.; Monaco, V.; Monti, M. Protein–DNA/RNA Interactions: An Overview of Investigation Methods in the -Omics Era. *J. Proteome Res.* **2021**, *20*, 3018–3030. [CrossRef] [PubMed]
15. Abdollahi, J.; Nouri-Moghaddam, B.; Ghazanfari, M. Deep Neural Network Based Ensemble learning Algorithms for the healthcare system (diagnosis of chronic diseases). *arXiv* **2021**, arXiv:2103.08182.
16. Kovatchev, B. A Century of Diabetes Technology: Signals, Models, and Artificial Pancreas Control. *Trends Endocrinol. Metab.* **2019**, *30*, 432–444. [CrossRef] [PubMed]
17. Facchinetti, A.; Sparacino, G.; Cobelli, C. Signal Processing Algorithms Implementing the "Smart Sensor" Concept to Improve Continuous Glucose Monitoring in Diabetes. *J. Diabetes Sci. Technol.* **2013**, *7*, 1308–1318. [CrossRef] [PubMed]
18. Bergman, R.N.; Ider, Y.Z.; Bowden, C.R.; Cobelli, C. Quantitative estimation of insulin sensitivity. *Am. J. Physiol.-Endocrinol. Metab.* **1979**, *236*, E667. [CrossRef]
19. Dalla Man, C.; Rizza, R.A.; Cobelli, C. Meal Simulation Model of the Glucose-Insulin System. *IEEE Trans. Biomed. Eng.* **2007**, *54*, 1740–1749. [CrossRef]
20. Gillette, K.; Gsell, M.A.; Prassl, A.J.; Karabelas, E.; Reiter, U.; Reiter, G.; Grandits, T.; Payer, C.; Štern, D.; Urschler, M.; et al. A Framework for the generation of digital twins of cardiac electrophysiology from clinical 12-leads ECGs. *Med. Image Anal.* **2021**, *71*, 102080. [CrossRef]
21. Bayer, J.; Prassl, A.J.; Pashaei, A.; Gomez, J.F.; Frontera, A.; Neic, A.; Plank, G.; Vigmond, E.J. Universal ventricular coordinates: A generic framework for describing position within the heart and transferring data. *Med. Image Anal.* **2018**, *45*, 83–93. [CrossRef]
22. Filippo, M.D.; Damiani, C.; Vanoni, M.; Maspero, D.; Mauri, G.; Alberghina, L.; Pescini, D. Single-cell Digital Twins for Cancer Preclinical Investigation. In *Metabolic Flux Analysis in Eukaryotic Cells*; Nagrath, D., Ed.; Springer: New York, NY, USA, 2020; Volume 2088, pp. 331–343.
23. Brunk, E.; Sahoo, S.; Zielinski, D.C.; Altunkaya, A.; Dräger, A.; Mih, N.; Gatto, F.; Nilsson, A.; Preciat Gonzalez, G.A.; Aurich, M.K.; et al. Recon3D enables a three-dimensional view of gene variation in human metabolism. *Nat. Biotechnol.* **2018**, *36*, 272–281. [CrossRef]
24. Chien, C.T.; Bartel, P.L.; Sternglanz, R.; Fields, S. The two-hybrid system: A method to identify and clone genes for proteins that interact with a protein of interest. *Proc. Natl. Acad. Sci. USA* **1991**, *88*, 9578–9582. [CrossRef] [PubMed]
25. Barrios-Rodiles, M.; Brown, K.R.; Ozdamar, B.; Bose, R.; Liu, Z.; Donovan, R.S.; Shinjo, F.; Liu, Y.; Dembowy, J.; Taylor, I.W.; et al. High-Throughput Mapping of a Dynamic Signaling Network in Mammalian Cells. *Science* **2005**, *307*, 1621–1625. [CrossRef]
26. Ewing, R.M.; Chu, P.; Elisma, F.; Li, H.; Taylor, P.; Climie, S.; McBroom-Cerajewski, L.; Robinson, M.D.; O'Connor, L.; Li, M.; et al. Large-scale mapping of human protein–protein interactions by mass spectrometry. *Mol. Syst. Biol.* **2007**, *3*, 89. [CrossRef]
27. Barabási, A.-L.; Gulbahce, N.; Loscalzo, J. Network medicine: A network-based approach to human disease. *Nat. Rev. Genet.* **2011**, *12*, 56–68. [CrossRef] [PubMed]
28. Newburger, D.E.; Bulyk, M.L. UniPROBE: An online database of protein binding microarray data on protein-DNA interactions. *Nucleic Acids Res.* **2009**, *37*, D77–D82. [CrossRef] [PubMed]
29. Castro-Mondragon, J.A.; Riudavets-Puig, R.; Rauluseviciute, I.; Lemma, R.B.; Turchi, L.; Blanc-Mathieu, R.; Lucas, J.; Boddie, P.; Khan, A.; Pérez, N.M.; et al. JASPAR 2022: The 9th release of the open-access database of transcription factor binding profiles. *Nucleic Acids Res.* **2022**, *50*, D165–D173. [CrossRef]
30. Batch, K.E.; Yue, J.; Darcovich, A.; Lupton, K.; Liu, C.C.; Woodlock, D.P.; El Amine, M.A.K.; Causa-Andrieu, P.I.; Gazit, L.; Nguyen, G.H.; et al. Developing a Cancer Digital Twin: Supervised Metastases Detection From Consecutive Structured Radiology Reports. *Front. Artif. Intell.* **2022**, *5*, 826402. [CrossRef] [PubMed]
31. Foster, J.C.; Taylor, J.M.G.; Ruberg, S.J. Subgroup identification from randomized clinical trial data. *Stat. Med.* **2011**, *30*, 2867–2880. [CrossRef] [PubMed]
32. Brookes, S.T.; Whitley, E.; Peters, T.J.; Mulheran, P.A.; Egger, M.; Davey Smith, G. Subgroup analyses in randomised controlled trials: Quantifying the risks of false-positives and false-negatives. *Health Technol. Assess.* **2001**, *5*, 1–56. [CrossRef]
33. Kehl, V.; Ulm, K. Responder identification in clinical trials with censored data. *Comput. Stat. Data Anal.* **2006**, *50*, 1338–1355. [CrossRef]
34. Gysi, D.M.; Do Valle, Í.; Zitnik, M.; Ameli, A.; Gan, X.; Varol, O.; Ghiassian, S.D.; Patten, J.J.; Davey, R.A.; Loscalzo, J.; et al. Network medicine framework for identifying drug-repurposing opportunities for COVID-19. *Proc. Natl. Acad. Sci. USA* **2021**, *118*, e2025581118. [CrossRef] [PubMed]

Disclaimer/Publisher's Note: The statements, opinions and data contained in all publications are solely those of the individual author(s) and contributor(s) and not of MDPI and/or the editor(s). MDPI and/or the editor(s) disclaim responsibility for any injury to people or property resulting from any ideas, methods, instructions or products referred to in the content.

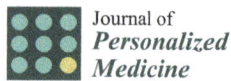

Article

The Influence of Slice Thickness, Sharpness, and Contrast Adjustments on Inferior Alveolar Canal Segmentation on Cone-Beam Computed Tomography Scans: A Retrospective Study

Julien Issa [1,2,*], Abanoub Riad [3,4], Raphael Olszewski [5,6,†] and Marta Dyszkiewicz-Konwińska [1,†]

1. Department of Diagnostics, Poznań University of Medical Sciences, Bukowska 70, 60-812 Poznan, Poland
2. Doctoral School, Poznań University of Medical Sciences, Bukowska 70, 60-812 Poznan, Poland
3. Department of Public Health, Faculty of Medicine, Masaryk University, 625 00 Brno, Czech Republic
4. Department of Oral and Maxillofacial Surgery, Justus-Liebig-University, 35392 Giessen, Germany
5. Department of Oral and Maxilofacial Surgery, Cliniques Universitaires Saint Luc, UCLouvain, Av. Hippocrate 10, 1200 Brussels, Belgium
6. Oral and Maxillofacial Surgery Research Lab (OMFS Lab), NMSK, Institut de Recherche Experimentale et Clinique, UCLouvain, Louvain-la-Neuve, 1348 Brussels, Belgium
* Correspondence: julien.issa@student.ump.edu.pl
† These authors contributed equally to this work.

Abstract: This retrospective study aims to investigate the impact of cone-beam computed tomography (CBCT) viewing parameters such as contrast, slice thickness, and sharpness on the identification of the inferior alveolar nerve (IAC). A total of 25 CBCT scans, resulting in 50 IACs, were assessed by two investigators using a three-score system (good, average, and poor) on cross-sectional images. Slice thicknesses of 0.25 mm, 0.5 mm, and 1 mm were tested, along with varying sharpness (0, 6, 8, and 10) and contrast (0, 400, 800, and 1200) settings. The results were statistically analyzed to determine the optimal slice thickness for improved visibility of IAC, followed by evaluating the influence of sharpness and contrast using the optimal thickness. The identified parameters were then validated by performing semi-automated segmentation of the IACs and structure overlapping to evaluate the mean distance. Inter-rater and intra-rater reliability were assessed using Kappa statistics, and inferential statistics used Pearson's Chi-square test. Inter-rater and intra-rater reliability for all parameters were significant, ranging from 69% to 83%. A slice thickness of 0.25 mm showed consistently "good" visibility (80%). Sharpness values of zero and contrast values of 1200 also demonstrated high frequencies of "good" visibility. Overlap analysis resulted in an average mean distance of 0.295 mm and a standard deviation of 0.307 mm across all patients' sides. The study revealed that a slice thickness of 0.25 mm, zero sharpness value, and higher contrast value of 1200 improved the visibility and accuracy of IAC segmentation in CBCT scans. The individual patient's characteristics, such as anatomical variations, decreased bone density, and absence of canal walls cortication, should be considered when using these parameters.

Keywords: diagnostic imaging; X-rays; cone-beam computed tomography; mandibular canal; tomography

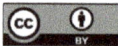

1. Introduction

The inferior alveolar canal (IAC) is an anatomical structure that carries the inferior alveolar nerve and blood vessels [1]. It originates at the mandibular foramen, passes through the mandibular body, and exits at the mental foramen [1,2]. In most cases, on conventional radiographs, IAC appears as a distinct radiolucent area bordered by superior and inferior radiopaque margins [3]. To mitigate the risk of potential nerve damage, it is essential to precisely identify the location of the IAC, particularly during procedures such as dental implant placement and extraction of impacted mandibular third molars [4,5]. This becomes even more crucial in cases of ridge atrophy [6]. The segmentation/tracing of the IAC can be more challenging in certain medical conditions, such as osteoporosis [7,8]. Lower bone density may significantly impede the visibility of the canal, especially in the mental foramen area. The precise location of the mental foramen can be an anatomical challenge due to its loop, which also requires clear identification on cross sections [9]. In this specific anatomical region, the nerve exhibits a propensity to approach the midline in closer proximity than the mental foramen itself. Moreover, the lack of cortication of the canal walls may make it difficult to mark its course and detect any changes in its path, as well as its furcation and additional branches [9–11].

Knowledge of the tools in tomography viewing software that can facilitate the process of determining the inferior alveolar canal is essential. Currently, the guidelines only include information on what cross sections the IAC could be assessed on [9]. Still, there are no additional recommendations on which parameters may facilitate the assessment of IAC on CBCT images. The segmentation/tracing of the IAC refers to the process of digitally outlining and delineating the boundaries of the IAC on digital radiographic images.

Cone-beam computed tomography (CBCT) provides high-resolution three-dimensional (3D) digital radiographic scans, making it an important tool for diagnosis and treatment planning [12]. CBCT imaging is based on a cone-shaped X-ray beam rotating around the patient's head, capturing multiple two-dimensional (2D) images [13]. These images are then reconstructed into 3D scans [13]. CBCT has shown satisfactory visibility of the IAC on cross-sectional images, surpassing the capabilities of conventional 2D radiographs [14–16].

CBCT images can be digitally modified to improve the visibility of anatomical structures. Modifications of the display settings can include slice thickness, sharpness, and contrast adjustments, among other parameters. Slice thickness refers to the thickness of each reconstructed image slice in the CBCT scan, with smaller thickness allowing for more detailed visualization but larger thickness yielding smoother scans [17,18]. Sharpness refers to the clarity and definition of the scanned structures on a CBCT scan [17]. It is influenced by factors such as detector resolution and reconstruction algorithms [17]. The contrast parameter in CBCT is used to quantify the variation in radiodensity or radiopacity among distinct anatomical features on a CBCT scan [17]. The scan contrast can be adjusted using windowing techniques [17]. Windowing defines the range of the pixel values that are visible on display, where a wider window reduces contrast, and a narrower window increases contrast [17,19].

While the expertise of the dentist is a crucial factor in IAC segmentation, optimizing CBCT settings can significantly enhance the consistency of the process. The knowledge of dentists regarding the fundamentals of dental tomography and the utilization of CBCT remains somewhat uncertain despite its widespread adoption in dentistry [20]. Hence, this retrospective study aims to bridge this gap by assessing the influence of CBCT basic view parameters, specifically contrast, slice thickness, and sharpness, on the segmentation/tracing of the IAC. This study also involves observers with varying levels of radiology training, typically representing the varying knowledge levels of a dentist using CBCT in their practice. To the best of our knowledge, this is the first retrospective study that employs this methodology. The findings from this study can provide practical insights for dentists using CBCT, in order to optimize their workflow and software settings for more accurate IAC segmentation during their clinical practice.

2. Materials and Methods

2.1. Data Acquisition

To conduct the study, CBCT scans of 25 patients (12 male and 13 female) aged 18 to 62 years were retrieved from the Poznan University of Medical Sciences database. All scans were performed between 2020 and 2021 and met the inclusion criteria outlined in Table 1.

Table 1. Inclusion criteria.

Inclusion Criteria	Exclusion Criteria
Patients aged 18 years old and above	Patients under 18 years old
Sufficient field of view (FOV) for visualizing the entire lower jaws	Insufficient FOV for visualizing the entire lower jaws
Dentulous or partially edentulous in the molar–premolar region	Edentulous in the molar–premolar region
CBCT scans without artifacts	CBCT scans with artifacts
Patients with periapical lesion not affecting the visibility of IAC	Patients with periapical lesion affecting the visibility of IAC

The scans were acquired using a Cranex 3D CBCT device (Soredex, USA) with an X-ray tube voltage of 90 kV, an X-ray tube current of 10 mA, and a voxel size of 0.25 mm. The field of view (FOV) ranged from 600 × 800 mm to 1600 × 1300 mm. The 25 scans were anonymized and stored in the Digital Imaging and Communications in Medicine (DICOM) file format. Since the IAC is present bilaterally, a total of 50 IACs were evaluated.

2.2. Evaluation

Romexis 6.2 software (Planmeca oy, Helsinki, Finland) was used to process the scans and generate 33 cross-sectional images (Figure 1) from each scan for further evaluation. This software was used as it facilitates the export of the segmented structure as a Standard Triangle Language (STL) file. Two independent investigators (an oral and maxillofacial radiologist with over ten years of experience and a trainee in oral and maxillofacial radiology with three years of experience) evaluated the images on an NEC MultiSync EA245WMi-2 display screen (Sharp NEC DisplaySolutions, Tokyo, Japan) under optimal ambient lighting conditions. The evaluation was repeated twice, with a 10-day interval. The investigators rated the visibility of the IAC based on a 3-score classification (good, average, and poor), as shown in Table 2. The Brightness value in Romexis 6.2 software (Planmeca oy, Helsinki, Finland) was fixed to 1808 by default.

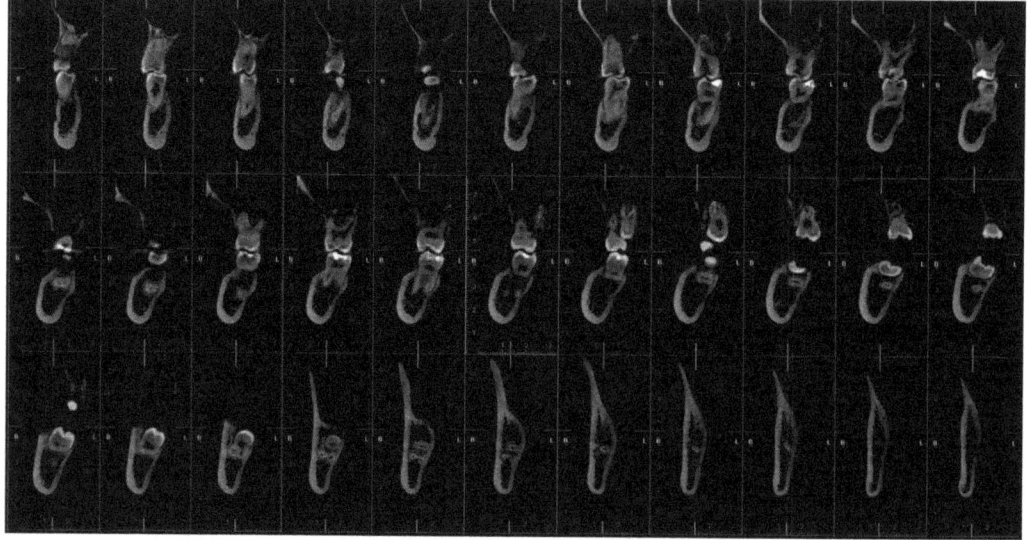

Figure 1. Snapshot of 33 cross-sectional images on Romexis 6.2 software (Planmeca oy, Helsinki, Finland): 0.25 mm thickness, sharpness, and contrast at zero.

Table 2. Three-score classification of IAC visibility.

Score	Description
Good	The cortical border of the IAC is well visible and distinguished from the surrounding structures in the 33 cross-sectional images
Average	The cortical border of the IAC is not visible and distinguished from the surrounding structures in less than 16 images (half of the images) of the 33 cross-sectional images
Poor	The cortical border of the IAC is not visible and distinguished from the surrounding structures in more than 16 images of 33 cross-sectional images

Slice thicknesses of 0.25 mm, 0.5 mm, and 1 mm were evaluated, with sharpness and contrast settings set to zero. The software's default configuration has sharpness and contrast set at zero, allowing us to test four different combinations. Subsequently, a rigorous statistical analysis was executed to pinpoint the optimal slice thickness value for achieving enhanced visibility of the IAC. Following this, the investigators examined the influence of varying sharpness values (6, 8, and 10) on IAC visibility using the slice thickness value that yielded the best results. Lastly, the impact of diverse contrast values (400, 800, and 1200) was assessed using the previously identified optimal combination of slice thickness and sharpness settings.

2.3. Evaluation of 3D Models

After obtaining the results, the recommended image display parameters value of slice thickness, sharpness, and contrast were applied on Romexis 6.2 (Planmeca oy, Helsinki, Finland). Using the IAC tracing option in Romexis 6.2 (Planmeca oy, Helsinki, Finland), the investigators independently conducted a semi-automated segmentation of the 50 IACs. This segmentation process was executed on a cross-sectional view with a fixed cylindrical diameter of 1.5 mm. The resulting segmentation data were then saved as individual STL files and subsequently exported to Cloud Compare v.2.13.alpha (open-source software available at http://www.cloudcompare.org/ accessed on 7 April 2023) for further analysis.

Cloud Compare was employed to perform a 3D registration, enabling the overlap and visualization of the segmented IACs produced by both investigators from the same scan. The objective of this process was to evaluate the accuracy of the segmentation performed by investigators with varying levels of expertise while adhering to the recommended parameters value. This evaluation focused on assessing the level of conformity between the segmented structures by analyzing volumetric deviations, thereby evaluating the practicality and effectiveness of the recommended parameter values.

In the initial steps of this assessment, a pre-registration process was carried out using the 3-point method within Cloud Compare v.2.13.alpha (open-source software available at http://www.cloudcompare.org/ accessed on 7 April 2023. For each segmented IAC, three points were strategically placed on each of the two obtained 3D models (STL file) at corresponding locations, specifically the mandibular foramen, molar, and premolar area. This step ensured the proper alignment of the 3D models in the spatial domain.

Following this alignment process, the 'compute cloud/mesh distance' function in Cloud Compare v.2.13.alpha (open-source software, http://www.cloudcompare.org/ accessed on 7 April 2023 was implemented. This function overlapped the two 3D models and generated numerical results, which included parameters like the mean distance and maximum distance (Figure 2). The software default setting for the overlap parameter was set at 100, indicating that the surfaces were configured to have full overlap, equivalent to 100% overlap, in this analysis.

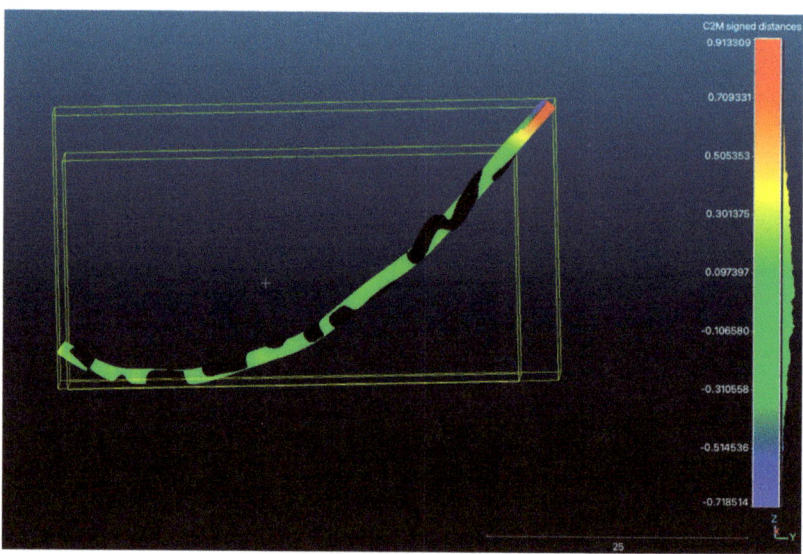

Figure 2. IAC overlapping and visualization of 3D comparison deviation chromatogram on Cloud Compare v.2.13.alpha (open-source software, http://www.cloudcompare.org/ accessed on 7 April 2023). The blue color represents the minus direction of deviation, the red color represents the plus direction of deviation, and the green color represents the average value.

2.4. Statistical Analysis

Statistical analysis was conducted using SPSS 29.0 (SPSS Inc., Chicago, IL, USA). Inter-rater and intra-rater reliability of the IAC visibility ratings were assessed using Kappa statistics, both between the two investigators and within each investigator, across the two evaluation sessions.

The inferential statistics were performed using Pearson's Chi-square test with a significance level of <0.05. To evaluate the degree of conformity between the structures represented by the volumetric deviations obtained from the segmentation of the IACs, the mean distance and standard deviation were computed, and the average was calculated.

3. Results

Table 3 presents the results of inter-rater and intra-rater reliability analysis of the operators for slice thickness, sharpness, and contrast. The findings indicate that the operators achieved a significant level of reliability for all three parameters. The inter-rater reliability percentages for slice thickness, sharpness, and contrast are 79%, 69%, and 76%, respectively. Meanwhile, the intra-rater reliability percentages for the same parameters are 83%, 83%, and 81%, respectively.

Table 3. The mean of inter-rater and intra-rater reliability for the evaluation of the evaluated parameters. SD, standard deviation.

	Inter-Rater Reliability		Intra-Rater Reliability	
	Mean	SD	Mean	SD
Slice thickness	0.790	0.126	0.829	0.084
Sharpness	0.687	0.103	0.834	0.105
Contrast	0.756	0.205	0.810	0.011

Table 4 indicates that the visibility of IAC was most consistently rated as "good" with a slice thickness of 0.25 mm, as 80% of the 50 IACs were rated as such. This is in comparison to 70% and 66% of IACs rated as "good" with slice thicknesses of 0.5 mm and 1 mm, respectively.

Table 4. The 0.25, 0.5, 1 mm slice thickness evaluation. Sharpness and contrast set at value 0.

Slice Thickness			Investigator 2			p-Value
			Good	Average	Poor	
0.25 mm		Good	40	1	0	
		Average	0	8	0	<0.001 *
		Poor	0	0	1	
0.5 mm	Investigator 1	Good	35	0	0	
		Average	2	12	0	<0.001 *
		Poor	0	0	1	
1 mm		Good	33	0	0	
		Average	3	13	0	<0.001 *
		Poor	0	0	1	

* Chi-square test, significance level (p-value) ≤ 0.05.

Similarly, Table 4 shows that the sharpness value of zero had the highest frequency of agreement among investigators in rating IAC visibility as "good" at 80%, followed closely by a sharpness value of 10 at 78% (Table 5). Sharpness values of 6 and 8 also had a high frequency of agreement at 76% (Table 5). In Table 6, the highest frequency of agreement among investigators for good visibility of IAC was found at a contrast value of 1200, with 82% of IACs rated as "good". A contrast value of 400 (Table 6) and 0 (Table 4) also had 80% of IACs rated as "good", while a contrast value of 800 (Table 6) had 76% of IACs rated as "good".

Table 5. The 6, 8, 10 sharpness value evaluation. Slice thickness set at 0.25 mm and contrast set at 0.

Sharpness			Investigator 2			p-Value
			Good	Average	Poor	
6		Good	38	2	1	
		Average	7	0	0	<0.001 *
		Poor	1	0	1	
8	Investigator 1	Good	38	2	1	
		Average	7	0	0	<0.001 *
		Poor	1	0	1	
10		Good	33	0	0	
		Average	3	13	0	<0.001 *
		Poor	0	0	1	

* Chi-square test, significance level (p-value) ≤ 0.05.

Table 7 presents the findings of the overlap analysis conducted by both investigators, focusing on the mean distance and standard deviation. The analysis was performed for each side (left and right) of the included patients. Across all patients' sides, the average mean distance and standard deviation values were determined to be 0.295 mm and 0.307 mm, respectively.

Table 6. The 400, 800, 1200 contrast value evaluation. Slice thickness set at 0.25 mm and sharpness set at value 0.

Contrast			Investigator 2			p-Value
			Good	Average	Poor	
400		Good	40	0	0	
		Average	1	7	0	<0.001 *
		Poor	0	1	1	
800	Investigator 1	Good	38	1	0	
		Average	2	6	0	<0.001 *
		Poor	0	0	3	
1200		Good	41	0	0	
		Average	0	7	0	<0.001 *
		Poor	0	0	2	

* Chi-square test, significance level (p-value) ≤ 0.05.

Table 7. Results of the overlapping analysis.

Patient	Side	Mean Distance	Standard Deviation
1	Right	0.342	0.310
	Left	0.267	0.291
2	Right	0.273	0.293
	Left	0.233	0.248
3	Right	0.268	0.267
	Left	0.223	0.243
4	Right	0.310	0.342
	Left	0.599	0.745
5	Right	0.323	0.336
	Left	0.812	0.851
6	Right	0.255	0.257
	Left	0.202	0.229
7	Right	0.225	0.240
	Left	0.174	0.209
8	Right	0.212	0.226
	Left	0.284	0.320
9	Right	0.389	0.363
	Left	0.384	0.353
10	Right	0.348	0.387
	Left	0.233	0.253
11	Right	0.198	0.235
	Left	0.235	0.245
12	Right	0.236	0.238
	Left	0.271	0.266
13	Right	0.463	0.441
	Left	0.251	0.270
14	Right	0.278	0.264
	Left	0.352	0.386
15	Right	0.313	0.305
	Left	0.266	0.251
16	Right	0.412	0.370
	Left	0.380	0.334
17	Right	0.329	0.299
	Left	0.314	0.346
18	Right	0.209	0.225
	Left	0.247	0.263
19	Right	0.291	0.251
	Left	0.284	0.253

Table 7. Cont.

Patient	Side	Mean Distance	Standard Deviation
20	Right	0.262	0.244
	Left	0.269	0.327
21	Right	0.301	0.296
	Left	0.295	0.333
22	Right	0.189	0.210
	Left	0.208	0.240
23	Right	0.174	0.201
	Left	0.224	0.241
24	Right	0.221	0.227
	Left	0.273	0.279
25	Right	0.420	0.550
	Left	0.242	0.246
Average		0.295	0.307

4. Discussion

The interpretation of dental radiography, especially concerning the segmentation of the IAC, is notably influenced by factors such as the acquisition parameters, image quality, and experience of the dentist. While the assessment of image quality is subjective and can vary among individuals, the primary goal is to ensure that the images provide sufficient information for clinical decision making. In this retrospective study, we aimed to investigate the impact of several CBCT view parameters, contrast, slice thickness, and sharpness on the accuracy of IAC segmentation.

Regarding slice thickness, our findings revealed that a slice thickness of 0.25 mm resulted in the highest frequency of IAC visibility rated as "good" by both investigators. This suggests that thinner slices enhance the visualization and differentiation of the cortical border of the IAC from surrounding structures, while a study by Pour et al. evaluated the effect of slice thickness (0.5 mm, 1 mm, 2 mm) on the visibility of IAC in CBCT images and concluded that slice thickness has no effect on the visibility of IAC [21]. In terms of sharpness, our study demonstrated that a sharpness value of zero exhibited the highest frequencies of agreement among investigators for rating IAC visibility as "good." This implies that a moderate level of sharpness contributes to better visualization of the IAC in CBCT scans. The evaluation of contrast values indicated that a contrast value of 1200 yielded the highest frequency of agreement among investigators for rating IAC visibility as "good." This implies that higher contrast values enhance the visibility of the IAC in CBCT scans.

A semi-automated segmentation of the IACs was performed to validate the identified parameters, followed by an overlap analysis. The mean distance to conformity is one of the metrics that can be used to quantitatively evaluate the overlapping comparison [22]. The results showed a mean distance of 0.295 ± 0.307, indicating a reasonable level of conformity between the volumetric deviations of the segmented structures. This validation confirms the reliability and accuracy of the identified parameters in enhancing IAC segmentation, irrespective of the evaluator's experience. Notably, the two investigators involved in the study had different levels of experience.

When applying these parameters, it is crucial to consider individual patient characteristics and specific clinical requirements. Factors such as patient age, sex, bone quality, and anatomical variations should be considered to ensure optimal image interpretation and clinical decision making. In a study by Miles et al. [23], the effect of age, gender, and location on the visibility of IAC was evaluated. The findings indicated that age had an impact on the visibility of the IAC, but this effect varied by location [23]. The first premolar region, specifically in the age range of 47–56, exhibited lower visibility compared to individuals aged over 65 [23]. Gender also played a significant role, with females generally having lower visibility than males, and the most pronounced difference was observed in the first premolar area [23].

Furthermore, other image settings such as field of view (FOV), bit depth, resolution, and the CBCT device brand should be considered. In a study by Kamburoğlu et al. [24], the Veraviewepocs 3D model X550 (J Morita Mfg. Corp., Kyoto, Japan) was found to provide the best image quality compared to the Iluma Ultra Cone-beam CT Scanner (3M Imtec, Ardmore, OK, USA), Kodak 9000 Extra-oral imaging system (Eastman Kodak Co, Rochester, NY, USA), and Vatech PanX-Duo3D_Pano/CBCT (Vatech, Seoul, Republic of Korea) [24]. Pour et al. [25] suggested that exporting mandibular CBCT images with a resolution of 0.32 mm and a 12-bit depth would yield good-to-moderate radiographic visibility of the IAC. Jasa et al. [26] conducted an in vitro study to assess the impact of exposure parameters and slice thickness on the visibility of clear and unclear IAC. The study revealed that detecting unclear IACs required higher exposure parameters or processing the images with thicker slices, whereas clear IACs could be adequately detected using lower exposure parameters [26].

In recent years, advancements in artificial intelligence (AI) have revolutionized the fields of oral and maxillofacial radiology. Numerous studies have explored the application of AI for IAC segmentation on both 2D and 3D radiographs, yielding promising results [27]. The integration of AI technology holds the potential to establish a globally standardized approach to dental reporting, providing support to dentists, streamlining their workflow, and ultimately leading to improved patient outcomes [27].

This pioneering retrospective study presents a unique approach, engaging observers of varying levels of radiology training in contrast to previous research. It demonstrates the potential utility of recommended parameters within image viewer software for achieving precise segmentation, regardless of the clinician or specialist's expertise. Furthermore, this study introduces an innovative method that involves 3D spatial overlap of the segmented IAC for validation of recommended parameter values. This method offers promising avenues for further research in the domain of oral and maxillofacial radiology, particularly in the context of IAC segmentation. This is especially significant, considering the limited existing literature in this field.

The presented study has a few limitations. The sample size was relatively small, which may limit the generalizability of the findings. Future studies would benefit from a more extensive and diverse patient population to further validate the identified parameters. Additionally, exploring the impact of using alternative CBCT devices or different image viewer software on the accuracy of IAC segmentation could provide valuable insights. Moreover, investigating the influence of other CBCT view parameters, such as field of view and exposure settings, could contribute to a more comprehensive understanding of their effects on IAC segmentation accuracy.

Future studies using different viewer software and exploring a range of parameters can contribute to the development of comprehensive guidelines for working with CBCT images. These guidelines can potentially assist practitioners in achieving precise evaluations, ultimately enhancing the diagnostic capabilities of CBCT in dentistry. It is worth noting that many dentists, despite utilizing CBCT in their practice, often lack comprehensive training and may not fully benefit from these advanced imaging techniques.

5. Conclusions

In conclusion, our study identified that thinner slice thickness (0.25 mm), zero sharpness value, and higher contrast value (1200) could enhance the visibility and accuracy of IAC segmentation in CBCT scans. However, individual patient characteristics of the bone pattern and specific clinical requirements should be considered when applying these parameters. The process of tracing IAC can be challenging and has no easily available gold standard.

Therefore, the findings from this study can serve as an initial step in establishing extended guidelines for IAC segmentation, improving the accuracy of this process on CBCT images. Further research with a larger sample size and using other software is recommended to validate and expand these findings.

Author Contributions: Conceptualization, J.I., R.O. and M.D.-K.; methodology, J.I. and M.D.-K.; formal analysis, J.I. and A.R.; investigation, J.I. and M.D.-K.; writing—original draft preparation, J.I. and A.R.; writing—review and editing, R.O. and M.D.-K. All authors have read and agreed to the published version of the manuscript.

Funding: Julien Issa is a participant in the STER Internationalization of Doctoral Schools Program from NAWA Polish National Agency for Academic Exchange No. PPI/STE/2020/1/00014/DEC/02. This work is supported by the Doctoral School of Poznan University of Medical Sciences through Young Scientists Grant No. SDUM-MGB 14/05/22.

Institutional Review Board Statement: The study was conducted in accordance with the Declaration of Helsinki. It was exempted from ethical approval due to its observational nature, and the data were anonymized.

Informed Consent Statement: Patient consent was waived due to the use of anonymized radiographs for the purposes of this retrospective study and the observational nature of the study.

Data Availability Statement: The data presented in this study are available on request from the corresponding author.

Conflicts of Interest: The authors declare no conflict of interest.

References

1. Derafshi, A.; Sarikhani, K.; Mirhosseini, F.; Baghestani, M.; Noorbala, R.; Kaboodsaz Yazdi, M. Evaluation of the Course of Inferior Alveolar Canal and its Relation to Anatomical Factors on Digital Panoramic Radiographs. *J. Dent.* **2021**, *22*, 213–218. [CrossRef]
2. Wolf, K.T.; Brokaw, E.J.; Bell, A.; Joy, A. Variant Inferior Alveolar Nerves and Implications for Local Anesthesia. *Anesth. Prog.* **2016**, *63*, 84–90. [CrossRef]
3. Juodzbalys, G.; Wang, H.L.; Sabalys, G. Anatomy of mandibular vital structures. Part I: Mandibular canal and inferior alveolar neurovascular bundle in relation with dental implantology. *J. Oral Maxillofac. Res.* **2010**, *1*, e2. [CrossRef] [PubMed]
4. Juodzbalys, G.; Wang, H.L.; Sabalys, G. Injury of the Inferior Alveolar Nerve during Implant Placement: A Literature Review. *J. Oral Maxillofac. Res.* **2011**, *2*, e1. [CrossRef] [PubMed]
5. Sarikov, R.; Juodzbalys, G. Inferior alveolar nerve injury after mandibular third molar extraction: A literature review. *J. Oral Maxillofac. Res.* **2014**, *5*, e1. [CrossRef]
6. Ulm, C.W.; Solar, P.; Blahout, R.; Matejka, M.; Watzek, G.; Gruber, H. Location of the mandibular canal within the atrophic mandible. *Br. J. Oral Maxillofac. Surg.* **1993**, *31*, 370–375. [CrossRef] [PubMed]
7. Chen, Y.; Liu, J.; Pei, J.; Liu, Y.; Pa, J. The Risk Factors that Can Increase Possibility of Mandibular Canal Wall Damage in Adult: A Cone-Beam Computed Tomography (CBCT) Study in a Chinese Population. *Med. Sci. Monit.* **2018**, *24*, 26–36. [CrossRef] [PubMed]
8. Jonasson, G.; Rythén, M. Alveolar bone loss in osteoporosis: A loaded and cellular affair? *Clin. Cosmet. Investig. Dent.* **2016**, *8*, 95–103. [CrossRef] [PubMed]
9. Fahd, A.; Temerek, A.T.; Kenawy, S.M. Validation of different protocols of inferior alveolar canal tracing using cone beam computed tomography (CBCT). *Dentomaxillofac. Radiol.* **2022**, *51*, 20220016. [CrossRef]
10. Weckx, A.; Agbaje, J.O.; Sun, Y.; Jacobs, R.; Politis, C. Visualization techniques of the inferior alveolar nerve (IAN): A narrative review. *Surg. Radiol. Anat.* **2016**, *38*, 55–63. [CrossRef] [PubMed]
11. Oliveira-Santos, C.; Souza, P.H.; de Azambuja Berti-Couto, S.; Stinkens, L.; Moyaert, K.; Rubira-Bullen, I.R.; Jacobs, R. Assessment of variations of the mandibular canal through cone beam computed tomography. *Clin. Oral Investig.* **2012**, *16*, 387–393. [CrossRef]
12. Shukla, S.; Chug, A.; Afrashtehfar, K.I. Role of Cone Beam Computed Tomography in Diagnosis and Treatment Planning in Dentistry: An Update. *J. Int. Soc. Prev. Community Dent.* **2017**, *7* (Suppl. 3), S125–S136. [CrossRef]
13. Venkatesh, E.; Elluru, S.V. Cone beam computed tomography: Basics and applications in dentistry. *J. Istanb. Univ. Fac. Dent.* **2017**, *51* (Suppl. 1), S102–S121. [CrossRef]
14. Saraydar-Baser, R.; Dehghani-Tafti, M.; Navab-Azam, A.; Ezoddini-Ardakani, F.; Nayer, S.; Safi, Y.; Shamloo, N. Comparison of the diagnostic value of CBCT and Digital Panoramic Radiography with surgical findings to determine the proximity of an impacted third mandibular molar to the inferior alveolar nerve canal. *J. Med. Life* **2015**, *8*, 83–89. [PubMed]
15. Jung, Y.H.; Cho, B.H. Radiographic evaluation of the course and visibility of the mandibular canal. *Imaging Sci. Dent.* **2014**, *44*, 273–278. [CrossRef]
16. Oliveira-Santos, C.; Capelozza, A.L.; Dezzoti, M.S.; Fischer, C.M.; Poleti, M.L.; Rubira-Bullen, I.R. Visibility of the mandibular canal on CBCT cross-sectional images. *J. Appl. Oral Sci.* **2011**, *19*, 240–243. [CrossRef] [PubMed]
17. Pauwels, R.; Araki, K.; Siewerdsen, J.H.; Thongvigitmanee, S.S. Technical aspects of dental CBCT: State of the art. *Dentomaxillofac. Radiol.* **2015**, *44*, 20140224. [CrossRef] [PubMed]
18. Chadwick, J.W.; Lam, E.W. The effects of slice thickness and interslice interval on reconstructed cone beam computed tomographic images. *Oral Surg. Oral Med. Oral Pathol. Oral Radiol. Endodontol.* **2010**, *110*, e37–e42. [CrossRef] [PubMed]

19. Coelho-Silva, F.; Martins, L.A.C.; Braga, D.A.; Zandonade, E.; Haiter-Neto, F.; de-Azevedo-Vaz, S.L. Influence of windowing and metal artefact reduction algorithms on the volumetric dimensions of five different high-density materials: A cone-beam CT study. *Dentomaxillofac. Radiol.* **2020**, *49*, 20200039. [CrossRef]
20. Brown, J.; Jacobs, R.; Levring Jäghagen, E.; Lindh, C.; Baksi, G.; Schulze, D.; Schulze, R. European Academy of DentoMaxilloFacial Radiology. Basic training requirements for the use of dental CBCT by dentists: A position paper prepared by the European Academy of DentoMaxilloFacial Radiology. *Dentomaxillofac. Radiol.* **2014**, *43*, 20130291. [CrossRef]
21. Pour, D.G.; Arzi, B.; Shamshiri, A.R. Assessment of slice thickness effect on visibility of inferior alveolar canal in cone beam computed tomography images. *Dent. Res. J.* **2016**, *13*, 527–531. [CrossRef] [PubMed]
22. Brock, K.K.; Mutic, S.; McNutt, T.R.; Li, H.; Kessler, M.L. Use of image registration and fusion algorithms and techniques in radiotherapy: Report of the AAPM Radiation Therapy Committee Task Group No. 132. *Med. Phys.* **2017**, *44*, e43–e76. [CrossRef] [PubMed]
23. Miles, M.S.; Parks, E.T.; Eckert, G.J.; Blanchard, S.B. Comparative evaluation of mandibular canal visibility on cross-sectional cone-beam CT images: A retrospective study. *Dentomaxillofac. Radiol.* **2016**, *45*, 20150296. [CrossRef] [PubMed]
24. Kamburoğlu, K.; Murat, S.; Kolsuz, E.; Kurt, H.; Yüksel, S.; Paksoy, C. Comparative assessment of subjective image quality of cross-sectional cone-beam computed tomography scans. *J. Oral Sci.* **2011**, *53*, 501–508. [CrossRef]
25. Pour, D.G.; Sedaghati, A.; Shamshiri, A.R. Effect of Resolution and Bit Depth on Inferior Alveolar Canal Visualization on Exported Mandibular Cone-Beam Computed Tomography Images. *J. Oral Maxillofac. Surg.* **2020**, *78*, 731–737. [CrossRef]
26. Jasa, G.R.; Shimizu, M.; Okamura, K.; Tokumori, K.; Takeshita, Y.; Weerawanich, W.; Yoshiura, K. Effects of exposure parameters and slice thickness on detecting clear and unclear mandibular canals using cone beam CT. *Dentomaxillofac. Radiol.* **2017**, *46*, 20160315. [CrossRef] [PubMed]
27. Issa, J.; Olszewski, R.; Dyszkiewicz-Konwińska, M. The Effectiveness of Semi-Automated and Fully Automatic Segmentation for Inferior Alveolar Canal Localization on CBCT Scans: A Systematic Review. *Int. J. Environ. Res. Public Health* **2022**, *19*, 560. [CrossRef]

Disclaimer/Publisher's Note: The statements, opinions and data contained in all publications are solely those of the individual author(s) and contributor(s) and not of MDPI and/or the editor(s). MDPI and/or the editor(s) disclaim responsibility for any injury to people or property resulting from any ideas, methods, instructions or products referred to in the content.

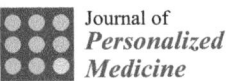

Article

Challenging ChatGPT 3.5 in Senology—An Assessment of Concordance with Breast Cancer Tumor Board Decision Making

Sebastian Griewing [1,2,3,*], Niklas Gremke [2], Uwe Wagner [2], Michael Lingenfelder [3], Sebastian Kuhn [1] and Jelena Boekhoff [2]

1. Institute for Digital Medicine, University Hospital Marburg, Philipps-University Marburg, Baldingerstraße, 35043 Marburg, Germany; sebastian.kuhn@uni-marburg.de
2. Department of Gynecology and Obstetrics, University Hospital Marburg, Philipps-University Marburg, Baldingerstraße, 35043 Marburg, Germany; gremken@staff.uni-marburg.de (N.G.); uwe.wagner@uk-gm.de (U.W.); jboekhof@med.uni-marburg.de (J.B.)
3. Institute for Healthcare Management, Chair of General Business Administration, Philipps-University Marburg, Universitätsstraße 24, 35037 Marburg, Germany; lingenfe@wiwi.uni-marburg.de
* Correspondence: griewin4@staff.uni-marburg.de; Tel.: +49-6421-58-67079

Abstract: With the recent diffusion of access to publicly available large language models (LLMs), common interest in generative artificial-intelligence-based applications for medical purposes has skyrocketed. The increased use of these models by tech-savvy patients for personal health issues calls for a scientific evaluation of whether LLMs provide a satisfactory level of accuracy for treatment decisions. This observational study compares the concordance of treatment recommendations from the popular LLM ChatGPT 3.5 with those of a multidisciplinary tumor board for breast cancer (MTB). The study design builds on previous findings by combining an extended input model with patient profiles reflecting patho- and immunomorphological diversity of primary breast cancer, including primary metastasis and precancerous tumor stages. Overall concordance between the LLM and MTB is reached for half of the patient profiles, including precancerous lesions. In the assessment of invasive breast cancer profiles, the concordance amounts to 58.8%. Nevertheless, as the LLM makes considerably fraudulent decisions at times, we do not identify the current development status of publicly available LLMs to be adequate as a support tool for tumor boards. Gynecological oncologists should familiarize themselves with the capabilities of LLMs in order to understand and utilize their potential while keeping in mind potential risks and limitations.

Keywords: artificial intelligence; large language models; gynecology; oncology; tumor board

1. Introduction

Medical research increasingly explores the application of artificial intelligence (AI) and novel machine learning methods that adaptively and automatically process heterogeneous health data to enable personalized medical treatment [1]. In light of modern health challenges, including the COVID-19 pandemic, deep and machine learning methods have been proven to facilitate medical decision making and provide benefits to patients and caregivers beyond the previously known non-medical areas of application of the technology [2–6]. Particularly for the diagnosis, treatment and follow-up of highly complex and chronic diseases, as is the case in oncology, there is growing interest in corresponding clinical applications of individualized precision medicine [7,8]. In view of the demographic development and rapid aging of the population in central Europe, a continuing increase in oncological disease is predicted [9]. In addition, methodological innovations such as patient-specific genomic sequencing are becoming accessible and cost-effective [10]. This leads to an almost exponential increase in oncology treatment data and medical knowledge through novel research opportunities [11]. While this treasure trove of oncological health data opens up a new dimension of scientific possibilities, it is beyond the capabilities of human cognitive processing and calls for the application of automated data computing [12,13].

Professionally trained clinical decision support systems (CDSSs), i.e., CancerLinq, OncoDoc or IBM Watson for Oncology, have proven their capability to process these data in large-scale retrospective, observational studies [14,15]. Nevertheless, the recent diffusion of access to public large language models (LLMs) takes the handling of AI-based applications for medical purposes to a new level. Since generative AI-based LLM ChatGPT was made available to the general public by OpenAI (San Francisco, CA, USA) in November 2022, the exploration of the collaboration between human cognition and intelligent machines has rapidly gained public interest. Swiftly, generative AI and LLMs have made their way into our daily lives, not stopping at how we manage our own health [16]. After just one year, questioning of ChatGPT's about personal health issues has become a normality for technology-savvy patients.

Initial pilot studies indicate acceptable accuracy of LLMs in clinical decision making and general medical knowledge throughout the clinical workflow [17]. With regard to breast cancer care, Rao et al. were able to provide evidence of the application of ChatGPT for radiology decision making and screening purposes, justifying its responsible use for radiology services [18]. The available studies argue for the evaluation of further use cases and greater accuracy before the implementation of LLMs in the clinical treatment process [18]. With respect to oncological treatment, research is exploring the consistency of publicly available LLMs and has intensified the discussion about the question whether AI-assisted decision making will change the way tumor boards are conducted [19–21]. In gyne-oncology, only two studies have investigated the performance of publicly available LLMs in breast cancer tumor board decision making [22,23]. While the authors advocate for the promising potential of LLMs in breast cancer tumor boards and clinical oncology, the scientific approach to handling the new technology is still in its infancy. Lukac et al. and Sorin et al. limited their study populations to a small number of randomly selected patient profiles; used a short input model that does not do justice to the information contained in the actual tumor board presentation; partially excluded high-complexity cases, i.e., primary distant metastasis; or neglected to distinguish between different breast cancer treatment options [22,23].

This explorative pilot study aims to extend the results reported by Lukac et al. and Sorin et al. to evaluate the concordance of treatment decisions made by the most prominent publicly available LLM, ChatGPT 3.5 by Open AI, with those of the multidisciplinary tumor board (MTB) of a gynecological oncology center in Germany. The study design is therefore based on patient profiles reflecting the patho- and immunomorphological diversity of primary breast cancer, including primary metastasis and precancerous tumor stages, and extends to a detailed and structured input model. In addition, the entire bandwidth of treatment options for breast cancer, including surgical re-excision, endocrine, chemotherapy, radiation therapy and genetic testing, is evaluated separately.

2. Patients and Methods

2.1. Patient Profiles

To capture the patho- and immunomorphological diversity of breast cancer in comprehensive manner, 20 patient profiles were designed by the head of the investigated gynecologic oncology center in orientation to the current immunohistochemical and molecular subtypes in accordance with the current breast cancer guidelines of the German Association of Gynecology and Obstetrics (DGGG) [24]. In addition, a differentiation by nodal status and postmenopausal status was performed for each subtype (P1–P20, as shown in Table 1).

Table 1. Generic patient profiles (P1–P20).

Patient Profiles				
Immunohistochemical and Molecular Subtype	Postmenopausal		Premenopausal	
	Nodal Negative	Nodal Positive	Nodal Negative	Nodal Positive
Luminal A	P1	P2	P3	P4
Luminal B	P5	P6	P7	P8
Her2 positive	P9	P10	P11	P12
Triple negative	P13	P14	P15	P16
DCIS	P17		P18	
DCIS with narrow resection margin	P19			
Inflammatory breast cancer				P20

Subsequently, the patient profiles were completed to include patient age, ECOG (Eastern Cooperative Oncology Group Performance Scale), previous illness, previous surgical treatment, birth history and oncological family history (as shown in Figures 1 and 2). Further diagnostic data were designed to the extent of pTNM classification, minimal resection margin (R0/R1, in mm), histological classification (non-special-type NST, invasive lobular, tubular or mucinous), grading (according to Bloom–Richardson–Elston score [25]), unilaterality versus bilaterality, and multifocality or -centricity. The data with regard to immunohistochemical and molecular subtyping were determined to the extent of hormonal status (estrogen receptor (ER), 0–100%; progesterone receptor (PR), 0–100%), Her2 status (immunohistology (IHC) or in situ hybridization (ISH)) and Ki-67 proliferation index (0–100%). For data security and compliance reasons, the profiles are fictitious and do not reflect actual patient cases. Based on this, we notified the university's ethics committee and were informed that ethical approval is not required.

P1-10	P1	P2	P3	P4	P5	P6	P7	P8	P9	P10
Patient Profiles	Postmenopausal Luminal A N-	Postmenopausal Luminal A N+	Premenopausal Luminal A N-	Premenopausal Luminal A N+	Postmenopausal Luminal B Her2- N-	Postmenopausal Luminal B Her2- N+	Premenopausal Luminal B Her2- N-	Premenopausal Luminal B Her2- N+	Postmenopausal Her2+ ER/PR- N-	Postmenopausal Her2+ ER/PR- N+
Age	62	61	50	45	62	58	40	35	58	65
Menopause Status	post	post	pre	pre	post	post	pre	pre	post	post
ECOG	0	0	1	1	0	1	0	0	1	2
Previous Illness	Bronchial asthma (no long-term therapy, acute therapy with inhaled corticosteroids and formoterol), arterial hypertension (with antihypertensive triple combination of diuretic, calcium antagonist and AT II antagonist)	Hypothyroidism (with L-thyroxine medication)	Relapsing remitting multiple sclerosis (last episode 5 years ago, no long-term medication)	HELLP Syndrome at first pregnancy at age of 34	Diabetes mellitus type 1, arterial hypertension (with ACE inhibitor medication), hemorrhoids	Crohn's disease (with continuous therapy with TNF-alpha inhibitors)	Deep vein thrombosis at age 25 while on contraceptive medication, heterozygous factor V Leiden	Colitis ulcerosa, Hashimoto-thyroiditis (with L-thyroxine medication)	COPD GOLD B (with inhaled long-acting muscarinic receptor antagonists and inhaled long-acting β2 sympathomimetics medication)	Atrial fibrillation (with direct oral anticoagulant and beta-blocker medication), pulmonary artery embolism at the age of 65 following immobilization during right-sided total hip arthroplasty
Previous surgical treatment	Transverse laparotomy for hysterectomy because of hypermenorrhea and uterine myomatosus at the age of 42, laparoscopic cholecystectomy at the age of 45, open appendectomy at the age of 29	Open cholecystectomy at the age of 35, breast-conserving tumorectomy for right-sided fibroadenoma at the age of 32, uterine curettage after early abortion at age of 20	Tonsillectomy in childhood, open appendectomy for complicated appendicitis without free perforation at the age of 27	Postpartum cardiomyopathy with intensive care ECMO support, Roux-Y gastric bypass for obesity (BMI 50) at the age of 32	Mamma abscess cleavage on the right side at the age of 35, open hemorrhoidectomy according to Milligan-Morgan at the age of 40	Bowel-sparing resection for ileum stenosis at the age of 35, open appendectomy at the age of 25, longitudinal laparotomy for mechanical ileus at the age of 55	Open appendectomy at the age of 28	Laparoscopy for cyst extirpation of left ovarian cyst at age 30	none	Right-sided total hip arthroplasty at the age of 65
Birth history	1 vaginal birth at age of 32, 1 cesarean at the age of 34, 1 early abortion at the age of 30	4 vaginal births at the age of 25, 27, 29 and 30, 1 early abortion at the age of 20	no prior birth	2 cesareans at the age of 34 and 38	4 vaginal births at the age of 18, 20, 26 and 30	no prior birth	1 vaginal birth at the age of 39	no prior birth	2 vaginal births at the age of 28 and 30	2 vaginal births at the age of 23 and 30 and 1 cesarean at the age of 35
Oncological family history	Maternal aunt with colon cancer at the age of 62	Maternal female cousin with hodgkin lymphoma at the age of 30	no prior oncological family history	Paternal uncle with prostate cancer at the age of 65	Paternal uncle with colon-cancer at the age of 40, paternal grandfather with colon-cancer at the age of 60, paternal cousin with colon cancer at the age of 35	Maternal grandmother with breast cancer at the age of 80	Sister-in-law with breast cancer at the age of 30	Paternal grandmother with breast cancer at the age of 70, paternal aunt with breast cancer at the age of 50, maternal uncle with pancreatic cancer at the age of 60	Maternal grandmother with endometrial cancer at the age of 75, mother with bile duct carcinoma at the age of 60	Sister with childhood acute lymphoblastic leukemia, father with gastric carcinoma at the age of 50
Previous surgical treatment	BCT+SLN right	BCT+SLN left	BCT+SLN right	BCT+SLN left	BCT+SLN right	BCT+SLN left	BCT+SLN left	BCT+SLN right	BCT+SLN left	MT+SLN right
TNM	pT1bN0MX	pT2c2pN1aM0	pT1apN0MX	pT1pN1aM0	pT3pN0M0	pT3(3)pN1aM0	pT2pN0M0	pT2pN1aM0	pT1apN0M0	pT3pN1aM0
Resection margin	R0, 5mm	R0, 6mm	R0, 1mm	R1 on lateral aspect	R0, 0.1mm	R0, 7mm	R1 on lateral aspect	R0, 2mm	R0, 0.05mm	R0, 10mm
Histological subtype	NST	Invasive-lobular	Mucinous	NST	Invasive-lobular	NST	Tubular	Invasive-lobular	NST	NST
Grading	G1	G1	G1	G2	G1	G2	G2	G3	G2	G2
UL/BL	Unilateral	Unilateral	Unilateral	Unilateral	Unilateral	Unilateral	Unilateral	Unilateral	Unilateral	Unilateral
MF/MC	Monofocal and -centric	Monocentric and multifocal, 2 foci	Monofocal and -centric	Monofocal and -centric	Monofocal and -centric	Monocentric and multifocal, 3 foci	Monofocal and -centric	Monofocal and -centric	Monofocal and -centric	Monofocal and -centric
ER	95%	85%	95%	100%	80%	75%	90%	75%	5%	0%
PR	80%	80%	90%	100%	75%	90%	50%	75%	1%	0%
Her2	Negative (IHC 0)	Negative (IHC 1+)	Negative (IHC 0)	Negative (IHC 0)	Negative (IHC 1+)	Negative (IHC 0)	Negative (IHC 2+, ISH negative)	Positive (IHC 3+)	Positive (ISH positive)	Positive (IHC 3+)
Ki-67	10%	15%	8%	10%	35%	28%	30%	40%	20%	35%

N+/-= nodal positive or negative, Her2+/-= Her2 positive or negative, BCT= breast-conserving tumorectomy, SLN= sentinellymphnodectomy, MT= mastectomy, UL/BL = uni- versus bilaterality, MF/MC= multifocality or -centricity, ER= estrogen receptor, PR= progesterone receptor, Her2= Her2 status, Ki-67= Ki-67-proliferation-index

Figure 1. Detailed patient profiles (P1–P10).

P11-20 Patient Profiles	P11 Premenopausal Her2-ER/PR-N-	P12 Premenopausal Her2+ ER/PR-N+	P13 Postmenopausal Triple Negative N-	P14 Postmenopausal Triple Negative N+	P15 Premenopausal Triple Negative N-	P16 Premenopausal Triple Negative N+	P17 Postmenopausal DCIS, clear resection margin	P18 Premenopausal DCIS, clear resection margin	P19 Postmenopausal DCIS, narrow resection margin	P20 Inflammatory Breast Cancer
Age	32	42	56	65	29	35	70	38	72	36
Menopause status	pre	pre	post	post	pre	pre	post	pre	post	pre
ECOG	0	0	0	1	0	0	2	0	1	0
Previous illness	Insulin-dependent gestational diabetes during the first pregnancy at the age of 20, postpartum depression at the age of 20	Pulmonary artery embolism after pelvic vein thrombosis at the age of 20, antiphospholipid syndrome with anticardiolipin antibodies (with permanent oral anticoagulation with phenprocoumon)	Insulin-dependent diabetes mellitus type 2, obesity with BMI of 43, obstructive sleep apnea syndrome, secondary arterial hypertension (with ACE inhibitor medication)	Addison's disease (currently under hydro- and fludrocortisone medication)	none	Paranoid schizophrenia (under stable condition with current olanzapine medication)	Arterial hypertension (with with AT II antagonist medication)	AV-node re-entry tachycardia (with beta-blocker medication)	Chronic lymphocytic leukaemia Stadium A	none
Previous surgical treatment	none	none	Abdominoplasty at the age of 50, bilateral mammary reduction mammoplasty for mammary hypertrophy at the age of 35	Total knee replacement on the left side at the age of 50	none	none	Vaginal hysterectomy with bilateral adnexectomy for uterine prolapse at the age of 55, transcatheter aortic-valve implantation due to aortic valve stenosis at the age of 69	none	Total shoulder arthroplasty on the left side	none
Birth history	1 vaginal birth at the age of 20	6 early abortions between the age of 20 and 26	3 vaginal births at the age of 20, 21 and 25	3 cesareans at the age of 25, 28 and 35	no prior birth	no prior birth	2 vaginal births at the age of 16 and 20	1 cesarean at the age of 36	1 vaginal birth at the age of 22	no prior birth
Oncological family history	Father with bronchial carcinoma at the age of 60, sister with osteosarcoma at the age of 18	Father with colon cancer at the age of 45, paternal grandmother with endometrial cancer at the age of 65, paternal uncle with urothelial carcinoma of the renal pelvis at the age of 55	Mother with breast cancer at the age of 40	Paternal grandmother with pancreatic cancer at the age of 59, maternal aunt with colon cancer at the age of 60	Mother with breast cancer at the age of 50, maternal grandmother with breast cancer at the age of 70	Maternal grandmother with endometrial cancer at age of 60, paternal uncle with rectum carcinoma at the age of 50	1 sister with peritoneal cancer at the age of 60, maternal grandmother with ovarian cancer at the age of 65	Paternal grandfather with prostate cancer at the age of 65, mother with chronic myeloid leukemia at the age of 70	Father with colon cancer at age 55	no cancer history
Previous surgical treatment	BCT+SLN left	BCT+SLN right	BCT+SLN left	none so far	none so far	none so far	MT right	BCT left and right	BCT+SLN left	none so far
TNM	pT2pN0M0	pT2pN1M0	pT1apN0M0	cT3pN+pM1 (OSS)	cT2bN0M0 on left side and cT1bcN0M0 on right side	cT2pN+pM1 (HEP)	pTis (size of the lesion 4.3 cm)	pTis on left and right side (size of the lesions: 2.3 cm on left side and 3.2 cm on right side)	pTis (size of lesion 1.5 cm)	cT4dpN+M0
Resection margin	R0, 4mm	R0, 2mm	R0, 1mm	not applicable	not applicable	not applicable	R0, 10mm	R0, 4 mm on left, 5 mm on right side	R0, 0.01mm	not applicable
Histological subtype	NST	NST	NST	NST	NST on left and right side	NST	not applicable	not applicable	not applicable	NST, inflammatory breast cancer with lymphangiosis carcinomatosa
Grading	G2	G3	G2	G3	G3	G3	not applicable	not applicable	not applicable	G3
UL/BL	Unilateral	Unilateral	Unilateral	Unilateral	Bilateral	Unilateral	Unilateral	Bilateral	Unilateral	Unilateral
MF/MC	Monofocal and -centric	Monofocal and -centric	Monofocal and -centric	not applicable	not applicable	not applicable	Monofocal and multicentric, 2 centers	Monofocal and -centric on left and right side	Monofocal and -centric	not applicable
ER	0%	0%	0%	0%	0% on left and right side	1%	95%	100% on left and right side	100%	5%
PR	0%	5%	0%	0%	0% on left and right side	2%	90%	100% on left and right side	100%	5%
Her2	Positive (ICH 3+)	Positive (ISH positive)	Negative (IHC 1+)	Negative (IHC 0)	Negative (IHC 0) on left and right side	Negative (IHC 1+)	not applicable	not applicable	not applicable	Positive (ISH positive)
Ki-67	65%	80%	40%	60%	70% left, 85% on right side	80%	not applicable	not applicable	not applicable	70%

N+/-= nodal positive or negative, Her2+/-= Her2 positive or negative, BCT= breast-conserving tumorectomy, SLN= sentinellymphnodectomy, UL/BL= uni- versus bilaterality, MF/MC= multicentricity or -centricity, ER= estrogen receptor, PR= progesterone receptor, Her2= Her2 status, Ki-67= Ki-67-proliferation-index

Figure 2. Detailed patient profiles (P11–P20).

2.2. Extended Input Model

The following extended input model was applied based on the aforementioned data from each patient profile. The structuring includes an introductory sentence, followed by basic profile-specific health data and the formulation of an oncological family history. Furthermore, the current surgical treatment of the tumor is stated, leading to a transition to detailed data about the lesion's patho- and immunomorphological characteristics. Lastly, the specific task (or challenge) is presented in connection with a clarification about the advisable treatment options (as shown in Figure 3).

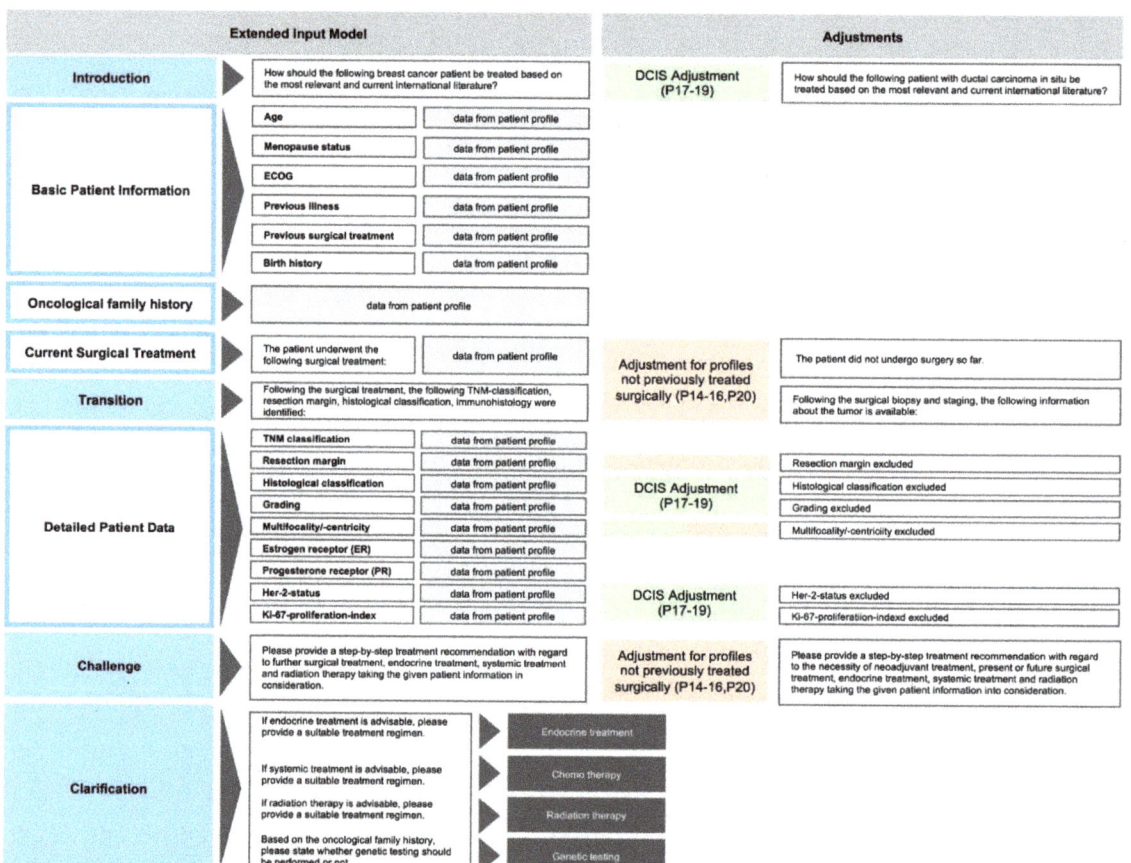

Figure 3. Extended input model.

Wording was slightly adjusted for patient profiles not previously treated surgically (P14–P16 and P20) and for cases of ductal carcinoma in situ (DCIS) (P17–P19).

2.3. Model Execution

Prior to model execution, a randomization of the profile sequence was executed (see File S1). Furthermore, a blinded version of the standardized input model without reference to the patient profile number was created. Afterwards, model execution was performed on 21 July 2023 by presenting one profile after another to the publicly available ChatGPT 3.5 (OpenAI LP, San Francisco, CA, USA). The study design focuses on testing the ChatGPT 3.5, as it is publicly available at no charge and, thus, primarily used by patients and healthcare professionals in a medical context at the present time. Correspondingly, the blinded version of the input model was translated to German using DeepL AI-based translation services (DeepL SE, Cologne, Germany), and the predefined patient profiles were discussed in the same randomized order by the actual multidisciplinary tumor board (MTB) of the investigated gynecologic oncology center on the same date. MTB participants were informed about the execution of an experiment without any information about the study design, and they were given the option to decline participation. Accordingly, they were instructed to treat patient cases and determine treatment decisions as they would in the regular course of tumor board decision making. On the specific date, the tumor board consisted of four specialized gyne-oncologists, two gynecologists, two oncologists, one human geneticist, one radiation physician, one pathologist and two gynecological residents. The head of the gynecologic oncology center under study did not participate in the study due to knowledge of the patient profiles.

2.4. Concordance Assessment

As specified in the input model, recommendations of the LLM and MTB were analyzed with respect to the treatment options of surgical treatment (ST), endocrine treatment (ET), systemic treatment or chemotherapy (CT), radiation therapy (RT) and genetic testing (GT). As such, they were measured in a bivariate manner (treatment option recommended = yes; not recommended = no). Concordance assessment of LLM and MTB treatment was performed in terms of descriptive statistical evaluation (in %) for each individual patient profile and for each subordinate treatment option separately. As LLMs are designed to generate a relative formulation, formulation of possible treatment was rated as recommended treatment.

3. Results

3.1. Treatment Recommendation Frequency

In total, 61 treatment recommendations were proposed by the LLM, and 48 were proposed by the MTB for the predefined patient profiles. The greatest difference in recommendation frequency results was obtained for GT (as shown in Table 2).

Table 2. Treatment recommendation frequency.

Treatment Option	ST		ET		CT		RT		GT	
Model Execution	LLM	MTB	LLM	MTB	LLM	MTB	LLM	MTB	LLM	MTB
Recommendation frequency	2	3	13	8	13	11	16	15	17	11

ST = surgical treatment; ET = endocrine treatment; CT = chemotherapy; RT = radiation therapy; GT = genetic testing.

3.2. Concordance Assessment Per Patient Profile

Concordance between LLM and MTB recommendations was registered for half of the patient profiles (CC_{Total} = 50.0%; 10 of 20 PP). Overall concordance for invasive breast cancer patients ($CC_{BreastCancer}$), excluding DCIS profiles P17 to 19 amounted to 58.8% (10 of 17 PP). Removing GT from the assessment resulted in full concordance (CC_{Total_NoGT}) for 68.4% (13 of 19 PP) of all PP and 81.25% (13 of 16 PP) for invasive breast cancer PP ($CC_{BreastCancer\_NoGT}$). PP 7 had to be excluded from the partial evaluation because the MTB recommended further testing using Endopredict® (Myriad Service GmbH, Munich, Germany) to assess the need for chemotherapy for the specific patient profile.

3.3. Concordance Assessment Per Treatment Option

The MTB recommended surgical re-excision (ST) for three, in comparison to two PP in the case of the LLM. Concordance for ET, CT, RT and GT amounted to CC_{ET} = 75.0% (15 of 20 PP), CC_{CT} = 94.5% (18 of 19 PP), CC_{RT} = 95.0% (19 of 20 PP) and CC_{GT} = 70.0% (14 of 20 PP) (as shown in Table 3). With regard to CT, PP 7 had to be removed from the assessment based on the aforementioned MTB decision on further breast cancer prognostic testing.

Table 3. Concordance assessment.

PP		ST	ET	CT	RT	GT	CC per PP
Postmenopausal Luminal A N−	1	yes	yes	yes	yes	no	no
Postmenopausal Luminal A N+	2	yes	yes	no	yes	no	no
Premenopausal Luminal A N−	3	yes	yes	yes	yes	yes	yes
Premenopausal Luminal A N+	4	yes	yes	yes	yes	yes	yes
Postmenopausal Luminal B Her2− N−	5	yes	yes	yes	yes	yes	yes
Postmenopausal Luminal B Her2− N+	6	yes	yes	yes	yes	no	no
Premenopausal Luminal B Her2− N−	7	yes	yes	n.a.	yes	no	no
Premenopausal Luminal B Her2+ N+	8	yes	yes	yes	yes	yes	yes
Postmenopausal Her2+ ER/PR− N−	9	yes	no	yes	yes	no	no
Postmenopausal Her2+ ER/PR− N+	10	yes	yes	yes	yes	no	no
Premenopausal Her2+ ER/PR− N-	11	yes	yes	yes	yes	yes	yes
Premenopausal Her2+ ER/PR− N+	12	yes	yes	yes	yes	yes	yes
Postmenopausal Triple Negative N−	13	yes	yes	yes	yes	yes	yes
Postmenopausal Triple Negative N+	14	yes	yes	yes	yes	yes	yes
Premenopausal Triple Negative N−	15	yes	yes	yes	yes	yes	yes
Premenopausal Triple Negative N+	16	yes	no	yes	yes	yes	no
Postmenopausal DCIS, clear resection margin	17	yes	no	yes	no	yes	no
Premenopausal DCIS, clear resection margin	18	yes	no	yes	yes	yes	no
Postmenopausal DCIS, narrow resection margin	19	no	no	yes	yes	yes	no
Inflammatory Breast Cancer	20	yes	yes	yes	yes	yes	yes
CC per TO		95.0%	75.0%	94.7%	95.0%	70.0%	50.0%

PP = patient profiles; yes = concordance between LLM and MTB; no = no concordance between LLM and MTB; PP = patient profile; ST = surgical treatment; ET = endocrine treatment; CT = chemotherapy; RT = radiation therapy; GT = genetic testing; CC per PP = concordance per patient profile; CC per TO = concordance per treatment option; N+/− = nodal positive or negative; Her2+/− = Her2 positive or negative; n.a. = not applicable.

3.4. Comparative Results of LLM and MTB Treatment Decisions

A direct comparison between the treatment recommendations of the LLM and MTB is presented in Table 4. Further details regarding qualitative treatment recommendations (i.e., aromatase inhibitor versus tamoxifen treatment in ET or specific chemotherapy regimen) are included in File S1.

Table 4. Comparative results.

PP		ST		ET		CT		RT		GT	
		LLM	MTB	LLM	MTB	LLM	MTB	LLM	MTB	LLM	MTB
Postmenopausal Luminal A N−	1	no	no	yes	yes	no	no	yes	yes	yes	no
Postmenopausal Luminal A N+	2	no	no	yes	yes	yes	no	yes	yes	yes	no
Premenopausal Luminal A N−	3	no	no	yes	yes	no	no	yes	yes	no	no
Premenopausal Luminal A N+	4	yes	yes	yes	yes	no	no	yes	yes	no	no
Postmenopausal Luminal B Her2− N−	5	no	no	yes	yes	no	no	yes	yes	yes	yes
Postmenopausal Luminal B Her2− N+	6	no	no	yes	yes	yes	yes	yes	yes	yes	no
Premenopausal Luminal B Her2− N−	7	yes	yes	yes	yes	yes	n.a.	yes	yes	yes	no
Premenopausal Luminal B Her2+ N+	8	no	no	yes	yes	yes	yes	yes	yes	yes	yes
Postmenopausal Her2+ ER/PR− N−	9	no	no	yes	no	yes	yes	yes	yes	yes	no
Postmenopausal Her2+ ER/PR− N+	10	no	no	no	no	yes	yes	yes	yes	yes	no
Premenopausal Her2+ ER/PR− N−	11	no	no	no	no	yes	yes	yes	yes	yes	yes
Premenopausal Her2+ ER/PR− N+	12	no	no	no	no	yes	yes	yes	yes	yes	yes
Postmenopausal Triple Negative N−	13	no	no	no	no	yes	yes	yes	yes	yes	yes
Postmenopausal Triple Negative N+	14	no	no	no	no	yes	yes	no	no	yes	yes
Premenopausal Triple Negative N−	15	no	no	no	no	yes	yes	no	no	yes	yes
Premenopausal Triple Negative N+	16	no	no	yes	no	yes	yes	no	no	yes	yes
Postmenopausal DCIS, clear resection margin	17	no	no	yes	no	no	no	yes	no	yes	yes
Premenopausal DCIS, clear resection margin	18	no	no	yes	no	no	no	yes	yes	yes	yes
Postmenopausal DCIS, narrow resection margin	19	no	yes	yes	no	no	no	yes	yes	no	no
Inflammatory Breast Cancer	20	no	no	no	no	yes	yes	no	no	yes	yes

PP = patient profiles; yes = treatment recommended; no = treatment not recommended; PP = patient profile; ST = surgical treatment; ET = endocrine treatment; CT = chemotherapy; RT = radiation therapy; GT = genetic testing; LLM = large language model; MTB = multidisciplinary tumor board.

4. Discussion

4.1. Main Findings

This observational study shows that ChatGPT 3.5, a publicly available LLM, can provide treatment recommendations for breast cancer patients that are consistent with multidisciplinary tumor board decision making of a gynecologic oncology center in Germany. This observation is important, as it adds to previous findings by applying an extended standardized input model, assessing a broader spectrum of patho- and immunomorphological breast cancer subtypes, including primary metastatic and precancerous tumor stages, in a structured manner, in addition to evaluating possible breast cancer treatment options separately. With CC_{Total} and $CC_{BreastCancer}$ amounting to 50.0% and 58.8%, respectively, the general level of concordance observed in this study lies in the middle of that reported in preceding studies by Lukac et al. and Sorin et al. The authors of these studies showed that the congruence of the chatbot's recommendations with those of the specific tumor board amounted to 70% (Sorin et. al.) and 16.05% (Lukac et al.) [22,23]. Once retrieving the GT option from assessment, as the necessity of genetic testing has not previously been measured equivalently by the colleagues, the study provides a total concordance level that matches the findings of Sorin et al. (CC_{Total_NoGT} = 68.4%). Furthermore, this level of accuracy meets the average performance of ChatGPT of 71.8% as measured by Rao et al. in their first-of-its-kind study that assessed the AI tool's potential use along the entire clinical workflow, including diagnostic workup, diagnosis and clinical management [17]. While Sorin et al. refrained from further distinguishment between treatment options, Lukac et al. did so without evaluating the concordance between these subgroups. Thus, this study adds to these previous findings by showing that concordance for individual treatment options, including ET, CT and RT (CC_{ET} = 75.0%, CC_{CT} = 94.5%, CC_{RT} = 95.0%), stands out considerably. However, compared to a professionally trained CDSS, i.e., Watson for Oncology, which has been proven to achieve overall concordance of up to 93% for breast cancer cases, we rate the LLM's performance as rather low [14,15].

4.2. Further Findings

4.2.1. Garbage in–Garbage Out

By applying an extended input model with detailed patient profiles (see Figures 1–3), this study demonstrates that the chatbot can only perform to the level of quality of the data it is fed. As such, it follows the principle of "garbage in–garbage out" for AI-enabled precision medicine applications [17,26]. While Lukac et al. argue that the chatbot does neglect neoadjuvant treatment, our extended input model contradicts this finding [23]. Once explicably asked to consider neoadjuvant treatment, ChatGPT 3.5 successfully identifies suitable situations for neoadjuvant treatment and provides detailed explanation, even mentioning a suitable chemotherapy regimen. Furthermore, our colleagues argue that the LLM does not include current or ongoing studies, which is based on the fact that ChatGPT 3.5 is limited to data published until September 2021. Thus, the LLM is not able to learn the latest science on oncology issues, so it needs to be trained on the latest standards in order to not fall back in "garbage out" situations. In the other hand, medical laypersons will have a hard time recognizing appropriate situations compared to oncology experts. In order not to fall into corresponding "garbage in–garbage out" situations, professionally trained CDSSs receive previously filtered high-quality data and literature as input for its computing process [14,15].

4.2.2. Lack of Consistency in Health Data Use

Although the study design presents an extended input model with a larger amount of detailed health data to the LLM, we must confirm the finding of our colleagues that ChatGPT partially fails to successfully and consistently take individual patient information into account. Thus, Lukac et al. stated that the LLM did not take age into consideration for systemic treatment in elderly patients [23]. Beyond that, extended input model applied herein provides the LLM with a detailed patient history on ECOG, previous illness, surgical history and birth history. Nevertheless, the chatbot did not apply this important background information to back up treatment decisions.

In contrast to this, the LLM successfully accessed the majority of the further provided health data, i.e., age and pre- or postmenopausal status were used to distinguish between aromatase inhibitor and selective estrogen receptor modulators or ovarian suppression by GnRH agonists, which confirms the findings of Sorin et al. and Lukac et al. [22,23]. As the extended input model explicitly asked for a suitable treatment regimen, the chatbot did provide correct medication (i.e., 2.5 mg letrozole p.o. daily) and treatment duration for some patient profiles. Novel findings of this study include the surgical treatment and minimal resection margin being commented on in terms of correctness and sufficiency, the necessity of re-excision being recognized for R1 situations and bilaterality being identified with successful distinguishment between left and right side. With regard to immunohistochemical and molecular subtypes, the LLM successfully took hormonal status, grading, Her2 status and Ki-67 proliferation index into account for treatment planning. Thus, it identified triple-negative cancer types; distinguished between Her2-positive and -negative situations, which resulted in the recommendation of targeted therapies (i.e., trastuzumab); and recognized primary metastatic situations. Furthermore, by providing an oncological family history for each patient profile, decision making with regard to genetic testing was tested to a novel extent. While Lukac et al. only acknowledged the LLM's potential to recognize the possibility of hereditary risk in a young patient with advanced breast cancer, this study's findings expand on this finding by showing its capacity to successfully interpret oncological family histories. Thus, the chatbot not only identifies a specific profile being prone to hereditary breast and ovarian cancer (HBOC) but also makes a differentiation for profiles with colorectal or endometrial disease, drawing a link to Lynch syndrome (i.e., P16 or P5).

By providing the extended health data to the LLM and explicitly requesting a suitable regimen for possible endocrine, radiation and chemotherapy treatment, the chatbot provided individualized treatment decisions for patient profiles in connection with a structured and detailed explanation. Furthermore, by confronting the LLM with diverse patient profiles, including high-complexity cases with primary metastasis, it showed potential to cover broader patho- and immunomorphological diversity of breast cancer in comparison to previous studies. Nevertheless, this study points out a lack of consistency in terms of when and how the LLM used the specific data.

4.2.3. Stepping into the Trip Trap

Another crucial limitation of the LLM becomes evident as it steps into predefined trip traps, resulting in raw treatment mistakes, which the MTB easily evaded. The chatbot recommended genetic testing based on a sister-in-law with breast cancer history (P7), stating the necessity of testing for BRCA 1 and 2 mutations. Furthermore, it neglected the necessity of re-excision for DCIS with a narrow resection margin of 0.01 mm (P19). Such fraudulent decisions hold the potential to adversely affect treatment decisions and negatively impact the patient's health situation. This confirms a critical challenge of natural language models in the context of breast cancer decision making. Regarding the notion of misalignment and hallucination, research recognizes a major challenge for LLMs, which tend to hallucinate unintended text, limiting their current level of development for use in real-world scenarios [27]. As the sister-in-law example shows, the stochastic nature of LLMs can be quickly exploited by misaligning simple designed inputs, resulting in fraudulent responses [28]. Although the performance of LLMs appears impressive when assessed superficially, it proves to be prone to misinterpretation and hallucinations despite being equipped with sufficient information, which limits its application in the medical context [17]. Even small errors in judgment can lead to significant treatment errors for breast cancer that pose a negative risk to a patient's health. The difference between 61 treatment recommendations from the LLM and the 48 from the MTB underlines the LLM's over-recommendation tendency, which ultimately may lead to overtreatment and lack of individualized treatment decision making, i.e., the chatbot recommended endocrine treatment for all DCIS profiles (P17-P19), as well as situations with low ER and PR positivity (P16 and P9), for invasive breast cancer, which are can-do decisions but not necessarily must-do. As one of the main motives of AI use is based on the adaptive automatic processing of heterogeneous health data to enable personalized medical treatment decisions, the current state of publicly available LLMs does not live up to this expectation [1].

4.3. Limitations and Suggestions for the Future

We acknowledge that this manuscript represents a pilot study that explores a novel scientific approach to the application of publicly available LLM ChatGPT 3.5 in the context of breast cancer care. Owing to the nature of explorative, small-scale pilot studies, the current study design includes a considerable number of limitations.

The present study design follows a single-center approach, which tests the LLM's performance against the decision making of a singular certified gynecologic oncology center in Germany. In order to enable the transferability and generalizability of the results, an extension to a multicenter and -national evaluation would be desirable. As such, the decisions of the investigated MTB are based on German standards according to the German Society of Gynecology and Obstetrics guidelines and may differ in an international comparison. Furthermore, this explorative study contains a limited number of patient profiles. Coherent to the testing of CDSS accuracy, the evaluation of LLMs should be extended to large-scale observational studies to allow for the assessment of statistical significance. This work is limited to testing of ChatGPT version 3.5. Follow-up studies should extend the study design to a comparability assessment by including the not-yet-freely available ChatGPT 4 or other LLMs. It remains important to note that due to the nature of a large language models, this observational study is limited to the qualitative interpretation of the LLM's wording and argumentation.

Nevertheless, the study design expands on preceding scientific work through the application of an extended input model and taking a broader spectrum of the patho- and immunohistological variety and treatment diversity of breast cancer care into consideration. Beyond that, we consider the scientific evaluation of publicly available LLMs to be necessary. Due to their diffusion of use in society, they are and will inevitably be used in medical contexts. At present, the scientific use and clinical application of LLMs are still in their infancy. This study has added to the specific setting of tumor board decision making. Nevertheless, the evaluation of further use cases throughout the clinical process are necessary to identify situations in which LLMs can create the greatest impact and benefits for patients and healthcare providers. We recognize that the qualities of LLMs will lead to them occupying a place in clinical medicine, but the optimal area of integration has yet to be defined.

5. Conclusions

As this pilot study explores the application of LLMs in oncological decision making, we also confronted the chatbot with the question of why it should, in perspective, be integrated in breast cancer tumor boards:

Authors: "Please provide a short argumentation of 100 words on why the use of ChatGPT should, in perspective, be integrated in breast cancer tumor boards?".

ChatGPT 3.5: "Integrating ChatGPT into breast cancer tumor boards offers invaluable benefits. Firstly, it ensures access to the latest medical knowledge, keeping oncologists up-to-date with rapidly evolving treatments and research. Secondly, ChatGPT can assist in analyzing complex patient data, improving diagnostic accuracy and treatment planning. Its ability to sift through vast medical literature and patient records swiftly aids in personalized care. Furthermore, it enhances communication within multidisciplinary teams, streamlining information sharing and decision-making. Overall, ChatGPT's integration empowers healthcare professionals with cutting-edge insights, potentially leading to more informed, efficient, and effective breast cancer care".

Technological advancement and further development of artificial intelligence (AI) and novel machine learning (ML) methods are projected to disrupt medical care and research by opening up a new dimension of personalized medical treatment decision making [8,11]. The abundance of health data driven by the rapid increase in medical knowledge and modern technological possibilities requires research-driven collaboration with human cognition and automated data processing. Furthermore, the ongoing diffusion of access and user acceptance of publicly available AI tools, including LLMs like ChatGPT, call for scientific monitoring of how to handle their application in medical care and research [26,29]. Few international studies have assessed the accuracy of LLMs for oncological decision making in comparison to MTBs. Although the technological readiness of public LLMs does not meet the level of accuracy required for individualized care decisions for breast cancer, previous studies have advocated for their potential as support tools for breast cancer tumor boards [23,30]. By challenging LLM ChatGPT 3.5 with an extended input model and detailed health data, this study adds to preceding findings and confirms the partial concordance of LLM and MTB decision making for a broader spectrum of care situations for breast cancer. Nevertheless, as the LLM makes considerably fraudulent decisions, which hold the potential to adversely affect treatment decisions and negatively impact the patient's health situation, we do not identify the current development status of publicly available LLMs to be adequate as support tools for tumor boards. Neither does the chatbot fulfill its own formulated qualities. In contrast, we reserve this area of high complexity and individualized treatment planning for oncological experts with, in perspective, increased support from professionally trained CDSSs [14,15]. Nevertheless, we acknowledge that LLMs will have a place in clinical medicine. Due to their explanatory power, they are powerful tools that can support patients along their care journey; inform and educate patients about their personal cancer diagnosis; facilitate physicians' access to relevant information by enhancing their up-to-date knowledge; and automate routine medical routine, i.e., automation of discharge summaries [17,22,30,31]. Gynecological oncologists should familiarize themselves with the capabilities of LLMs in order to understand and utilize their potential while keeping in mind potential risks and limitations.

Supplementary Materials: The following supporting information can be downloaded at: https://www.mdpi.com/article/10.3390/jpm13101502/s1, File S1: Protocols of the Reponses of the LLM and MTB.

Author Contributions: Conceptualization, S.G. and J.B.; Methodology, S.G., J.B., N.G.; Software, S.G., J.B. and N.G.; Validation, S.G., J.B. and N.G.; Formal Analysis, S.G., J.B. and N.G.; Investigation, S.G., J.B. and N.G; Resources, M.L., U.W. and S.K.; Data Curation, J.B. and N.G.; Writing—Original Draft Preparation, S.G.; Writing—Review and Editing, J.B., N.G. and S.K.; Visualization, S.G.; Supervision, M.L., U.W. and S.K.; Project Administration, M.L., U.W. and S.K. All authors have read and agreed to the published version of the manuscript.

Funding: The authors declare that no funds, grants or other support were received during the preparation of this manuscript. Open access funding is provided by the Open Access Publishing Fund of Philipps-Universität Marburg with the support of the Deutsche Forschungsgemeinschaft (DFG, German Research Foundation). S.G. and N.G. were supported by the Clinician Scientist program (SUCCESS-program) of Philipps-University of Marburg and the University Hospital of Giessen and Marburg.

Data Availability Statement: The data presented in this study are available in File S1.

Conflicts of Interest: The authors declare no conflict of interest.

References

1. Quazi, S. Artificial intelligence and machine learning in precision and genomic medicine. *Med. Oncol.* **2022**, *39*, 120. [CrossRef] [PubMed]
2. Ghaderzadeh, M.; Aria, M.; Asadi, F. X-Ray equipped with artificial intelligence: Changing the COVID-19 diagnostic paradigm during the pandemic. *Biomed. Res. Int.* **2021**, *2021*, 9942873. [CrossRef]

3. Ghaderzadeh, M.; Asadi, F.; Jafari, R.; Bashash, D.; Abolghasemi, H.; Aria, M. Deep convolutional neural network-based computer-aided detection system for COVID-19 using multiple lung scans: Design and implementation study. *J. Med. Internet Res.* **2021**, *23*, e27468. [CrossRef] [PubMed]
4. Garavand, A.; Behmanesh, A.; Aslani, N.; Sadeghsalehi, H.; Ghaderzadeh, M. Towards siagnostic aided systems in coronary artery disease detection: A comprehensive multiview survey of the state of the art. *Int. J. Intell. Syst.* **2023**, *2023*, 6442756. [CrossRef]
5. Gheisari, M.; Ebrahimzadeh, F.; Rahimi, M.; Moazzamigodarzi, M.; Liu, Y.; Pramanik, P.; Heravi, M.A.; Mehbodniya, A.; Ghaderzadeh, M.; Feylizadeh, M.R.; et al. Deep learning: Applications, architectures, models, tools, and frameworks: A comprehensive survey. *CAAI Trans. Intell. Technol.* **2023**, *8*, 581–606. [CrossRef]
6. Zheng, Q.; Tian, X.; Yu, Z.; Jiang, N.; Elhanashi, A.; Saponara, S.; Yu, R. Application of wavelet-packet transform driven deep learning method in PM2.5 concentration prediction: A case study of Qingdao, China. *Sustain. Cities Soc.* **2023**, *92*, 104486. [CrossRef]
7. Fertig, E.J.; Jaffee, E.M.; Macklin, P.; Stearns, V.; Wang, C. Forecasting cancer: From precision to predictive medicine. *Med* **2021**, *2*, 1004–1010. [CrossRef]
8. Rösler, W.; Altenbuchinger, M.; Baeßler, B.; Beissbarth, T.; Beutel, G.; Bock, R.; von Bubnoff, N.; Eckardt, J.N.; Foersch, S.; Loeffler, C.M.L.; et al. An overview and a roadmap for artificial intelligence in hematology and oncology. *J. Cancer Res. Clin. Oncol.* **2023**, *149*, 7997–8006. [CrossRef]
9. Europe's Cancer Beating Plan: A New EU Approach to Prevention, Treatment and Care. Available online: https://ec.europa.eu/commission/presscorner/detail/en/ip_21_342 (accessed on 22 September 2023).
10. Tarawneh, T.S.; Rodepeter, F.R.; Teply-Szymanski, J.; Ross, P.; Koch, V.; Thölken, C.; Schäfer, J.A.; Gremke, N.; Mack, H.I.D.; Gold, J.; et al. Combined focused next-generation sequencing assays to guide precision oncology in solid tumors: A retrospective analysis from an institutional molecular tumor board. *Cancers* **2022**, *14*, 4430. [CrossRef]
11. Barker, A.D.; Lee, J.S.H. Translating "big data" in oncology for clinical benefit: Progress or paralysis. *Cancer Res.* **2022**, *82*, 2072–2075. [CrossRef]
12. Bhattacharya, T.; Brettin, T.; Doroshow, J.H.; Evrard, Y.A.; Greenspan, E.J.; Gryshuk, A.L.; Hoang, T.T.; Lauzon, C.B.V.; Nissley, D.; Penberthy, L.; et al. AI meets exascale computing: Advancing cancer research with large-scale high performance computing. *Front. Oncol.* **2019**, *9*, 984. [CrossRef]
13. Stahlberg, E.A.; Abdel-Rahman, M.; Aguilar, B.; Asadpoure, A.; Beckman, R.A.; Borkon, L.L.; Bryan, J.N.; Cebulla, C.M.; Chang, Y.H.; Chatterjee, A.; et al. Exploring approaches for predictive cancer patient digital twins: Opportunities for collaboration and innovation. *Front. Digit. Health* **2022**, *4*, 1007784. [CrossRef]
14. Zhao, X.; Zhang, Y.; Ma, X.; Chen, Y.; Xi, J.; Yin, X.; Kang, H.; Guan, H.; Dai, Z.; Liu, D.; et al. Concordance between treatment recommendations provided by IBM Watson for Oncology and a multidisciplinary tumor board for breast cancer in China. *Jpn. J. Clin. Oncol.* **2020**, *50*, 852–858. [CrossRef] [PubMed]
15. Somashekhar, S.P.; Sepúlveda, M.J.; Puglielli, S.; Norden, A.D.; Shortliffe, E.H.; Rohit Kumar, C.; Rauthan, A.; Arun Kumar, N.; Patil, P.; Rhee, K.; et al. Watson for Oncology and breast cancer treatment recommendations: Agreement with an expert multidisciplinary tumor board. *Ann. Oncol.* **2018**, *29*, 418–423. [CrossRef] [PubMed]
16. Xue, V.W.; Lei, P.; Cho, W.C. The potential impact of ChatGPT in clinical and translational medicine. *Clin. Transl. Med.* **2023**, *13*, e1216. [CrossRef] [PubMed]
17. Rao, A.; Pang, M.; Kim, J.; Kamineni, M.; Lie, W.; Prasad, A.K.; Landman, A.; Dreyer, K.; Succi, M.D. Assessing the utility of ChatGPT throughout the entire clinical workflow: Development and usability study. *J. Med. Internet Res.* **2023**, *25*, e48659. [CrossRef]
18. Rao, A.; Kim, J.; Kamineni, M.; Pang, M.; Lie, W.; Dreyer, K.J.; Succi, M.D. Evaluating GPT as an adjunct for radiologic decision making: GPT-4 Versus GPT-3.5 in a breast imaging pilot. *J. Am. Coll. Radiol.* **2023**. [CrossRef]
19. Ali, R.; Tang, O.Y.; Connolly, I.D.; Zadnik Sullivan, P.L.; Shin, J.H.; Fridley, J.S.; Asaad, W.F.; Cielo, D.; Oyelese, A.A.; Doberstein, C.E.; et al. Performance of ChatGPT and GPT-4 on neurosurgery written board examinations. *Neurosurgery* **2023**. [CrossRef]
20. Vela Ulloa, J.; King Valenzuela, S.; Riquoir Altamirano, C.; Urrejola Schmied, G. Artificial intelligence-based decision-making: Can ChatGPT replace a multidisciplinary tumour board? *Br. J. Surg.* **2023**, *110*, 1543–1544. [CrossRef]
21. Hamamoto, R.; Koyama, T.; Kouno, N.; Yasuda, T.; Yui, S.; Sudo, K.; Hirata, M.; Sunami, K.; Kubo, T.; Takasawa, K.; et al. Introducing AI to the molecular tumor board: One direction toward the establishment of precision medicine using large-scale cancer clinical and biological information. *Exp. Hematol. Oncol.* **2022**, *11*, 82. [CrossRef]
22. Sorin, V.; Klang, E.; Sklair-Levy, M.; Cohen, I.; Zippel, D.B.; Balint Lahat, N.; Konen, E.; Barash, Y. Large language model (ChatGPT) as a support tool for breast tumor board. *NPJ Breast Cancer* **2023**, *9*, 44. [CrossRef] [PubMed]
23. Lukac, S.; Dayan, D.; Fink, V.; Leinert, E.; Hartkopf, A.; Veselinovic, K.; Janni, W.; Rack, B.; Pfister, K.; Heitmeir, B.; et al. Evaluating ChatGPT as an adjunct for the multidisciplinary tumor board decision-making in primary breast cancer cases. *Arch. Gynecol. Obstet.* **2023**. [CrossRef]
24. Interdisciplinary Evidenced-Based Practice Guideline for the Early Detection, Diagnosis, Treatment and Follow-Up of Breast Cancer Long Version 4.4, May 2021, AWMF Registration Number: 032/045OL. Available online: https://www.leitlinienprogramm-onkologie.de/leitlinien/mammakarzinom (accessed on 22 September 2023).

25. Bloom, H.J.; Richardson, W.W. Histological grading and prognosis in breast cancer; a study of 1409 cases of which 359 have been followed for 15 years. *Br. J. Cancer* **1957**, *11*, 359–377. [CrossRef]
26. Compton, C. Getting to personalized cancer medicine: Taking out the garbage. *Cancer* **2007**, *110*, 1641–1643. [CrossRef] [PubMed]
27. Ji, Z.; Lee, N.; Frieske, R.; Yu, T.; Su, D.; Xu, Y.; Ishii, E.; Bang, Y.; Dai, W.; Madotto, A.; et al. Survey of hallucination in natural language generation. *ACM Comput. Surv.* **2023**, *55*, 1–38. [CrossRef]
28. Perez, F.; Ribeiro, I. Ignore previous prompt: Attack techniques for language models. *arXiv* **2022**. [CrossRef]
29. De Angelis, L.; Baglivo, F.; Arzilli, G.; Privitera, G.P.; Ferragina, P.; Tozzi, A.E.; Rizzo, C. ChatGPT and the rise of large language models: The new AI-driven infodemic threat in public health. *Front. Public Health* **2023**, *11*, 1166120. [CrossRef]
30. Sorin, V.; Barash, Y.; Konen, E.; Klang, E. Large language models for oncological applications. *J. Cancer Res. Clin. Oncol.* **2023**, *149*, 9505–9508. [CrossRef]
31. Patel, S.B.; Lam, K. ChatGPT: The future of discharge summaries? *Lancet Digit. Health* **2023**, *5*, e107–e108. [CrossRef] [PubMed]

Disclaimer/Publisher's Note: The statements, opinions and data contained in all publications are solely those of the individual author(s) and contributor(s) and not of MDPI and/or the editor(s). MDPI and/or the editor(s) disclaim responsibility for any injury to people or property resulting from any ideas, methods, instructions or products referred to in the content.

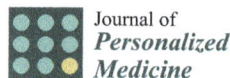

Perspective

Comprehensive Deciphering the Complexity of the Deep Bite: Insight from Animal Model to Human Subjects

Nezar Watted [1,2,3], Iqbal M. Lone [4], Osayd Zohud [4], Kareem Midlej [4], Peter Proff [5] and Fuad A. Iraqi [3,4,5,*]

1. Center for Dentistry Research and Aesthetics, Jatt 45911, Israel; nezar.watted@gmx.net
2. Department of Orthodontics, Faculty of Dentistry, Arab America University, Jenin 919000, Palestine
3. Gathering for Prosperity Initiative, Jatt 45911, Israel
4. Department of Clinical Microbiology and Immunology, Sackler Faculty of Medicine, Tel-Aviv University, Tel Aviv 69978, Israel; iqbalzoo84@gmail.com (I.M.L.); osaydzohud@mail.tau.ac.il (O.Z.); kareem.milej@gmail.com (K.M.)
5. University Hospital of Regensburg, Department of Orthodontics, University of Regensburg, 93053 Regensburg, Germany; pter.proff@klinik.uni-regensburg.de
* Correspondence: fuadi@tauex.tau.ac.il

Abstract: Deep bite is a malocclusion phenotype, defined as the misalignment in the vertical dimension of teeth and jaws and characterized by excessive overlap of the upper front teeth over the lower front teeth. Numerous factors, including genetics, environmental factors, and behavioral ones, might contribute to deep bite. In this study, we discuss the current clinical treatment strategies for deep bite, summarize the already published findings of genetic analysis associated with this complex phenotype, and their constraints. Finally, we propose a comprehensive roadmap to facilitate investigations for determining the genetic bases of this complex phenotype development. Initially, human deep bite phenotype, genetics of human deep bite, the prevalence of human deep bite, diagnosis, and treatment of human deep bite were the search terms for published publications. Here, we discuss these findings and their limitations and our view on future strategies for studying the genetic bases of this complex phenotype. New preventative and treatment methods for this widespread dental issue can be developed with the help of an understanding of the genetic and epigenetic variables that influence malocclusion. Additionally, malocclusion treatment may benefit from technological developments like 3D printing and computer-aided design and manufacture (CAD/CAM). These technologies enable the development of personalized surgical and orthodontic guidelines, enhancing the accuracy and effectiveness of treatment. Overall, the most significant results for the patient can only be achieved with a customized treatment plan created by an experienced orthodontic professional. To design a plan that meets the patient's specific requirements and expectations, open communication between the patient and the orthodontist is essential. Here, we propose to conduct a genome-wide association study (GWAS), RNAseq analysis, integrating GWAS and expression quantitative trait loci (eQTL), micro and small RNA, and long noncoding RNA analysis in tissues associated with deep bite malocclusion in human, and complement it by the same approaches in the collaborative cross (CC) mouse model which offer a novel platform for identifying genetic factors as a cause of deep bite in mice, and subsequently can then be translated to humans. An additional direct outcome of this study is discovering novel genetic elements to advance our knowledge of how this malocclusion phenotype develops and open the venue for early identification of patients carrying the susceptible genetic factors so that we can offer early prevention and treatment strategies, a step towards applying a personalized medicine approach.

Keywords: deep bite; clinical treatment strategies; genetics of deep bite; animal model; genomics approaches

Citation: Watted, N.; Lone, I.M.; Zohud, O.; Midlej, K.; Proff, P.; Iraqi, F.A. Comprehensive Deciphering the Complexity of the Deep Bite: Insight from Animal Model to Human Subjects. *J. Pers. Med.* **2023**, *13*, 1472. https://doi.org/10.3390/jpm13101472

Academic Editor: Daniele Giansanti

Received: 5 September 2023
Revised: 27 September 2023
Accepted: 6 October 2023
Published: 8 October 2023

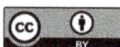

Copyright: © 2023 by the authors. Licensee MDPI, Basel, Switzerland. This article is an open access article distributed under the terms and conditions of the Creative Commons Attribution (CC BY) license (https://creativecommons.org/licenses/by/4.0/).

1. Introduction

The term "malocclusion", which refers to the misalignment of upper and lower teeth and jaws and is a widespread dental condition affecting millions of people worldwide, can negatively affect oral health, including limiting function such as the ability to eat, speak, and practice good oral hygiene [1]. Malocclusion can also affect how one looks and lead to a loss of confidence and self-esteem [1]. Genetic, environmental, and developmental factors are among malocclusion's multifactorial and complex causes [2]. Dental research has made significant strides toward understanding the molecular causes of malocclusion, with genetics and genomics shedding light on particular genes and signaling pathways that affect jaw development, tooth eruption, and completion of tooth root development. It is still difficult to fully comprehend the complex interactions between genetic and environmental factors that lead to malocclusion [3].

A deep bite is a common orthodontic problem when the upper front teeth overlap the lower front teeth excessively (Figure 1). This condition can cause various issues, including difficulty in the function of biting and chewing, speech problems, and even jaw pain.

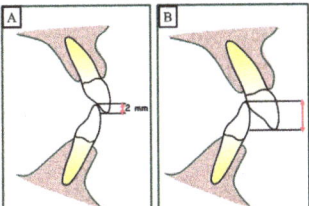

Figure 1. Definition of an overbite as a vertical relationship or the distance between the maxillary central incisor and the opposing mandibular central incisor. (**A**) shows a physiological overbite of 2–3 mm, and a deep bite caused when overbite increased by more than 3 mm is shown in (**B**).

The deep bite can be underlined and defined by different types including skeletal deep bite, dentoaleolar deep bite, and a combination of skeletal and dentoalveolar deep bite (Figure 2).

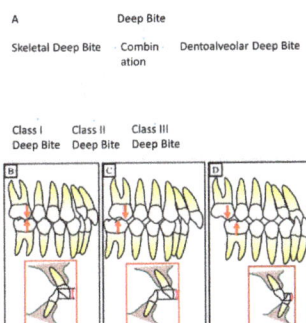

Figure 2. The different types of deep bite. (**A**) shows a diagram to illustrate the different types of deep bites. (**B**) shows a deep bite with Class I. (**C**) shows deep bite with Class II, and (**D**) shows a deep bite with Class III.

It is known that the type of skeletal deep bite is caused by growth disturbance in the vertical dimension and is called anterior growth. The interbasal angle between the base of the maxilla and the base of the mandible decreases due to the anterior rotation of the mandible during growth. Accordingly, the soft tissue structures develop and adapt to "soft tissue go with the bone". The result as a phenotype is *"short face syndrome"*. The skeletal deep bite can occur in all angle classes, as shown in Figure 3.

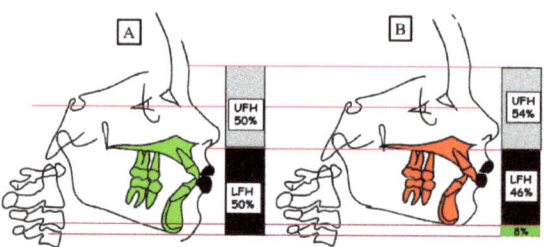

Figure 3. Schematic representation of the vertical dimension for a physiological overbite (**A**) and skeletal deep bite (**B**). (**A**) Physiological vertical dimension; harmonious relation between the upper facial height (UFH 50%) and lower facial height (LFH 50%). (**B**) A skeletal deep bite because of the anterior rotation of the mandible. There is a decreased lower facial height (LFH 46%) compared to the upper face height (UFH 54%).

The deep bite defined by dental malformation is caused in the vertical dimension. Elongation, teeth that usually erupted too far, or tooth migration result in a significant vertical overlap of the front teeth. This is usually not associated with profile changes in the vertical dimension, as shown in Figure 4.

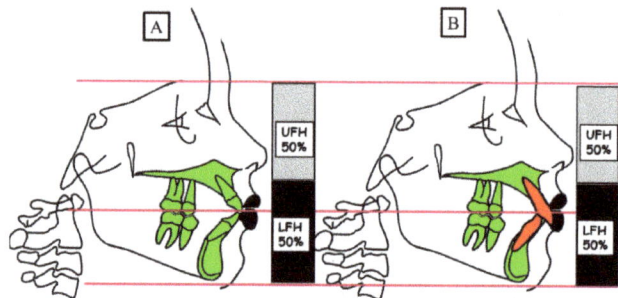

Figure 4. Schematic representation of the vertical dimension for a physiological overbite (**A**) and dentoalveolar deep bite (**B**). (**A**) Physiological vertical dimension; harmonious relation between the upper facial height (UFH 50%) and lower facial height (LFH 50%). (**B**) A dentoalveolar deep bite because of the elongation of the front teeth; harmonious relation between the upper facial height (UFH 50%) and lower facial height (LFH 50%).

Finally, the deep bite may be caused by a combination of skeletal and dentoalveolar dysgnathy. In this case, the patient's phenotype and profile exhibits a disharmony in vertical dimension *"short face syndrome"*, as shown in Figure 5.

A deep bite can be caused by various factors, including genetics, environmental and behavioral factors [4]. While environmental factors such as thumb sucking, tongue-thrusting, and prolonged pacifier use can contribute to the development of deep bites, there is also evidence to suggest that genetics may play a role [4]. Several studies have identified specific genes that may be associated with the development of deep bite. Many researchers have identified specific genes that may be associated with the development of deep bite, such as the IRF6 and BMP4 genes [2,5]. Other studies have suggested that variations in genes related to bone growth and development, such as the RUNX2 and COL1A1 genes, may also play a role in the development of deep bite [6]. Overall, while environmental factors can contribute to the development of deep bite, there is evidence to suggest that genetics may also play a vital role. Further research is needed to identify specific genes and genetic pathways that are involved in the development of this malocclusion.

With the aid of animal models, the molecular analysis of malocclusion has been dramatically enhanced. With the help of these models, researchers can examine how environmental and genetic factors affect the development of misaligned teeth and test various preventative and therapeutic strategies. Because of their small size, simplicity in breeding, and genetic resemblance to humans, mice are one of the most commonly used animal models [7]. The collaborative cross (CC) mouse is an effective tool for researching complex genetic traits like malocclusion. CC mice are bred to produce a genetically diverse population to increase their genetic variation. This mouse population is a great model for research on the genetic causes of malocclusion because it has a distinctive and varied array of genetic variants [7]. The CC mouse population has previously been used to study complex genetic traits like body weight, and metabolic disorders [8]. The genetic diversity of CC mice offers a powerful tool to comprehend the genetic components of malocclusion and enables researchers to pinpoint genetic variants that contribute to complex traits [9,10].

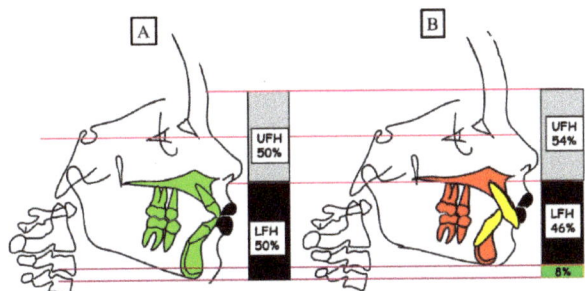

Figure 5. Schematic representation of the vertical dimension for a physiological overbite (**A**) and the combination of skeletal and dentoalveolar deep bite (**B**). (**A**) Physiological vertical dimension; harmonious relation between the upper facial height (UFH 50%) and lower facial height (LFH 50%). (**B**) A skeletal and dentoalveolar deep bite because of the anterior rotation of the mandible and elongation of the front teeth. There is a decreased lower facial height (LFH 46%) compared to the upper face height (UFH 54%).

1.1. Etiology

Epigenetic factors, such as DNA methylation, histone modification, and microRNA regulation, can also play a role in malocclusion development. Epigenetic changes can alter gene expression patterns and influence the development of the teeth and jaws. For example, studies have shown that DNA methylation patterns are altered in patients with malocclusion, and these changes can affect gene expression patterns involved in jaw growth and tooth eruption [11]. Additionally, epigenetic changes can be influenced by environmental factors such as diet, stress, and exposure to toxins. For example, studies have shown that maternal stress during pregnancy can alter DNA methylation patterns in the offspring, potentially leading to craniofacial abnormalities and malocclusion [12].

In summary, the genetic causes of malocclusion involve variations in genes and signaling pathways that are involved in jaw growth, tooth eruption, and dental occlusion. Epigenetic factors, such as DNA methylation and microRNA regulation, can also play a role in malocclusion development. Understanding the genetic and epigenetic factors that contribute to malocclusion can inform the development of new prevention and treatment strategies for this common dental problem.

There are numerous unnoticed skeletal or dental irregularities under a deep bite malocclusion. Therefore, it is essential to understand that a deep bite is not a disease, but rather a clinical expression of an underlying skeletal or dental irregularity. Skeletal or dental overbites are influenced by environmental, genetic, or a mix of environmental and genetic variables during development. Skeletal deep bites are typically characterized by (1) a growing mismatch between the mandibular and maxillary jawbones, (2) convergent rotation of the jaw bases, and/or (3) a deficient mandibular ramus height. Particularly in the lower portion of the face, the anterior facial height is frequently tiny in such circumstances. The incisors' supraocclusion (overeruption), on the other hand, is indicated by dental deep bites [13] or infraocclusion (undereruption) of the molars or a combination of the two [14]. Alterations to the tooth morphologies, early loss of permanent teeth leading to a lingual collapse of the maxillary or mandibular anterior teeth, mesiodistal breadth of anterior teeth, and age-related natural deepening of the bite are other factors that might have an impact on this condition.

Also known as "acquired deep bites", deep bites are mainly brought on by environmental factors. It is a well-known fact that there is a dynamic equilibrium of forces between the structures around the teeth, specifically the tongue, the buccinator, the mentalis, and the orbicularis oris muscles, and the occlusal forces that help in the balanced development and maintenance of the occlusion. A malocclusion can be caused by any environmental factor that upsets this dynamic balance; the instances include:

1. A tongue protrusion to the side or an improper tongue position that causes the back teeth to be infraoccluding;
2. Abrasive tooth wear or erosion of the occlusal surface;
3. The posterior teeth's anterior tips pointing toward the extraction sites;
4. Continually sucking one's thumb.

To create a thorough diagnosis and treatment plan for each patient and achieve the best possible skeletal, dental, and esthetic outcomes, it is necessary to investigate the etiology of deep bites carefully.

1.2. Deep Bite Prevalence

Increased overbite, or deep bite, is defined as a vertical overlap of the incisors that is perpendicular to the occlusal plane and is quantified in millimeters (mm), proportionately (incisor overlap %), or subjectively (lower incisor contact with upper arch or palate). According to Nielsen (1991), skeletal origins of deep bite (low mandibular plane angle, decreased lower face height) and dentoalveolar origins (overeruption of the teeth) are the two most typical categories [15]. According to threshold values used, ethnic group, and gender, deep bite prevalence ranges from 8.4 to 51.5% and 5.9 to 15.9% of cases of palatal impingement and non-traumatic tooth contact have been documented [16–18]. Comparing Class II malocclusion to Class I malocclusion, Lux et al. (2009) found a strong correlation between the two and higher overbite [18]. A deep bite may be connected to Class II Division 2, which has a prevalence of 5.3% and is a less common malocclusion [19]. According to the literature, Upadhyay et al. (2008), angle Class I and II Division 2 malocclusions both exhibit an elevated overbite in conjunction with retrusive incisors [20].

2. Methods

2.1. Literature Search for Research on the Genetics of Deep Bite Development

The 2009 checklist, the GRADE criteria, and the PRISMA recommendations for systematic meta-analyses and reviews were all followed in this investigation. We searched for articles that discussed the genetic or epigenetic components of deep bite between the early 1990s and May 2023. We identified studies that met the following inclusion criteria: (1) original study or meta-analysis; (2) English-language writing; (3) deep bite in humans; (4) genetics of deep bite in humans; (5) prevalence of deep bite in humans; and (6) diagnosis and treatment of deep bite in humans. The following studies were disqualified from consideration: histopathologic, in vitro, or computational studies; transcriptomic or expression studies without epigenetic/genotyping analysis; reports focusing on other conditions and malocclusions that were merely discussed; and reports for which we lacked access to the full text or that were written in a different language. Using the search engines PubMed (National Library of Medicine) and Google Scholar (https://scholar.google.com, accessed on 1 April 2023), a study was conducted in the months of April and May 2023 using the terms "human deep bite", "genetics of human deep bite", "prevalence of human deep bite", "diagnosis of human deep bite", and "treatment of human deep bite". Three authors independently evaluated the titles and abstracts, evaluated the database search results, and considered carefully examining the work. Any disagreements were resolved through consensus during the title/abstract or complete article review rounds. Each qualifying study in this systematic review was formally assessed. Separately evaluated by the authors were the included studies' quality evaluation and bias risk.

2.2. Clinical Records and Ethical Statement

The demographic and clinical information for the analysis is obtained from the patient's orthodontic records. The gender, date of birth, age at treatment initiation, suggested treatment regimen, including extraction and non-extraction of premolars, and length of active orthodontic treatment. To estimate total treatment duration, the starting date is defined as the date of first molar band placement or first direct bonding, and the completion date is defined as the date of orthodontic retainer delivery. All clinical photos were obtained after signing a consent form by the patients to access their data.

2.3. Growth Considerations

There is general agreement that treating patients who are still developing makes correcting their deep bite easier and more stable than treating individuals who have stopped growing significantly [21]. It is generally beneficial to treat such patients at a phase of vigorous mandibular growth since growth tends to increase the vertical relationship between the maxillae and the mandible. Because condylar growth enables dentoalveolar growth during the growing period, tooth eruption can be induced in the posterior segments but repressed in the anterior. Even more so in a patient with a hypodivergent skeletal arrangement, the posterior occlusion prevents such a movement in adults. If such a tooth movement is carried out, its stability is really in doubt since it alters the physiology of the muscles, which raises the risk of recurrence. Fixed or removable appliances are required to produce the best treatment outcomes in these malocclusions and others where growth stimulation is no longer viable. Surgical intervention can be necessary for some patients with severe skeletal deformity.

2.4. Assessment of the Vertical Dimension

Varlık et al. (2013) recommended incisor intrusion as the best treatment for deep bite correction [22]; however, Mapare et al. [23] and others decided to treat the bulk of their patients with premolar and molar eruption. Instead of relying solely on anecdotal evidence, it is crucial to carefully analyze how extrusive or intrusive mechanics may change a patient's vertical facial height, which may then have an impact on how the maxilla and mandible are related anteriorly and posteriorly.

The interocclusal space, often known as the freeway [24], is the space between the occlusal or incisal surfaces of the mandibular and maxillary teeth when the jaw is in the physiological rest position. Between 2 and 4 mm is typical. More incredible options for correction occur when there is a larger-than-normal free space because vertical alveolar development can be guided. Increasing the lower facial height or face convexity, for instance, can cure the deep bite and enhance facial esthetics in Class II, Division 2 patients with a hypodivergent facial pattern, redundant lips, and a flat mandibular plane angle. The point A–point B discrepancy and an abnormally broad lower face would be accentuated in most other Class II malocclusions, though, and increasing the vertical dimension is not necessarily desirable in these cases.

2.5. Soft Tissue Evaluation

For deep bite correction in the modern era, "soft tissue relationships" are a critical diagnostic tool. When deciding whether to keep, intrude, or extrude the maxillary incisors relative to the upper lip, the clinician must always take the location of the teeth concerning the position of the lips into consideration. Dynamic smile analysis is becoming more popular than static grin photography for evaluating malocclusions and creating effective treatment regimens for their repair as the emphasis on smile esthetics and smile design grows [25].

During the initial assessment, the possibility of incisal exposure should be taken into account in three distinct clinical settings: speaking, a smile, and a relaxed lip position. An acceptable amount of incisor exposure in a relaxed lip position is between 2 and 4 mm, including the incisal margins. In a smile, the typical incisor exposure is about two thirds that of the upper incisor, according to Drummond and Capelli (2016) (Figure 6). Additionally, they stated that while females may have 1 to 2 mm of gingival exposure, most men's grins do not reveal any gingiva on the upper lip. The treatment strategy should concentrate on either posterior extrusion (if the vertical parameters permit it) or lower incisor intrusion if this criterion is met and a deep bite is still present (Figure 7). A selective intrusion of the upper incisors may be necessary if the occlusal plane is "significantly" below the ideal since this would display excessive gingiva (Figure 8). Since several separate facial muscles are used during the speech, incisor exposure may provide additional information. The "interlabial gap" is a crucial additional consideration. It would not be advisable to perform posterior extrusive mechanics on patients with a significant interlabial gap since this could make the patient's appearance worse by widening the interlabial gap. A widening of the interlabial gap can lead to several additional issues, including the inability to close the lips naturally and related functional issues. Comparably, posterior extrusive mechanics may be preferable in people who have redundant upper and lower lips or no interlabial gap but have an extreme overbite.

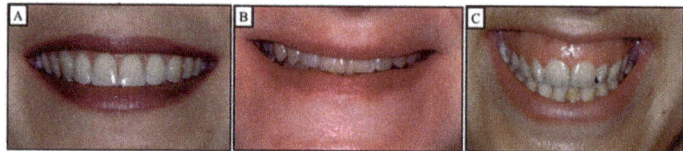

Figure 6. The different types of smiles. (**A**) shows an "Average smile"; the typical incisor exposure is 75–100% of the front tooth length. (**B**) shows a low smile; the typical incisor exposure is less than 75% of the front tooth length. (**C**) shows a "high smile"; the typical incisor exposure is more than 100% of the front tooth length with the appearance of the gingiva more than 2 mm.

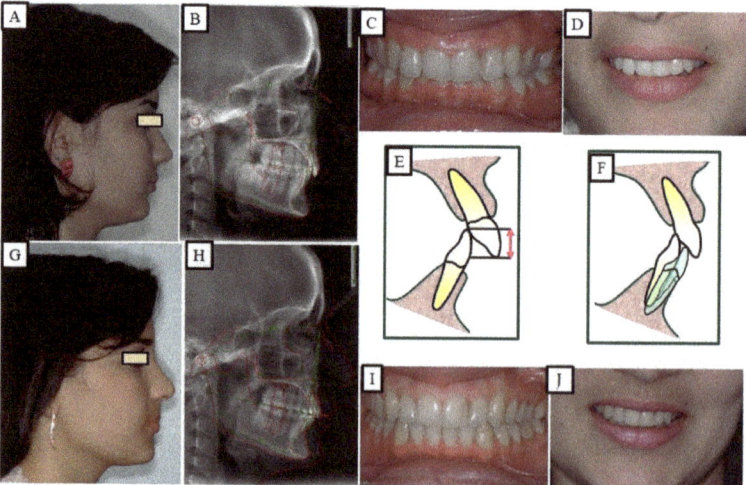

Figure 7. A patient with a deep bite. The treatment was achieved via the intrusion of the mandibular anterior teeth and simultaneous extrusion of the posterior teeth. (**A–E**) show before orthodontic treatment and show an average smile; therefore, the intrusion was performed in the mandibular anterior teeth. (**F–J**) show after orthodontic treatment.

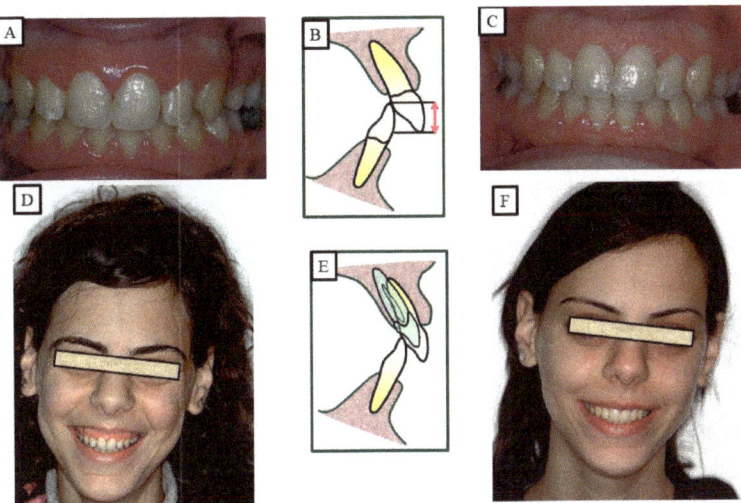

Figure 8. A patient with a deep bite and gummy smile, and the treatment was achieved by the intrusion of the maxillary anterior teeth. (**A–C**) show before orthodontic treatment, where the patient showed a high smile; therefore, the intrusion was performed in the maxillary anterior teeth. As a result of the intrusion and minimal gingivectomy, the gammy smile was significantly reduced or eliminated. (**D–F**) show after orthodontic treatment.

The incisors can also be flared (proclinated), which essentially hides deep bites. Patients who were born with retroclined incisors (Class II, Division 2 cases), for example, benefit from it the most. To reduce the danger of root resorption, gingival recession, and bone dehiscence, quick labial tipping of mandibular incisors must be avoided, particularly on a small symphysis with doubtful labio-lingual breadth of the alveolar bone [26]. Unwanted face esthetics are another possible contraindication.

2.6. Clinical Treatment of Deep Bite

Several studies have been conducted to investigate the genetic factors that contribute to this malocclusion [27]. The treatment of deep bite depends on various factors, including the severity and type of malocclusion, the patient's age and overall health, and other individualized considerations. The accompanying treatment approach and several etiologic factors will influence how deep bite correction is administered. However, as was already noted, there are three different techniques to cure deep bite malocclusions: intrusion of the upper and lower incisors, extrusion of the upper and lower posterior teeth, or a combination of the two. Similarly, orthodontic treatment is also the primary treatment for deep bite. The goal of treatment is to realign the teeth and jaws to achieve a more even bite. This may involve using braces, clear aligners, or other orthodontic appliances to move the teeth into the correct position. In more severe cases, orthognathic surgery may be necessary to correct the underlying skeletal issue causing the deep bite (Figure 9).

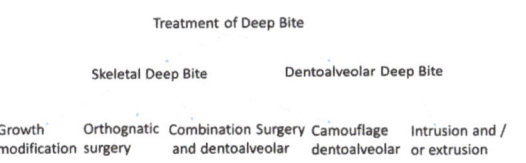

Figure 9. Diagram to illustrate the different types of treatment of deep bite; treatment variants of deep bite depending on age, stage of growth, cause of deep bite, function, and aesthetics.

According to Proffit and Fields [17], deep bites are the most typical malocclusion in children and adults. "Overbite more than 5 mm is found in nearly 20% of the children and 13% of the adults", claims [17]. If the patient does not want repair for aesthetic reasons, subjects with minor deep bites usually do not need to be corrected. Although it is a clinical issue, a significant overbite should be treated with orthodontic or orthosurgical intervention. According to Amarnath et al. [28], a severe overbite can damage the incisive papilla, wear down the teeth, disrupt mastication, affect the temporomandibular joint, and wear down the gums. A deep bite can be corrected using a variety of orthodontic techniques. The etiology of malocclusion and an analysis of the critical variables must be considered while choosing a treatment plan for each patient, as presented in Figures 10–14. One of the most significant issues facing orthodontists is the maintenance of a deep bite that has been repaired. Relapses following treatment are frequent when appropriate etiologic factor identification is not performed.

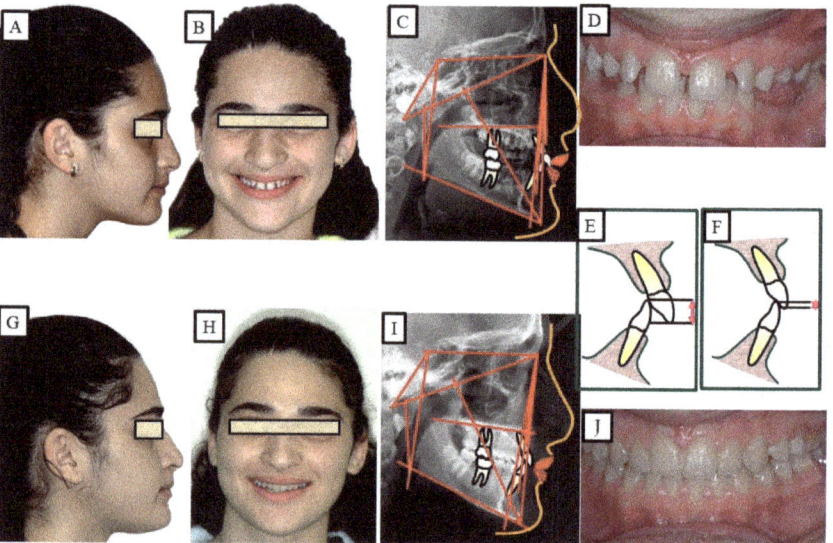

Figure 10. A young patient with dentoalveolar deep bite and average smile. The deep bite is corrected by the intrusion of the front teeth (especially the front of the lower jaw) and the extrusion of the posterior teeth. (**A**–**E**) show the case before orthodontic treatment, while (**F**–**J**) show after orthodontic treatment.

Moreover, technological advancements, such as 3D printing and computer-assisted design and manufacturing (CAD/CAM), are promising in treating malocclusion. These technologies for facilitate the creation of customized orthodontic appliances and surgical guides, thereby improving treatment precision and efficiency. Overall, a personalized treatment plan developed by a qualified orthodontic specialist is essential for achieving the best possible outcomes for the patient. Close consideration of the patient's age, overall health, and the severity and type of malocclusion is vital for successful treatment. Therefore, open communication between the patient and the orthodontist is crucial to create a plan that suits the patient's unique needs and expectations.

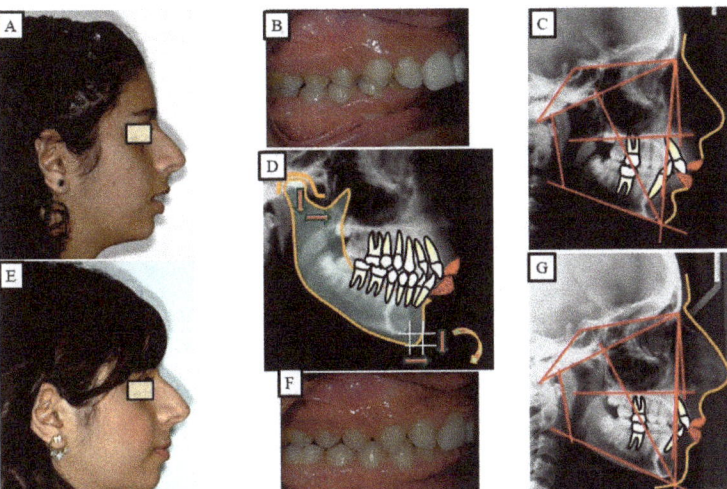

Figure 11. A young patient with Class II dysgnathy and deep bite (skeletal) in growing age. The correction of the deep skeletal bite is performed by influencing growth vertical; the condyle is the growth center. (**A–E**) show before orthodontic treatment. (**D**) shows a simulation of mandibular displacement through growth modification, a change in mandibular position due to growth in all dimensions. (**E–G**) show after orthodontic treatment.

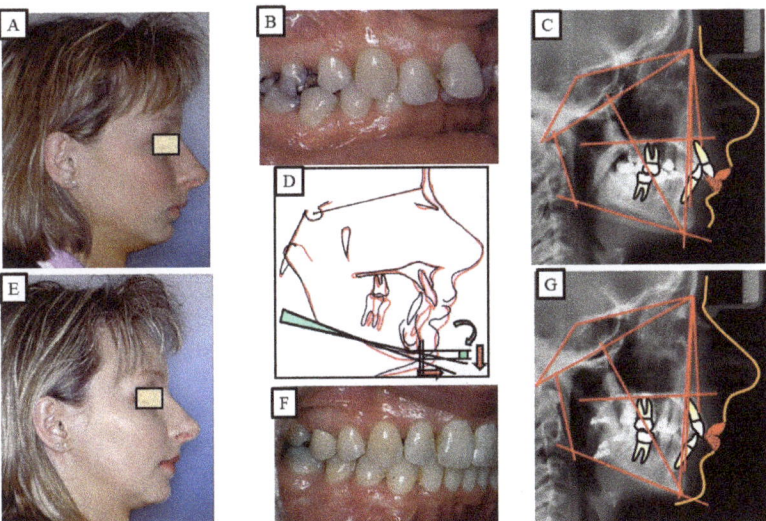

Figure 12. An adult patient with Class II dysgnathy and deep bite (skeletal). The correction of skeletal Class II and the skeletal deep bite is performed via combined orthodontic surgical treatment. Posterior rotation of the mandible during surgical mandibular advancement caused bite elevation and lengthening of the lower facial height. (**A–C**) show orthodontic surgical treatment. (**D**) shows the over-positioning of the pre-treatment (black) and post-treatment (red) radiographs due to the changes in sagittal and vertical dimensions. The surgical rotation of the mandible caused the opening of the mandibular angle, which led to the lengthening of the lower facial height. (**E–G**) show after orthodontic treatment.

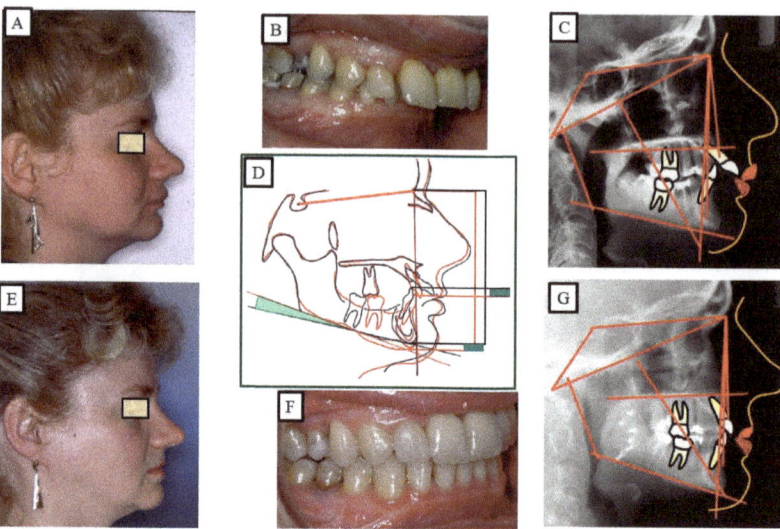

Figure 13. An adult patient with Class II dysgnathy and deep bite (skeletal and dentoalveolar). The correction of skeletal Class II and skeletal deep bite is performed via intrusion of the frontal teeth and combined orthodontic surgical treatment. Posterior rotation of the mandible during surgical mandibular advancement caused bite elevation and lengthening of the lower facial height. (**A–C**) show before orthodontic surgical treatment. (**D**) shows the over-positioning of the pre-treatment (black) and post-treatment (red) radiographs due to the changes in the sagittal and vertical dimensions. The surgical rotation of the mandible caused the opening of the mandibular angle, which led to the lengthening of the lower facial height. (**E–G**) show after orthodontic treatment.

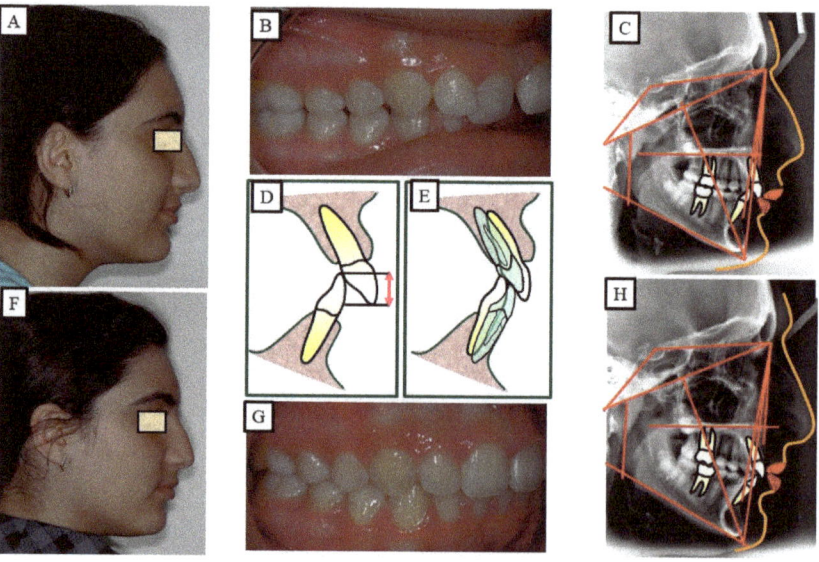

Figure 14. An adult patient with Class II dysgnathy and deep bite (skeletal and dentoalveolar). The correction of skeletal Class II and the skeletal deep bite is performed via camouflage therapy, intrusion and protrusion of the frontal teeth, and extraction of the posterior teeth. (**A–D**) show before orthodontic surgical treatment, while (**E–H**) show after orthodontic treatment.

2.7. Utilizing Mouse Models and Collaborative Cross Populations to Explore Phenotypes of Deep Bite

Dental conditions such as deep bite can significantly impact an individual's oral health and quality of life. Exploration the underlying genetic and environmental factors contributing to these conditions are crucial for developing effective treatment strategies. Mouse has shown similar vulnerability to numerous infections and environmental factors to humans; therefore, many restrictions in studies of human populations can be overcome. Mouse models and collaborative cross populations have emerged as valuable tools for studying complex traits and uncovering the intricate mechanisms involved in dental disorders. This article explores how these innovative approaches can shed light on the phenotypes of deep bite, offering new insights into their etiology and potential therapeutic interventions [29].

Unveiling the Genetic Basis Mouse models provide a powerful platform for investigating the genetic factors contributing to deep bite. By manipulating specific genes or introducing mutations, researchers can create mice with dental phenotypes resembling these conditions. Studying these models allows researchers to identify candidate genes involved in the development and maintenance of dental occlusion. Furthermore, by utilizing knockout or knock-in mouse models, scientists can investigate the effects of specific genes and their interactions on dental morphology and occlusal relationships [30].

Standard laboratory mouse lines, however, contain little genetic variety and are therefore only marginally relevant for researching diverse genetic manifestations within complex disorders. To address this, the collaborative cross (CC), genetically varied recombinant inbred mouse lines were created. The CC mouse lines were developed to be an emerging technique for precise genomic mapping and characterization of the genetic components behind complex phenotypes, focusing on critical importance to human health. The requirement to simulate genetic diversity led to the formation of the mouse CC genetic reference population (GRP). This one-of-a-kind GRP source is a large panel of recombinant inbred (RI) strains created particularly for complex trait research from a genetically heterogeneous group of eight founder breeds [7,8,10] suggesting a strength over any previously reported approach [9]. This unique resource is a large panel of recombinant inbred (RI) strains derived from a genetically diverse set of eight founder strains and designed specifically for complex trait analysis [9,31], and suggests a power than any reported approaches earlier [32–35]. The founder strains are genetically varied, comprising three wild generated strain founders (CAST/Ei, PWK/PhJ, and WSB/EiJ) and five common laboratory strains (A/J, C57BL/6J, 129S1/SvImJ, NOD/LtJ, and NZO/HiLtJ). The substantial genetic variation of the final group of CC mice is a result of this divergence. An entirely different genetic mosaic can be created in a new CC line by altering the sequence of the founder strains during the outbreed mating stage. As a result, each CC line's genetic component is distinct and has genotypes that are stable and well known. Compared to previous mouse sets, this genetic reference population (GRP) contains a comparatively high degree of recombination events (4.4 million SNPS segregate between the founders), two times the number of genetic differences present in the normal human population (about 36 million SNPs). The latest QTL assessment stimulation research utilizing the CC population revealed that the mapped interval's resolution may be less than one Mb [32–35].

Collaborative cross (CC) populations offer a unique opportunity to dissect the complex nature of deep bite. The CC is a panel of genetically diverse recombinant inbred mouse strains derived from multiple founder strains. This diversity enables researchers to study the effects of genetic variation on phenotypic variability. By phenotyping the dental occlusion of CC mice, researchers can identify genetic loci associated with deep bite traits. Subsequent mapping studies can pinpoint specific genomic regions and candidate genes contributing to the observed phenotypes, facilitating a deeper understanding of the underlying biology [36]. In addition to genetic factors, environmental influences play a critical role in developing dental occlusion abnormalities. The CC mouse genetic reference population (GRP) allows researchers to investigate gene–environment interactions by subjecting CC mice to various environmental conditions or exposures. By manipulating factors such as diet, mechanical loading, or hormonal influences, researchers can evaluate how these external variables interact with genetic predispositions to affect dental occlusion. This multifaceted approach provides insights into the complex interplay between genetic and environmental factors in the development of deep bite and open bite.

It should be possible to run GWAS on CC breeds, identify crucial quantitative trait loci (QTL), discover candidate genes, and define modifiers for the key genes linked to the Deep bite features while under minimal levels of external sources of variance. It is strongly believed that the tremendous genetic diversity of the CC mice strains offers a good foundation for finding novel genetic loci connected to these described traits and going forward with confirmation utilizing conditional knockout techniques and mouse knockout genes.

The knowledge gained from mouse models and CC populations can be translated into human dentistry, improving diagnostic and therapeutic strategies. Understanding the genetic and environmental factors underlying deep bite in mouse models enables researchers to identify potential biomarkers and genetic risk factors in humans. These findings may inform the development of targeted interventions and personalized treatment approaches. Furthermore, mouse models allow for preclinical testing of novel therapeutic interventions, such as gene therapies or pharmacological treatments, before translating them into clinical trials [29,37]. The workflow diagram for the generation of system genetic datasets of cellular, molecular, and clinical trait data combined to analyze various correlations between malocclusion and deep bite phenotypes in human and mouse models are represented in Figure 15.

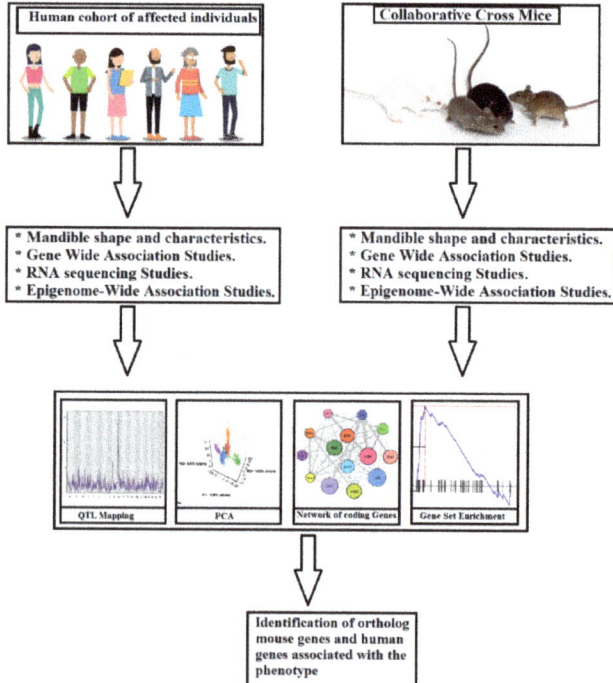

Figure 15. Workflow for creating system genetic databases from the extremely heterogeneous CC population, whose propensity to develop deep bite malocclusion may vary greatly. To check for deep bite malocclusion, mice are examined. Then, different associations between malocclusion and deep bite characteristics are analyzed using a combination of cellular, molecular, and clinical trait data. The regulatory genomic areas are implicated in phenotypic variation in both in vitro and in vivo monitored traits and can be identified using QTL mapping by merging SNP genotype data from each CC lineage. Finding susceptibility genes linked to the emergence of deep bite in humans may be possible by combining data with later candidate gene association studies in humans.

3. Discussion

Excessive vertical overlapping of the mandibular incisors by the maxillary incisors in a centric occlusion is also known as a deep bite or deep overbite. The normal overbite is between one and three millimeters, and the incisal margins of the lower teeth should touch the upper teeth's cingulum or just above it. According to Sreedhar and Baratam (2009), the average overbite is roughly 30%, or one third, of the mandibular incisors' clinical crown height because of variations in their length [38]. Numerous researchers have examined the skeletal and dental patterns associated with deep bite malocclusion. Deep bite malocclusion was found to be associated with a decreased gonial angle, a deep curve of the spee, a smaller posterior maxilla, a downward rotation of the palatal plane, and a more forward position of the ramus, according to research by Fattahi et al. (2014), who examined the morphologic factors in deep bite and patients [14]. Alveolar and skeletal dimensions related to overbites and reduced facial height were evaluated by Beckmann et al. [39]. They hypothesized that a deeper bite was associated with decreased lower facial height, bigger anterior alveolar and basal regions, and retroinclination of the maxillary incisors [39]. In their 2004 study, Bydass et al. examined how overbite and overjet were affected by the depth of the spee curve. Because of the lower anterior teeth that protruded, there was an increase in overbite in the deep curve of the spee [40]. According to Ceylan and Eroz (2001), an overbite can change how the mandible and maxilla look and is linked to a smaller gonial angle [41]. In participants with a deep bite and a normal overbite, Al-Zubaidi and Obaidi (2006) measured the lower facial height (LFH) [42]. They discovered no variations in the LFH, maxillary and mandibular anterior alveolar, and basal height between the two groups. El-Dawlatly et al. (2012) assessed skeletal and dental parameters in patients with deep bite malocclusion. They demonstrated that deep bite has a multi-factorial etiology, with the exaggerated curve of spee and a decreased gonial angle being the main contributing factors [43]. Naumann et al. (2000) investigated the vertical elements of overbite alteration in a longitudinal study. Their study revealed that skeletal elements had a more significant impact on overbite modification than dental elements and that the mandible had a more significant impact on overbite modification than the maxilla [44].

According to earlier research, the maxillary dentoalveolar region is where a deep bite and a typical bite vary. Dentoalveolar morphology of the upper and lower jaws, according to Betzenberger et al. [45], was the cause of overbite alterations. This study aims to identify the most common dental and skeletal contributing variables to deep bite malocclusion and the effects of skeletal and dentoalveolar characteristics on deep bite malocclusion. Undoubtedly, practitioners are better equipped to provide the most effective care when fully aware of the dental and skeletal causes of deep bite malocclusion [45].

To enable any future reconstructive dental surgery, reduce increased tooth wear, and lessen tissue stress from tooth contact, treatment of deep bite malocclusion is advised [46]. When malocclusion returns years after the conclusion of treatment, patients may request a second opinion or start to doubt the value of their previous therapy. Thus, stability over the long run appears to be more crucial than the actual outcome. Even in cases that have received the best care possible, relapse—a dentoalveolar and skeletal change that occurs after orthodontic treatment and returns the mouth to its original malocclusion—is frequently seen [47]. These alterations are attributed to natural restoration of force homeostasis [17], periodontal remodeling [48], growth, or normal/abnormal development (Iseri and Solow (1996)). Some investigators (Al Yami et al. (1999)) found a constant relapse of all malocclusion characteristics and the loss of around one third of the orthodontic treatment outcome over a ten-year period of follow-up [49]. Thus, one of orthodontics' greatest challenges is maintaining the stability of the orthodontic outcome.

Dental deep bite cases are said to have relapsed if their overbite increases after therapy is complete. Deep bite malocclusions are said to be prone to relapse in a number of writers [50]. A sample with a deep bite and retroclined incisors was evaluated by Lapatki et al. (2004), who discovered 20% vertical relapse on average two years after treatment. In research examining samples with different malocclusions, a number of conclusions involving deep bite relapse are documented [51]. A total of 21 out of 31 cases in which the spee curve in a Class II Division 1 sample was examined showed a steady relapse over the years or decades [52]. In a similar vein, a Class II Division 2 sample from Canut and Arias (1999) discovered a positive connection between years out of retention and overbite relapse [53]. Despite using removable retention for a year, 80% of patients with short facial types experienced a rise in overbite 2 years after treatment was finished [54].

Growth [55], function [56], and incisor overeruption [57] are some of the factors that might contribute to the formation of a deep bite and may also do so in the case of a relapse. Pre-treatment severity of malocclusion and relapse were not significantly correlated, and mandibular intercanine width, overbite, overjet, mandibular incisor irregularity, or arch length were not able to predict relapse, according to Preston et al. [58]. No matter the method of treatment, the authors discovered a much higher prevalence of relapse in patients whose dentitions had not fully leveled at the end of the procedure. Different relapse rates regardless of the method of treatment were not demonstrated by a number of authors [58]. An overbite relapse was linked in one research to mandibular incisors that protruded after orthodontic treatment. It is currently not possible to anticipate an individual's risk of relapse following deep bite therapy because there is neither a systematic review of deep bite retention, stability, or relapse, nor is there any way to determine if a person would experience either.

A significant overbite is one of the issues that orthodontists address the most commonly. According to Sonnesen and Svensson [59], deep bite has been linked to aberrant mandibular function, TMJ issues, and may harm mandibular development. Horiuchi et al. [60] have identified a similar association. Because of this, correcting a deep bite is frequently a crucial part of orthodontic care. It is commonly acknowledged that correcting a deep bite on a patient who is still growing is easier and more stable than trying to do it on someone who has stopped growing significantly [61]. Invasion of the occlusal highway and the correction's opposition to the robust, mature jaw musculature, which is less adaptable to elongation, have both been identified as causes for the greater relapse potential in adults [62]. Additionally, any tooth movement affects the functional equilibrium that is established during growth and maturity [63]. Through the process of growth and development, the skeletodental and soft-tissue components structurally adapt to one another to create a functionally balanced condition [64]. A shift in the mandibular muscular balance takes place because widening the bite is typically performed via protrusion of posterior teeth [13]. If the correction is to stay stable, either the musculature must adjust in some way to its new functional resting length or the bone arrangement must alter. There are various places in the mandible that have been proven to be able to respond to environmental challenges; it is possible that compensatory development will occur in these sites.

After receiving orthodontic treatment for a moderate deep bite, there was little evidence of vertical relapse 12 years later. If the incisor overlap increased by more than 50% during the follow-up, it was considered a relapse. At long-term follow-up, 90% of the patients displayed normal vertical relations, while 10% of them displayed relapse with a modest median increase of 6.7%. The prevalence and severity of deep bite relapse were relatively low and clinically negligible in instances with mild dentoalveolar deep bite that had undergone effective treatment, retention by fixed retainers, and a temporary removable upper plate.

When facial types were evaluated, a recent study indicated that individuals with high angles had a decreased propensity to relapse than patients with normal or low angles [65]. The relatively lengthy treatment period suggests that the majority of the periodontal remodeling [66] had already occurred at the time of debonding, and it is not anticipated that it would have significantly contributed to the relapse. Treatment options include fixed appliances with or without extraction, removable appliances with or without extractions, and in more severe cases, maxillofacial surgery to treat the deep bite [67]. There have been numerous therapeutic approaches and combinations employed, including maxillofacial surgery, as presented in Figures 12 and 13. There are three possible ways to level the arch/curve of spee and treat deep bite malocclusion with orthodontics: (1) lower and/or upper incisor intrusion [68]; (2) labial inclination of the incisors (pseudo-intrusion); and (3) extrusion of posterior teeth possibly associated with a clockwise rotation of the mandible, which would increase lower face height [47]. According to Bernstein et al. [52], this hypothetical clockwise rotation does not always appear to take place. The available literature cannot be used to draw any conclusions about the efficacy of treating Class II Division 2 malocclusion in children [69]. Different treatment approaches and combinations were used to stabilize deep bites.

The development of skeletal structures is somewhat influenced by the environment and partially by genetics, as this article has shown. It is therefore impossible to discount the significance of the hereditary foundation of malocclusions. The practice of genetically supported orthodontics has advanced significantly. However, because most malocclusions and dental malformations are polygenic, it is very difficult to identify the hereditary basis of these conditions. The mapping of inherited conditions pertaining to dentofacial development has been possible because to the information provided by the human genome project. To accurately identify all the unique genes responsible for each type of skeletal diversity, additional genetic research is necessary. A genetic correction of genetically regulated abnormalities and malocclusions may be possible in the near future due to the field's rapid advancement.

Author Contributions: Conceptualization, F.A.I., P.P. and N.W.; Methodology, I.M.L., O.Z. and K.M.; Validation, F.A.I.; Investigation, I.M.L., O.Z., K.M. and N.W.; Resources, F.A.I., P.P. and N.W; Data Curation, I.M.L., O.Z. and K.M.; Writing—Original Draft Preparation, O.Z. and I.M.L.; Writing—Review and Editing, P.P., N.W. and F.A.I.; Supervision, F.A.I., P.P. and N.W.; Project Administration, F.A.I.; Funding Acquisition, F.A.I., P.P. and N.W. All authors have read and agreed to the published version of the manuscript.

Funding: This study was supported by a core fund from Tel Aviv University, Arab American University in Jenin, and the University Hospital of Regensburg.

Institutional Review Board Statement: Ethical review and approval were waived for this study since there was no intervention procedure involved with patients or biological sample collection. However, we used ICS from patients for using their cephalometric images.

Informed Consent Statement: Informed consent was obtained from all subjects involved in the study.

Data Availability Statement: Not applicable.

Conflicts of Interest: The authors declare no conflict of interest.

References

1. Achmad, H.; Noor Armedina, R.; Timokhina, T.; Goncharov, V.V.; Sitanaya, R.; Riyanti, E. Literature Review: Problems of Dental and Oral Health Primary School Children. *Indian J. Forensic Med. Toxicol.* **2021**, *15*, 4146–4162. [CrossRef]
2. Neela, P.K.; Atteeri, A.; Mamillapalli, P.K.; Sesham, V.M.; Keesara, S.; Chandra, J.; Monica, U.; Mohan, V. Genetics of Dentofacial and Orthodontic Abnormalities. *Glob. Med. Genet.* **2020**, *7*, 95. [CrossRef]
3. Moreno Uribe, L.M.; Miller, S.F. Genetics of the Dentofacial Variation in Human Malocclusion. *Orthod. Craniofac. Res.* **2015**, *18*, 91. [CrossRef] [PubMed]
4. Zebrick, B.; Teeramongkolgul, T.; Nicot, R.; Horton, M.J.; Raoul, G.; Ferri, J.; Vieira, A.R.; Sciote, J.J. ACTN3 R577X Genotypes Associate with Class II and Deepbite Malocclusions. *Am. J. Orthod. Dentofacial. Orthop.* **2014**, *146*, 603–611. [CrossRef] [PubMed]
5. Soni, R.; Vivek, R.; Srivastava, A.; Singh, A.; Srivastava, S.; Chaturvedi, T.P. Van Der Woude Syndrome Associated with Hypodontia: A Rare Clinical Entity. *Case Rep. Dent.* **2012**, *2012*, 1–3. [CrossRef]
6. Doraczynska-Kowalik, A.; Nelke, K.H.; Pawlak, W.; Sasiadek, M.M.; Gerber, H. Genetic Factors Involved in Mandibular Prognathism. *J. Craniofacial Surg.* **2017**, *28*, e422–e431. [CrossRef] [PubMed]
7. Lone, I.M.; Midlej, K.; Ben Nun, N.; Iraqi, F.A. Intestinal Cancer Development in Response to Oral Infection with High-Fat Diet-Induced Type 2 Diabetes (T2D) in Collaborative Cross Mice under Different Host Genetic Background Effects. *Mamm. Genome* **2023**, *34*, 56–75. [CrossRef] [PubMed]
8. Lone, I.M.; Iraqi, F.A. Genetics of Murine Type 2 Diabetes and Comorbidities. *Mamm. Genome* **2022**, *33*, 421–436. [CrossRef] [PubMed]
9. Lone, I.M.; Ben Nun, N.; Ghnaim, A.; Schaefer, A.S.; Houri-Haddad, Y.; Iraqi, F.A. High-Fat Diet and Oral Infection Induced Type 2 Diabetes and Obesity Development under Different Genetic Backgrounds. *Anim. Model. Exp. Med.* **2023**, *6*, 131–145. [CrossRef]

10. Ghnaim, A.; Lone, I.M.; Ben Nun, N.; Iraqi, F.A. Unraveling the Host Genetic Background Effect on Internal Organ Weight Influenced by Obesity and Diabetes Using Collaborative Cross Mice. *Int. J. Mol. Sci.* **2023**, *24*, 8201. [CrossRef]
11. Huh, A.; Horton, M.J.; Cuenco, K.T.; Raoul, G.; Rowlerson, A.M.; Ferri, J.; Sciote, J.J. Epigenetic Influence of KAT6B and HDAC4 in the Development of Skeletal Malocclusion. *Am. J. Orthod. Dentofac. Orthop.* **2013**, *144*, 568–576. [CrossRef]
12. Kundakovic, M.; Jaric, I. The Epigenetic Link between Prenatal Adverse Environments and Neurodevelopmental Disorders. *Genes* **2017**, *8*, 104. [CrossRef]
13. Bardideh, E.; Tamizi, G.; Shafaee, H.; Rangrazi, A.; Ghorbani, M.; Kerayechian, N. The Effects of Intrusion of Anterior Teeth by Skeletal Anchorage in Deep Bite Patients; A Systematic Review and Meta-Analysis. *Biomimetics* **2023**, *8*, 101. [CrossRef] [PubMed]
14. Fattahi, H.; Pakshir, H.; Afzali Baghdadabadi, N.; Shahian Jahromi, S.; Afzali Baghdadabadi, N. Skeletal and Dentoalveolar Features in Patients with Deep Overbite Malocclusion. *J. Dent.* **2014**, *11*, 629.
15. Nielsen, I.L. Vertical Malocclusions: Etiology, Development, Diagnosis and Some Aspects of Treatment. *Angle Orthod.* **1991**, *61*, 247–260. [PubMed]
16. Tausche, E.; Luck, O.; Harzer, W. Prevalence of Malocclusions in the Early Mixed Dentition and Orthodontic Treatment Need. *Eur. J. Orthod.* **2004**, *26*, 237–244. [CrossRef] [PubMed]
17. Proffit, W.R.; Fields, H.W.; Larson, B.; Sarver, D.M. *Contemporary Orthodontics-e-Book*; Elsevier Health Sciences: Amsterdam, The Netherlands, 2018.
18. Lux, C.J.; Dücker, B.; Pritsch, M.; Komposch, G.; Niekusch, U. Occlusal Status and Prevalence of Occlusal Malocclusion Traits among 9-Year-Old Schoolchildren. *Eur. J. Orthod.* **2009**, *31*, 294–299. [CrossRef]
19. Ota, K.; Arai, K. Prevalence and Patterns of Tooth Agenesis in Angle Class II Division 2 Malocclusion in Japan. *Am. J. Orthod. Dentofac. Orthop.* **2015**, *148*, 123–129. [CrossRef]
20. Upadhyay, M.; Nagaraj, K.; Yadav, S.; Saxena, R. Mini-Implants for En Masse Intrusion of Maxillary Anterior Teeth in a Severe Class II Division 2 Malocclusion. *J. Orthod.* **2008**, *35*, 79–89. [CrossRef] [PubMed]
21. Huang, G.J.; Bates, S.B.; Ehlert, A.A.; Whiting, D.P.; Chen, S.S.H.; Bollen, A.M. Stability of Deep-Bite Correction: A Systematic Review. *J. World Fed. Orthod.* **2012**, *1*, e89–e96. [CrossRef]
22. Varlik, S.K.; Alpakan, Ö.O.; Türköz, Ç. Deepbite Correction with Incisor Intrusion in Adults: A Long-Term Cephalometric Study. *Am. J. Orthod. Dentofac. Orthop.* **2013**, *144*, 414–419. [CrossRef] [PubMed]
23. Mapare, S.; Mundada, R.; Karra, A.; Agrawal, S.; Mahajan, S.; Tadawalkar, A. Extraction or Nonextraction in Orthodontic Cases: A Review. *J. Pharm. Bioallied Sci.* **2021**, *13*, 2–5.
24. Vinnakota, D.N.; Kanneganti, K.C.; Pulagam, M.; Karnati, P.K.R. Freeway Space Determination Using Lateral Profile Photographs: A Pilot Study. *J. Indian Prosthodont. Soc.* **2016**, *16*, 242–247. [CrossRef]
25. Mahn, E.; Sampaio, C.S.; Pereira da Silva, B.; Stanley, K.; Valdés, A.M.; Gutierrez, J.; Coachman, C. Comparing the Use of Static versus Dynamic Images to Evaluate a Smile. *J. Prosthet. Dent.* **2020**, *123*, 739–746. [CrossRef]
26. Mazurova, K.; Kopp, J.B.; Renkema, A.M.; Pandis, N.; Katsaros, C.; Fudalej, P.S. Gingival Recession in Mandibular Incisors and Symphysis Morphology-a Retrospective Cohort Study. *Eur. J. Orthod.* **2018**, *40*, 185–192. [CrossRef]
27. Cakan, D.G.; Ulkur, F.; Taner, T.U. The Genetic Basis of Facial Skeletal Characteristics and Its Relation with Orthodontics. *Eur. J. Dent.* **2012**, *6*, 340–345. [CrossRef] [PubMed]
28. Bc, A. Clinical Overview of Deep Bite Management. *Int. J. Contemp. Dent.* **2010**, *1*, 30.
29. Lone, I.M.; Zohud, O.; Nashef, A.; Kirschneck, C.; Proff, P.; Watted, N.; Iraqi, F.A. Dissecting the Complexity of Skeletal-Malocclusion-Associated Phenotypes: Mouse for the Rescue. *Int. J. Mol. Sci.* **2023**, *24*, 2570. [CrossRef] [PubMed]
30. Carver, E.A.; Oram, K.F.; Gridley, T. Craniosynostosis in Twist Heterozygous Mice: A Model for Saethre-Chotzen Syndrome. *Anat. Rec.* **2002**, *268*, 90–92. [CrossRef]
31. Zohud, O.; Lone, I.M.; Midlej, K.; Obaida, A.; Masarwa, S.; Schröder, A.; Küchler, E.C.; Nashef, A.; Kassem, F.; Reiser, V.; et al. Towards Genetic Dissection of Skeletal Class III Malocclusion: A Review of Genetic Variations Underlying the Phenotype in Humans and Future Directions. *J. Clin. Med.* **2023**, *12*, 3212. [CrossRef] [PubMed]
32. Iraqi, F.A.; Mahajne, M.; Salaymah, Y.; Sandovski, H.; Tayem, H.; Vered, K.; Balmer, L.; Hall, M.; Manship, G.; Morahan, G.; et al. The Genome Architecture of the Collaborative Cross Mouse Genetic Reference Population. *Genetics* **2012**, *190*, 389–401. [CrossRef]
33. Levy, R.; Mott, R.F.; Iraqi, F.A.; Gabet, Y. Collaborative Cross Mice in a Genetic Association Study Reveal New Candidate Genes for Bone Microarchitecture. *BMC Genom.* **2015**, *16*, 1013. [CrossRef]
34. Lone, I.M.; Zohud, O.; Midlej, K.; Proff, P.; Watted, N.; Iraqi, F.A. Skeletal Class II Malocclusion: From Clinical Treatment Strategies to the Roadmap in Identifying the Genetic Bases of Development in Humans with the Support of the Collaborative Cross Mouse Population. *J. Clin. Med.* **2023**, *12*, 5148. [CrossRef] [PubMed]
35. Dorman, A.; Baer, D.; Tomlinson, I.; Mott, R.; Iraqi, F.A. Genetic Analysis of Intestinal Polyp Development in Collaborative Cross Mice Carrying the Apc Min/+ Mutation. *BMC Genet.* **2016**, *17*, 1–11.
36. Iraqi, F.A.; Churchill, G.; Mott, R. The Collaborative Cross, Developing a Resource for Mammalian Systems Genetics: A Status Report of the Wellcome Trust Cohort. *Mamm. Genome* **2008**, *19*, 379–381. [CrossRef] [PubMed]
37. Yehia, R.; Lone, I.M.; Yehia, I.; Iraqi, F.A. Studying the Pharmagenomic Effect of Portulaca Oleracea Extract on Anti-Diabetic Therapy Using the Collaborative Cross Mice. *Phytomedicine Plus* **2023**, *3*, 100394. [CrossRef]
38. Sreedhar, C.; Baratam, S. Deep Overbite—A Review (Deep Bite, Deep Overbite, Excessive Overbite). *Ann. Essences Dent.* **2009**, *I*, 8–25. [CrossRef]

39. Beckmann, S.H.; Kuitert, R.B.; Prahl-Andersen, B.; Segner, D.; The, R.P.; Tuinzing, D.B. Alveolar and Skeletal Dimensions Associated with Lower Face Height. *Am. J. Orthod. Dentofac. Orthop.* **1998**, *113*, 498–506. [CrossRef]
40. Baydaş, B.; Yavuz, I.; Atasaral, N.; Ceylan, I.; Dağsuyu, I.M. Investigation of the Changes in the Positions of Upper and Lower Incisors, Overjet, Overbite, and Irregularity Index in Subjects with Different Depths of Curve of Spee. *Angle Orthod.* **2004**, *74*, 349–355.
41. Ceylan, I.; Eröz, Ü.B. The Effects of Overbite on the Maxillary and Mandibular Morphology. *Angle Orthod.* **2001**, *71*, 110–115.
42. Al-Zubaidi, S.; Obaidi, H. The Variation of the Lower Anterior Facial Height and Its Component Parameters among the Three over Bite Relationships (Cephalometric Study). *Al-Rafidain Dent. J.* **2006**, *6*, 106–113. [CrossRef]
43. El-Dawlatly, M.M.; Fayed, M.M.S.; Mostafa, Y.A. Deep Overbite Malocclusion: Analysis of the Underlying Components. *Am. J. Orthod. Dentofac. Orthop.* **2012**, *142*, 473–480. [CrossRef] [PubMed]
44. Naumann, S.A.; Behrents, R.G.; Buschang, P.H. Vertical Components of Overbite Change: A Mathematical Model. *Am. J. Orthod. Dentofac. Orthop.* **2000**, *117*, 486–495. [CrossRef] [PubMed]
45. Betzenberger, D.; Ruf, S.; Pancherz, H. The Compensatory Mechanism in High-Angle Malocclusions: A Comparison of Subjects in the Mixed and Permanent Dentition. *Angle Orthod.* **1999**, *69*, 27–32. [PubMed]
46. Silness, J.; Johannessen, G.; Røynstrand, T. Longitudinal Relationship between Incisal Occlusion and Incisal Tooth Wear. *Acta Odontol. Scand.* **1993**, *51*, 15–21. [CrossRef] [PubMed]
47. Danz, J.C.; Greuter, C.; Sifakakis, L.; Fayed, M.; Pandis, N.; Katsaros, C. Stability and Relapse after Orthodontic Treatment of Deep Bite Cases—A Long-Term Follow-up Study. *Eur. J. Orthod.* **2014**, *36*, 522–530. [CrossRef] [PubMed]
48. Ackerman, J.L.; Proffit, W.R. Soft Tissue Limitations in Orthodontics: Treatment Planning Guidelines. *Angle Orthod.* **1997**, *67*, 327–336.
49. Al Yami, E.A.; Kuijpers-Jagtman, A.M.; Van't Hof, M.A. Orthodontic Treatment Need Prior to Treatment and 5 Years Postretention. *Community Dent. Oral Epidemiol.* **1998**, *26*, 421–427. [CrossRef]
50. Piancino, M.G.; Tortarolo, A.; Di Benedetto, L.; Crincoli, V.; Falla, D. Chewing Patterns and Muscular Activation in Deep Bite Malocclusion. *J. Clin. Med.* **2022**, *11*, 1702. [CrossRef]
51. Lapatki, B.G.; Klatt, A.; Schulte-Mönting, J.; Stein, S.; Jonas, I.E. A Retrospective Cephalometric Study for the Quantitative Assessment of Relapse Factors in Cover-Bite Treatment. *J. Orofac. Orthop./Fortschritte Der Kieferorthopadie* **2004**, *65*, 475–488. [CrossRef]
52. Bernstein, R.L.; Preston, C.B.; Lampasso, J. Leveling the Curve of Spee with a Continuous Archwire Technique: A Long Term Cephalometric Study. *Am. J. Orthod. Dentofac. Orthop.* **2007**, *131*, 363–371. [CrossRef]
53. Canut, J.A.; Arias, S. A Long-Term Evaluation of Treated Class II Division 2 Malocclusions: A Retrospective Study Model Analysis. *Eur. J. Orthod.* **1999**, *21*, 377–386. [CrossRef]
54. Zaher, A.R.; Bishara, S.E.; Jakobsen, J.R. Posttreatment Changes in Different Facial Types. *Angle Orthod.* **1994**, *64*, 425–436. [PubMed]
55. Baccetti, T.; Franchi, L.; McNamara, J.A. Longitudinal Growth Changes in Subjects with Deepbite. *Am. J. Orthod. Dentofac. Orthop.* **2011**, *140*, 202–209. [CrossRef] [PubMed]
56. Sciote, J.J.; Horton, M.J.; Rowlerson, A.M.; Ferri, J.; Close, J.M.; Raoul, G. Human Masseter Muscle Fiber Type Properties, Skeletal Malocclusions, and Muscle Growth Factor Expression. *J. Oral Maxillofac. Surg.* **2012**, *70*, 440–448. [CrossRef]
57. Lowe, A.A.; Santamaria, J.D.; Fleetham, J.A.; Price, C. Facial Morphology and Obstructive Sleep Apnea. *Am. J. Orthod. Dentofac. Orthop.* **1986**, *90*, 484–491. [CrossRef]
58. Preston, C.B.; Maggard, M.B.; Lampasso, J.; Chalabi, O. Long-Term Effectiveness of the Continuous and the Sectional Archwire Techniques in Leveling the Curve of Spee. *Am. J. Orthod. Dentofac. Orthop.* **2008**, *133*, 550–555. [CrossRef]
59. Sonnesen, L.; Svensson, P. Temporomandibular Disorders and Psychological Status in Adult Patients with a Deep Bite. *Eur. J. Orthod.* **2008**, *30*, 621–629. [CrossRef] [PubMed]
60. Horiuchi, Y.; Horiuchi, M.; Soma, K. Treatment of Severe Class II Division 1 Deep Overbite Malocclusion without Extractions in an Adult. *Am. J. Orthod. Dentofac. Orthop.* **2008**, *133*, S121–S129. [CrossRef]
61. Daokar, S.; Agrawal, G. Deep Bite Its Etiology, Diagnosis and Management: A Review. *J. Orthod. Endod.* **2016**, *2*, 4. [CrossRef]
62. Mew, J.R.C. The Postural Basis of Malocclusion: A Philosophical Overview. *Am. J. Orthod. Dentofac. Orthop.* **2004**, *126*, 729–738. [CrossRef]
63. Masella, R.S.; Meister, M. Current Concepts in the Biology of Orthodontic Tooth Movement. *Am. J. Orthod. Dentofac. Orthop.* **2006**, *129*, 458–468. [CrossRef] [PubMed]
64. Cheong, Y.W.; Lo, L.J. Facial Asymmetry: Etiology, Evaluation, and Management. *Chang. Gung Med. J.* **2011**, *34*, 341–351. [PubMed]
65. Pollard, D.; Akyalcin, S.; Wiltshire, W.A.; Rody, W.J. Relapse of Orthodontically Corrected Deepbites in Accordance with Growth Pattern. *Am. J. Orthod. Dentofac. Orthop.* **2012**, *141*, 477–483. [CrossRef] [PubMed]
66. Kilic, N.; Oktay, H.; Ersoz, M. Effects of Force Magnitude on Relapse: An Experimental Study in Rabbits. *Am. J. Orthod. Dentofac. Orthop.* **2011**, *140*, 44–50. [CrossRef] [PubMed]
67. Hans, M.G.; Kishiyama, C.; Parker, S.H.; Wolf, G.R.; Noachtar, R. Cephalometric Evaluation of Two Treatment Strategies for Deep Overbite Correction. *Angle Orthod.* **1994**, *64*, 265. [PubMed]

68. Ng, J.; Major, P.W.; Heo, G.; Flores-Mir, C. True Incisor Intrusion Attained during Orthodontic Treatment: A Systematic Review and Meta-Analysis. *Am. J. Orthod. Dentofac. Orthop.* **2005**, *128*, 212–219. [CrossRef]
69. Millett, D.T.; Cunningham, S.J.; O'Brien, K.D.; Benson, P.E.; de Oliveira, C.M. Orthodontic Treatment for Deep Bite and Retroclined Upper Front Teeth in Children. *Cochrane Database Syst. Rev.* **2018**, *2018*, CD005972. [CrossRef]

Disclaimer/Publisher's Note: The statements, opinions and data contained in all publications are solely those of the individual author(s) and contributor(s) and not of MDPI and/or the editor(s). MDPI and/or the editor(s) disclaim responsibility for any injury to people or property resulting from any ideas, methods, instructions or products referred to in the content.

Perspective

Narrating the Genetic Landscape of Human Class I Occlusion: A Perspective-Infused Review

Iqbal M. Lone [1], Osayd Zohud [1], Kareem Midlej [1], Obaida Awadi [2], Samir Masarwa [2], Sebastian Krohn [3], Christian Kirschneck [3], Peter Proff [3], Nezar Watted [2,4,5] and Fuad A. Iraqi [1,3,5,*]

[1] Department of Clinical Microbiology and Immunology, Sackler Faculty of Medicine, Tel-Aviv University, Tel Aviv 69978, Israel; iqbalzoo84@gmail.com (I.M.L.); osaydzohud@mail.tau.ac.il (O.Z.); kareemmidlej@mail.tau.ac.il (K.M.)

[2] Center for Dentistry Research and Aesthetics, Jatt 45911, Israel; awadi.obaida@gmail.com (O.A.); sameer.massarwa@gmail.com (S.M.); nezar.watted@gmx.net (N.W.)

[3] Department of Orthodontics, University Hospital of Regensburg, University of Regensburg, 93053 Regensburg, Germany; sebastian.krohn@klinik.uni-regensburg.de (S.K.); christian.kirschneck@klinik.uni-regensburg.de (C.K.); peter.proff@klinik.uni-regensburg.de (P.P.)

[4] Department of Orthodontics, Faculty of Dentistry, Arab America University, Jenin 919000, Palestine

[5] Gathering for Prosperity Initiative, Jatt 45911, Israel

* Correspondence: fuadi@tauex.tau.ac.il

Abstract: This review examines a prevalent condition with multifaceted etiology encompassing genetic, environmental, and oral behavioral factors. It stands as a significant ailment impacting oral functionality, aesthetics, and quality of life. Longitudinal studies indicate that malocclusion in primary dentition may progress to permanent malocclusion. Recognizing and managing malocclusion in primary dentition is gaining prominence. The World Health Organization ranks malocclusions as the third most widespread oral health issue globally. Angle's classification system is widely used to categorize malocclusions, with Class I occlusion considered the norm. However, its prevalence varies across populations due to genetic and examination disparities. Genetic factors, including variants in genes like MSX1, PAX9, and AXIN2, have been associated with an increased risk of Class I occlusion. This review aims to provide a comprehensive overview of clinical strategies for managing Class I occlusion and consolidate genetic insights from both human and murine populations. Additionally, genomic relationships among craniofacial genes will be assessed in individuals with Class I occlusion, along with a murine model, shedding light on phenotype–genotype associations of clinical relevance. The prevalence of Class I occlusion, its impact, and treatment approaches will be discussed, emphasizing the importance of early intervention. Additionally, the role of RNA alterations in skeletal Class I occlusion will be explored, focusing on variations in expression or structure that influence craniofacial development. Mouse models will be highlighted as crucial tools for investigating mandible size and prognathism and conducting QTL analysis to gain deeper genetic insights. This review amalgamates cellular, molecular, and clinical trait data to unravel correlations between malocclusion and Class I phenotypes.

Keywords: Class I occlusion (CIO); prevalence; quantitative trait loci (QTL) mapping; genome-wide association study (GWAS); epigenetics-wide association study (EWAS); micro and small RNA analysis

1. Introduction

Malocclusion is an atypical arrangement of teeth or a relationship between dental arches that falls outside the normal range [1]. Malocclusion has a complex etiology that includes genetic, environmental, and hazardous oral behaviors [2]. Malocclusion is a complicated facial skeleton developmental condition affecting the jaws, tongue, and face muscles [3] and stands as one of the three primary illnesses that impair human oral functionality, aesthetics, social interactions, and health-related quality of life [4,5]. Prior longitudinal research has shown that primary dentition malocclusion may lead to permanent dental malocclusion [6,7]. Malocclusion, if left untreated, can progress, ranging from moderate to severe, with variable effects on aesthetics and functionality [8]. Research centered on the early identification and management of malocclusion during primary dentition is becoming increasingly prevalent.

According to the World Health Organization, malocclusions are the third most widespread oral health issue, trailing behind dental caries and periodontal diseases [9]. Skeletal abnormalities and malocclusions are diverse disorders that afflict people all over the globe, impairing aesthetics and language function and reducing quality of life [10]. In 1899, Angle established his categorization of occlusions based on the relationship between the buccal groove of the mandibular first permanent molar and the mesiobuccal cusp of the maxillary first permanent molar. Angle Class I occlusion (CIO) is considered the ideal occlusion and is an orthodontic treatment goal for sagittal occlusal anomalies, as shown in Figure 1. This classification is considered one of the most used methods for identifying malpositions of molar relationships [11]. This prevalence varies widely between different populations and ethnicities and is clinically heterogeneous. This variation is likely due to genetic and examination variations in different studies [12,13]. Class I prevalence is considered the most frequent occlusion class globally, ranging from 34.9% to 93.6% in different populations [14–17]. Like any other malocclusion, Class I occlusions have complicated causes, which are frequently linked to environmental, genetic, and social issues [18]. There is a wide range of published primary research data and reports on Class I occlusion prevalence; the reason for this may be differences in ethnic groups, age groups, registration procedures, and classifications of malocclusions [19].

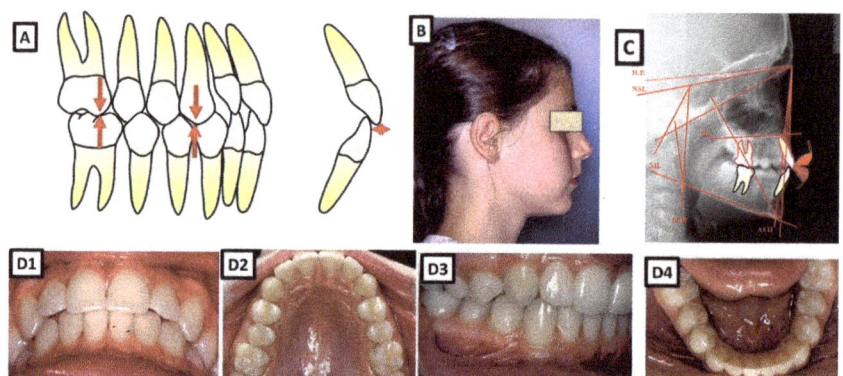

Figure 1. A biometric photo and images of a patient with Class I. In a Class I molar relationship, the mesiobuccal cusp of the maxillary first permanent molar occludes with the buccal groove of the mandibular first molar (**A**). In this definition, the malposition of the teeth, except for the first molars, is not included. (**B–D**) show clinical examples, where (**B**) shows extraoral, (**C**) cephalometric, and (**D1–D4**) intraoral for dental and skeletal Class I without dentoalveolar malposition of the teeth in both jaws.

The genetics and epigenetics of this condition have been the subject of numerous studies in recent years. Research has suggested that Class I occlusion has a complex etiology, with genetic and environmental factors playing a role [20]. Studies have identified several genetic variants associated with an increased occurrence of Class I occlusion, including those in genes involved in craniofacial development such as *MSX*1, *PAX*9, and *AXIN*2 [21]. Additionally, studies have also shown that epigenetic changes, such as DNA methylation and histone modifications, can also play a role in the development of Class I occlusion by affecting the expression of genes involved in craniofacial development [22]. Several genetic variants have been identified as being associated with an increased risk of Class I occlusion.

These include single nucleotide polymorphisms (SNPs) in genes involved in craniofacial development. One of them is *MSX1*, a gene that codes for a transcription factor that plays a role in developing the craniofacial skeleton and teeth. Studies have found that SNPs in *MSX1* are associated with an increased risk of Class I occlusion [23]. *EDA* (ectodysplasin A) and *XEDAR* (X-linked ectodermal dysplasia receptor gene) are suggested to be associated with Class I dental-crowding patients [23]. *PAX9* also codes for a transcription factor and is involved in the development of the craniofacial skeleton and teeth. Studies have found that SNPs in PAX9 are associated with an increased risk of Class I occlusion and other dental anomalies, such as hypodontia [24]. The *AXIN2* gene regulates the Wnt signaling pathway, which is essential for craniofacial development. Studies have found that SNPs in *AXIN*2 are associated with an increased risk of Class I occlusion [24].

Other genes that have been identified as associated with Class I occlusion include *ESRRB* [25], *FGF3* [26], *FGF4* [27], *FGF9* [27], *GREM*2 [28], *IRF6* [29], *JAG1* [29], *LHX8* [30], and *TWIST*1 [31]. It's important to note that most studies on this topic have been conducted on specific populations; the results may not be generalizable to other populations. Additional investigation is required to comprehend the genetic basis of Class I occlusion and how it may vary among different populations.

The primary objective of this review is to provide an overview of the various clinical strategies employed to manage these intricate phenotypes. Additionally, we aim to compile and condense the existing body of knowledge concerning the genetic aspects of Class I occlusion (CIO) in both human and mouse populations.

The report aims to assess genomic relationships among putative craniofacial genes among individuals with Class I occlusion in combination with a murine model. The study characterizes craniofacial skeletal phenotypes in patients with Class I occlusion and generates genetic data on craniofacial genes/loci to identify phenotype–genotype associations of clinical relevance. Several research findings have suggested anterior–posterior and vertical variance in individuals exhibiting Class I occlusion and a certain type of skeletal malocclusion. Prospective research ought to investigate soft-tissue variances to learn more about the genetic basis of skeletal and soft-tissue anomalies in individuals with Class I occlusion. Assessing the genotype–phenotype correlations will help us better comprehend the biological control of postnatal facial development and will guide therapeutic practice to increase the effectiveness of therapy for individuals with occlusion. In addition, we reviewed studies using a mouse model to examine the genetic foundation of mandible dimensions and prognathism.

2. Literature Search

We conducted a comprehensive review of peer-reviewed articles in the PubMed and Google Scholar search engines, using the terms "human and mice Class I occlusion", "genetics of human and mice Class I occlusion", "QTL mapping and gene associated with human and mice Class I occlusion", "prevalence of Class I occlusion", and "treatment of Class I occlusion".

The literature search was performed between January and April 2023 in the PubMed and Google Scholar search engines, and original articles indexed from early 1990 to January 2023 defining molecular characteristics of skeletal deformities and occlusions were searched for and selected. We found suitable papers based on the inclusion criteria listed below: (1) original research or systematic review, (2) written in English, (3) human Class I occlusion, (4) genetics of human Class I occlusion, (5) QTL analysis and gene linkage with Class I occlusion in humans, and (6) prevalence of Class I occlusion. The exclusion criteria were as follows: (1) transcriptomic or expression analysis without epigenetic/genotyping analysis, (2) articles focused on other diseases in which occlusions were merely mentioned, and (3) articles whose full-text versions were not available to us or that were written in other languages.

Three researchers separately assessed the search record. They reviewed the titles and abstracts and performed a thorough examination of the articles. Any disagreements were addressed by consensus by evaluating either the title/abstract review or the entire manuscript. This method included official reviews of all qualified studies. The selected studies' quality and possibility of bias risk were appraised alone by the contributors. In cases where disagreements arose among the researchers regarding the inclusion or exclusion of a particular manuscript, a consensus-based approach was employed. The process involved open discussions among the researchers to evaluate the manuscript in question. Any differences in opinion were thoroughly examined, and the researchers worked collaboratively to reach a consensus decision. This consensus-building process was applied to both the title/abstract review phase and the evaluation of the entire manuscript. To maintain transparency and rigor in our methodology, all qualified studies underwent formal reviews, and the selected studies' quality and potential risk of bias were assessed independently by each contributing researcher. This collaborative and systematic approach ensured that only the most relevant and high-quality studies were included in our review.

3. Prevalence of Class I Occlusion

The frequency of Class I occlusion varies by country, gender, and age group. Several researchers have previously reported the incidence of occlusion in Saudi people [32–34]. The current study was motivated by little documented information on the prevalence of occlusion features within different cohorts. As a result, having data on occlusion is critical for estimating the total need for therapy. Shaw et al. developed the Index of Treatment Need (IOTN) in the United Kingdom, and due to its straightforwardness and practicality [35], it is broadly acknowledged and regarded as a technique for assessing therapy needs [36–38]. Various researchers in various countries have broadly validated the IOTN index's legitimacy and consistency [35,39–41]. Occlusion epidemiological studies not only aid orthodontic therapy strategy but also provide a genuine investigation avenue for identifying environmental and inherited factors that contribute to the genesis of occlusion [42]. In addition, such investigations promise to help with understanding the necessary resources and preventative measures, as well as establishing appropriate healthcare programs. The current study assessed the incidence of occlusion and orthodontic therapy requirements.

The illness burden of occlusion among preschoolers varies significantly worldwide, with incidence rates varying from 26.0% in India [19] to 87.0% in Brazil [43]. Several provinces and cities across mainland China have conducted epidemiological studies on primary dentition occlusion. The Chinese Stomatological Association (CSA) conducted the most recent and most thorough investigation in Chinese children more than two decades ago, revealing a malocclusion rate of 51.84% in Chinese children [44]. Nonetheless, the poll took place in merely 12 regions throughout China. Per our understanding, there is a scarcity of detailed and crucial data about the prevalence of occlusion in deciduous dentition. The current study aims to raise awareness among policymakers and healthcare practitioners on the epidemiological and medical characteristics of occlusion, setting the basis for efficient occlusion avoidance and management in initial dentition.

4. Clinical Outcomes of the Phenotype and Clinical Records

The demographic and medical data for the study were obtained from the patient's orthodontic records, including gender; date of birth; age at treatment initiation; suggested treatment regimen, including extraction and non-extraction of premolars; and length of active orthodontic treatment. To calculate total therapy duration, the starting date was defined as the date of the first molar band placement or first direct bonding, and the completion date was defined as the date of orthodontic retainer delivery.

5. Dental Cast Analysis

5.1. Mandibular Crowding Assessment

The quantity of mandibular crowding is computed by subtracting the arch perimeter (circumference measured from the mesial of one permanent first molar to its antimere) from the total of the mesiodistal widths of all permanent mandibular teeth except molars [45].

5.2. Occlusal Index Computation

The occlusal index is determined using the weighted Peer Assessment Rating (PAR index) established by Ahmad et al. [46], which involves the assessment of five occlusal aspects (posterior occlusion, overjet, overbite, midline, and maxillary tooth displacements) with well-defined measurement criteria (Table 1). The PAR index calculation 30 scores were recorded as follows:

1. Posterior Occlusion

In the original PAR index, posterior occlusion is defined as the area between the contact spot between the canine tooth's rear and the first permanent molar's front. The posterior dental link is scored in three spatial planes: anteroposterior, vertical, and transverse deviations, as shown in Table 1. The results are added together and then doubled. Each posterior segment, whether on the right or left side, is captured separately.

2. Overjet

Positive or negative overjet is the horizontal relationship or the distance between the most protruding maxillary central incisor and the opposing mandibular central incisor. Throughout this measurement, the scale is aligned with the occlusal level and radially aligned with the arch axis. The overjet amount was translated to a value via Table 1, after which it was multiplied by 5.

3. Overbite

Overbite is measured in millimeters as a vertical relationship or the distance between the maxillary central incisor and the opposing mandibular central incisor or the degree of open bite, using the tooth with the most significant overlap as a reference. The score was obtained from Table 1, after which it was multiplied by 3.

4. Midline

The score from Table 1 was used to determine the discrepancy of the maxillary midline with the lower central incisors, and it was then multiplied by 3.

5. Maxillary Tooth Displacement

Only in the maxillary anterior region are movements like crowding, spacing, and impacted teeth noted. These occlusal characteristics are noted using the shortest distance between contact points of neighboring teeth parallel to the occlusal plane. The criteria listed in Table 1 are used to convert these measurements into scores, which are then added. When less than 4 mm of space is available for a tooth, it is deemed impacted.

The term "Initial PAR" (PARi) was assigned to the PAR index when calculated from the pre-treatment impressions. Conversely, the term "Final PAR" (PARf) was used when the index was computed based on the post-treatment impressions. The PAR score was calculated by assigning marks to the dental relationships that are intra-arch (such as crowding) and inter-arch (such as overbite, overjet, crossbite, and midline), as well as by using an ordinal scale with an average value of 0. The more significant the value achieved with these indicators, the more serious the malocclusion. Every measurement within the primary and last castings was measured utilizing an electronic instrument.

Table 1. Criteria applied to score each component of the Peer Assessment Rating (PAR index).

Occlusal Relationships	Discrepancy	Score	Weight	
Anteroposterior	Good interdigitation—Class I, II, or III	0	2	Posterior Occlusion
	Less than half of premolar width	1		
	Half of premolar width	2		
Vertical	No discrepancy in intercuspation	0	2	
	Posterior open bite on at least two teeth greater than 2 mm	1		
Transverse	No crossbite	0	2	
	Crossbite tendency	1		
	Single tooth in crossbite	2		
	More than one tooth in crossbite	3		
	More than one tooth in scissor bite	4		
Positive	0–3 mm	0	5	Overjet
	3.1–5 mm	1		
	5.1–7 mm	2		
	7.1–9 mm	3		
	Greater than 9 mm	4		
Negative	No discrepancy	0	5	
	One or more teeth edgetoedge	1		
	One single tooth in crossbite	2		
	Two teeth in crossbite	3		
	More than two teeth in crossbite	4		
Negative	No open bite	0	3	Overbite
	Open bite less than and equal to 1 mm	1		
	Open bite 1.1–2 mm	2		
	Open bite 2.1–3 mm	3		
	Open bite greater than or equal to 4 mm	4		
Positive	Less than or equal to 1/3 coverage of lower incisor	0	3	
	Greater than 1/3 but less than 2/3 coverage of lower incisor	1		
	Greater than 2/3 coverage of lower incisor	2		
	Greater than or equal to full coverage of lower incisor	3		
Crowding	0–1 mm displacement	0	1	Displacement
	1.1–2 mm displacement	1		
	2.1–4 mm displacement	2		
Spacing Impaction	4.1–8 mm displacement	3		
	Greater than 8 mm	4		
	Impacted teeth	5		
Midline	Coincident and up to 1/4 lower incisor width	0	3	
	Deviated 1/4 to 1/2 lower incisor width	1		
	Deviated more than 1/2 lower incisor width	2		

5.3. Assessing Changes in Occlusal Discrepancy

By dividing PARf values by PARi values, the occlusal discrepancy changes brought about by each treatment regimen were computed (PARi—PARF). The index's numerical decline accounted for occlusal alterations specifically caused by the treatment plan [47,48]. Additionally, the proportion of PAR decrease during therapy (PcPAR) was measured to confirm the degree of recovery compared to the original degree of occlusion [47,48]. The mathematical formula shown below was used to calculate this:

$$PcPAR = (PARi - PARf)/PARi * 100$$

5.4. Treatment Efficiency (TE) Index

The highest variation in the occlusal index obtained during the shortest duration of treatment is considered efficient. The subsequent equation, where the denominator represents the overall treatment duration, was used to compute this [49].

$$TE = PcPAR/TIME$$

5.5. Treatment for Class I Occlusion

Since patients often have a favorable soft-tissue environment and harmonious skeletal features, except in bimaxillary cases, Class I occlusions are treated to correct dentoalveolar malpositions of the teeth. Although these dental issues are not specific to Class I occlusion and are observed in other malocclusions, they are described in this study. These dental issues include gaps, tooth malposition (rotation, infraocclusion, supraocclusion, tipping), crowding, impacted teeth, ectopic teeth, crossbites, deep bites, and open bites, as presented in Figure 2. Because the problem is purely dentoalveolar and not skeletal, the treatment will also be dentoalveolar with different devised strategies, as presented in Figures 3–9.

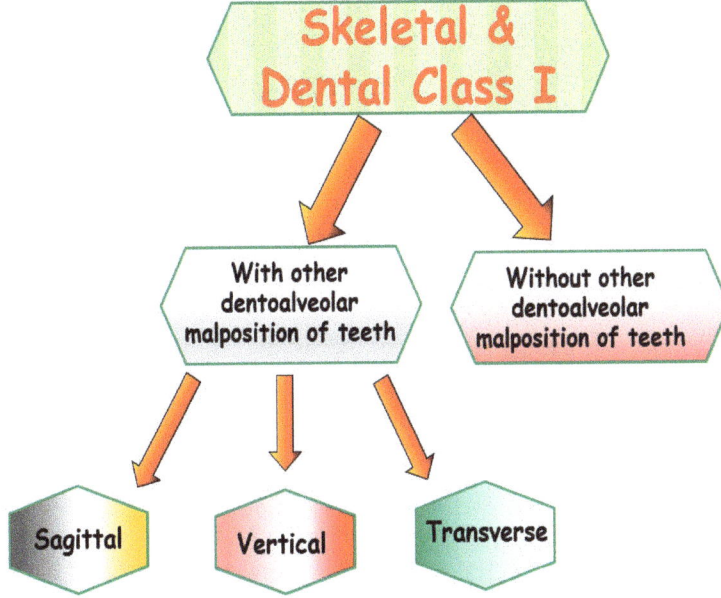

Figure 2. Schematic representation of the possible occurrence of Class I occlusion with or without dentoalveolar malposition of the teeth in all dimensions (sagittal, vertical, and transversal).

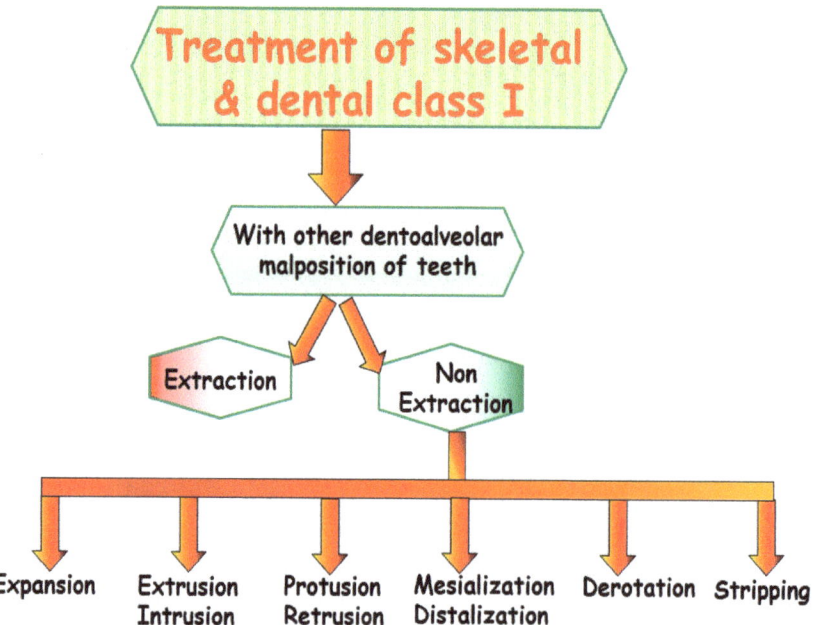

Figure 3. Schematic representation of the treatment options under consideration of the dentofacial aesthetics and function.

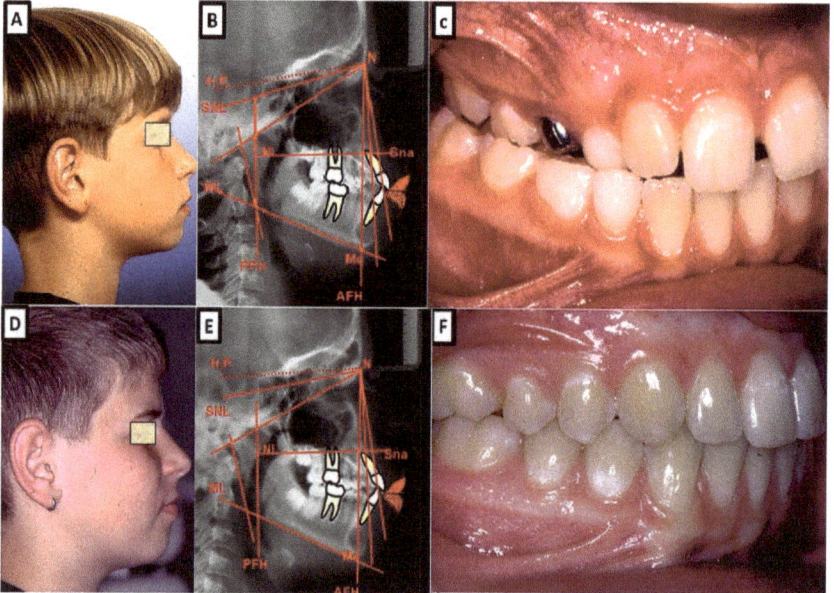

Figure 4. Biometric photo and images of a patient with a Class I occlusion with a transverse problem in the maxilla on the right side (crossbite). The treatment was carried out by transverse up righting of the teeth. (**A–C**) are before treatment, and (**D–F**) are after treatment.

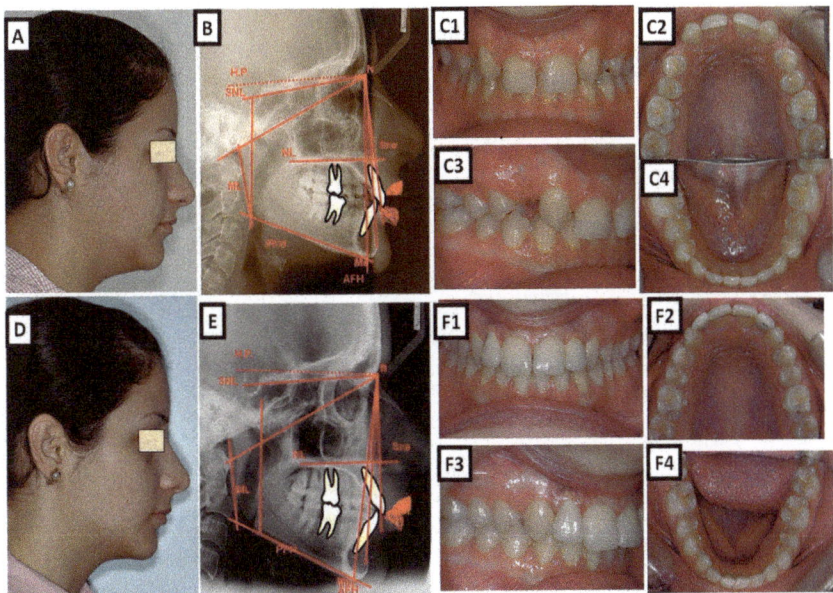

Figure 5. Biometric photo and images of a patient with a Class I occlusion with a vertical problem (deep bite), crowding, and teeth malposition. (**A–C**) are before treatment, and (**D–F**) are after treatment.

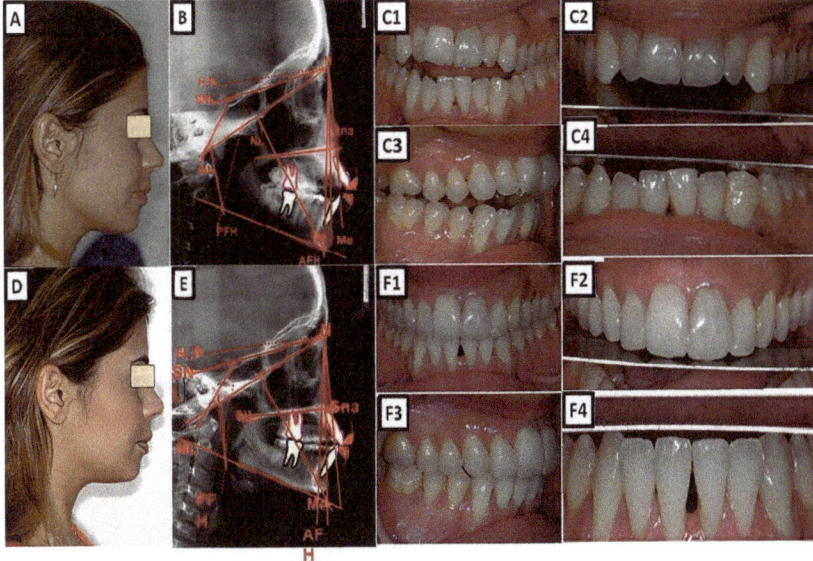

Figure 6. A Abiometric photo and images of a patient with a Class I occlusion with other malpositions of the teeth in the three dimensions: transverse (lateral crossbite), sagittal (increased overjet), vertical (open bite), and crowding. The treatment was performed with a fixed appliance; the front teeth were extruded. (**A–C**) show before treatment, and (**D–F**) are after treatment.

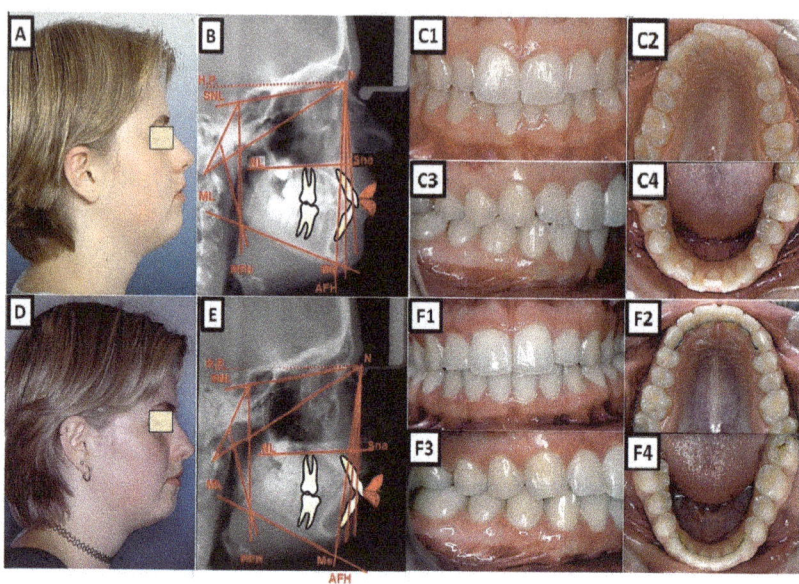

Figure 7. A biometric photo and images of a patient with a Class I occlusion with a dentoalveolar malposition of the teeth and crowding. The treatment was carried out with a fixed appliance. The space was created by approximal enamel reduction. (**A–C**) show before treatment, and (**D–F**) are after treatment.

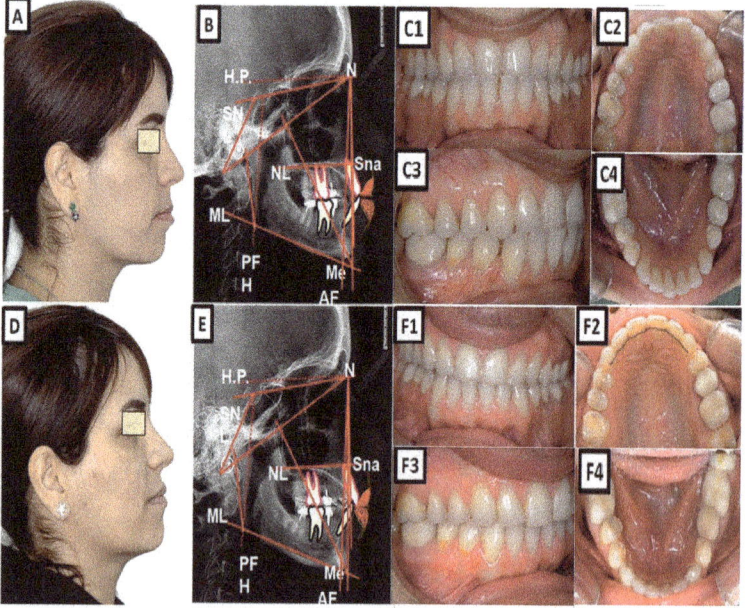

Figure 8. A biometric photo and images of a patient with a Class I occlusion with a sagittal malposition of the frontal teeth (frontal crossbite), crowding, and other teeth malpositions. The frontal crossbite was corrected by protrusion of the upper incisors. (**A–C**) show the case before treatment, and (**D–F**) are after treatment.

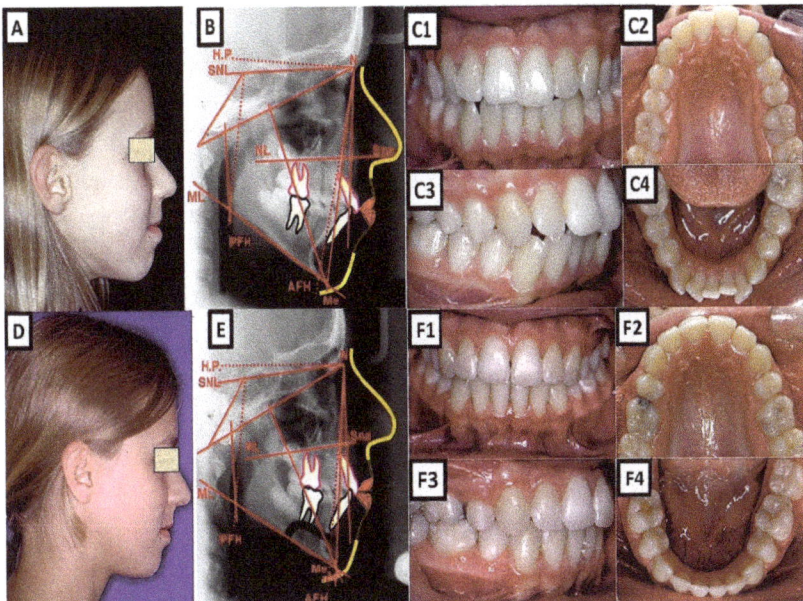

Figure 9. Biometric photo and images of a patient with a Class I occlusion with crowding and other teeth malpositions. The upper and the lower incisors are protruded. For the treatment, four premolars were extracted to retrude the upper and lower incisors and to resolve the crowding. (**A–C**) show the case before treatment, and (**D–F**) are after treatment.

5.6. Spacing and Crowding

The patient's skeletal profile, the kind of occlusion, the degree of crowding, the angle of the teeth, the amount of accessible space, and the amount of space required for occlusion correction all play a role in deciding how to close excessive spaces or relieve crowding.

5.7. Spacing

Supernumeraries, early tooth loss, microdontia, frenal attachment to the incisive papilla, and congenitally absent teeth can all cause spacing. If possible, the reason for the space should be removed; for instance, a frenectomy is necessary if a median diastema is brought on by a big labial frenum. To assess the existence of supernumeraries in cases with a median diastema, a periapical radiograph is typically also required.

5.8. Primary Dentition

Active treatment is not recommended for primary teeth with excessive gaps, based on monitoring.

5.9. Mixed Dentition

Depending on the patient's age, the cause of the spacing, and its severity, spacing can be monitored in mild situations. When the upper canines erupt, the mild divergence and increased space between the upper incisors between the ages of 7 and 12 is considered normal (the "ugly duckling" period). Premature loss of posterior teeth, especially primary second molars, might be a problem during the mixed dentition stage since there is a chance that the permanent first molars may move posteriorly. In these circumstances, the space must be maintained to allow the eruption of permanent successors. The transpalatal arch, lower lingual holding arch, and Nance holding appliance are a few examples of space maintainers. This also aims at preventing a midline shift in the early loss of deciduous canines.

5.10. Permanent Dentition

If there is a favorable soft-tissue environment and no serious skeletal abnormalities, excessive gaps can be corrected with clear aligners. With permanent appliances, space closure is also simple to carry out. If the space is caused by tooth loss, one alternative is to use fixed appliances to make enough room, depending on the periodontal health, for an implant or bridge. To obtain the best results in microdontia and peg laterals, a combination of orthodontic and restorative treatment is recommended.

5.11. Crowding

Crowding is caused by a size difference between the teeth and dental arches. There are numerous techniques to offer the necessary room for the treatment of crowding, such as arch expander equipment or extraction to gain large spaces and active open-coil springs for acquiring minor spaces.

5.12. Primary Dentition

Early-stage crowding results from a lack of primate spaces and indicates that crowding will happen in permanent dentition. The emergence of permanent teeth must also be closely watched, making regular checkups crucial.

5.13. Mixed Dentition

Phase I treatment helps to make room in numerous different ways when there is mild to moderate crowding that leads to ectopic eruption or impaction of permanent teeth. The incisors are grouped by partial fixed appliance therapy, or 2×4, in mild situations. After enough room has been made, a fixed lingual retainer is affixed to the palate of the incisors to stop relapse after the fixed appliances are removed. To maintain the space, space maintainers are bonded, and the eruption of the permanent dentition is tracked. This early intervention aims to stop severe crowding in the permanent dentition, stop ectopic eruptions, and stop the need to remove permanent teeth to make room once growth has stopped. An expander plate, such as a quick maxillary expander or a gradual maxillary expander (quad helix), is used to widen narrow arches before the growth spurt. After enough room has been created with the use of an expander, this form of therapy can be utilized in conjunction with partial braces to align the newly erupted teeth.

5.14. Permanent Dentition

A series of aligners can correct mild to moderate crowding when there are no skeletal differences. The use of a detachable appliance can result in the tipping of just one or two teeth. For detachable appliances to work best, high patient compliance is required. Extractions are recommended after the initial growth surge and in situations of extreme congestion. An orthodontist is always the one to decide whether to extract a tooth. The degree of anchorage required heavily influences whether people need space maintainers. Therefore, extractions are always thoughtfully designed with enough anchoring in adults.

5.15. RNA Alterations in Skeletal Class I Occlusion

RNA variation refers to variations in the expression or structure of RNA molecules that can affect their function [50]. In the context of skeletal Class I occlusion, RNA variation can refer to variations in the expression or structure of RNA molecules that are involved in the development of the craniofacial skeleton and teeth, which can affect the formation of the jaw and teeth and contribute to the development of skeletal Class I occlusion [29]. There have been several studies that have identified specific RNAs that are altered in skeletal Class I occlusion [51]. However, it is important to note that most of these studies have been conducted on specific populations, and the results may not be generalizable to other populations. In addition, most of the studies focus on specific genes and pathways, and more studies are required to properly comprehend the role of RNA in the formation of skeletal Class I occlusion.

Previous studies have shown that changes in the expression of specific genes can affect the development of the craniofacial skeleton and teeth and may contribute to the development of skeletal Class I occlusion [29]. For example, changes in the expression of genes involved in the Wnt signaling pathway, such as *AXIN2*, can affect craniofacial development and influence the formation of skeletal Class I occlusion [52]. In addition to changes in gene expression, variations in the structure of RNA molecules can also affect their function [53]. For example, variations in the structure of microRNAs (miRNAs), small non-coding RNA molecules that regulate gene expression, have been shown to affect craniofacial development and most likely will contribute to the development of skeletal Class I occlusion [54].

A study found that miR-29 is downregulated in the gingival tissue of individuals with skeletal Class I occlusion and that this downregulation is associated with an increase in the expression of the target genes*COL1A1* and *MMP13*, which are involved in the regulation of bone remodeling [55]. In addition, miR-31 is downregulated in the gingival tissue of individuals with skeletal Class I occlusion, and this downregulation is associated with an increase in the expression of the target gene*TWIST1*, which is involved in regulating craniofacial development [56]. Further, miR-124 was found to be downregulated in the gingival tissue of individuals with skeletal Class I occlusion, and this downregulation is associated with an increase in the expression of the target gene*Dlx5*, which is involved in the regulation of tooth development [57].

5.16. A Mouse Model for Studying Mandible Size, Prognathism, and QTL Analysis

Mouse models have been widely used to study the genetics and epigenetics of skeletal Class I occlusion [31,32,58]. These models allow researchers to manipulate specific genes or environmental factors better to understand their role in the development of this condition. One common approach is to generate mouse models with specific genetic mutations in genes associated with skeletal Class I occlusion. For example, researchers have generated mice with mutations in the *MSX1*, *PAX9*, and *AXIN2* genes, among others, and observed changes in craniofacial development and tooth formation like those seen in human patients with skeletal Class I occlusion [59–61]. Another approach is to use mouse models to study the effects of environmental factors on the development of skeletal Class I occlusion. For example, researchers have used mouse models to study the consequences of maternal nutrition in the formation of the craniofacial bone and teeth and have observed changes in craniofacial development and tooth formation that are similar to those seen in human patients with skeletal Class I occlusion [62,63].

Mouse models have also been used to study the epigenetic mechanisms involved in developing skeletal Class I occlusion. For example, researchers have used mouse models to study the effects of DNA methylation and histone modifications on gene activity involved in craniofacial development and have observed changes in craniofacial development and tooth formation that are similar to those seen in human patients with skeletal Class I occlusion [64]. Several QTLs for skeletal Class I occlusion have been identified using linkage and association studies in human and animal models. These studies have identified regions of the genome associated with an increased risk of skeletal Class I occlusion and other occlusal traits, such as tooth size and shape and certain craniofacial features [30]. The QTL was identified for skeletal Class I occlusion and other occlusal traits on chromosome 7. In mice, the identified region on chromosome 7 was associated with a significant reduction in overbite, which is a characteristic of skeletal Class I occlusion. Further, a region on chromosome 8 in mice was identified as associated with differences in dental dimensions and morphology. The workflow diagram for generating systems genetics datasets of cellular, molecular, and clinical trait data combined to analyze various correlations between malocclusion and Class I phenotypes is represented in Figure 10.

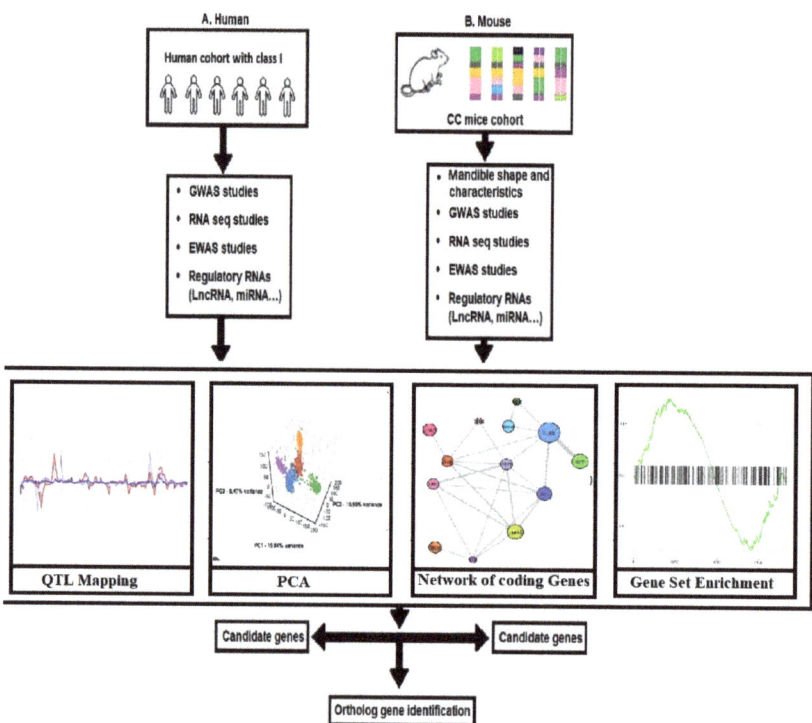

Figure 10. The process for creating systems genetics datasets encompassing cellular, molecular, and clinical trait data is outlined in the workflow. These datasets are amalgamated to facilitate the analysis of correlations between malocclusion and Class I phenotypes. By integrating SNP genotype data, the regulatory genomic regions linked to phenotypic variation are identified. Furthermore, using QTL mapping, specific traits monitored in vitro and in vivo can be pinpointed. Combining these data with subsequent candidate gene association studies conducted in human populations can unveil susceptibility genes linked to the onset of Class I occlusion in individuals.

5.17. *The Collaborative Cross-Mouse Population—A Potent Resource for Systemic Genetic Analysis of Class I Occlusion*

Traditional laboratory mouse strains, on the other hand, possess limited genetic diversity, which makes them less suitable for investigating genetic variations in intricate traits. To overcome this limitation, the collaborative cross (CC) was introduced, generating a novel set of highly genetically diverse recombinant inbred mouse strains. The CC mouse strains were established as a novel resource to enable precise mapping and recognition of the genetic elements responsible for intricate phenotypes, with a specific emphasis on those relevant to human health. The establishment of the collaborative cross genetic reference population (GRP) of mice was driven by the necessity to simulate genetic diversity. This unique genetic reference population (GRP) resource consists of a substantial collection of recombinant inbred (RI) strains. These strains were derived from a genetically diverse selection of eight founding strains, intentionally designed for in-depth analysis of complex traits [65–68], offering an advantage over any previously documented method [69].

This distinctive resource comprises many recombinant inbred (RI) strains. These strains were generated from a genetically varied pool of eight founder strains, explicitly focusing on facilitating the analysis of complex traits and implying a potency surpassing any previously reported methodologies [70]. The group of eight founder strains demonstrates significant genetic diversity, encompassing five widely used laboratory strains (A/J,

C57BL/6J, 129S1/SvImJ, NOD/LtJ, NZO/HiLtJ) and three wild-derived strains (CAST/Ei, PWK/PhJ, WSB/EiJ). This divergence in their phylogenetic origins dramatically contributes to the extensive genetic variation observed within the resulting population of collaborative cross mice.

The CC mouse is a GRP that exhibits a twofold increase in genetic variations, encompassing more than 36 million SNPs. These variations mirror those found within the natural human population, Additionally, it demonstrates a relatively elevated frequency of recombination events in comparison to other mouse sets, with 4.4 million SNPs segregating between the founders [70–72]. A recent study involving QTL analysis using the CC population indicated that the mapped interval resolution could potentially be less than 1 Mb [70–76].

The expansion of the genetic map within the CC population is approximately fourfold, leading to a proportionally enhanced precision in QTL map positioning. Given the inbred origin of all genetic traits, each QTL's genetic variance is amplified. Moreover, the phenotyping of numerous individuals within each line helps to diminish environmental sources of variance. Compared to conventional F2 mapping populations, this approach significantly multiplies the mapping power of the recombinant inbred line (RIL) set.

CC strains should provide a distinct chance to conduct GWAS and map significant quantitative trait loci (QTL) and subsequently identify candidate genes, as well as mapping modifiers for significant genes associated with Class I traits, while lowering the surrounding obstacles. There is a firm conviction that the substantial genetic diversity present in the founding strains of the CC mouse population offers a robust foundation for uncovering new genetic loci associated with these specific phenotypes. This framework further enables the validation process using mouse knockout genes and conditional knockout methodologies.

5.18. The Forthcoming Focus Entails the Creation of an Innovative Model Aimed at Mapping Major and Modifier Genes Linked to Skeletal Class I Malocclusion Using the Collaborative Cross (CC) Model

Systems genetics presents a promising avenue for comprehending the intricate array of biological factors that underlie complex traits within genetically diverse populations. This approach harnesses an array of experimental and statistical techniques to meticulously quantify phenotypes—including transcript, protein, and metabolite levels—within these genetically segregated populations, which exhibit anticipated variations for the traits of interest. Systems genetics investigations have provided an initial holistic perspective of the intricate molecular framework behind complex traits. Such studies are invaluable for pinpointing genes, pathways, and networks that are the foundation for common diseases. In this context, we propose harnessing the capabilities of the CC lines to map genes associated with Class I. Our proposal involves conducting a conventional exploration of candidate genes linked to Class I via GWAS, building upon the successful precedent established by prior publications [65–76].

The initial comprehensive exploration of the genetic basis for Class I characteristics has been facilitated through systems genetics analysis, a methodology that aids in identifying genes, signaling pathways, and networks responsible for prevalent disorders. This investigation involves merging data related to cellular, molecular, and clinical aspects to examine the associations among various Class I occlusion phenotypes. By amalgamating SNP genotype data from each CC lineage, regulatory genomic regions implicated in phenotypic variability in both in vitro and in vivo monitored traits are identified. The potential identification of susceptibility genes associated with the onset of Class I occlusion in humans can be achieved by combining data with subsequent investigations in the association of candidate genes in humans.

This experimental design presents the opportunity for parallel in vitro/in vivo screening, bolstered by the development of high-throughput assessment technologies and computational methodologies, leading to a better understanding of how diverse genetic alterations collectively impact the initiation and severity of Class I occlusion. Validated gene–gene interactions and gene–environment networks can be harnessed to inform risk assessment for Class II malocclusion prevention or identify pharmaceutical targets in human systems. Through systems genetics, a comprehensive grasp of the disease's biology and severity will likely be attained by deciphering the mechanisms of the genetic loci (QTL and genes) uncovered in genome-wide association studies (GWAS) that contribute to susceptibility to Class I occlusion.

Currently, there is extensive molecular research underway concerning regulatory RNAs, encompassing gene expression, DNA methylation, small and microRNA, and long non-coding RNA profiles across a range of diseases. However, to our knowledge, minimal research exists regarding the status of these molecules in the context of skeletal Class II malocclusion. In light of this, we propose that exploring these regulatory RNAs in this condition holds significant promise and will contribute to a more profound comprehension of the molecular underpinnings of the disease.

The workflow diagram presented in Figure 10 outlines the process for generating systems genetics datasets comprising cellular, molecular, and clinical trait data. These datasets are amalgamated to analyze the correlations between Class I phenotypes. The integration of human and mouse approaches, coupled with the application of identification, screening, and exclusion methods, is depicted in the diagram. This systematic approach is a roadmap to facilitate a comprehensive investigation into the intricate mechanisms underlying Class I occlusion.

In conclusion, gaining insight into how the genetic loci (QTL and genes) identified through genome-wide association studies (GWAS) contribute to the susceptibility of Class I phenotypes, in conjunction with the utilization of systems genetics, is poised to enhance our comprehension of both the biology and the nature of the disease.

6. Discussion

This study aims to provide a comprehensive understanding of Class I occlusion. The kinds of occlusion in teenage age groups have been described in numerous studies published in the literature from various nations. Though this is the case, comparisons of the findings from these studies are challenging due to differences in the age and size of the study populations and the methodologies used to record occlusal connections. According to reports, the prevalence of malocclusion varies by gender, age, and nation. There havenot been enough investigations to gauge the prevalence [32–34]. One of the most straightforward techniques for recording occlusion is calculating the overall frequency of occlusion and the requirement for orthodontic treatment. It is more common to have Angle's Class I occlusion and less common to have Angle's Class III occlusion. The results show that Class III malocclusion is the least common malocclusion, with Angle's Class I and Class II ranking first and second, respectively. According to Al-Emran et al. and Al-Balkhi and Zahrani, Class I, Class II division 1, and Class III malocclusions are the most prevalent in the Saudi population [77,78].

Understanding global epidemiological data aids in establishing priorities for occlusion treatment and the resources needed in terms of work capacity, skills, agility, and materials to be used. To organize the logical planning of orthodontic preventative and therapeutic actions, national public health agencies should be aware of the incidence of occlusion features. Furthermore, evaluations of occlusion prevalence by various groups and geographical regions may reveal the existence of distinct genetic and environmental causes. A precise global picture of the prevalence of occlusion in primary, mixed, and permanent dentitions was produced by this systematic review. Our review found no appreciable variations in male and female occlusion rates, with more than half of children and adolescents worldwide experiencing one type of occlusion. Except for one continent, none of the world's continents had a reduction in this high incidence to below 50%. The significant number of papers (n = 81) and high level of methodological quality across all included studies provide strong support for the epidemiological relevance of occlusion, according to this review.

The prevalence of occlusion is highest in early childhood during the era of deciduous teeth (54%), and it remains stable during permanent dentition (54%). These prevalence figures show that occlusion is a significant issue for oral health and a financial burden for the families of affected children and public dental health programs. Health policymakers, pediatricians, and dentists should be encouraged to carry out preventive or early diagnosis and develop appropriate treatment strategies because it may be possible to prevent the onset of occlusion from the earliest age (i.e., by avoiding poor oral habits in children) [79,80].

Understanding the type of occlusion and how severe it is will assist in determining whether the group under study requires dental orthodontic treatment and how their oral health is. The current study will also help create customized programs for treating and promoting oral health. According to other observations, refugees are more prone to several ailments, including dental [81]. According to recent studies [82–84], refugees have a greater incidence of dental caries and poor oral hygiene than host populations. Untreated dental conditions can cause tooth decay or loss, influencing poor eating patterns and lower quality of life [81]. The most common treatment offered to refugee children, according to a prior study, is extraction, which is a sign of poor oral hygiene and a tendency for refugees to seek dental care late during their sickness, usually for emergency treatment [82–85]. These results, however, might point to a lack of restorative treatment services due to low funding and a delay in access to dental care [82–85].

The prevalence of deciduous dentition occlusion is depicted in this meta-analysis in a more precise and thorough manner. According to statistics, various occlusions affect roughly 45.5% of children in mainland China. In addition, significant heterogeneity was found between provinces, which may result from varying criteria, ethnic backgrounds, age ranges, registration processes, or environmental and genetic factors [86,87]. Class I occlusion has the highest predicted occurrence among the two Angle classifications. It is helpful to think about a systematic review of occlusion prevalence among Iranian children that found that poor hygiene and healthcare combined with excessive sugar consumption, which results in caries and the early loss of deciduous teeth, increased the prevalence of Class I occlusion [88]. In addition to genetics, mandibular protrusion and improper feeding practices, like supine nursing, increased the likelihood of occlusion [89]. In Class II malocclusion, a low prevalence rate of 7.97% was noted.

Patients with Class I occlusion who received either four premolar extractions or no treatment should be included in the samples. Since the compatibility of groups for the degree of the initial occlusion will lessen the potential of bias, attention should be on this particular type of occlusion. According to earlier studies, the degree of the initial anteroposterior mismatch influences the length of the treatment and its effectiveness [49,90]. There is less chance of confounding and selection bias because the distribution of sex, age, PARi, and mandibular crowding is consistent between groups. The degree to which genetic variance among individuals can explain variations in their attributes is determined by the degree of heritability [91]. The genetic predisposition to malocclusion susceptibility is supported by a number of data sources. Numerous dental and facial traits, such as mid- and lower facial dimensions, dental spacing, arch dimensions, and Bolton-type tooth size differences, have moderate to high heritability proportions (>60%) documented. On the other hand, overbite (53%) and overjet (28%) have lower heritability, suggesting a larger vulnerability to environmental variables [92,93].

7. Conclusions

In this narrative and perspective paper, we have embarked on a comprehensive exploration of Class I occlusion, shedding light on the diverse aspects of this intriguing dental phenomenon. As we delved into the literature, it became evident that although a wealth of research exists on various forms of occlusion, comparing findings across studies remains a challenge. This is primarily due to differences in the age and size of study populations and the methodologies used to document occlusal connections. Furthermore, the prevalence of malocclusion is subject to variations based on factors such as gender, age, and geographical location, leading to complexities in drawing universal conclusions.

Our findings indicated that Angle's Class I occlusion is the most prevalent, followed by Class II, whereas Class III malocclusion is the least common. Understanding global epidemiological data is crucial to establishing priorities in occlusion treatment and the allocation of resources, including workforce, skills, agility, and materials. National public health agencies must be informed about the prevalence of occlusion characteristics to strategically plan orthodontic preventative and therapeutic interventions. Furthermore, analyzing occlusion prevalence across diverse demographic groups and regions may reveal distinct genetic and environmental factors that contribute to its occurrence.

Of particular interest is the observation that occlusion prevalence peaks during early childhood with deciduous teeth (54%) and remains stable during permanent dentition (54%). These prevalence figures underscore the critical role of occlusion in oral health and its economic implications for families and public health programs. This insight calls for proactive measures, such as preventive strategies and early diagnosis, to address occlusion-related issues, including children's oral habits.

Additionally, our study highlights the challenges faced by vulnerable populations, such as refugees, who often experience higher rates of dental conditions. These disparities necessitate increased attention from health policymakers, pediatricians, and dentists to develop targeted strategies for prevention, diagnosis, and treatment.

This narrative review and perspective paper offers a multifaceted exploration of Class I occlusion, drawing from diverse sources and perspectives. By unraveling the complexities of occlusion, we aim to contribute to the broader discourse on oral health, inform public health policies, and inspire future research endeavors in this fascinating field.

Author Contributions: Conceptualization, F.A.I., P.P. and N.W.; methodology, I.M.L., O.Z., K.M., O.A., S.M., S.K. and C.K.; validation, F.A.I.; investigation, I.M.L., O.Z., K.M., N.W., O.A., S.M., S.K. and C.K.; resources, F.A.I., P.P., N.W., S.K. and C.K.; data curation, I.M.L., O.Z. and K.M.; writing—original draft preparation, O.Z. and I.M.L.; writing—review and editing, P.P., N.W. and F.A.I.; supervision, F.A.I., P.P. and N.W.; project administration, F.A.I.; funding acquisition, F.A.I., P.P. and N.W. All authors have read and agreed to the published version of the manuscript.

Funding: This study was supported by a core fund from Tel Aviv University, Arab American University in Jenin, and the University Hospital of Regensburg.

Institutional Review Board Statement: Ethical review and approval were waived for this study since there was no intervention procedure involving patients or biological sample collection. However, we used ICS from patients to use their cephalometric images.

Informed Consent Statement: Informed consent was obtained from all subjects involved in the study.

Data Availability Statement: Not applicable.

Conflicts of Interest: The authors declare no conflict of interest.

References

1. Gupta, D.K.; Singh, S.P.; Utreja, A.; Verma, S. Prevalence of Malocclusion and Assessment of Treatment Needs in β-Thalassemia Major Children. *Prog. Orthod.* **2016**, *17*, 7. [CrossRef]
2. Heimer, M.V.; Tornisiello Katz, C.R.; Rosenblatt, A. Non-Nutritive Sucking Habits, Dental Malocclusions, and Facial Morphology in Brazilian Children: A Longitudinal Study. *Eur. J. Orthod.* **2008**, *30*, 580–585. [CrossRef]
3. Peres, K.G.; Barros, A.J.D.; Peres, M.A.; Victoria, C.G. Effects of Breastfeeding and Sucking Habits on Malocclusion in a Birth Cohort Study. *Rev. Saude Publica* **2007**, *41*, 343–350. [CrossRef] [PubMed]
4. Marques, L.S.; Pordeus, I.A.; Ramos-Jorge, M.L.; Filognio, C.A.; Filognio, C.B.; Pereira, L.J.; Paiva, S.M. Factors Associated with the Desire for Orthodontic Treatment among Brazilian Adolescents and Their Parents. *BMC Oral Health* **2009**, *9*, 34. [CrossRef]
5. Tak, M.; Nagarajappa, R.; Sharda, A.J.; Asawa, K.; Tak, A.; Jalihal, S.; Kakatkar, G. Prevalence of Malocclusion and Orthodontic Treatment Needs among 12–15 Years Old School Children of Udaipur, India. *Eur. J. Dent.* **2013**, *7*, S045–S053. [CrossRef] [PubMed]
6. Onyeaso, C.O.; Isiekwe, M.C. Occlusal Changes from Primary to Mixed Dentitions in Nigerian Children. *Angle Orthod.* **2008**, *78*, 64–69. [CrossRef]

7. Legovic, M.; Mady, L. Longitudinal Occlusal Changes from Primary to Permanent Dentition in Children with Normal Primary Occlusion. *Angle Orthod.* **1999**, *69*, 264–266.
8. Dimberg, L.; Lennartsson, B.; Arnrup, K.; Bondemark, L. Prevalence and Change of Malocclusions from Primary to Early Permanent Dentition: A Longitudinal Study. *Angle Orthod.* **2015**, *85*, 728–734. [CrossRef]
9. Alhammadi, M.S.; Halboub, E.; Fayed, M.S.; Labib, A.; El-Saaidi, C. Global Distribution of Malocclusion Traits: A Systematic Review. *Dent. Press J. Orthod.* **2018**, *23*, 40.e1. [CrossRef] [PubMed]
10. Claudino, D.; Traebert, J. Malocclusion, Dental Aesthetic Self-Perception and Quality of Life in a 18 to 21 Year-Old Population: A Cross Section Study. *BMC Oral Health* **2013**, *13*, 3. [CrossRef]
11. Gravely, J.F.; Johnson, D.B. Angle's Classification of Malocclusion: An Assessment of Reliability. *Br. J. Orthod.* **2016**, *1*, 79–86. [CrossRef]
12. Garbin, A.J.Í.; Perin, P.C.P.; Garbin, C.A.S.; Lolli, L.F. Malocclusion Prevalence and Comparison between the Angle Classification and the Dental Aesthetic Index in Scholars in the Interior of São Paulo State—Brazil. *Dental Press J. Orthod.* **2010**, *15*, 94–102. [CrossRef]
13. Gelgör, İ.E.; Karaman, İ.A.; Ercan, E. Prevalence of Malocclusion Among Adolescents In Central Anatolia. *Eur. J. Dent.* **2007**, *1*, 125–131. [CrossRef] [PubMed]
14. Lew, K.K.; Foong, W.C. Horizontal Skeletal Typing in an Ethnic Chinese Population with True Class III Malocclusions. *Br. J.Orthod.* **1993**, *20*, 19–23. [CrossRef] [PubMed]
15. Khan, M.; Fida, M. Assessment of Psychosocial Impact of Dental Aesthetics. *J. Coll. Physicians Surg. Pak.* **2008**, *18*, 559.
16. Mtaya, M.; Brudvik, P.; Åstrøm, A.N. Prevalence of Malocclusion and Its Relationship with Socio-Demographic Factors, Dental Caries, and Oral Hygiene in 12- to 14-Year-Old Tanzanian Schoolchildren. *Eur. J. Orthod.* **2009**, *31*, 467–476. [CrossRef]
17. Cenzato, N.; Nobili, A.; Maspero, C. Prevalence of Dental Malocclusions in Different Geographical Areas: Scoping Review. *Dent. J.* **2021**, *9*, 117. [CrossRef]
18. Debnath, S. Preliminary Studies on the Inhibition Potential of Indian Domestic Curd against Coliforms, an Emerging Periodontal Pathogen. *J. Indian Soc. Periodontol.* **2017**, *21*, 357–365. [CrossRef]
19. Dhar, V.; Jain, A.; Van Dyke, T.E.; Kohli, A. Prevalence of Gingival Diseases, Malocclusion and Fluorosis in School-Going Children of Rural Areas in Udaipur District. *J. Indian Soc. Pedod. Prev. Dent.* **2007**, *25*, 103–105. [CrossRef]
20. Cakan, D.G.; Ulkur, F.; Taner, T.U. The Genetic Basis of Facial Skeletal Characteristics and Its Relation with Orthodontics. *Eur. J. Dent.* **2012**, *6*, 340. [CrossRef]
21. Gupta, P.; Chaturvedi, P.; Sharma, V. Expressional Analysis of MSX1 (Human) Revealed Its Role in Sagittal Jaw Relationship. *J. Clin. Diagn. Res.* **2017**, *11*, 71–77. [CrossRef] [PubMed]
22. Huh, A.; Horton, M.J.; Cuenco, K.T.; Raoul, G.; Rowlerson, A.M.; Ferri, J.; Sciote, J.J. Epigenetic Influence of KAT6B and HDAC4 in the Development of Skeletal Malocclusion. *Am. J. Orthod. Dentofac. Orthop.* **2013**, *144*, 568–576. [CrossRef] [PubMed]
23. Zeng, B.; Zhao, Q.; Li, S.; Lu, H.; Lu, J.; Ma, L.; Zhao, W.; Yu, D. Novel EDA or EDAR Mutations Identified in Patients with X-Linked Hypohidrotic Ectodermal Dysplasia or Non-Syndromic Tooth Agenesis. *Genes* **2017**, *8*, 259. [CrossRef] [PubMed]
24. Koskinen, S.; Keski-Filppula, R.; Alapulli, H.; Nieminen, P.; Anttonen, V. Familial Oligodontia and Regional Odontodysplasia Associated with a PAX9 Initiation Codon Mutation. *Clin. Oral Investig.* **2019**, *23*, 4107–4111. [CrossRef] [PubMed]
25. Casado, P.L.; Quinelato, V.; Cataldo, P.; Prazeres, J.; Campello, M.; Bonato, L.L.; Aguiar, T. Dental Genetics in Brazil: Where We Are. *Mol. Genet. Genom. Med.* **2018**, *6*, 689. [CrossRef] [PubMed]
26. Dizak, P.; Burnheimer, J.; Deeley, K.; Vieira, A.R. Malocclusion May Be Attributed to Variation among 10 Genes. *Open J. Stomatol.* **2021**, *11*, 263–269. [CrossRef]
27. Xiong, X.; Li, S.; Cai, Y.; Chen, F. Targeted Sequencing in FGF/FGFR Genes and Association Analysis of Variants for Mandibular Prognathism. *Medicine* **2017**, *96*, e7240. [CrossRef]
28. Kantaputra, P.N.; Pruksametanan, A.; Phondee, N.; Hutsadaloi, A.; Intachai, W.; Kawasaki, K.; Ohazama, A.; Ngamphiw, C.; Tongsima, S.; Ketudat Cairns, J.R.; et al. ADAMTSL1 and Mandibular Prognathism. *Clin. Genet.* **2019**, *95*, 507–515. [CrossRef]
29. Gershater, E.; Li, C.; Ha, P.; Chung, C.H.; Tanna, N.; Zou, M.; Zheng, Z. Genes and Pathways Associated with Skeletal Sagittal Malocclusions: A Systematic Review. *Int. J. Mol. Sci.* **2021**, *22*, 13037. [CrossRef]
30. Jaruga, A.; Ksiazkiewicz, J.; Kuzniarz, K.; Tylzanowski, P. Orofacial Cleft and Mandibular Prognathism—Human Genetics and Animal Models. *Int. J. Mol. Sci.* **2022**, *23*, 953. [CrossRef]
31. Da Fontoura, C.S.G.; Miller, S.F.; Wehby, G.L.; Amendt, B.A.; Holton, N.E.; Southard, T.E.; Allareddy, V.; Moreno Uribe, L.M. Candidate Gene Analyses of Skeletal Variation in Malocclusion. *J. Dent. Res.* **2015**, *94*, 913–920. [CrossRef] [PubMed]
32. AlQarni, M.A.; Banihuwaiz, A.H.; Alshehri, F.D.; Alqarni, A.S.; Alasmari, D.S. Evaluate the Malocclusion in Subjects Reporting for Orthodontic Treatment among Saudi Population in Asser Region. *J. Int. Oral Health* **2014**, *6*, 42. [PubMed]
33. Zohud, O.; Lone, I.M.; Midlej, K.; Obaida, A.; Masarwa, S.; Schröder, A.; Küchler, E.C.; Nashef, A.; Kassem, F.; Reiser, V.; et al. Towards Genetic Dissection of Skeletal Class III Malocclusion: A Review of Genetic Variations Underlying the Phenotype in Humans and Future Directions. *J. Clin. Med.* **2023**, *12*, 3212. [CrossRef] [PubMed]
34. Aldrees, A.M. Pattern of Skeletal and Dental Malocclusions in Saudi Orthodontic Patients. *Saudi Med. J.* **2012**, *33*, 315–320.
35. Shaw, W.C.; Richmond, S.; O'Brien, K.D.; Brook, P.; Stephens, C.D. Quality Control in Orthodontics: Indices of Treatment Need and Treatment Standards. *Br. Dent. J.* **1991**, *170*, 107–112. [CrossRef]

36. Abdullah, M.S.B.; Rock, W.P. Assessment of Orthodontic Treatment Need in 5,112 Malaysian Children Using the IOTN and DAI Indices. *Community Dent. Health* **2001**, *18*, 242–248.
37. Grzywacz, I. Orthodontic Treatment Needs and Indications Assessed with IONT. *Ann. Acad. Medicae Stetin.* **2004**, *50*, 115–122.
38. Kolawole, K.A.; Otuyemi, O.D.; Jeboda, S.O.; Umweni, A.A. The Need for Orthodontic Treatment in a School and Referred Population of Nigeria Using the Index of Orthodontic Treatment Need (IOTN). *Odontostomatol. Trop.* **2008**, *31*, 11–19.
39. Esa, R.; Razak, I.A.; Allister, J.H. Epidemiology of Malocclusion and Orthodontic Treatment Need of 12–13-Year-Old Malaysian Schoolchildren. *Community Dent. Health* **2001**, *18*, 31–36.
40. Järvinen, S. Indexes for Orthodontic Treatment Need. *Am. J. Orthod. Dentofac. Orthop.* **2001**, *120*, 237–239. [CrossRef]
41. Beglin, F.M.; Firestone, A.R.; Vig, K.W.L.; Beck, F.M.; Kuthy, R.A.; Wade, D. A Comparison of the Reliability and Validity of 3 Occlusal Indexes of Orthodontic Treatment Need. *Am. J. Orthod. Dentofac. Orthop.* **2001**, *120*, 240–246. [CrossRef] [PubMed]
42. Hassan, R.; Rahimah, A. Occlusion, Malocclusion and Method of Measurements-an Overview. *Arch. Orofac. Sci.* **2007**, *2*, 3–9.
43. Leite-Cavalcanti, A.; Medeiros-Bezerra, P.K.; Moura, C. Breast-Feeding, Bottle-Feeding, Sucking Habits and Malocclusion in Brazilian Preschool Children [Aleitamento Natural, Aleitamento Artificial, Hábitos de Sucção e Maloclusões Em Pré-EscolaresBrasileiros]. *Rev. Salud Publica* **2007**, *9*, 194–204. [PubMed]
44. Fu, M.; Zhang, D.; Wang, B.; Deng, Y.; Wang, F.; Ye, X. The Prevalence of Malocclusion in China—An Investigation of 25,392 Children. *Chin. J. Stomatol.* **2002**, *37*, 371–373.
45. Devakrishnan, D.; Gnansambandam, V.; Kandasamy, S.; Sengottuvel, N.; Kumaragurubaran, P.; Rajasekaran, M. Comparative Study of Tooth Size and Arch Dimensions in Class I Crowded, Proclined Malocclusion and Class I Normal Occlusion. *J. Pharm. Bioallied Sci.* **2021**, *13*, S783. [CrossRef]
46. Ahmad, N.; Fida, M. Orthodontic Treatment Outcome Assessment Using Peer Assessment Rating (PAR) Index. *Pak. Oral Dent. J.* **2010**, *30*.
47. Leon-Salazar, V.; Janson, G.; Henriques, J.F.C. Influence of Initial Occlusal Severity on Time and Efficiency of Class i Malocclusion Treatment Carried out with and without Premolar Extractions. *Dent. Press J. Orthod.* **2014**, *19*, 38–49. [CrossRef]
48. Ishida, E.; Kunimatsu, R.; Medina, C.C.; Iwai, K.; Miura, S.; Tsuka, Y.; Tanimoto, K. Dental and Occlusal Changes during Mandibular Advancement Device Therapy in Japanese Patients with Obstructive Sleep Apnea: Four Years Follow-Up. *J. Clin. Med.* **2022**, *11*, 7539. [CrossRef]
49. Miyajima, K.; McNamara, J.A.; Kimura, T.; Murata, S.; Iizuka, T. Craniofacial Structure of Japanese and European-American Adults with Normal Occlusions and Well-Balanced Faces. *Am. J. Orthod. Dentofac. Orthop.* **1996**, *110*, 431–438. [CrossRef]
50. Vihinen, M. Systematics for Types and Effects of RNA Variations. *RNA Biol.* **2021**, *18*, 481. [CrossRef]
51. Jiang, Q.; Mei, L.; Zou, Y.; Ding, Q.; Cannon, R.D.; Chen, H.; Li, H. Genetic Polymorphisms in FGFR2 Underlie Skeletal Malocclusion. *J. Dent. Res.* **2019**, *98*, 1340–1347. [CrossRef]
52. Shimomura, T.; Kawakami, M.; Tatsumi, K.; Tanaka, T.; Morita-Takemura, S.; Kirita, T.; Wanaka, A. The Role of the Wnt Signaling Pathway in Upper Jaw Development of Chick Embryo. *Acta Histochem. Cytochem.* **2019**, *52*, 19. [CrossRef] [PubMed]
53. Singh, K.P.; Miaskowski, C.; Dhruva, A.A.; Flowers, E.; Kober, K.M. Mechanisms and Measurement of Changes in Gene Expression. *Biol. Res. Nurs.* **2008**, *20*, 369–382. [CrossRef] [PubMed]
54. Suzuki, A.; Yoshioka, H.; Liu, T.; Gull, A.; Singh, N.; Le, T.; Zhao, Z.; Iwata, J. Crucial Roles of MicroRNA-16-5p and MicroRNA-27b-3p in Ameloblast Differentiation Through Regulation of Genes Associated With Amelogenesis Imperfecta. *Front. Genet.* **2022**, *13*, 788259. [CrossRef] [PubMed]
55. Yan, L.; Liao, L.; Su, X. Role of Mechano-Sensitive Non-Coding RNAs in Bone Remodeling of Orthodontic Tooth Movement: Recent Advances. *Prog. Orthod.* **2022**, *23*, 1–21. [CrossRef] [PubMed]
56. Jin, Y.; Long, D.; Li, J.; Yu, R.; Song, Y.; Fang, J.; Yang, X.; Zhou, S.; Huang, S.; Zhao, Z. Extracellular Vesicles in Bone and Tooth: A State-of-Art Paradigm in Skeletal Regeneration. *J. Cell. Physiol.* **2019**, *234*, 14838–14851. [CrossRef] [PubMed]
57. Xin, Y.; Liu, Y.; Li, J.; Liu, D.; Zhang, C.; Wang, Y.; Zheng, S. A Novel LncRNA Mediates the Delayed Tooth Eruption of Cleidocranial Dysplasia. *Cells* **2022**, *11*, 2729. [CrossRef]
58. Lone, I.M.; Zohud, O.; Nashef, A.; Kirschneck, C.; Proff, P.; Watted, N.; Iraqi, F.A. Dissecting the Complexity of Skeletal-Malocclusion-Associated Phenotypes: Mouse for the Rescue. *Int. J. Mol. Sci.* **2023**, *24*, 2570. [CrossRef] [PubMed]
59. Kist, R.; Watson, M.; Wang, X.; Cairns, P.; Miles, C.; Reid, D.J.; Peters, H. Reduction of Pax9 Gene Dosage in an Allelic Series of Mouse Mutants Causes Hypodontia and Oligodontia. *Hum. Mol. Genet.* **2005**, *14*, 3605–3617. [CrossRef]
60. Lammi, L.; Arte, S.; Somer, M.; Järvinen, H.; Lahermo, P.; Thesleff, I.; Pirinen, S.; Nieminen, P. Mutations in AXIN2 Cause Familial Tooth Agenesis and Predispose to Colorectal Cancer. *Am. J. Hum. Genet.* **2004**, *74*, 1043. [CrossRef]
61. Mitsui, S.N.; Yasue, A.; Masuda, K.; Naruto, T.; Minegishi, Y.; Oyadomari, S.; Noji, S.; Imoto, I.; Tanaka, E. Novel Human Mutation and CRISPR/Cas Genome-Edited Mice Reveal the Importance of C-Terminal Domain of MSX1 in Tooth and Palate Development. *Sci. Rep.* **2016**, *6*, 38398. [CrossRef] [PubMed]
62. Lanham, S.A.; Bertram, C.; Cooper, C.; Oreffo, R.O.C. Animal Models of Maternal Nutrition and Altered Offspring Bone Structure—Bone Development across the Lifecourse. *Eur. Cell Mater.* **2011**, *22*, 321–332. [CrossRef]
63. Vora, S.R. Mouse Models for the Study of Cranial Base Growth and Anomalies. *Orthod. Craniofac. Res.* **2017**, *20*, 18–25. [CrossRef]
64. Nishio, C.; Huynh, N. Skeletal Malocclusion and Genetic Expression: An Evidence-Based Review. *J. Dent. Sleep Med.* **2016**, *3*, 57–63. [CrossRef]

65. Lone, I.M.; Midlej, K.; Nun, N.B.; Iraqi, F.A. Intestinal cancer development in response to oral infection with high-fat diet-induced Type 2 diabetes (T2D) in collaborative cross mice under different host genetic background effects. *Mamm. Genome* **2023**, *34*, 56–75. [CrossRef] [PubMed]
66. Lorè, N.I.; Sipione, B.; He, G.; Strug, L.J.; Atamni, H.J.; Dorman, A.; Mott, R.; Iraqi, F.A.; Bragonzia, A. Collaborative Cross Mice Yield Genetic Modifiers for Pseudomonas Aeruginosa Infection in Human Lung Disease. *mBio* **2020**, *11*, e00097-20. [CrossRef]
67. Lone, I.M.; Iraqi, F.A. Genetics of Murine Type 2 Diabetes and Comorbidities. *Mamm. Genome* **2022**, *33*, 421–436. [CrossRef]
68. Yehia, R.; Lone, I.M.; Yehia, I.; Iraqi, F.A. Studying the Pharmagenomic effect of Portulaca oleracea extract on anti-diabetic therapy using the Collaborative Cross mice. *Phytomed. Plus* **2023**, *3*, 100394. [CrossRef]
69. Churchill, G.A.; Airey, D.C.; Allayee, H.; Angel, J.M.; Attie, A.D.; Beatty, J.; Beavis, W.D.; Belknap, J.K.; Bennett, B.; Berrettini, W.; et al. The Collaborative Cross, a Community Resource for the Genetic Analysis of Complex Traits. *Nat. Genet.* **2004**, *36*, 1133–1137. [CrossRef]
70. Churchill, G.A. Recombinant Inbred Strain Panels: A Tool for Systems Genetics. *Physiol. Genom.* **2007**, *31*, 174–175. [CrossRef]
71. Durrant, C.; Tayem, H.; Yalcin, B.; Cleak, J.; Goodstadt, L.; Pardo-Manuel De Villena, F.; Mott, R.; Iraqi, F.A. Collaborative Cross Mice and Their Power to Map Host Susceptibility to Aspergillus Fumigatus Infection. *Genome Res.* **2011**, *21*, 1239–1248. [CrossRef] [PubMed]
72. Iraqi, F.A.; Mahajne, M.; Salaymah, Y.; Sandovski, H.; Tayem, H.; Vered, K.; Balmer, L.; Hall, M.; Manship, G.; Morahan, G.; et al. The Genome Architecture of the Collaborative Cross Mouse Genetic Reference Population. *Genetics* **2012**, *190*, 389–401. [CrossRef]
73. Levy, R.; Mott, R.F.; Iraqi, F.A.; Gabet, Y. Collaborative Cross Mice in a Genetic Association Study Reveal New Candidate Genes for Bone Microarchitecture. *BMC Genom.* **2015**, *16*, 1013. [CrossRef]
74. Lone, I.M.; Zohud, O.; Midlej, K.; Proff, P.; Watted, N.; Iraqi, F.A. Skeletal Class II Malocclusion: From Clinical Treatment Strategies to the Roadmap in Identifying the Genetic Bases of Development in Humans with the Support of the Collaborative Cross Mouse Population. *J. Clin. Med.* **2023**, *12*, 5148. [CrossRef] [PubMed]
75. Lone, I.M.; Nun, N.B.; Ghnaim, A.; Schaefer, A.S.; Houri-Haddad, Y.; Iraqi, F.A. High-fat diet and oral infection induced type 2 diabetes and obesity development under different genetic backgrounds. *Anim. Models Exp. Med.* **2023**, *6*, 131–145. [CrossRef]
76. Dorman, A.; Binenbaum, I.; Abu-ToamihAtamni, H.J.; Chatziioannou, A.; Tomlinson, I.; Mott, R.; Iraqi, F.A. Genetic Mapping of Novel Modifiers for Apc Min Induced Intestinal Polyps' Development Using the Genetic Architecture Power of the Collaborative Cross Mice. *BMC Genom.* **2021**, *22*, 566. [CrossRef]
77. Al-Balkhi, K.; Al-Zahrani, A. The Pattern of Malocclusions in Saudi Arabian Patients Attending for Orthodontic Treatment at the College of Dentistry, King Saud University, Riyadh. *Saudi Dent. J.* **1994**, *6*, 138–144.
78. Al-Emran, S.; Wisth, P.J.; Böe, O.E. Prevalence of Malocclusion and Need for Orthodontic Treatment in Saudi Arabia. *Community Dent. Oral Epidemiol.* **1990**, *18*, 253–255. [CrossRef]
79. Lione, R.; Buongiorno, M.; Laganà, G.; Cozza, P.; Franchi, L. Early Treatment of Class III Malocclusion with RME and Facial Mask: Evaluation of Dentoalveolar Effects on Digital Dental Casts. *Eur. J. Paediatr. Dent. Off. J. Eur. Acad. Paediatr. Dent.* **2015**, *16*, 217–220.
80. D'Apuzzo, F.; Grassia, V.; Quinzi, V.; Vitale, M.; Marzo, G.; Perillo, L. Paediatric Orthodontics Part 4: SEC III Protocol in Class III Malocclusion. *Eur. J. Paediatr. Dent.* **2019**, *20*, 330. [CrossRef]
81. Al Naasan, Z.; Broadbent, J.M.; Duncan, W.J.; Smith, M.B. Perceptions of Tailored Oral Health Education Resources among Former Refugees. *N. Z. Dent. J.* **2022**, *118*.
82. Salim, N.A.; ElSa'aideh, B.B.; Maayta, W.A.; Hassona, Y.M. Dental Services Provided to Syrian Refugee Children in Jordan: A Retrospective Study. *Spec. Care Dent.* **2020**, *40*, 260–266. [CrossRef]
83. Salim, N.A.; Maayta, W.A.; Hassona, Y.; Hammad, M. Oral Health Status and Risk Determinants in Adult Syrian Refugees in Jordan. *Community Dent. Health* **2021**, *38*, 53–58. [CrossRef] [PubMed]
84. Salim, N.A.; Maayta, W.; ElSa'aideh, B.B. The Oral Health of Refugees: Issues and Challenges Arising from a Case Series Analysis. *Community Dent. Oral Epidemiol.* **2020**, *48*, 195–200. [CrossRef] [PubMed]
85. Salim, N.A.; Shaini, F.J.; Sartawi, S.; Al-Shboul, B. Oral Health Status and Dental Treatment Needs in Syrian Refugee Children in Zaatari Camp. *J. Refug. Stud.* **2021**, *34*, 2492–2507. [CrossRef]
86. Vázquez-Nava, F.; Quezada-Castillo, J.A.; Oviedo-Treviño, S.; Saldivar-González, A.H.; Sánchez-Nuncio, H.R.; Beltrán-Guzmán, F.J.; Vázquez-Rodríguez, E.M.; Vázquez Rodríguez, C.F. Association between Allergic Rhinitis, Bottle Feeding, Non-Nutritive Sucking Habits, and Malocclusion in the Primary Dentition. *Arch. Dis. Child.* **2006**, *91*, 836–840. [CrossRef] [PubMed]
87. Góis, E.G.O.; Ribeiro, H.C.; Vale, M.P.P.; Paiva, S.M.; Serra-Negra, J.M.C.; Ramos-Jorge, M.L.; Pordeus, I.A. Influence of Nonnutritive Sucking Habits, Breathing Pattern and Adenoid Size on the Development of Malocclusion. *Angle Orthod.* **2008**, *78*, 647–654. [CrossRef]
88. Akbari, M.; Lankarani, K.B.; Honarvar, B.; Tabrizi, R.; Mirhadi, H.; Moosazadeh, M. Prevalence of Malocclusion among Iranian Children: A Systematic Review and Meta-Analysis. *Dent. Res. J. (Isfahan)* **2016**, *13*, 387. [CrossRef] [PubMed]
89. Warren, J.J.; Levy, S.M.; Nowak, A.J.; Tang, S. Non-Nutritive Sucking Behaviors in Preschool Children: A Longitudinal Study. *Pediatr. Dent.* **2000**, *22*, 187–191. [PubMed]
90. Janson, G.; Nakamura, A.; Barros, S.E.; Bombonatti, R.; Chiqueto, K. Efficiency of Class i and Class Ii Malocclusion Treatment with Four Premolar Extractions. *J. Appl. Oral Sci.* **2014**, *22*, 522–527. [CrossRef]

91. Ghnaim, A.; Lone, I.M.; Ben Nun, N.; Iraqi, F.A. Unraveling the Host Genetic Background Effect on Internal Organ Weight Influenced by Obesity and Diabetes Using Collaborative Cross Mice. *Int. J. Mol. Sci.* **2023**, *24*, 8201. [CrossRef] [PubMed]
92. Naini, F.B.; Moss, J.P. Three-dimensional assessment of the relative contribution of genetics and environment to various facial parameters with the twin method. *Am. J. Orthod. Dentofac. Orthop.* **2004**, *126*, 655–665. [CrossRef] [PubMed]
93. Moreno Uribe, L.M.; Miller, S.F. Genetics of the dentofacial variation in human malocclusion. *Orthod. Craniofacial Res.* **2015**, *18*, 91–99. [CrossRef] [PubMed]

Disclaimer/Publisher's Note: The statements, opinions and data contained in all publications are solely those of the individual author(s) and contributor(s) and not of MDPI and/or the editor(s). MDPI and/or the editor(s) disclaim responsibility for any injury to people or property resulting from any ideas, methods, instructions or products referred to in the content.

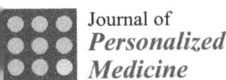

Article

Navigating the Landscape of Personalized Medicine: The Relevance of ChatGPT, BingChat, and Bard AI in Nephrology Literature Searches

Noppawit Aiumtrakul [1], Charat Thongprayoon [2,*], Supawadee Suppadungsuk [2,3], Pajaree Krisanapan [2,4], Jing Miao [2], Fawad Qureshi [2] and Wisit Cheungpasitporn [2]

1 Department of Medicine, John A. Burns School of Medicine, University of Hawaii, Honolulu, HI 96813, USA; noppawit@hawaii.edu
2 Division of Nephrology and Hypertension, Department of Medicine, Mayo Clinic, Rochester, MN 55905, USA; supawadee.sup@mahidol.ac.th (S.S.); pajareek@tu.ac.th (P.K.); miao.jing@mayo.edu (J.M.); qureshi.fawad@mayo.edu (F.Q.); cheungpasitporn.wisit@mayo.edu (W.C.)
3 Chakri Naruebodindra Medical Institute, Faculty of Medicine Ramathibodi Hospital, Mahidol University, Samut Prakan 10540, Thailand
4 Department of Internal Medicine, Faculty of Medicine, Thammasat University, Pathum Thani 12120, Thailand
* Correspondence: thongprayoon.charat@mayo.edu

Abstract: Background and Objectives: Literature reviews are foundational to understanding medical evidence. With AI tools like ChatGPT, Bing Chat and Bard AI emerging as potential aids in this domain, this study aimed to individually assess their citation accuracy within Nephrology, comparing their performance in providing precise. Materials and Methods: We generated the prompt to solicit 20 references in Vancouver style in each 12 Nephrology topics, using ChatGPT, Bing Chat and Bard. We verified the existence and accuracy of the provided references using PubMed, Google Scholar, and Web of Science. We categorized the validity of the references from the AI chatbot into (1) incomplete, (2) fabricated, (3) inaccurate, and (4) accurate. Results: A total of 199 (83%), 158 (66%) and 112 (47%) unique references were provided from ChatGPT, Bing Chat and Bard, respectively. ChatGPT provided 76 (38%) accurate, 82 (41%) inaccurate, 32 (16%) fabricated and 9 (5%) incomplete references. Bing Chat provided 47 (30%) accurate, 77 (49%) inaccurate, 21 (13%) fabricated and 13 (8%) incomplete references. In contrast, Bard provided 3 (3%) accurate, 26 (23%) inaccurate, 71 (63%) fabricated and 12 (11%) incomplete references. The most common error type across platforms was incorrect DOIs. Conclusions: In the field of medicine, the necessity for faultless adherence to research integrity is highlighted, asserting that even small errors cannot be tolerated. The outcomes of this investigation draw attention to inconsistent citation accuracy across the different AI tools evaluated. Despite some promising results, the discrepancies identified call for a cautious and rigorous vetting of AI-sourced references in medicine. Such chatbots, before becoming standard tools, need substantial refinements to assure unwavering precision in their outputs.

Keywords: literature review; nephrology references; ChatGPT; Bing Chat; Bard AI; accuracy; personalized medicine; precision medicine

Citation: Aiumtrakul, N.; Thongprayoon, C.; Suppadungsuk, S.; Krisanapan, P.; Miao, J.; Qureshi, F.; Cheungpasitporn, W. Navigating the Landscape of Personalized Medicine: The Relevance of ChatGPT, BingChat, and Bard AI in Nephrology Literature Searches. *J. Pers. Med.* 2023, *13*, 1457. https://doi.org/10.3390/jpm13101457

Academic Editor: Daniele Giansanti

Received: 10 September 2023
Revised: 29 September 2023
Accepted: 29 September 2023
Published: 30 September 2023

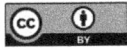

Copyright: © 2023 by the authors. Licensee MDPI, Basel, Switzerland. This article is an open access article distributed under the terms and conditions of the Creative Commons Attribution (CC BY) license (https://creativecommons.org/licenses/by/4.0/).

1. Introduction

The digital era has brought about transformative changes in various aspects of our lives, with the medical field being no exception [1,2]. Within the vast expanse of medical literature, scholars, clinicians, and medical professionals rely heavily on evidence-based studies to formulate decisions, guidelines, and recommendations for patients [3]. Literature reviews play an instrumental role in this process, often serving as the cornerstone to understanding the ever-expanding universe of medical evidence [4]. However, while the volume of information is expanding, so is the need for efficient tools to extract relevant knowledge.

The growing number of published articles has led to a substantial increase in the references that physicians and researchers must stay updated with. As of 2020, there were over 30 million articles indexed in PubMed alone, with an estimated addition of a million entries each year [5]. This exponential growth makes the task of manually extracting, comparing, and verifying references not only laborious but also prone to human errors [6]. In this context, AI-powered platforms are emerging as potential aides for literature reviews [7]. Contemporary innovations have introduced platforms such as ChatGPT [8], Bing Chat [9] and Bard AI [10]. These tools are not just digital cataloging systems but smart engines that claim to understand and retrieve precise information. The allure of such platforms lies in their ability to rapidly sift through vast data sets, potentially offering precise references that would take humans considerably longer to extract [11,12].

The emergence of ChatGPT, a creation of OpenAI, introduces promising prospects spanning a variety of domains, with a pronounced emphasis on the enrichment of healthcare education [13]. This AI framework not only highlights its advanced acumen in information retrieval but also adeptly addresses syntactical inaccuracies, thereby serving as a valuable resource for literature evaluations and the composition of scholarly manuscripts [8]. In a parallel vein, Bing Chat, a product of Microsoft, emerges as an AI-driven conversational agent capable of engendering inventive and novel content, spanning the spectrum from poetic compositions and narratives to code snippets, essays, musical compositions, satirical renditions of celebrities, and visual representations [9]. Akin to its counterparts, Bard AI, the brainchild of Google, assumes its stance as a formidable entity within the domain of AI models, having undergone rigorous training on an expansive corpus encompassing textual and code-oriented knowledge culled from diverse sources, including literary works and academic articles [10]. The transformative potential of these technological tools in revolutionizing the paradigm of information retrieval is evident; however, their precision, particularly in terms of adhering to meticulous citation protocols, remains subject to meticulous examination.

The accuracy of citations within scholarly discourse is far from being a mere ritualistic practice; rather, it holds a pivotal role. These references provide a conduit for readers to retrace the steps back to original sources, thereby ensuring the veracity of derived conclusions and recommendations firmly anchored in authentic research endeavors. The presence of even minute inaccuracies within references can cast a shadow of doubt over the entirety of a scholarly paper, thereby undermining both its credibility and the integrity of the author [14]. This holds critical importance, especially in specialized fields such as Nephrology, where medical treatments have far-reaching effects on patient health and general well-being, including risks such as kidney failure or allograft rejection or failure. A single incorrect reference carries the risk of initiating misunderstandings, which could eventually lead to less than ideal or even harmful clinical decisions. The present investigation, therefore, is conceived with the overarching aim of unraveling the precision exhibited by these emergent AI entities in the realm of citations, particularly within the highly specialized terrain of Nephrology.

The purpose of this study is to assess the citation accuracy of AI models including ChatGPT (versions 3.5 and 4.0) [15], Bing Chat, and Bard AI in retrieving and validating references for academic research in nephrology.

2. Materials and Methods

2.1. Search Strategy and Criteria

We used three distinct AI chatbots to perform literature searches in nephrology, including (1) ChatGPT, (2) Bing Chat, and (3) Bard AI. To ensure the comparability of these chatbots, we standardized the criteria for evaluating their performance based on search results' relevance, comprehensiveness, and the timeliness of the articles retrieved. ChatGPT is a large language model developed by OpenAI and integrates both GPT-3.5 [16] and GPT-4.0 models [15] that comprehend and generate human-like responses through text. Bing Chat is powered by GPT-4.0 and incorporated into the Microsoft Edge browser, which has another capability to generate images and innovative content [9]. Bard AI, a robust Large Language Model (LLM) developed by Google based on Pathways Language Model 2 (PaLM2) and trained on an expansive collection of text and code that exhibits creative content design.

On 1 August 2023, we generated the prompt to ask AI chatbots to provide 20 references in Vancouver style, a commonly used citation style in academic writing in each Nephrology topics; The topics were chosen to reflect a comprehensive understanding of the field and were pre-determined through a review of the most common nephrology subjects discussed in existing literature. (1) general nephrology, (2) glomerular disease, (3) hypertension, (4) acute kidney injury, (5) chronic kidney disease, (6) end-stage kidney disease, (7) electrolyte disorders, (8) acid-base disturbances, (9) kidney stones, (10) hemodialysis, (11) peritoneal dialysis and (12) kidney transplantation. There was slight difference between the prompts used for each individual AI chatbot as we modified the prompt to optimize their responses; "please provide 20 references in Vancouver style and links of the most updated literatures regarding (Nephrology topic)" for ChatGPT, "provide Vancouver references with DOI of 20 articles on (Nephrology topic)" for Bing Chat, and "20 updated references regarding (Nephrology topic) in Vancouver style" for Bard AI. We used only GPT-3.5 model for ChatGPT because GPT-4.0 was unable to provide actual references but it solely provided examples of references despite our attempt to modify the prompt used. We documented five key components of provided references: (1) author name, (2) publication title, (3) journal title, (4) publication year or issue and (5) digital object identifier (DOI). This categorization was performed to ensure the verification process adhered to a uniform criterion for all three chatbots, facilitating a balanced assessment.

We verified the existence and accuracy of the references using several medical literature databases. The databases were selected based on their reputability and coverage in the field of nephrology. We initially used the provided DOI to search for its corresponding references in PubMed [5], the widely recognized database in biomedical literatures. If we could not find the reference in PubMed or we had incomplete or missing DOI, we used Google Scholar [17] or Web of Science [18] as additional databases for comprehensive search. We used University of Hawaii library website [19] and google search to check references of textbook or book chapter.

We categorized the validity of the provided references from the AI chatbot into following groups; (1) incomplete, (2) fabricated, (3) inaccurate, and (4) accurate. These categories were defined to allow for the precise characterization of the search results, which is crucial for determining the reliability and utility of AI-generated references. Reference was defined as incomplete when the provided reference information was inadequate to verify its existence in aforementioned medical databases. Reference was defined as fabricated when we could not find the reference in the database. Reference was defined as existing but inaccurate when we could identify the reference in the database but at least one of five reference components were incorrect. Reference was defined as existing and accurate when we could identify the reference in the database and all of five reference components were correct. A flow diagram of the research methodology was Illustrated in Figure 1 and the example of an assessment of references was illustrated in Figure 2.

To assess both the magnitude and directionality of linear relationships among different performance indicators of the chatbots, we computed Pearson correlation coefficients. The Pearson correlation method was chosen for its sensitivity to linear associations, making it well-suited for our dataset, which we ascertained met the assumptions of linearity, normality, and homoscedasticity. In these matrices, individual cells contain the computed Pearson coefficients, which are bounded between -1 and 1. The closer a coefficient is to 1, the stronger the positive linear relationship, indicating that an increase in one performance metric is likely paralleled by an increase in another. In contrast, a coefficient value nearing -1 reveals a strong negative relationship, meaning that a rise in one metric typically results in a decline in another. These boundaries are strict and allow for nuanced interpretation: a value of exactly 1 or -1 would signify a perfect linear relationship, positive or negative respectively, although such a result is exceedingly rare in practical applications. Coefficients approximating zero signify weak or negligible linear relationships, implying that changes in one variable are not systematically accompanied by changes in another. The use of Pearson correlation analysis in this context is instrumental for pinpointing specific performance metrics that may be most amenable to enhancements, thereby aiding in targeted optimization of chatbot functionalities.

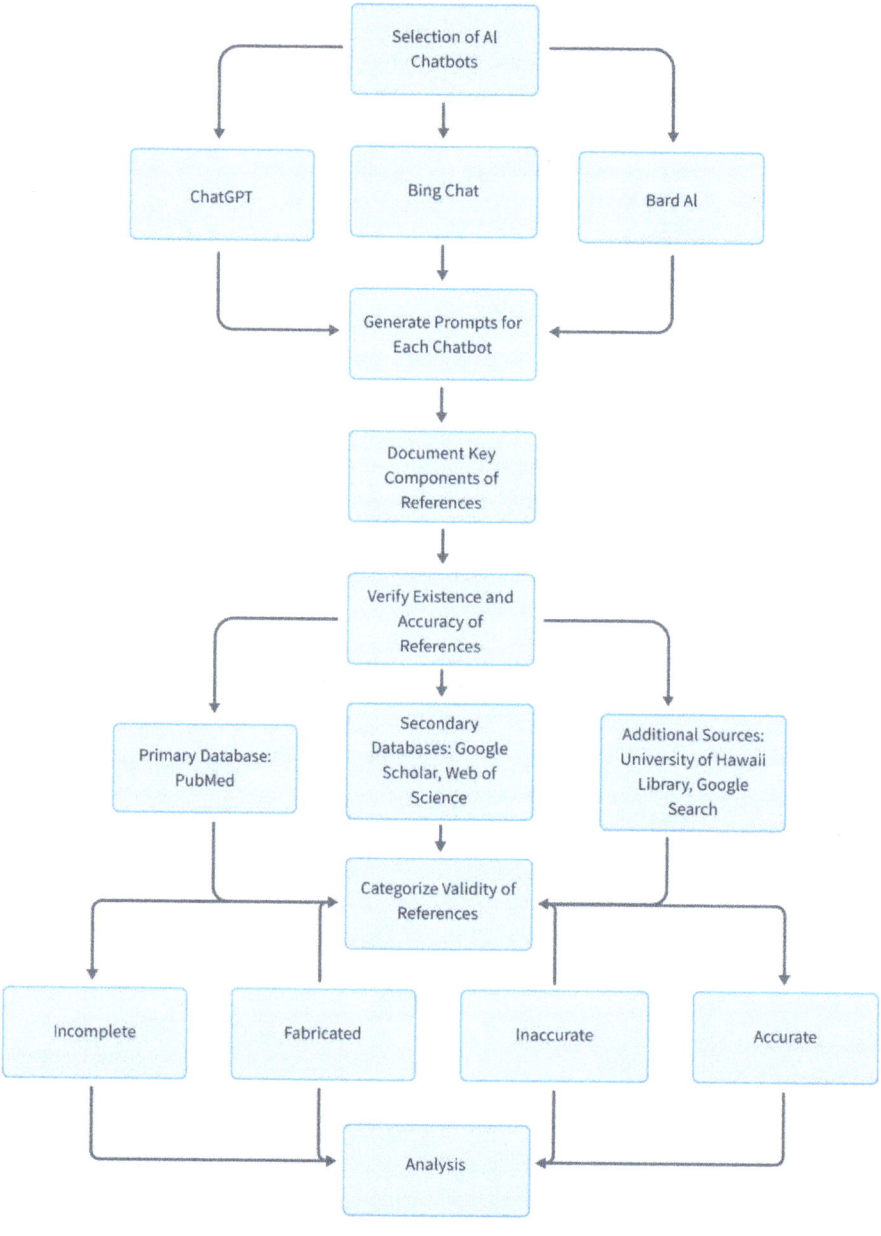

Figure 1. Flow diagram of using AI chatbots for literature search and assessment of validity.

9. Kidney Disease: Improving Global Outcomes (KDIGO) CKD-MBD Update Work Group. KDIGO 2017 clinical practice guideline update for the diagnosis, evaluation, prevention, and treatment of chronic kidney disease-mineral and bone disorder (CKD-MBD). Kidney Int Suppl. 2017 Jul;7(1):1-59. doi: 10.1016/j.kisu.2017.04.001.

10. McCullough KP, Morgenstern H, Saran R, Herman WH, Robinson BM. Projecting ESRD incidence and prevalence in the United States through 2030. J Am Soc Nephrol. 2019 May;30(5):127-135. doi: 10.1681/ASN.2018070736.

11. Hecking M, Bieber BA, Ethier J, Kautzky-Willer A, Sunder-Plassmann G, Säemann MD, Hörl WH, Jardine AG, Marchetti P, Seitz-Polski B, Tordoir J, Chazot C, Levin NW, Fouque D, Lamacchia O, Wanner C, Wiecek A, Moissl U, Pascual J, Floege J, Cannata-Andía JB, Pipili C, Zaoui P, London G, Zoccali C, Caskey FJ, Postorino M, Canaud B. Sex-Specific Differences in Hemodialysis Prevalence and Practices and the Male-to-Female Mortality Rate: The Dialysis Outcomes and Practice Patterns Study (DOPPS). PLoS Med. 2014 Oct 28;11(10):e1001750. doi: 10.1371/journal.pmed.1001750.

12. Wetmore JB, Li S, Molony JT, Liu J, Yan S, Gilbertson DT, Collins AJ. Relationship between elevated pulse pressure and outcomes in patients with CKD: a multicenter prospective cohort study. Am J Kidney Dis. 2016 Mar;67(3):448-56. doi: 10.1053/j.ajkd.2015.08.020.

13. van der Sande FM, Kooman JP, Ieunissen KML, van der Sande FM, Kooman JP, Ieunissen KML. [Hemodialysis: past, present, and future]. Ned Tijdschr Geneeskd. 2018;162:D2751. Dutch.

14. Saran R, Bragg-Gresham JL, Rayner HC, Goodkin DA, Keen ML, Van Dijk PC, Kurokawa K, Piera L, Saito A, Fukuhara S, Young EW, Held PJ, Port FK. Nonadherence in hemodialysis: associations with mortality, hospitalization, and practice patterns in the DOPPS. Kidney Int. 2003 Feb;64(1):254-62. doi: 10.1046/j.1523-1755.2003.00064.x.

15. Weinhandl ED, Nieman KM, Gilbertson DT, Collins AJ. Hospitalization in the year preceding initiation of maintenance hemodialysis, 1996-2010. Am J Kidney Dis. 2015 Apr;65(4): 594-602. doi: 10.1053/j.ajkd.2014.11.017.

Figure 2. Demonstration of citation assessment regarding hemodialysis topic. The non-highlighted texts represent accurate parts. The blue highlights represent incorrect parts. The pink highlights indicate fabricated references.

2.2. Statistical Analysis

We reviewed the references and excluded duplicated reference from the same AI chatbot before analysis. We presented the validity of the provided references as counts with percentages and compared among AI chatbots using Chi-squared test. p-value < 0.05 was considered statistically significant. IBM SPSS statistics version 26 was used for all statistical analyses.

The calculations of Pearson correlation coefficients involved generating correlation matrices, executed with Python's Seaborn library—a tool that efficiently interfaces with Pandas for data structuring and Matplotlib for graphical output.

3. Results

Although each AI chatbots was expected to provide 240 references (20 references in each of 12 nephrology topics), 41 (17%), 65 (29%) and 39 (26%) references provided by ChatGPT, Bing Chat and Bard, respectively, were found as duplicated references, while 17 (7%) references from Bing Chat and 89 (37%) references from Bard were absent.

A total of 199 (83%), 158 (66%) and 112 (47%) unique references were provided from ChatGPT, Bing Chat and Bard, respectively. ChatGPT provided 76 (38%) accurate, 82 (41%) inaccurate, 32 (16%) fabricated and 9 (5%) incomplete references. Bing Chat provided 47 (30%) accurate, 77 (49%) inaccurate, 21 (13%) fabricated and 13 (8%) incomplete references. In contrast, Bard provided 3 (3%) accurate, 26 (23%) inaccurate, 71 (63%) fabricated and 12 (11%) incomplete references. The proportion of existing references were similar between ChatGPT and Bing Chat, but ChatGPT provided higher proportion of accurate references. Bard had the highest proportion of fabricated and incomplete references. There were statistically significant differences in proportion of accurate, inaccurate and fabricated references between ChatGPT and Bard, and between Bing Chat and Bard. However, the validity between ChatGPT and Bing Chat did not significantly differ (Table 1 and Figure 3).

Table 1. Validity of provided references from ChatGPT, Bing Chat and Bard AI.

	ChatGPT-3.5 (n = 199)	Bing Chat (n = 158)	Bard (n = 112)	*p*-Value
Accurate	76 (38.2%) *	47 (29.8%) **	3 (2.7%) *,**	<0.001
Inaccurate	82 (41.2%) *	77 (48.7%) **	26 (23.2%) *,**	<0.001
Fabricated	32 (16.1%) *	21 (13.3%) **	71 (63.4%) *,**	<0.001
Incomplete	9 (4.5%)	13 (8.2%)	12 (10.7%)	0.11

* Significant difference between ChatGPT-3.5 and Bard $p < 0.05$. ** Significant difference between Bing Chat and Bard $p < 0.05$.

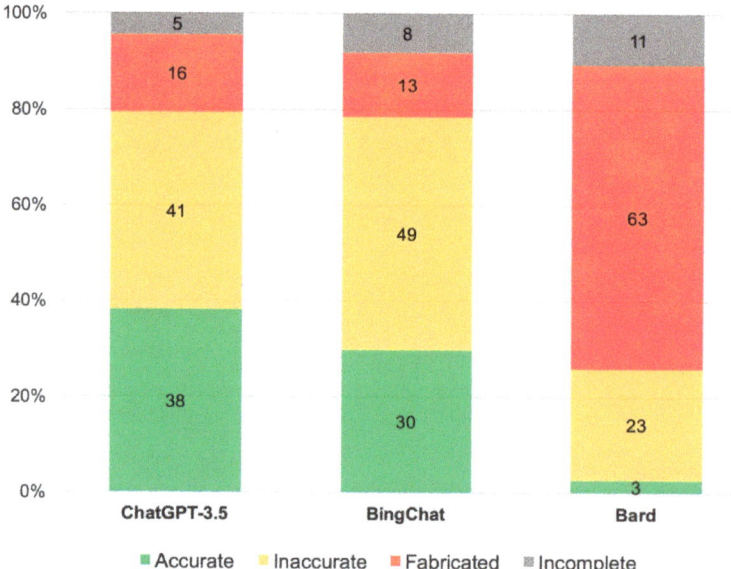

Figure 3. Comparison of validity in providing literature between ChatGPT, Bing Chat and Bard AI.

When we assessed the reason for inaccurate references, DOI was the most common inaccurate component in references provided by ChatGPT and Bing Chat, followed by author name, publication year/issue, journal title, and reference title. In contrast, author name was the most common reason inaccurate component in references provided by Bard, followed by DOI, publication year/issue, journal title, and reference title. Significant differences of all inaccuracy domains were found between ChatGPT and Bard, and between Bing Chat and Bard, while ChatGPT and Bing Chat were not statistically different (Table 2 and Figures 4 and 5).

Table 2. Types of inaccuracy detected among the inaccurate references between ChatGPT, Bing Chat and Bard AI.

	ChatGPT-3.5 (n = 82)	Bing Chat (n = 77)	Bard (n = 26)	*p*-Value
Inaccurate DOI	74 (90.3%) *	68 (88.3%) **	18 (69.2%) *,**	0.02
Inaccurate title	4 (4.9%) *	2 (2.6%) **	7 (26.9%) *,**	<0.001
Inaccurate author	18 (22.0%) *	13 (16.9%) **	19 (73.1%) *,**	<0.001
Inaccurate journal/book	10 (12.2%) *	6 (7.8%) **	8 (30.8%) *,**	0.010
Inaccurate year/issue	14 (17.1%) *	7 (9.1%) **	15 (57.7%) *,**	<0.001

* Significant difference between ChatGPT-3.5 and Bard $p < 0.05$. ** Significant difference between Bing Chat and Bard $p < 0.05$.

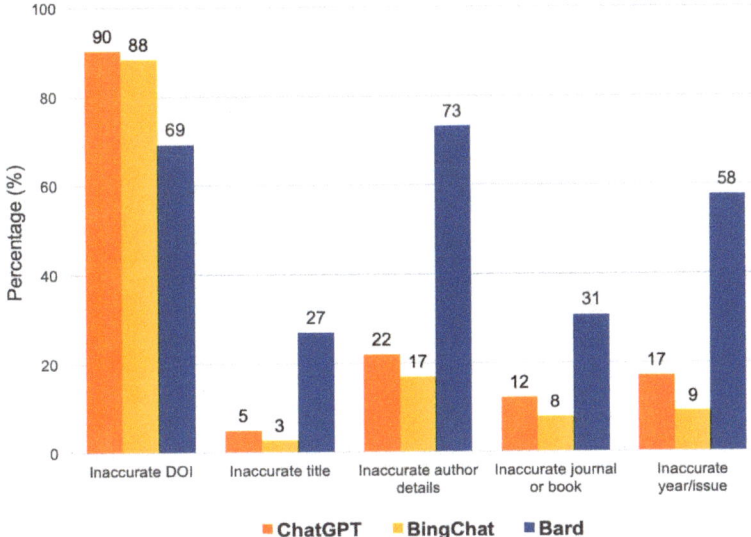

Figure 4. Percentages of each type of inaccuracy among the inaccurate references of ChatGPT, Bing Chat and Bard AI.

3.1. Correlation Analysis

3.1.1. Validity Metrics

Accurate vs. Inaccurate: A negative correlation of −0.92 suggests that as the accuracy of a chatbot increases, the inaccuracy decreases.

Inaccurate vs. Incomplete: A high positive correlation (0.99) is observed, indicating that chatbots that inaccurate information are also likely to provide incomplete answers (Figure 6).

3.1.2. Incorrect Information Metrics

Missing DOI vs. Wrong DOI: A strong negative correlation of −0.75 implies that chatbots that often miss DOIs are less likely to provide wrong DOIs.

Wrong Author vs. Wrong Journal/Book: A negative correlation of −0.58 suggests that if a chatbot frequently gets the author wrong, it is less likely to get the journal or book wrong (Figure 7).

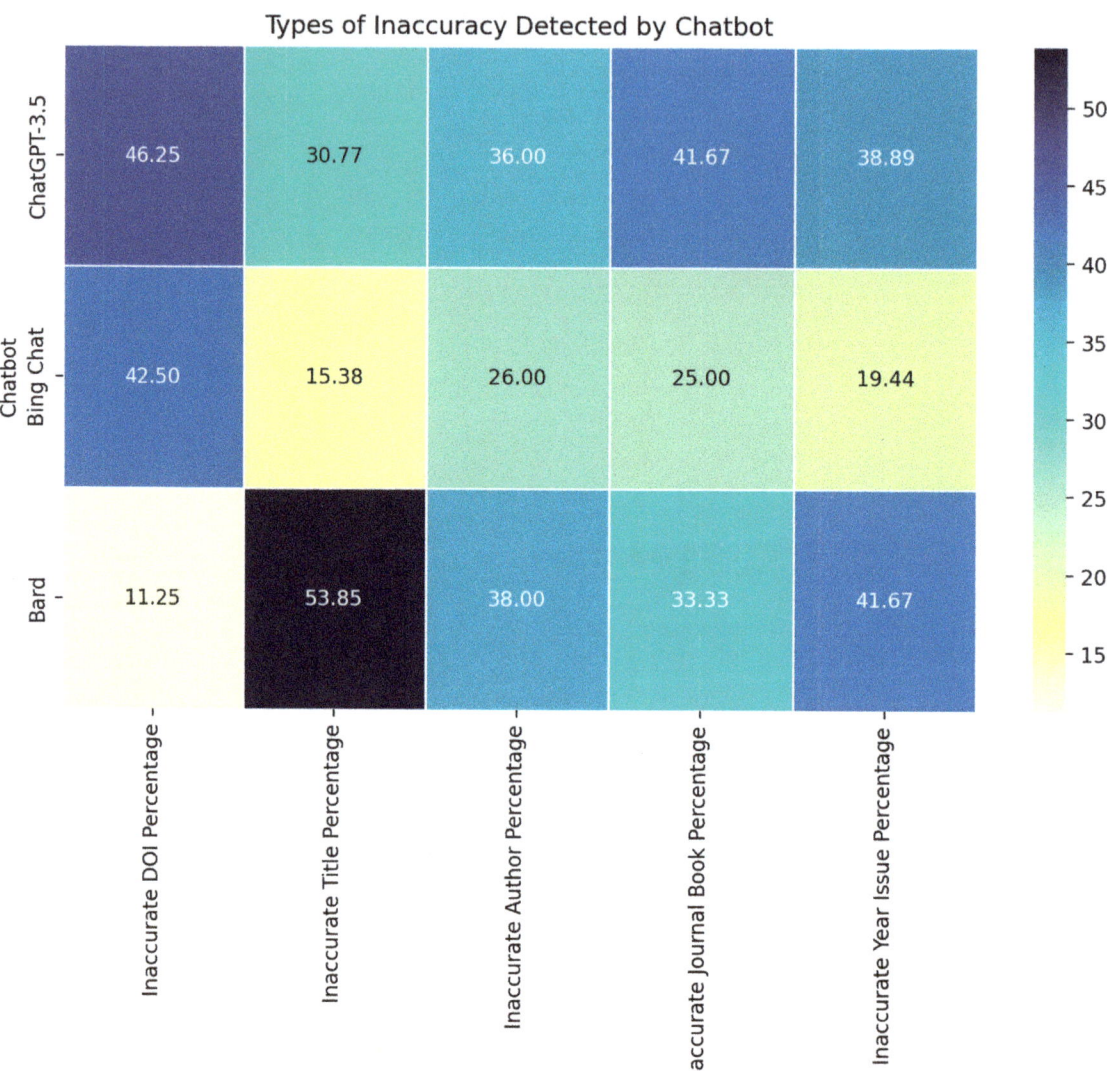

Figure 5. Heatmap visualizing the types of inaccuracies detected among the references provided by each chatbot. The rows represent the chatbots: ChatGPT-3.5, Bing Chat, and Bard. The columns represent the types of inaccuracies: DOI, Title, Author, Journal/Book, and Year/Issue. The intensity of the color indicates the magnitude of the inaccuracy, with darker shades representing higher percentages.

3.1.3. Missed and Duplicate Metrics

Missed vs. Duplicate: A strong negative correlation of -1 suggests that chatbots that miss information are unlikely to produce duplicate information (Figure 8).

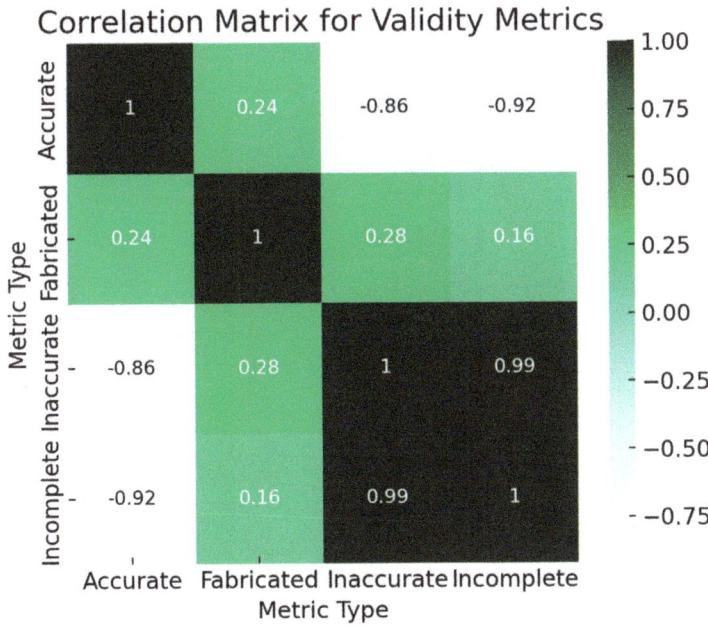

Figure 6. Correlation Matrix for Validity Metrics.

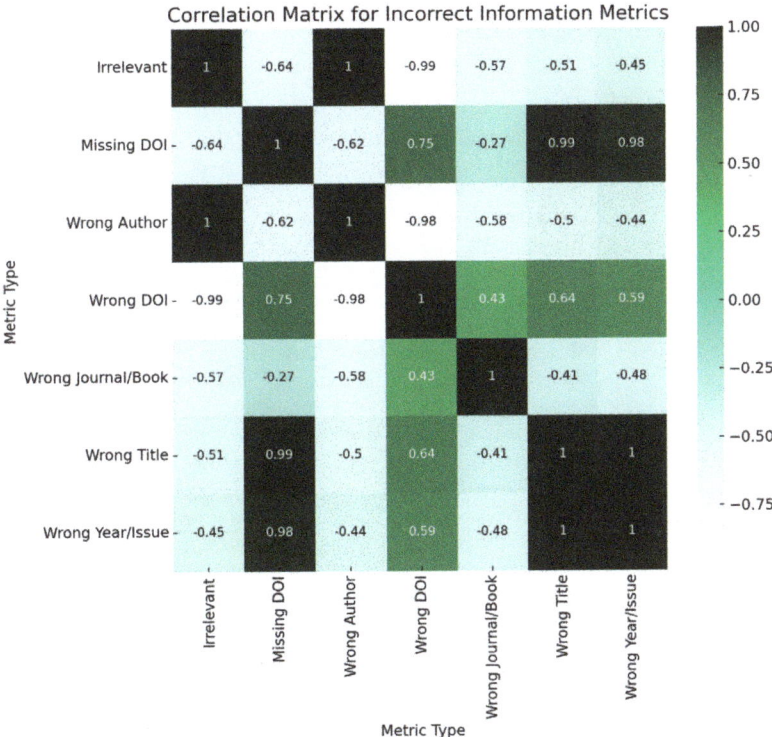

Figure 7. Correlation Matrix for Incorrect Information Metrics.

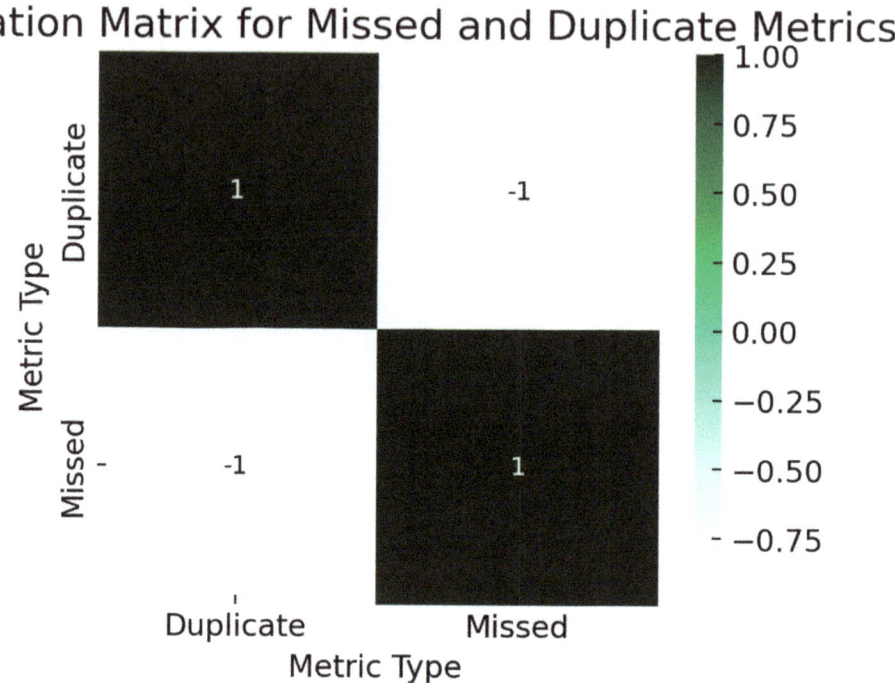

Figure 8. Correlation Matrix for Missed and Duplicate Metrics.

4. Discussion

The advancement of AI within the medical field has led to substantial transformations [20,21], including assisting in the specialized diet supports [22,23], prevention of potential allergic reactions [24,25], detection of prescription errors [26], extraction of drug interactions from the literature [27], and particularly concerning literature reviews [28,29]. As the production of medical evidence continues to grow at an accelerated rate, the need for effective tools to sift through and analyze pertinent information has become critically important. In response to this need, AI-powered platforms such as ChatGPT, Bing Chat, and Bard AI have emerged as potential aids in literature reviews [11,12,29]. The findings of this study, however, demonstrate varying degrees of reliability and validity exhibited by the three generative AI chatbots, namely ChatGPT-3.5, Bing Chat and Bard, when tasked with providing references pertaining to Nephrology subjects. It is important to recognize that the utilization of AI chatbots for generating dependable and valid references is accompanied by certain limitations and challenges, encompassing concerns such as the generation of fabricated, inaccurate and incomplete references.

The study outcomes delineate distinctive patterns regarding citation accuracy within the purview of AI tools. ChatGPT emerges with the highest precision at 38%, emblematic of its adherence to established citation protocols. This, however, coexists with a notable proportion of erroneous references at 41%. In contrast, Bing Chat demonstrates an alternative pattern, characterized by a preponderance of inaccurate references (49%) alongside a relatively diminished occurrence of entirely accurate references (30%). However, the validity of ChatGPT and Bing Chat in providing Nephrology references were not significantly different. Bard AI, conversely, exhibits the highest incidence of fabricated references (63%) and incomplete references (11%), suggesting an avenue for enhancement in its reference generation mechanism. It is pertinent to underscore that the discordances identified, including the misallocation of DOIs, underscore the criticality of scrupulous attention to minutiae within the medical realm, where even minor inaccuracies bear substantial consequences.

The study's findings underscore the heterogeneity in citation accuracy among the evaluated AI tools. While each tool showcased certain strengths, such as ChatGPT's higher accuracy rate, the discrepancies identified emphasize the need for careful and rigorous vetting of AI-sourced references in the medical field. The precision and authenticity of references hold critical significance, especially considering the potential consequences of medical decisions that rely on these sources. The substantial discrepancies observed in citation accuracy among these AI chatbots reveal that they may not consistently meet the rigorous standards demanded by the medical realm. ChatGPT's relatively high accuracy, even with its considerable inaccuracies, signifies a degree of potential utility, but the prevalence of incorrect and fabricated references remains a pressing concern.

In terms of optimizing chatbot performance for specific needs, several strategic considerations emerge from the data. If accuracy is of utmost importance, ChatGPT-3.5 stands out as the most reliable choice, although it would benefit from targeted improvements in areas like DOI accuracy. BingChat, on the other hand, offers a different set of trade-offs: it generates less fabricated information but is more prone to inaccuracies. Therefore, it could serve as a viable option where the fabrication of data is a primary concern. The analysis strongly suggests avoiding the experimental version of Bard as of 1 August 2023, for tasks requiring high reliability, given its alarming rates of both fabricated and inaccurate information. Additionally, each chatbot has identifiable weak areas—ChatGPT-3.5 with incorrect DOIs and BingChat with missing DOIs, for instance. These weaknesses could be mitigated through secondary verification systems. When it comes to handling duplicates and missed responses, ChatGPT-3.5 offers the most favorable profile, despite a 17.08% duplication rate. For those prioritizing quality over quantity, the data indicate that focusing on further optimizing ChatGPT-3.5 is the most effective approach. Advanced methods, such as machine learning algorithms, could be employed to refine its performance in specific areas like DOI accuracy. Finally, for those open to unconventional strategies, exploring ensemble methods that combine the strengths of different chatbots could be a worthwhile avenue for research. While speculative, such an approach could result in a more robust and versatile chatbot solution.

Medical research is a cornerstone of evidence-based practice, where even minor errors can have profound consequences on patient care, clinical decisions, and scientific advancement [30]. The findings of this study serve as a warning against premature reliance on AI-generated references in the medical domain. The presence of inaccuracies, fabrications, and incomplete references is untenable, as these undermine the integrity of scholarly work and compromise the trust placed in medical research. Consequently, policies and guidelines need to be developed to ensure the responsible and ethical integration of AI tools in medical research processes. These policies should emphasize the need for rigorous validation and vetting of AI-generated references before their incorporation into clinical decision-making or research publications.

The correlation analysis revealed several noteworthy aspects that could significantly inform strategies for optimizing chatbot performance. First, there's a clear trade-off in validity; a chatbot that excels in accuracy tends to produce less inaccurate information. However, such bots might still fabricate or provide incomplete information, necessitating caution. Second, specific risk areas were identified. For instance, chatbots that frequently miss DOIs are less prone to providing incorrect DOIs, and vice versa. This insight could be invaluable for implementing targeted validation strategies. Moreover, the correlation between missed and duplicated information suggests another layer of complexity. While chatbots that frequently miss information are unlikely to produce duplicates, the correlation is strong, thus requiring strategic monitoring. This monitoring could focus on specific error types that a chatbot is prone to making. For example, a chatbot that often produces incorrect information may also be susceptible to delivering incomplete responses. Lastly, the correlations offer avenues for customization and fine-tuning of chatbot behavior. Knowing a bot's strengths and weaknesses in particular areas enables the implementation of specialized validation or correction systems. As an example, if a chatbot is generally accurate but frequently errs in DOI references, a secondary validation system could be introduced specifically to check and correct DOI information. This approach allows for the leveraging of the chatbot's strengths while mitigating its weaknesses.

The integration of AI tools in the medical field introduces complex ethical considerations [28,29,31–33]. As evidenced by this study, the inaccuracies and fabrications in AI-generated references could potentially lead to misinterpretation, misinformation, and misguided medical decisions. Therefore, it is imperative to establish robust ethical frameworks and policy guidelines that guide the responsible use of AI chatbots in generating references for medical research. Such policies should prioritize patient safety, research integrity, and the advancement of medical knowledge. To address these concerns, regulatory bodies and professional organizations should collaborate to develop guidelines that mandate thorough validation and scrutiny of AI-generated references before they are incorporated into research papers, clinical guidelines, or medical recommendations. These guidelines could stipulate the necessity of human oversight, validation by domain experts, and cross-referencing with established databases. Furthermore, ethical considerations should extend to the transparency of AI-generated content. Users should be informed when references are AI-generated, allowing them to assess the reliability and credibility of the sources. This transparency aligns with the principles of informed consent and empowers readers to make informed judgments about the validity of the information presented.

5. Limitations

This study bears several limitations that warrant acknowledgment.

- AI platforms: Our assessment exclusively focused solely on ChatGPT (GPT-3.5 and GPT-4.0), Bing Chat, and Bard AI, excluding other emerging AI platforms that may exhibit distinct citation accuracy profiles.
- Lack of clinical implications: We did not explore the downstream impact of reference inaccuracies on downstream research, clinical decision-making, or patient outcomes, which could provide crucial insights into the practical implications of AI-generated references in the medical domain.
- Limited citation assessment: While the study accounted for discrepancies in citation elements such as DOIs and author names, we did not investigate potential errors in other bibliographic elements, such as the accuracy of the Vancouver format or page ranges. This omission could underestimate the full scope of inaccuracies present in AI-generated references.
- Variability due to updates: The AI models used in this study are subject to updates and modifications. The investigation was conducted with specific versions of AI models, and as these models undergo continuous refinement, their citation accuracy may evolve.
- Scope: The study's sample size of Nephrology topics and AI-generated references might not fully capture the breadth of medical literature or the complexity of citation accuracy in other medical specialties. The study's exclusive focus on AI chatbots limits the exploration of potential variations in citation accuracy among different AI-powered tools, such as summarization algorithms or natural language processing applications.
- Validity of databases: The assessment of AI-generated references relied on cross-referencing with established databases, assuming the accuracy of these databases. Any errors or discrepancies present in the reference databases could influence the study's findings and conclusions.
- Chatbot Extensions and Web Search: As the technological landscape evolves, chatbots are increasingly being equipped with the ability to integrate extensions and external resources, including web search functions. While this feature augments the utility of chatbots, it simultaneously introduces another layer of complexity in terms of citation accuracy and source validation. There is an imperative for future studies to critically evaluate the accuracy and reliability of references generated through these additional features.

6. Conclusions

This study underscores the foundational significance of unwavering research fidelity within the intricate domain of Nephrology. While the potential of AI tools for streamlining literature reviews is evident, the identified discrepancies call for a cautious and meticulous approach in their utilization. The medical community's commitment to precision demands that even minor inaccuracies remain unacceptable. As the potential for AI tools to revolutionize medical research and practice persists, it is essential to refine and fortify these chatbots before they can be confidently embraced as standard tools.

Author Contributions: Conceptualization, N.A., C.T., S.S., P.K., J.M., F.Q. and W.C.; Data curation, N.A. and W.C.; Formal analysis, N.A., C.T., F.Q. and W.C.; Funding acquisition, C.T. and W.C.; Investigation, N.A., C.T., S.S. and W.C.; Methodology, N.A., C.T., S.S., P.K., J.M., F.Q. and W.C.; Project administration, N.A., C.T., J.M. and W.C.; Resources, N.A., C.T., S.S. and W.C.; Software, N.A., C.T. and W.C.; Supervision, C.T., S.S., P.K., J.M., F.Q. and W.C.; Validation, N.A., C.T., S.S., J.M. and W.C.; Visualization, N.A., C.T. and W.C.; Writing—original draft, N.A., C.T. and W.C.; Writing—review & editing, N.A., C.T., S.S., P.K., J.M., F.Q. and W.C. The responses, demonstrations, and figures presented in this manuscript were created using AI chatbots, including with the utilization of ChatGPT (GPT-3.5), an AI language model developed by OpenAI,. Bing Chat (GPT-4.0) generated by Microsoft, and Bard AI built on PaLM operated by Google. The flow diagram and mind map showcased in this manuscript were designed using Whimsical. Visualizations were designed using Data Interpreter. All authors have read and agreed to the published version of the manuscript.

Funding: This research received no external funding.

Institutional Review Board Statement: The study was conducted and approved by the Institutional Review Board (or Ethics Committee) of Mayo Clinic Institute Review Broad (IRB number 23-005661, 30 June 2023).

Informed Consent Statement: Not applicable.

Data Availability Statement: Data Availability Statements are available in the original publication, reports, and preprints that were cited in the reference citation.

Acknowledgments: The manuscript presents a research study that employed AI chatbots for its investigations. Notably, it incorporated the use of ChatGPT versions GPT-3.5 and GPT-4.0, both developed by OpenAI. Additionally, the study made use of Bing Chat, a product of Microsoft, and Bard AI, which is based on the PaLM architecture and is a Google initiative. The manuscript also features a flow diagram crafted using Whimsical. The other contents of this manuscript were generated by the authors and did not employ AI systems for writing purposes. All content written in this manuscript results from the authors' contributions.

Conflicts of Interest: The authors declare no conflict of interest. All authors had access to the data and played essential roles in writing of the manuscript.

References

1. Blanco-Gonzalez, A.; Cabezon, A.; Seco-Gonzalez, A.; Conde-Torres, D.; Antelo-Riveiro, P.; Pineiro, A.; Garcia-Fandino, R. The Role of AI in Drug Discovery: Challenges, Opportunities, and Strategies. *Pharmaceuticals* **2023**, *16*, 891. [CrossRef] [PubMed]
2. Salim, H. Living in the digital era: The impact of digital technologies on human health. *Malays. Fam. Physician* **2022**, *17*, 1. [CrossRef] [PubMed]
3. Djulbegovic, B.; Guyatt, G.H. Progress in evidence-based medicine: A quarter century on. *Lancet* **2017**, *390*, 415–423. [CrossRef]
4. Cooper, C.; Booth, A.; Varley-Campbell, J.; Britten, N.; Garside, R. Defining the process to literature searching in systematic reviews: A literature review of guidance and supporting studies. *BMC Med. Res. Methodol.* **2018**, *18*, 85. [CrossRef]
5. National Library of Medicine. PubMed. Available online: https://pubmed.ncbi.nlm.nih.gov/ (accessed on 20 August 2023).
6. Kuper, A. Literature and medicine: A problem of assessment. *Acad. Med.* **2006**, *81*, S128–S137. [CrossRef] [PubMed]
7. Temsah, O.; Khan, S.A.; Chaiah, Y.; Senjab, A.; Alhasan, K.; Jamal, A.; Aljamaan, F.; Malki, K.H.; Halwani, R.; Al-Tawfiq, J.A.; et al. Overview of Early ChatGPT's Presence in Medical Literature: Insights From a Hybrid Literature Review by ChatGPT and Human Experts. *Cureus* **2023**, *15*, e37281. [CrossRef]
8. OpenAI. Introducing ChatGPT. Available online: https://openai.com/blog/chatgpt (accessed on 20 August 2023).
9. Edge, M. Bing Chat. Available online: https://www.microsoft.com/en-us/edge/features/bing-chat?form=MT00D8 (accessed on 20 August 2023).

10. Google. An Important Next Step on Our AI Journey. Available online: https://blog.google/technology/ai/bard-google-ai-search-updates/ (accessed on 20 August 2023).
11. Wagner, M.W.; Ertl-Wagner, B.B. Accuracy of Information and References Using ChatGPT-3 for Retrieval of Clinical Radiological Information. *Can. Assoc. Radiol. J.* **2023**. [CrossRef]
12. King, M.R. Can Bard, Google's Experimental Chatbot Based on the LaMDA Large Language Model, Help to Analyze the Gender and Racial Diversity of Authors in Your Cited Scientific References? *Cell. Mol. Bioeng.* **2023**, *16*, 175–179. [CrossRef]
13. Miao, J.; Thongprayoon, C.; Cheungpasitporn, W. Assessing the Accuracy of ChatGPT on Core Questions in Glomerular Disease. *Kidney Int. Rep.* **2023**, *8*, 1657–1659. [CrossRef]
14. Barroga, E.F. Reference accuracy: Authors', reviewers', editors', and publishers' contributions. *J. Korean Med. Sci.* **2014**, *29*, 1587–1589. [CrossRef]
15. OpenAI. GPT-4 Is OpenAI's Most Advanced System, Producing Safer and More Useful Responses. Available online: https://openai.com/gpt-4 (accessed on 20 August 2023).
16. OpenAI. ChatGPT-3.5. Available online: https://chat.openai.com/ (accessed on 20 August 2023).
17. Google. Google Scholar. Available online: https://scholar.google.co.th/ (accessed on 26 August 2023).
18. Clarivate. Web of Science. Available online: https://www.webofscience.com/wos/author/search (accessed on 26 August 2023).
19. University of Hawai'i at Manoa Library. Available online: https://manoa.hawaii.edu/library/ (accessed on 26 August 2023).
20. Yeung, A.W.K.; Kulnik, S.T.; Parvanov, E.D.; Fassl, A.; Eibensteiner, F.; Volkl-Kernstock, S.; Kletecka-Pulker, M.; Crutzen, R.; Gutenberg, J.; Hoppchen, I.; et al. Research on Digital Technology Use in Cardiology: Bibliometric Analysis. *J. Med. Internet Res.* **2022**, *24*, e36086. [CrossRef]
21. Li, J.O.; Liu, H.; Ting, D.S.J.; Jeon, S.; Chan, R.V.P.; Kim, J.E.; Sim, D.A.; Thomas, P.B.M.; Lin, H.; Chen, Y.; et al. Digital technology, tele-medicine and artificial intelligence in ophthalmology: A global perspective. *Prog. Retin. Eye Res.* **2021**, *82*, 100900. [CrossRef] [PubMed]
22. Qarajeh, A.; Tangpanithandee, S.; Thongprayoon, C.; Suppadungsuk, S.; Krisanapan, P.; Aiumtrakul, N.; Garcia Valencia, O.A.; Miao, J.; Qureshi, F.; Cheungpasitporn, W. AI-Powered Renal Diet Support: Performance of ChatGPT, Bard AI, and Bing Chat. *Clin. Pract.* **2023**, *13*, 1160–1172. [CrossRef]
23. Lee, C.; Kim, S.; Kim, J.; Lim, C.; Jung, M. Challenges of diet planning for children using artificial intelligence. *Nutr. Res. Pract.* **2022**, *16*, 801–812. [CrossRef] [PubMed]
24. Dumitru, M.; Berghi, O.N.; Taciuc, I.A.; Vrinceanu, D.; Manole, F.; Costache, A. Could Artificial Intelligence Prevent Intraoperative Anaphylaxis? Reference Review and Proof of Concept. *Medicina* **2022**, *58*, 1530. [CrossRef]
25. Segura-Bedmar, I.; Colon-Ruiz, C.; Tejedor-Alonso, M.A.; Moro-Moro, M. Predicting of anaphylaxis in big data EMR by exploring machine learning approaches. *J. Biomed. Inform.* **2018**, *87*, 50–59. [CrossRef]
26. Levivien, C.; Cavagna, P.; Grah, A.; Buronfosse, A.; Courseau, R.; Bezie, Y.; Corny, J. Assessment of a hybrid decision support system using machine learning with artificial intelligence to safely rule out prescriptions from medication review in daily practice. *Int. J. Clin. Pharm.* **2022**, *44*, 459–465. [CrossRef]
27. Zhang, T.; Leng, J.; Liu, Y. Deep learning for drug-drug interaction extraction from the literature: A review. *Brief. Bioinform.* **2020**, *21*, 1609–1627. [CrossRef]
28. Bhattacharyya, M.; Miller, V.M.; Bhattacharyya, D.; Miller, L.E. High Rates of Fabricated and Inaccurate References in ChatGPT-Generated Medical Content. *Cureus* **2023**, *15*, e39238. [CrossRef]
29. Hill-Yardin, E.L.; Hutchinson, M.R.; Laycock, R.; Spencer, S.J. A Chat(GPT) about the future of scientific publishing. *Brain Behav. Immun.* **2023**, *110*, 152–154. [CrossRef]
30. Garattini, S.; Jakobsen, J.C.; Wetterslev, J.; Bertele, V.; Banzi, R.; Rath, A.; Neugebauer, E.A.; Laville, M.; Masson, Y.; Hivert, V.; et al. Evidence-based clinical practice: Overview of threats to the validity of evidence and how to minimise them. *Eur. J. Intern. Med.* **2016**, *32*, 13–21. [CrossRef] [PubMed]
31. Alkaissi, H.; McFarlane, S.I. Artificial Hallucinations in ChatGPT: Implications in Scientific Writing. *Cureus* **2023**, *15*, e35179. [CrossRef]
32. Garcia Valencia, O.A.; Suppadungsuk, S.; Thongprayoon, C.; Miao, J.; Tangpanithandee, S.; Craici, I.M.; Cheungpasitporn, W. Ethical Implications of Chatbot Utilization in Nephrology. *J. Pers. Med.* **2023**, *13*, 1363. [CrossRef] [PubMed]
33. Garcia Valencia, O.A.; Thongprayoon, C.; Jadlowiec, C.C.; Mao, S.A.; Miao, J.; Cheungpasitporn, W. Enhancing Kidney Transplant Care through the Integration of Chatbot. *Healthcare* **2023**, *11*, 2518. [CrossRef] [PubMed]

Disclaimer/Publisher's Note: The statements, opinions and data contained in all publications are solely those of the individual author(s) and contributor(s) and not of MDPI and/or the editor(s). MDPI and/or the editor(s) disclaim responsibility for any injury to people or property resulting from any ideas, methods, instructions or products referred to in the content.

Article

AI-Driven Decision Support for Early Detection of Cardiac Events: Unveiling Patterns and Predicting Myocardial Ischemia

Luís B. Elvas [1,2,*], Miguel Nunes [1], Joao C. Ferreira [1,2], Miguel Sales Dias [1] and Luís Brás Rosário [3]

1. ISTAR, Instituto Universitário de Lisboa (ISCTE-IUL), 1649-026 Lisbon, Portugal; miguel_bonacho@iscte-iul.pt (M.N.); jcafa@iscte-iul.pt (J.C.F.); miguel.dias@iscte-iul.pt (M.S.D.)
2. Inov Inesc Inovação—Instituto de Novas Tecnologias, 1000-029 Lisbon, Portugal
3. Faculty of Medicine, Lisbon University, Hospital Santa Maria/CHULN, CCUL, 1649-028 Lisbon, Portugal; lsrosario@medicina.ulisboa.pt
* Correspondence: luis.elvas@iscte-iul.pt

Abstract: Cardiovascular diseases (CVDs) account for a significant portion of global mortality, emphasizing the need for effective strategies. This study focuses on myocardial infarction, pulmonary thromboembolism, and aortic stenosis, aiming to empower medical practitioners with tools for informed decision making and timely interventions. Drawing from data at Hospital Santa Maria, our approach combines exploratory data analysis (EDA) and predictive machine learning (ML) models, guided by the Cross-Industry Standard Process for Data Mining (CRISP-DM) methodology. EDA reveals intricate patterns and relationships specific to cardiovascular diseases. ML models achieve accuracies above 80%, providing a 13 min window to predict myocardial ischemia incidents and intervene proactively. This paper presents a Proof of Concept for real-time data and predictive capabilities in enhancing medical strategies.

Keywords: cardiovascular diseases; myocardial infarction; pulmonary thromboembolism; aortic stenosis; stenosis cardiology; exploratory data analysis; artificial intelligence; machine learning; data mining; prediction

1. Introduction

Cardiovascular diseases are the leading cause of mortality worldwide. In 2020, cardiovascular diseases (CVDs) accounted for 17.9 million deaths, or 32% of all global deaths [1,2]. CVDs are also a leading cause of hospitalization and disability. Addressing these complexities requires innovative approaches that empower medical practitioners to make informed decisions, leading to improved patient outcomes and more effective healthcare strategies [2]. Notably, a study by Oxford Population Health's Health Economics Research Centre unveiled that in 2021, cardiovascular diseases incurred a cost of EUR 282 billion in the European Union (EU) economy [3]. This economic burden emphasizes the urgent need for innovative approaches that enhance medical decisions and healthcare strategies, ultimately improving patient outcomes.

In modern medical practice, physicians are confronted with intricate clinical scenarios that demand timely and data-driven interventions [4]. In the realm of Intensive Care Units, the ability to harness comprehensive patient data for insightful decisions has the potential to dramatically impact patient care and enhance healthcare quality [5]. In the current medical practice, patients have several physiologic parameters monitored—e.g., Heart Rate, Blood Pressure, Oxymetry, Body Temperature—that raise alarms when pre specified thresholds are crossed, which prompts diagnostic or therapeutic interventions. In this sense, patient care is triggered after the fact, as if a car driver were driving looking at the rear mirror. This is in contrast with other sciences and work practices, for example, Meteorology, where prediction drives Agriculture or Navigation decisions, based on data-driven models.

The intersection of medical technology and data science has opened new avenues for tackling disease prediction. Machine learning, a subset of artificial intelligence, promises to unravel intricate patterns within vast datasets. Its modeling techniques, capable of extracting meaningful insights from complex clinical information, coupled with its predictive prowess, could reshape how cardiac diseases are diagnosed, treated, and even forecasted and prevented.

Machine learning techniques (ML) offer a transformative paradigm in cardiovascular healthcare, enabling the integration of diverse data sources to unveil hidden correlations, prognostic markers, and emerging risk factors [6]. This technology has the potential to empower clinicians with predictive tools that can anticipate adverse cardiac events, enabling early interventions and personalized treatment strategies. Early diagnosis and intervention are essential for improving the outcomes of patients with CVDs [7]. This is where machine learning can play a valuable role that can be used to analyze large amounts of data and identify patterns that would be difficult to detect by human experts [8]. ML has been shown to be effective in predicting CVDs, even in patients who have no symptoms [9]. The precision of these models holds the potential to improve patient care, reduce hospitalizations, and mitigate the long-term impact of cardiac diseases [9].

Our approach showcases the capabilities unlocked through structured health database analysis from a real-world problem. In our quest to advance cardiovascular healthcare, our study adopts an innovative approach that underscores both privacy and collaboration. Importantly, these data were homomorphically encrypted to uphold privacy and confidentiality standards. The application of Data Sharing Agreements (DSAs) ensures responsible and compliant data sharing practices, safeguarding patient information [10].

Our commitment to enhance cardiovascular healthcare is mapped in a central research question: "How can fusion of Exploratory Data Analysis (EDA) techniques and predictive Machine Learning models assist medical staff in accurate clinical decision-making, and facilitate timely medical interventions of a preventive nature?". This pivotal question guides our exploration into harnessing data-driven methodologies to drive innovative solutions in the context of cardiac care.

The core objectives of our study are two-fold, aligning seamlessly with the holistic nature of our research question. Firstly, we endeavor to unravel intricate patterns within the multi-syndrome dataset from Hospital Santa Maria through meticulous EDA. This analytical journey offers insights into disease-specific trends, risk factors, and underlying relationships, thereby equipping medical professionals with a deeper understanding of cardiovascular diseases for enhanced diagnosis, prognosis, and treatment strategies. Secondly, we are dedicated to harnessing the predictive power of machine learning models to anticipate myocardial ischemia. By utilizing the knowledge gained from our exploratory analysis, we aim to develop intelligent predictive models capable of forecasting cardiac incidents with a high degree of accuracy. This predictive capability has the potential to empower healthcare practitioners to implement preemptive measures, enabling timely interventions that significantly impact patient outcomes.

Our main objective, as directed by physicians, was to explore and extract knowledge from patient data related to three specific diseases: myocardial infarction, pulmonary thromboembolism, and aortic stenosis, because they serve as useful comparators for COVID-19 (coronavirus disease 2019), the newly emerged disease.

This paper illustrates the potential of AI-driven approaches to health data analysis. While we focus on myocardial infarction, pulmonary thromboembolism, and aortic stenosis for illustrative purposes, the underpinning principle is universally applicable, including for patients diagnosed with COVID-19. With structured, annotated and well-prepared data (including physiological data), these methodologies can be extended to address any other diseases, harnessing the power of data and technology to pioneer enhanced healthcare.

In summary, our paper charts a path towards addressing cardiovascular diseases by leveraging data analysis and predictive machine learning models. By harmonizing advanced technology with medical insights, we equip clinicians with the tools to aid them in making informed accurate decisions, pre-empt risk situations, and optimize patient care and clinical outcomes. In the rapidly advancing field of cardiovascular healthcare, our study is a significant contribution, providing data-driven evidence-based insights that have implications for improved patient outcomes.

2. State of the Art

In this section, we went through the existing body of knowledge in the realm of artificial intelligence (AI) applications within cardiovascular diseases. We followed the PRISMA methodology (Preferred Reporting Items for Systematic Reviews and Meta-Analysis) [11], not merely as a matter of convention, but to illuminate the path we have forged in pursuit of our research objectives. We recognize the potential for questions to arise regarding the integration of this comprehensive literature review into our broader study. Therefore, it is essential to clarify the rationale and significance of our approach.

The literature review within this study serves a dual role that is both foundational and contextual. We utilize it to identify research gaps and limitations that have guided the formulation of our research questions. Furthermore, it places our study within the broader landscape of AI-driven healthcare, offering readers a glimpse into the evolution and current state of the art. One of our primary objectives in conducting this literature review was to identify critical research gaps and limitations in existing studies. These gaps, as illuminated through our systematic review process, have played a pivotal role in shaping the specific research questions addressed in this article. Our intention is not to overshadow the primary focus of our research but to underscore the significance of our contributions by addressing unresolved questions in the field.

2.1. Search Strategy and Inclusion Criteria

Conducted in July 2023, this literature review focused solely on articles and reviews written in English, published in journals between 2018 and 2023, sourced from the Scopus and Web of Science Core Collection databases. We removed any duplicated articles to ensure data integrity.

To ensure clarity in our search, we constructed a comprehensive search query encompassing the concepts of "Machine Learning", "Artificial Intelligence", or "Data Mining" applied to the context of "Decision Support System", "Data Analytics", or "Data Analysis". This search was specifically targeted at the population of "Hospital Data" or "Health Data", with additional filtering based on "Cardiology" or "Cardiovascular Disease". We ended up with the following query "("Machine Learning" OR "Artificial Intelligence" OR "Data Mining") AND ("Decision Support System" OR "Data Analytic" OR "Data Analysis") AND ("Hospital Data" OR "Health Data") AND ("Cardiology" OR "Cardiovascular Disease")".

2.2. Results

The application of the mentioned query to the said Core Collection databases retrieved 21 papers. After the acquisition of such papers, we followed the PRISMA workflow, as depicted in Figure 1, illustrating our analysis of the reviewed articles.

Our goal was to investigate the application of Artificial Intelligence (AI) or machine learning in Health Data, with a specific focus on heart diseases. Throughout our literature review, we came across various topics related to this subject, and Table 1 summarizes the key themes found in each document. Without surprise, Heart Disease Prediction emerged as a prominent topic in this field, and the Internet of Things (IoT) also played a significant role in data acquisition, enabling further analysis. Additionally, the Risk Assessment of heart diseases or mortality was prevalent in the studies that were examined.

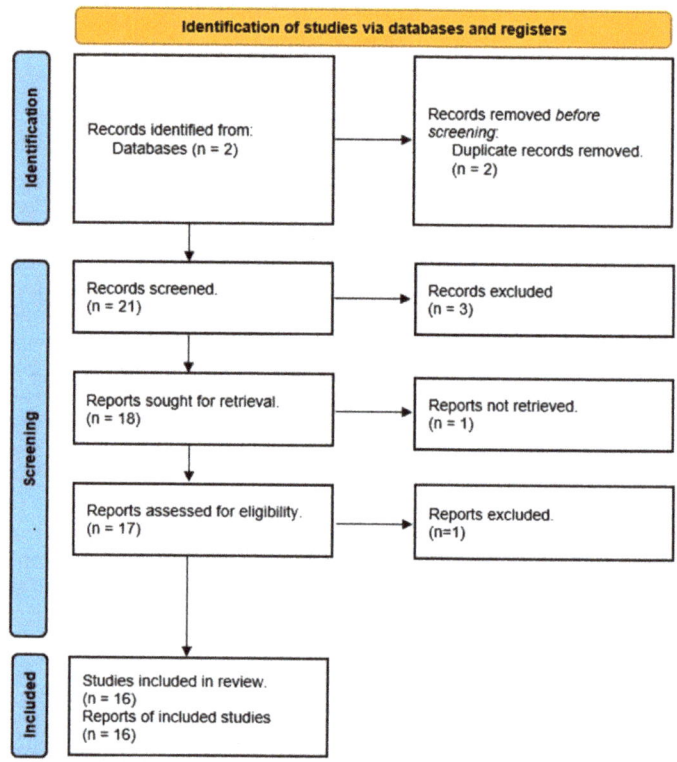

Figure 1. PRISMA workflow diagram.

Table 1. Topics found in literature review.

Topic	Reference	Number of Documents
Heart Disease Prediction	[12–20]	9
IoT	[12–16,21,22]	7
Risk Assessment	[16–19]	4
Big Data	[13,20]	2
Mortality Prediction	[19]	1
Recommender Systems	[23–25]	3
Clustering	[26]	1
Blockchain	[15]	1

A more detailed review of each document is also presented next, where article [27] discusses the significance of data integration and introduces a diagnosis recommender system designed to assist physicians. In the same topic, ref. [26] presents a recommender-system solution that utilizes clustering techniques for each disease partition, including angina, non-cardiac chest pain, silent ischemia, and myocardial infarction.

Study [15] proposes the integration of Blockchain with AI to strengthen both technologies and create a novel solution that serves the objective of providing improvements in cardiovascular medicine.

Articles [12–14,21] use IoT sensors to capture data and then use data to predict and diagnose heart diseases with very promising results. Refs. [20,28] discuss the development of an optimized feature-selection algorithm designed to predict heart diseases at an early stage. Work [29] also discuss the development of a heart disease prediction model (on benchmarking datasets). Article [17] proposes the development of a machine learning algorithm to predict myocardial infarction diagnosis using electronic health record data readily available during Emergency Department assessments. Work [22] is a state of the art for using the Internet of Things with quantum dots in medicine. This integration offers advanced disease detection and personalized treatments through precise data collection. Healthcare benefits from the Artificial Intelligence-aided IoT, which securely transmits patient data for tailored solutions.

Work [18] discusses the establishment of early warning models to assess and prevent diseases such as stroke, heart failure, and renal failure. The authors of [16] utilize IoT biosensors in a machine learning-based risk-assessment approach. Ref. [19] focuses on predicting the mortality risk of patients during or shortly after cardiac surgery using machine learning techniques for cardiac risk assessment.

The authors of [23] present a comprehensive review that delves into the history of artificial intelligence in medicine, exploring its contemporary and future applications in adult and pediatric cardiology, with a focus on selected concentrations. The review also addresses the existing barriers to implementing these advanced technologies. Furthermore, the article concludes by discussing the notable advantages of having a recommender system in place. Such a system would not only enhance workflow efficiency but also provide physicians with more time to spend with their patients, leading to increased job satisfaction. As a result, patients are expected to experience improved satisfaction as they benefit from more face-to-face time with their physicians.

Globally, there is a concerted effort to maximize the advantages of artificial intelligence in medicine [23], aiming to assist physicians in achieving better performance and enhance patients' experiences during hospitalization. However, we found a gap in the post-diagnosis phase. Following a patient's hospitalization, they are connected to numerous medical devices and our study centers on the analysis of select data gathered from these devices, aiming to assist physicians in comprehending typical patient behavior post-diagnosis. Distinguishing itself from previous research, our primary emphasis lies in maximizing the utility of existing hospital medical devices and harnessing the resultant data in the post-diagnosis phase. Our objective is twofold: first, to identify patterns during the post-diagnosis phase that could aid physicians in better evaluating patients' progress; second, we propose predicting potential cardiological complications that may arise during the hospitalization period and impact patients' well-being.

3. Methodology

In the pursuit of our research objectives, we employed a systematic-approach CRISP-DM to guide the development of our study. Leveraging the comprehensive patient data from Hospital Santa Maria, we followed a structured methodology to uncover insights and develop predictive models. Our database, integral to this study, includes data from 512,764 patients and contains continuous clinical signals such as Temperature, Blood Oxygen Level (SpO2), Heart Rate, and Arterial Blood Pressure. This dataset, comprising 138 tables and occupying 75 gigabytes of data, was provided under the framework of the FCT project DSAIPA/AI/0122/2020 AIMHealth—Mobile Applications Based on Artificial Intelligence [11]. The availability of the database for research was approved by the Ethical Committee of the Faculty of Medicine of Lisbon, one of the project partners.

These patients were selected from the Medical Intensive Care Units of Hospital de Santa Maria, the largest Portuguese Public Hospital, located in Lisbon. They were already diagnosed with specific diseases, and we chose to identify or forecast myocardial ischemia, a daunting complication, in three specific diseases—Acute Myocardial Infarction, Pulmonary Thromboembolism, and Aortic Stenosis—that represent a spectrum of Cardiovascular Diseases (CVDs).

This approach was informed by industry-standard frameworks like the Cross-Industry Standard Process for Data Mining (CRISP-DM) [24]. The utilization of such methodologies ensures a rigorous and well-organized process, aligning with best practices while allowing us to focus on the medical significance and practical implications of our findings. Building upon a doctoral research initiative, Data Sharing Agreements were meticulously crafted and signed. The implementation of homomorphic encryption, initially explored in a previously published paper [10], imparted an additional layer of academic rigor and depth to our methodology.

The combination of systematic methodologies, comprehensive patient data, advanced ML techniques, and ethical considerations forms the robust foundation of our research, enabling us to pursue a deeper understanding of cardiovascular diseases and their predictive modeling.

By leveraging CRISP-DM, we aimed to develop models that are not only accurate but also meaningful for medical professionals navigating the complexities of cardiovascular healthcare. Within CRISP-DM, we divided our efforts into two key areas: (1) exploratory data analysis (EDA) and (2) machine learning (ML) predictive models. This division allowed us not only to conduct a comprehensive evaluation of the data and gain a more thorough understanding of each disease, but also to structure this study effectively.

3.1. Exploratory Data Analysis

In Section 4 of our study, we conducted EDA for decision support purposes, during which we analyzed each disease individually. This phase of our methodology aimed to uncover critical insights into the progression of myocardial ischemia within the context of three specific diseases: Acute Myocardial Infarction, Pulmonary Thromboembolism, and Aortic Stenosis. By thoroughly examining the data through EDA, we laid the foundation for our subsequent ML modeling efforts.

3.2. Machine Learning Predictive Models

Section 5 of our study marked the application of ML models to the diseases under study. This phase involved the implementation and evaluation of predictive models to identify or forecast myocardial ischemia within the specified diseases. By harnessing the power of advanced ML techniques, we sought to provide clinicians with valuable tools for making informed, accurate decisions, preempting risk situations, and optimizing patient care and clinical outcomes in the rapidly advancing field of cardiovascular healthcare.

4. Exploratory Data Analysis for Decision Support

With a firm commitment to elevating patient outcomes and enhancing medical strategies, this chapter embarks on a journey through the vast expanse of patient data collected from Hospital Santa Maria. By employing exploratory data analysis (EDA) techniques, we uncover hidden relationships, correlations, and trends that have the potential to redefine clinical decision making in cardiovascular healthcare. This expedition seeks to reveal nuanced intricacies that can significantly shape the course of patient care.

During the EDA phase, our primary objective was to unveil insights and hidden patterns within the data that hold the promise of aiding in early treatment or risk assessment. We concentrated on identifying patient profiles and recurrent patterns in frequently measured physiological data, along with examination results. This phase forms the bedrock of our research, providing a comprehensive understanding of disease-specific trends and risk factors that underpin the subsequent predictive models.

Our primary focus was on a table called RT_Data, which contains real-time data collected during patients' hospital stays. This valuable table encompasses physiological data, vital signs, and information gathered from medical devices. Among all the variables, a few were selected by physicians to study their behavior and examine if there are any relevant patterns for each disease. It is crucial to emphasize that while numerous columns were available, our physicians' colleagues meticulously handpicked the most pertinent ones for our disease study. The most commonly recorded physiological variables, Heart Rate, Respiratory Rate, Arterial systolic Blood Pressure, Arterial Diastolic Blood Pressure and Mean Arterial Pressure, were chosen as they reflect the momentaneous function of the cardiovascular and respiratory systems and their reflex regulation (see Table 2).

Table 2. RT-Data DB table composition.

Variable Name	Variable Description
RTDATADBOID	Database Object ID for each collection of real-time data
CREATIONDATE	Date and time of real-time data collection
RESPIRATION RATE FROM EKG	Respiration Rate Value
ST SEGMENT LEAD V5	ST segment deviation from baseline in the ECG Leads V5
ST SEGMENT LEAD V4	ST segment deviation from baseline in the ECG Leads V4
ST SEGMENT LEAD V3	ST segment deviation from baseline in the ECG Leads V3
ST SEGMENT LEAD V2	ST segment deviation from baseline in the ECG Leads V2
ST SEGMENT LEAD V1	ST segment deviation from baseline in the ECG Leads V1
ST SEGMENT LEAD AVF	ST segment deviation from baseline in the ECG Leads aVF
ST SEGMENT LEAD AVR	ST segment deviation from baseline in the ECG Leads aVR
ST SEGMENT LEAD AVL	ST segment deviation from baseline in the ECG Leads aVL
ST SEGMENT LEAD III	ST segment deviation from baseline in the ECG Leads III
MEAN ARTERIAL PRESSURE 2	Mean Arterial Pressure Value
DIASTOLIC PRESSURE (ART.) 2	Diastolic Pressure Value
SYSTOLIC PRESSURE (ART.) 2	Systolic Pressure Value
HEART RATE	Heart Rate Value

Additionally, we conducted a thorough examination of the diagnostic table (see Table 3), which played a crucial role in our analysis. This table provided essential details regarding the prescribed diagnoses for each patient, allowing us to filter and concentrate specifically on the diagnoses corresponding to the selected diseases: myocardial infarction, pulmonary thromboembolism, and aortic stenosis.

Table 3. Diagnoses DB table composition.

Variable Name	Variable Description
DIAGDBOID	Database Object ID for each diagnosis
DIAGDESC	Description of each diagnosis
DIAGTYPEDESC	List of diagnoses
DIAGCODE	Code associated with a particular diagnosis in the list of diagnoses

To construct comprehensive patient profiling, we gathered additional information from the patients table in Table 4, and also from the patient's admission table in Table 5. The patient's table enabled us to collect information about individual characteristics, while the patient's admission table provided details about patient's weight, height, and the time of their hospitalization. Furthermore, we consulted a separate table that stored information about medical tests including the name of the test, the date it was conducted, and the results of the test (Table 6).

By combining these diverse sources of data, our objective was to create a holistic view of each patient's medical journey and gain valuable insights into their conditions, treatment progress, and overall health. Table 7 provides a summary of the utilized database tables along with their respective rationales, aimed at enhancing the understanding of the material by the readers.

Table 4. Patient DB table composition.

Variable Name	Variable Description
PATIENTDBOID	Database Object ID for each patient
BIRTHDATE	Patient birth date
BLOODGROUP	Patient blood group
SEX	Patient gender
ETHNICITY	Patient ethnicity

Table 5. Admission DB table composition.

Variable Name	Variable Description
ADMISSIONDBOID	Database Object ID for each admission
STARTED	Admission start datetime
ENDED	Admission end datetime
WEIGHT	Admission weight
HEIGHT	Admission height

Table 6. Laboratory test DB table composition.

Variable Name	Variable Description
LABTESTDBOID	Database Object ID for each Laboratory Test
STARTED	Datetime of test realization
ANALYSISDESC	Name of analysis component
VALUE	Result for analysis component

Table 7. Summary of utilized DB tables and their description.

DB Table	Description	No. Observations
Patients	Obtain personal information to build a patient profile	512,764
Admission	How long a patient was hospitalized	1,159,139
Diagnoses	Filter by desired diseases	126,126
LabTests	Extract date and result from specific exams	8,043,764
RT_Data	Real-time data monitored during patients' hospitalization	30,404,477

As shown in Table 7, we were presented with a considerable volume of data generated by a real hospital. This untapped data reserve possessed the inherent potential to significantly enhance physicians' performance and patient care. By utilizing advanced analytical techniques, these surplus data could be transformed into valuable insights, offering a wealth of information that can aid physicians in making more informed and accurate clinical decisions.

To ensure our analysis focused on the desired diseases, we began by refining the diagnosis table to include only the diagnoses that corresponded to our three target diseases. However, this process proved to be more complex than initially anticipated due to the hospital's non-standardized data collection and generation practices. The diagnostic entries exhibited variations in formatting, including the use of abbreviations, mixed cases (uppercase and lowercase), and inconsistent naming conventions.

After applying our filtering criteria, all the selected entries underwent crucial validation and verification by our team's physicians. Their thorough review provided an additional layer of scrutiny and assurance, enabling us to confidently proceed with our analysis.

Next, we proceeded to retrieve all the information about patients and admissions of patients who had been diagnosed with at least one of the remaining entries in the filtered diagnoses table. To ensure a holistic analysis, we extended our data-acquisition phase to encompass the real-time data. We narrowed down this table to include only the patients identified in the previous steps. For each disease, we began by merging all the information collected about patients and admissions, and the real-time data into a (python) Pandas DataFrame that we will now refer to as the "Hospitalization Dataset". Subsequently, we created additional variables, including the patients' age, duration of admission in days, and time of admission in minutes at each observation of the real-time data collection.

Additionally, we retrieved medical-examination data from the LabTests table. Specifically, for all three diseases, we obtained patients' exam results for Troponin and N-terminal prohormone of brain natriuretic peptide (NT-proBNP) levels and we joined that information with patients' and admissions data for each one of the three diseases, resulting in a dataset that we will refer to as the "Medical Tests Dataset". Troponin and NT-proBNOP are biological markers specific to cardiac lesion and/or strain. Troponin is a cardiac-specific protein released when myocardium cells are injured. NT-proBNP is a pro hormone released by the heart upon volume or pressure overload. Troponin is a marker of ischemia, so it correlates with ST deviation, while NT-proBNP is from heart failure congestion. After collecting all the medical test data related to NT-proBNP, we conducted an examination of the data within our CRISP-DM data preparation stage. We performed various procedures, such as removing duplicate entries and ensuring that the tests were conducted during the patient's hospitalization period. Additionally, we eliminated tests with implausible results, such as values of 0 or negative values. Despite these efforts, upon analyzing the data for each disease, we regret to report that the number of valid tests remained extremely low and insignificant for us to proceed with further analysis. As a result, the Medical Tests Dataset only included Troponin Tests and their corresponding results for each disease. The NT-proBNP data set did not have enough data to perform a valid analysis.

Overall, we began our individual analyses with two distinct datasets for each disease. The first dataset, referred to as "Hospitalization Dataset", incorporated information about patients, admissions and real-time data measured throughout their hospitalization. The second dataset, named "Medical Tests Dataset", comprised patient, admission, and test result information for Troponin. As our data preparation (acquisition, cleaning and filtering) phase was finally completed, we proceeded to better study and understand each disease.

4.1. Myocardial Infarction

4.1.1. Hospitalization Dataset

Our EDA for Myocardial Infarction included a dataset of 260 patients. Among them, 57 patients were female, and 203 patients were male. This dataset consisted of 368,285 observations, with each observation representing a real-time data collection record for an individual patient. The age range of patients diagnosed with Myocardial Infarction varied from 16 years (the youngest patient) to 88 years (the oldest patient). In terms of data collection, we observed that one patient had the highest number of real-time data collection records, with a total exceeding 23,000. This patient was hospitalized for approximately two and a half months.

Then, we performed common data preparation procedures, such as removing duplicate entries and addressing missing values. After performing the aforementioned procedures, we proceeded to analyze certain parameters such as Heart Rate and Respiratory Rate, as they are the vital signs usually collect for this disease, since their variation can determine Ischemia.

In our initial descriptive statistics approach, we grouped the heart rate measurements by extracting the hourly pattern of each measurement. Our objective was to investigate whether the time of day had any influence on the frequency of heart rate readings. To further enrich the graph's information, we also incorporated the gender variable to assess any significant differences, as shown in Figure 2.

Observing Figure 2, several notable patterns emerge. Firstly, it is evident that women tend to have higher rates of tachycardia compared to men. Additionally, an intriguing observation is that the average heart rate appears to be higher during the nighttime period compared to the daytime period. This fact prompted us to expand our analysis by incorporating the day of admission as an additional grouping factor for heart rate measurements. By including this level of grouping alongside the hour and minute of each measurement, our aim was to explore potential trends or variations in heart rate patterns throughout the duration of the patients' admission days, as depicted in Figure 3.

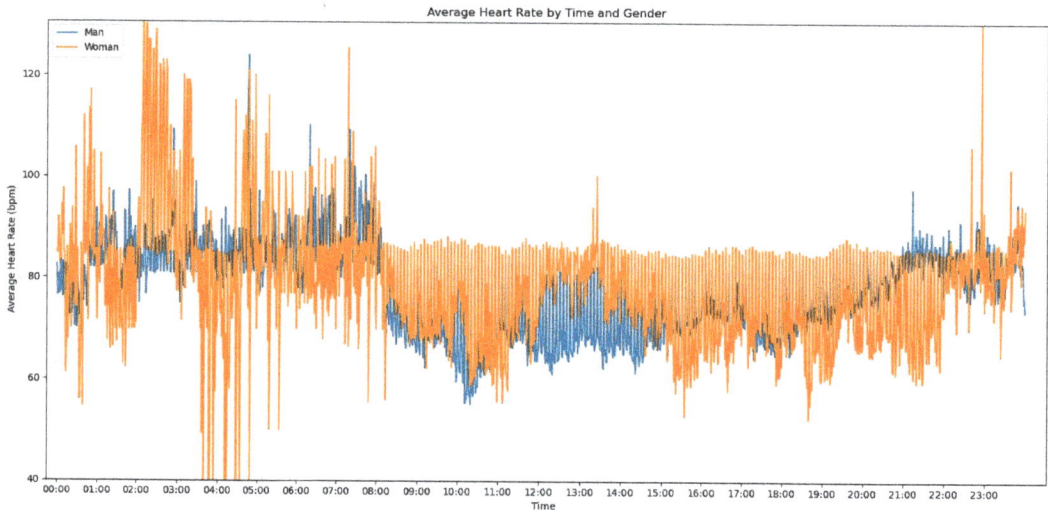

Figure 2. Average Heart Rate by time and gender.

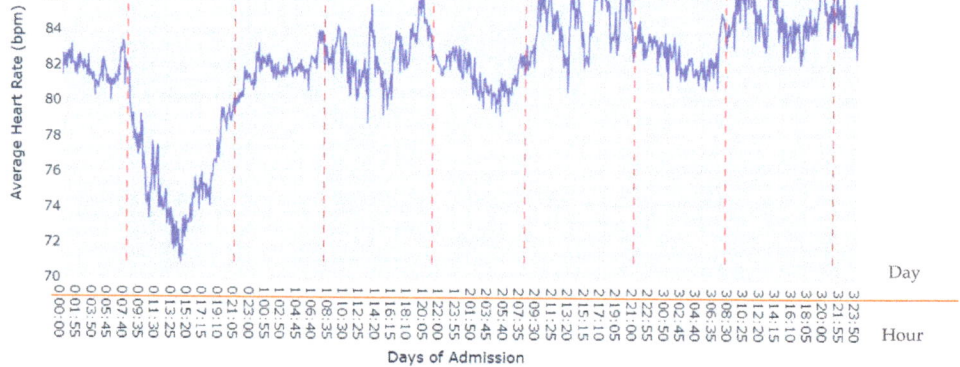

Figure 3. Average Heart Rate in the initial 4 days of admission by daytime and nighttime period.

As we can see in Figure 3, during the first 24 h of admission into the hospital, there is a decline in the patients' average heart rate values during the daytime period. From 8 am until lunchtime, the values progressively decrease, and from lunchtime until the start of the nighttime period, they increase. In the subsequent days of admission, the average value oscillates between the 80s bpm during both the day and nighttime, with no noticeable differences. So, that phenomenon in the first 24 h of admission lead us to another analysis where we explored with more detail the evolution of heart rate during that period of admission. To accomplish this, we utilized the average values based on minutes of admission, focusing specifically on the time span from minute 1 to minute 1440, which corresponds to the first 24 h of admission. This analysis allowed us to explore how the heart rate changes over this crucial initial period of hospitalization, as seen in Figure 4.

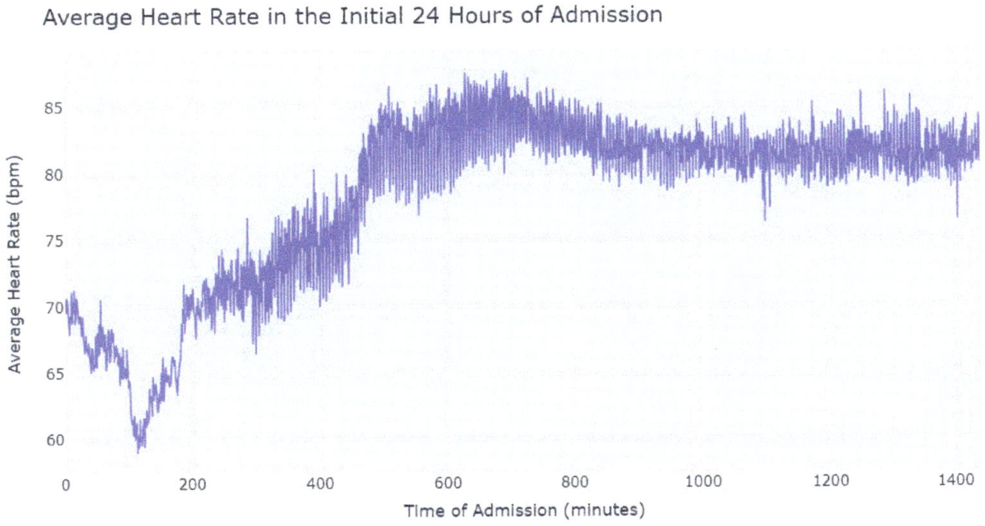

Average Heart Rate in the Initial 24 Hours of Admission

Figure 4. Average Heart Rate in the initial 24 h of admission.

It's notable to observe in Figure 4 that the average heart rate progressively decreases until around 2 h after admission starts; this happens since patients with a Myocardial Infarction undergo angioplasty in the first hour.

This marks the lowest average heart rate, after which it begins to increase progressively, eventually stabilizing between 80 and 85 after 8 h of admission. This behavior of the average heart rate could possibly be influenced by medication or medical procedures (such as percutaneous coronary intervention), and once their effects take place, the value tends to stabilize.

Shifting our focus, another measure chosen to evaluate patients' conditions was the Respiration Rate (taken from thoracic impedance from EKG). Initially, we had more than 47,000 observations with this measure recorded. However, after ensuring that the value was greater than 0, we were left with only about 39,000 records. Out of these, 36,000 measurements were taken during the first 24 h of hospital admission. As a result, we focused our analysis on this subset of data, as depicted in Figure 5.

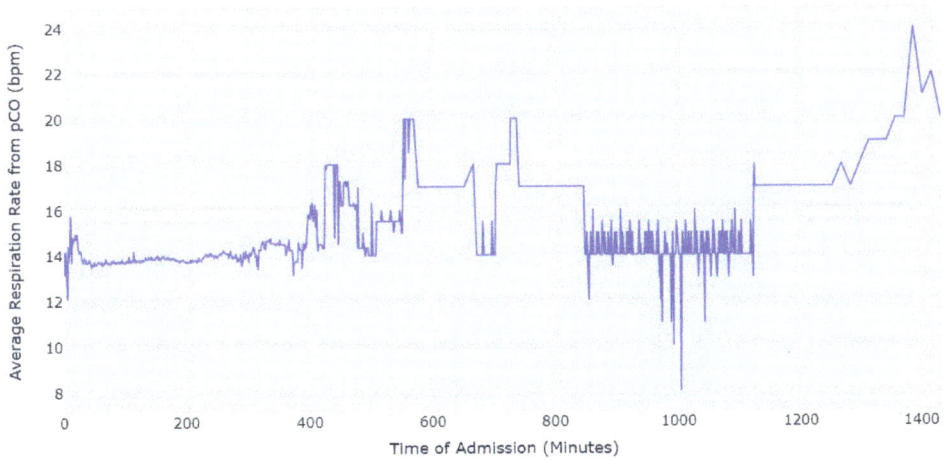

Figure 5. Average Respiration Rate for first 24 h of admission.

As we can see in Figure 5, the average value of the respiration rate during the first 24 h of admission (1440 min) oscillates between 12 and 20, with a decrease to 8 occurring close to 17 h after the admission start. Subsequently, there is an increase in the average value, which is observed close to the 24 h mark since the admission start.

4.1.2. Medical Tests Dataset

Shifting our focus to the dataset of medical exams, we conducted an analysis to comprehend the progression of Troponin over time. Specifically, we examined 1546 observations of Troponin exams.

After removing duplicate entries and applying specific filters to ensure the inclusion of only relevant exams conducted during the hospitalization period, we successfully eliminated all tests that were not administered during the specified timeframe. As a result of these two procedures, our dataset was refined, consisting now of 1348 records for Troponin. To analyze the Troponin exams more effectively, we grouped them based on the average values per day of admission, Figure 6.

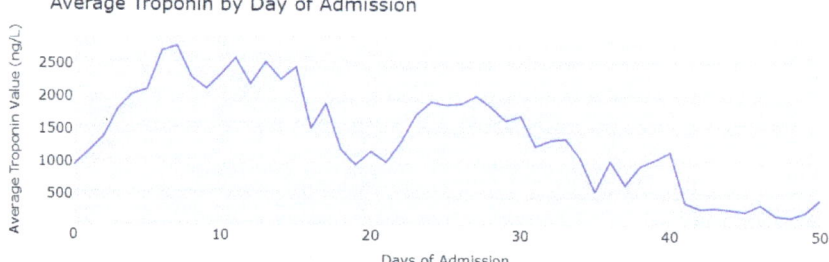

Figure 6. Average Troponin values by day of admission.

The average value of Troponin starts at 1000 ng/L and exhibits a tendency to increase during the initial days of admission, reaching a peak of more than 2500 ng/L on the 7th day, followed by an oscillating but progressively decreasing pattern. For healthy individuals, Troponin values are expected to be lower than 14 ng/L for healthy people, and it is evident that for patients diagnosed with myocardial infarction, these values never return to the considered normal range even after more than 1 month from the start of their hospital admission.

4.2. Pulmonary Thromboembolism

4.2.1. Hospitalization Dataset

For the pulmonary thromboembolism disease, we had a total of 48 patients, consisting of 28 males and 20 females. The age range of the patients spanned from 0 years to 91 years, with the longest hospitalization duration lasting for 322 days. The dataset with real-time data consisted of 87,760 observations, with each row representing a real-time data collection instance for an individual patient.

As in the previous disease, we handled duplicates by removing them, and any instances of missing values were addressed by exclusion, ensuring the data's integrity remained intact.

Furthermore, we conducted an analysis of heart rate and respiration rate measures to identify patterns that could assist physicians in understanding the evolution of these parameters. The objective was to provide valuable insights into how these vital signs change over time and enable healthcare professionals to take appropriate actions based on a patient's individual evolution compared to the typical behavior observed in the majority of patients. Once again, we commenced our analysis by examining heart rate patterns across hours and genders, with the aim of identifying intriguing trends, as shown Figure 7.

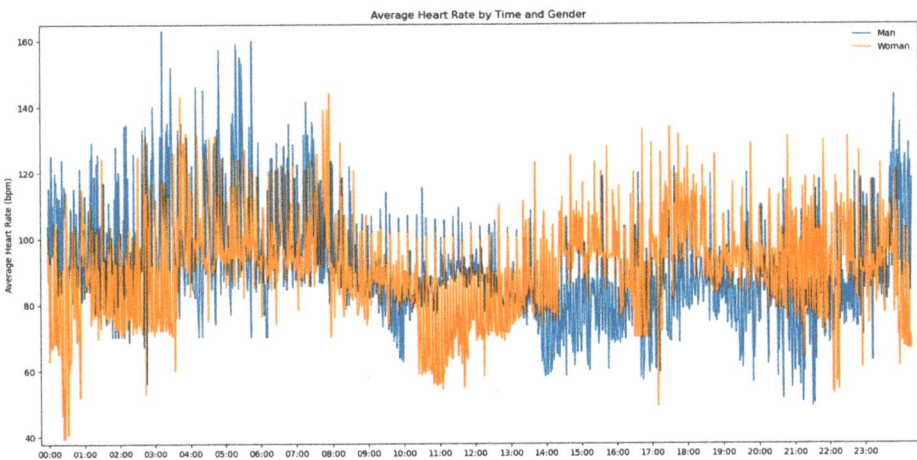

Figure 7. Average Heart Rate by time and gender.

Figure 7 shows a distinction from myocardial infarction. The average Heart Rate values tend to be tachycardic, and there is no significant difference between men and women, even during the daytime or nighttime periods. The values oscillate between 60 bpm and 140 bpm, with men having a few average heart rate values above 140 bpm during the nighttime period.

Then, we proceed our analysis by grouping Heart Rate values based on their day of admission and the specific hour and minute, computing the average value for each group, as seen in Figure 8. Subsequently, we plotted the resulting graph to examine any discernible patterns. Our primary objective was to investigate whether a similar pattern, as observed in Myocardial Infarction cases, would emerge. Specifically, we were interested in determining whether there was a notable minimum average heart rate during the daytime period of day 0, which could be indicative of a common trend in both conditions.

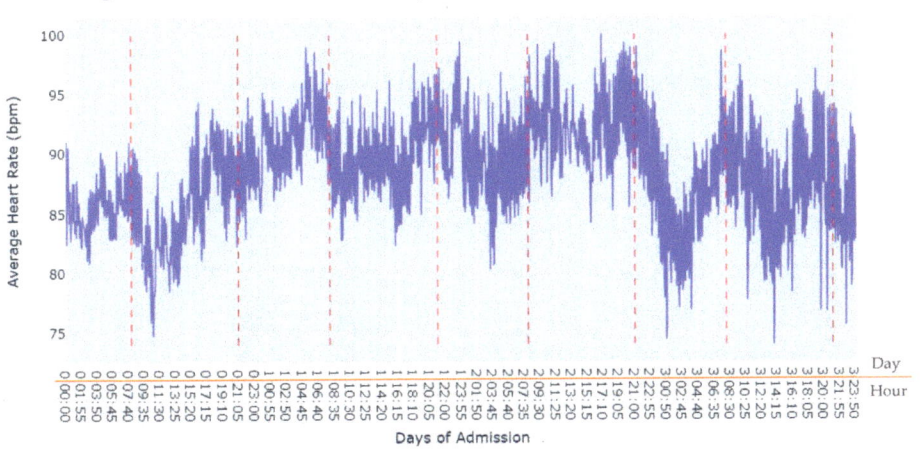

Figure 8. Average Heart Rate in the initial 4 days of admission by daytime and nighttime periods.

As depicted in Figure 8, the behavior of Heart Rate in this disease does not exhibit similarities with Myocardial Infarction. The values, rather, indicate signs of tachycardia, but there is no significant discernible pattern observed during different days of admission.

Additionally, we conducted an analysis of the first 24 h of admission to investigate whether there were any instances of minimum or decreasing average heart rate values, Figure 9. The purpose was to ascertain whether such occurrences could be attributed to specific medical procedures or medication administered to the patient upon admission to the hospital.

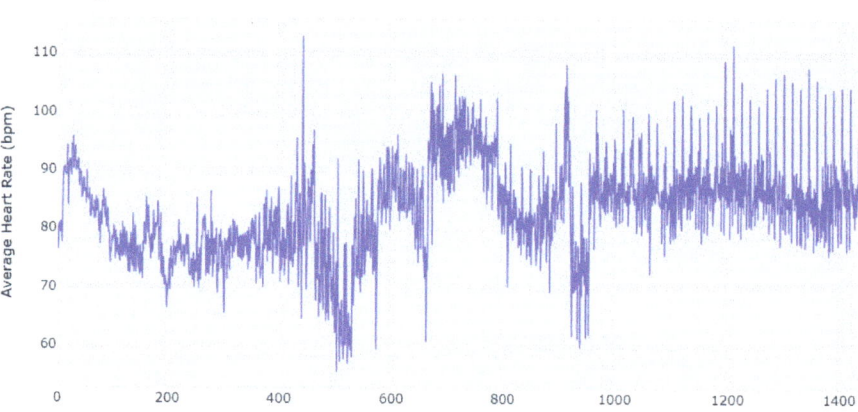

Figure 9. Average Heart Rate in the initial 24 h of admission.

In Figure 9, we can observe the same trend shown in Figure 8. The average heart rate values of patients diagnosed with pulmonary thromboembolism exhibit significant fluctuations. Patients frequently experience tachycardia, where heart rate values during the first 24 h can oscillate widely, ranging from under 60 to over 110 beats per minute (bpm).

Shifting our focus to the Respiration Rate, we had more than 6500 valid observations. To ensure data integrity, we performed certain procedures, such as removing observations where the value of the respiration rate was equal to or lower than 0 (impossible values in this context). By applying these data cleaning procedures, we aimed to maintain the accuracy and reliability of the dataset for further analysis. Figure 10 presents the average respiration rate from EKG in the first 24 h of admission.

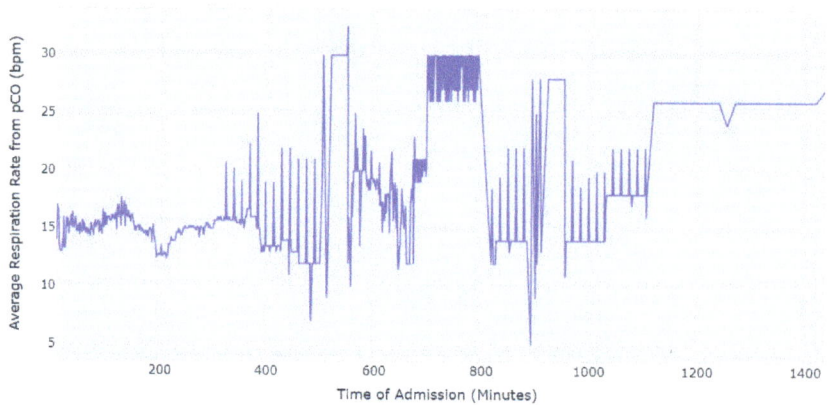

Figure 10. Average Respiration Rate for first 24 h of admission.

After approximately 5 h of hospitalization, the average value of respiration rate starts to exhibit significant fluctuations. During the initial 5 h, the average value remains relatively stable, around 15. However, after this period, the average respiration rate shows oscillations, varying between 5 and 30 in certain instances. This observation suggests that the respiration rate tends to become more erratic as the time since admission progresses.

4.2.2. Medical Tests Dataset

In terms of medical tests, we conducted a review to ensure we had a significant number of Troponin tests performed on patients diagnosed with pulmonary thromboembolism. The same procedures described in myocardial infarction were applied to ensure we had only relevant and valid tests and after careful examination, we aimed to retain 219 tests out of the total 244. Then, we grouped Troponin values based on the day of admission when the examination was conducted, and calculated the average value for each day, which is shown in Figure 11.

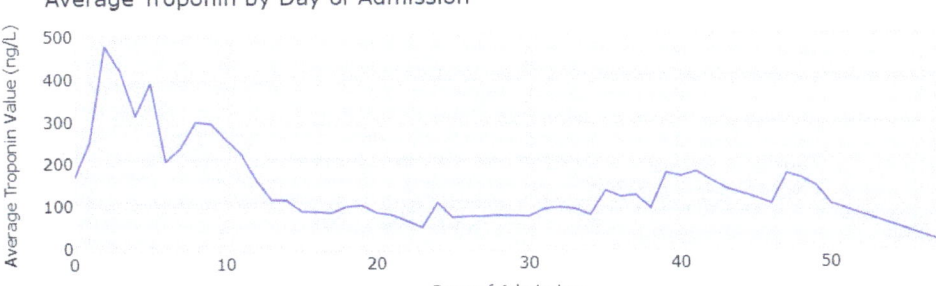

Figure 11. Average Troponin values by day of admission.

As observed in Figure 11, the average value of troponin initially increases, similarly to what is seen in myocardial infarction cases. However, after two days of admission, it starts to decrease with occasional minor increases. Notably, the highest average value of Troponin recorded was slightly below 500 ng/L, which contrasts with myocardial infarction cases where values reached 2500 ng/L.

4.3. Aortic Stenosis

4.3.1. Hospitalization Dataset

As with the previous diseases, we began by presenting some descriptive statistics of the data under study. The dataset comprised 794,694 observations of real-time data collected from 660 patients, where 370 were male and 290 female. The ages of the patients ranged from 0 years to 93 years. Notably, the patient with the longest hospitalization period was admitted for 925 days, from 9 February 2017 to 23 August 2019.

After applying the same procedures as before, we conducted an analysis of the heart rate and respiration rate signals.

As this disease had a substantial number of patients, with a relatively even distribution among genders, we first examined the average heart rate based on the hour and minute of measurement, as well as considering the patients' gender; see Figure 12.

We can notice almost no difference between the genders in terms of the average heart rate values. The analysis indicates that both male and female patients with this disease exhibit similar trends in their heart rate patterns. It is also intriguing to observe a pattern that was previously noted in myocardial infarction but is not as prominent in pulmonary thromboembolism. The average heart rate values tend to be lower during the daytime period compared to the nighttime period, where the highest value from the daytime period almost corresponds to the lowest average heart rate value from the nighttime period.

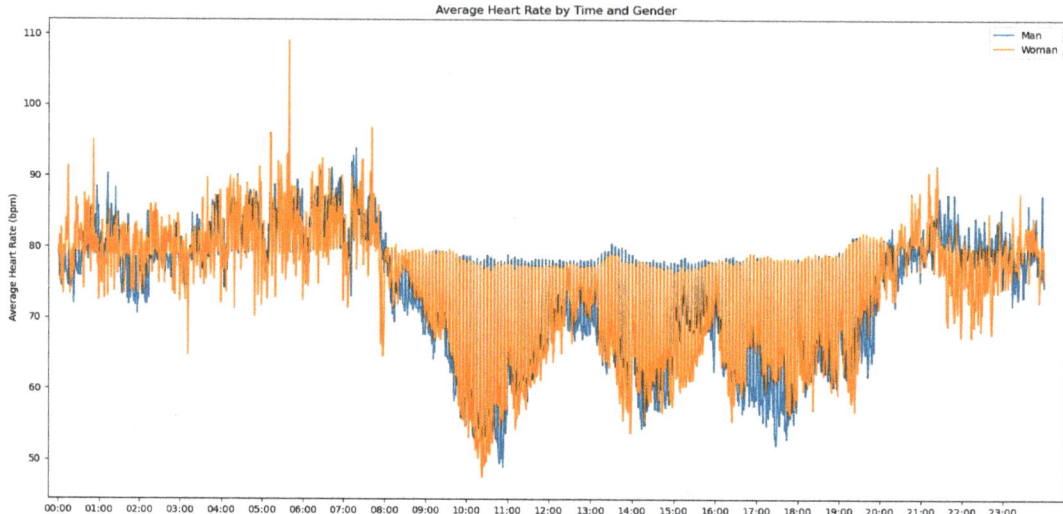

Figure 12. Average Heart Rate by time and gender.

This fact led us to investigate the influence of the daytime period on the average heart rate values, the results of which are shown in Figure 13. By analyzing the heart rate data during daytime periods, we sought to discern potential patterns or variations that could shed light on how this specific time of day may impact the average heart rate in patients.

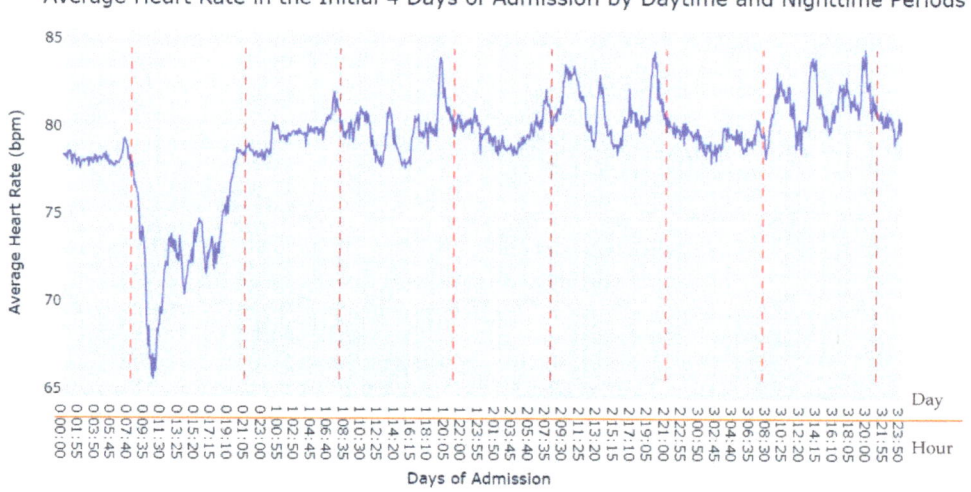

Figure 13. Average Heart Rate in the initial 4 days of admission by daytime and nighttime periods.

Aortic stenosis exhibits a similar behavior to myocardial infarction. Those suffering from myocardial infarction are submitted to Angioplasty while patients suffering from aortic stenosis are admitted and in the next day have a scheduled procedure Transcutaneous Aortic Valve Implantation (TAVI) with sedation and or anesthesia. On the first day of admission (day 0), during the daytime period, the lowest average value of their heart rate is noted. From 8 am onwards, their heart rate starts decreasing (when they are submitted to

TAVI), and throughout the daytime period, it never reaches the average value of heart rate seen during the nighttime period on the first day of admission. Subsequently, in the following days, the heart rate values show greater stability, both within each day and between the daytime and nighttime periods. Even in comparison with pulmonary thromboembolism, most of the data for aortic stenosis exhibits remarkable stability, except for the observed phenomenon on the first day of admission. The heart rate values demonstrate a consistent pattern over time, indicating relatively steady and consistent behavior in most cases. Our efforts were then focused on studying the first 24 h of admission, as depicted in Figure 14, to understand if it showed a similar behavior to myocardial infarction, where the average heart rate decreases and reaches its lowest value approximately one and a half hours after the admission starts.

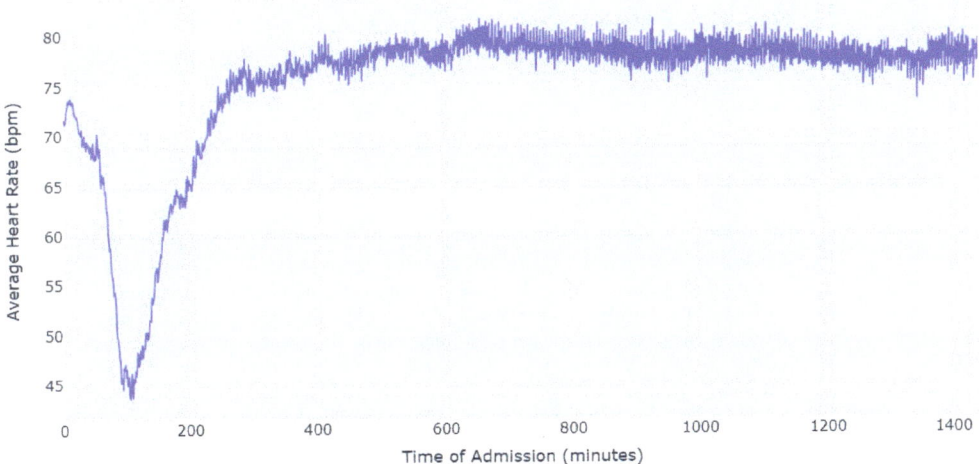

Figure 14. Average Heart Rate in the initial 24 h of admission.

Once again, Figure 14 presents a behavior quite like myocardial infarction in aortic stenosis patients. The average heart rate starts decreasing after admission and reaches its lowest value at approximately 2 h. Subsequently, the heart rate gradually increases until it reaches around 75 bpm. Over the remainder of the first 24 h, the average heart rate remains stable, fluctuating between 75 and 80 bpm. This consistent and characteristic pattern of heart rate changes in the initial 24 h of admission resembles the behavior typically seen in myocardial infarction cases. The behavior of heart rate in aortic stenosis and myocardial infarction is quite similar when compared to pulmonary thromboembolism, where tachycardia is more prevalent globally. However, unlike in the former cases, there is not a significant gradual decrease or increase in heart rate values.

Shifting our focus to the Respiration Rate, we analyzed the values from the first 24 h of admission, Figure 15. Out of the total 63,000 observations, a substantial majority of 57,000 observations were specifically from the first 24 h of admission.

Once again, we observed new evidence of a behavior similar to myocardial infarction in aortic stenosis patients. The average values of Respiration Rate rarely exceeded the limits considered normal for healthy individuals, which typically fall within the range of 12 to 20 breaths per minute. Pulmonary thromboembolism did not exhibit a markedly different behavior, but it did surpass the anticipated values on multiple occasions.

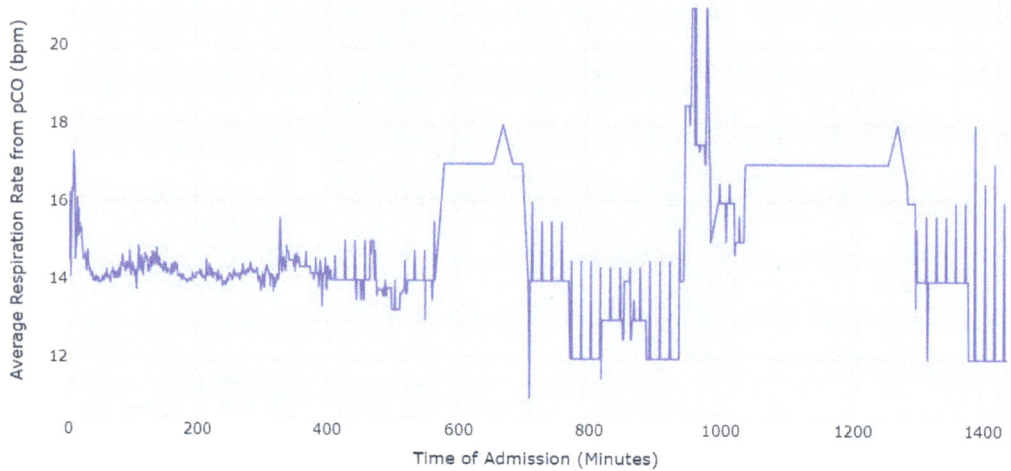

Figure 15. Average Respiration Rate for first 24 h of admission.

4.3.2. Medical Tests Dataset

Analyzing the Troponin tests, we first filtered these exams to ensure they were conducted within the hospitalization period. Out of the total Troponin tests, 2872 exams were considered valid and were included in the analysis. Then, we followed a similar approach to before by grouping the values of tests based on the admission day when they were conducted. Subsequently, we calculated the average value of Troponin for each day, as seen in Figure 16.

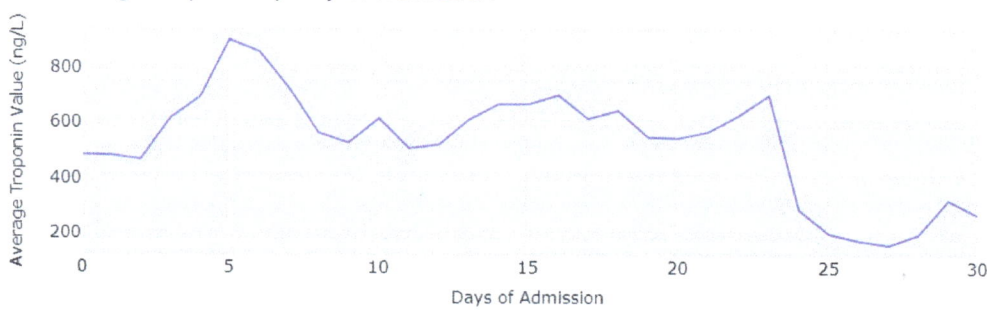

Figure 16. Average Troponin value by day of admission.

Conversely, the values of Troponin in aortic stenosis patients across the day of admission are not similar to Troponin figures in myocardial infarction patients, contrasting in their heart rate and respiration rate. In aortic stenosis, the average Troponin value reaches its highest point after 5 days of admission and then gradually decreases but remains relatively stable until the 24th day of admission. Unlike myocardial infarction, the Troponin values in aortic stenosis patients never reach levels as high as 1000 ng/L. Even when compared with pulmonary thromboembolism, the behavior of troponin differs. In aortic stenosis cases, the highest value is only reached after 5 days, whereas in pulmonary thromboembolism, it occurs earlier. By the 12th day, troponin levels in pulmonary thromboembolism drop below 200 ng/L, whereas in aortic stenosis, this value is only achieved after 25 days of admission. The distinct behavior of Troponin in aortic stenosis patients is noticeably different.

5. Machine Learning Predictive Models—Myocardial Ischemia Prediction

Moving beyond the Exploratory Data Analysis, our focus shifted to the machine learning (ML) modeling phase, where our aim was to predict myocardial ischemia. This predictive capability allows us to anticipate critical events and provide physicians with the tools necessary for early interventions. The overarching purpose of our data analysis was to aid physicians in making well-informed and accurate decisions, ultimately enhancing patient outcomes, and elevating the overall quality of care.

To initiate our predictions, we employed the Hospitalization Dataset for each of the three diseases. This dataset includes variables known as ST Segment Lead that are represented as float values, which can be either positive or negative. Myocardial ischemia can be detected using ST segment modification, this being an established marker of cardiac injury without cellular death. It may happen as part of an unfavorable evolution of the disease or therapeutic insufficiency. We evaluated these values using the ST-segment-T wave criteria [25], which is suggestive of myocardial ischemia (MI). The criteria for ST-elevation and ST-depression are distinct, and for each variable under study, specific rules were applied to determine the presence of myocardial ischemia. For each disease, we analyzed each record and verified whether, according to the values of our ST-Segment variables and the aforementioned criteria, myocardial ischemia was present or not. A Boolean variable was created to represent the phenomena. Table 8 presents the number of observations (rows) in the Hospitalization Dataset, the number of diagnosed patients, the number of patients that had MI and the number of observations with myocardial ischemia for each disease under study. Please note that these patients were admitted to the hospital with cardiac diseases and were measured with a non-regular frequency of 1–5 min, which could explain the higher number of cases of myocardial ischemia.

Table 8. Presence of myocardial ischemia (MI) for each disease.

Disease	No. Observations	No. Patients	Patients' w/MI	No. Observations w/MI
Myocardial Infarction	368,285	260	254	144,273
Pulmonary Thromboembolism	87,760	48	22	17,357
Aortic Stenosis	794,694	660	649	394,967

Starting our predictions, the initial idea was to utilize shift variables to attempt a prediction of whether a patient would experience myocardial ischemia in the future. For each ST variable, the Heart Rate variable and the MI variable, we selected the past values (lag) based on the autocorrelation of the patient with the most observations. Since the dataset contained multiple records for various patients, it was crucial to check the autocorrelation for only one patient to ensure accurate predictions of myocardial ischemia based on shift values for that specific patient. We performed this procedure for each one of the three diseases under study, utilizing the respective Hospitalization Dataset. Autocorrelation, in essence, quantifies the extent of similarity between a variable and its past values across various time intervals. The interdependence over time within the dataset can substantially impact the performance of a model. A noticeable autocorrelation could suggest a strong temporal relationship between ST Segment measurements or MI occurrences at different points in time. This indicates that the current ST Segment value could potentially be influenced by its own historical values. In the domain of predictive modeling, autocorrelation plays a pivotal role in refining the accuracy of predictions. This phenomenon enables us to utilize past values effectively to formulate forecasts for the future.

Based on the observations in Figure 17 and the autocorrelation graphs for all ST Segment variables, Heart Rate and MI, we selected a lag of 13 and created the respective shifted variables. It is important to note that lag 13 could represent 13 min or more, considering the irregular frequency of data collection, which could range from 1 to 5 min.

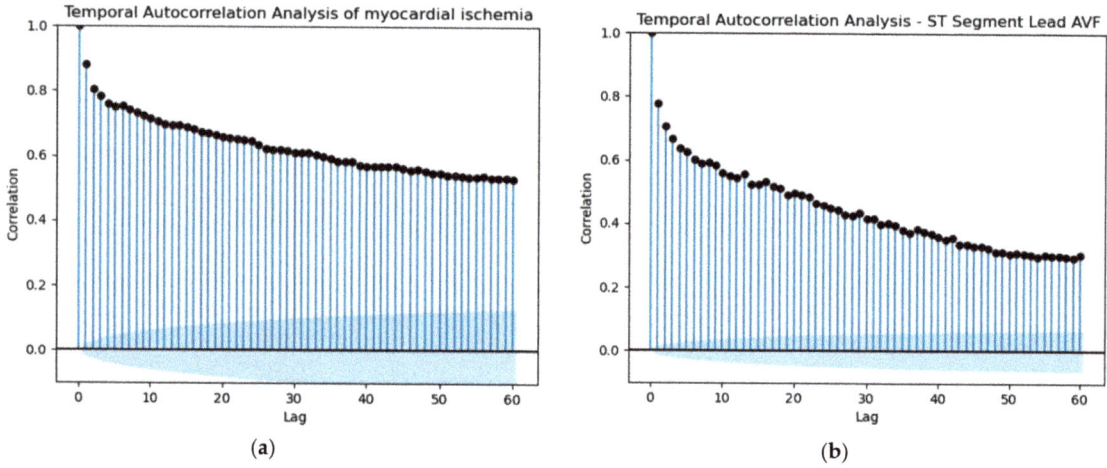

Figure 17. Here we represent as an example the autocorrelation plots for the variables myocardial ischemia and ST Segment Lead AVF, where (**a**) represents the autocorrelation for myocardial ischemia and (**b**) represents the autocorrelation for ST segment Lead AVF.

Categorical variables, such as ethnicity, sex, or blood group, were converted into dummy variables. Afterward, we calculated the correlation between each variable and our target variable, myocardial ischemia, and selected the ones with the highest correlation, as shown in Table 9. Of these selected variables, Troponin was discarded since it has no predictive value; as troponin is an indicator of cellular necrosis, it is not included in the analysis of ischemia (since it only appears a posteriori).

Table 9. Variables used in models by disease.

Myocardial Infarction	Pulmonary Thromboembolism	Aortic Stenosis	Global Model
Height	Height	Shift_Myocardial_Ischemia	Age
Age	Weight	Shift_Heart_Rate	Shift_Myocardial_Ischemia
Shift_Myocardial_Ischemia	Age	Shift_Segment_Lead_AVL	Shift_Segment_Lead_AVL
Shift_Segment_Lead_AVL	Shift_Myocardial_Ischemia	Shift_Segment_Lead_AVR	Shift_Segment_Lead_III
Shift_Segment_Lead_AVF	Shift_Heart_Rate	Myocardial_Ischemia	Ethnicity_Caucasian
Shift_Segment_Lead_III	Shift_Segment_Lead_AVL		Myocardial_Ischemia
Ethnicity_Caucasian	Shift_Segment_Lead_AVF		
Myocardial_Ischemia	Shift_Segment_Lead_III		
	Ethnicity_Caucasian		
	Sex_Female		
	Myocardial_Ischemia		

In addition to this selection, we also included PatientDboid (the primary key for the patients DB table), to conduct further analysis. We also combined all the data from the hospitalization datasets for the three diseases to create a global model. The same procedures were conducted as with each individual disease.

For each disease, after selecting the variables to include in the model, we decided to split the data between train and test sets based on patients. We randomly selected one patient within the top five with the most rows for each disease and used them for the test set, while excluding them from the training set. Afterward, we dropped the PatientDboid column and created separate sets of X and Y for both the training and test datasets. For the global model, we randomly split the data into training and test sets using an 80–20 proportion. The algorithms we employed for the machine learning modeling were Random Forest, Naïve Bayes, and Neural Network. We constructed a Neural Network with two hidden layers, each consisting of 1024 and 512 neurons, respectively. The activation function used in both hidden layers was ReLU (Rectified Linear Unit), while the output layer employed the Sigmoid activation function. For optimization, we utilized the Adam optimizer and the binary cross-entropy loss function.

Table 10 presents the results, highlighting the best-performing algorithm for each disease. We evaluated the performance of each algorithm using all four standard classification evaluation metrics (F1-Score, Accuracy, Precision, Recall). Additionally, the table includes the number of records in the training and test sets for each disease.

Table 10. Performance of algorithms by disease.

Disease	Algorithm	F1-Score	Accuracy	Precision	Recall
Myocardial Infarction	Random Forest	0.81	0.82	0.81	0.80
# Train Set: 356,905	Naive Bayes	0.81	0.82	0.81	0.81
# Test Set: 8023	Neural Network	0.86	0.82	0.86	0.86
Pulmonary Thromboembolism	Random Forest	0.92	0.94	0.92	0.91
# Train Set: 80,685	Naive Bayes	0.73	0.75	0.73	0.82
# Test Set: 6595	Neural Network	0.87	0.94	0.87	0.87
Aortic Stenosis	Random Forest	0.83	0.87	0.84	0.83
# Train Set: 778,744	Naive Bayes	0.83	0.86	0.83	0.83
# Test Set: 9365	Neural Network	0.91	0.87	0.91	0.92
Global Model	Random Forest	0.86	0.86	0.86	0.86
# Train Set: 990,756	Naïve Bayes	0.84	0.84	0.84	0.84
# Train Set: 247,690	Neural Network	0.84	0.85	0.84	0.83

As evident from the results in Table 10, the best-performing algorithms achieved impressive scores close to 90% for each evaluation metric, indicating their good predictive capabilities in identifying myocardial ischemia with a time lag of 13. These highly promising outcomes offer strong encouragement for the subsequent stages of implementation, as the algorithms demonstrated the potential to assist physicians in real time in providing timely advice regarding myocardial ischemia occurrence and forecast in patients.

When comparing the global model with the disease-specific models, the results are not as impressive, if we think of the first case. However, the global model is more versatile as it is not solely trained on data from one disease. It is also important to mention that each model can be applied to patients with any disease, with the only requirement being the data specified in Table 9 for the chosen model. These innovative results underscore the significance of further steps in refining and deploying the algorithms in clinical settings. The potential benefits of such predictive models are immense, as they can aid healthcare professionals in proactively managing, forecasting and offering personalized care to patients at risk of myocardial ischemia.

6. Discussion

In this section, we engage in a comprehensive discussion of the findings and implications of our study, while also acknowledging the limitations and ethical considerations inherent in AI-driven healthcare research.

In the context of our research question, "how can fusion of Exploratory Data Analysis (EDA) techniques and predictive machine learning models assist medical staff in accurate clinical decision-making and facilitate timely medical interventions of a preventive nature?", we presented charts for our use cases in three specific diseases—acute myocardial infarction, pulmonary thromboembolism and aortic stenosis—that represent a range of studied CVDs. We employed machine algorithms to predict MI within a 13 min window, for patients diagnosed with these studied diseases. The implementation of a global model with all the patients (without filtering by disease), where we achieved 86% for each evaluation metric, demonstrates its ability to generalize. The best result for predicting MI was achieved when trained and evaluated for patients suffering from Pulmonary Thromboembolism and Aortic Stenosis. Our ability to forecast myocardial ischemia incidents with these levels of accuracy, particularly within a 13 min window, holds promising implications for timely medical interventions and improved patient outcomes.

As with any research endeavor, it is essential to acknowledge the limitations of our study. We confronted the challenges posed by the lack of standardization in data collection procedures and the prevalence of unstructured clinical information in Electronic Medical Records. These limitations impacted the accuracy and generalizability of our predictive models, and we recognize the need for ongoing efforts to enhance data quality and standardization.

The use of AI in healthcare necessitates a robust consideration of ethical implications. We acknowledge our access to the clinical data of patients admitted to the Intensive Care Units of Hospital de Santa Maria, in the framework of FCT project DSAIPA/AI/0122/2020 AIMHealth, and the work [10], where DSAs were signed and homomorphic encryption was implemented. These ethical safeguards protected patient privacy and confidentiality while enabling critical research.

In the spirit of continuous improvement, we will engage in self-critique by identifying areas for enhancement and future research directions. Our exploration of myocardial ischemia prediction, while promising, remains a singular facet of AI applications in cardiovascular healthcare. We advocate for a broader exploration of AI's potential in addressing various cardiovascular diseases, and on behalf of the study that was conducted [10], we will focus on further enhancing the robustness and generalizability of our predictive models by integrating data from multiple hospitals and medical institutions. This collaborative approach aims to encompass a broader patient population and provide a more comprehensive understanding of cardiovascular diseases.

7. Conclusions

Our exploratory data analysis of the three studied diseases enables physicians to grasp patterns in Heart Rate, Respiration Rate, and Troponin values. Going forward, they can compare data from new patients with the established behavioral norms derived from previous patients diagnosed with the same disease. We believe that this approach enables physicians to gain a more profound understanding of the recovery status and spend more time with patients that show different behaviors. For future work, we suggest conducting an analysis of additional medical tests, such as NT-proBNP.

In our study, it is also noteworthy to observe that aortic stenosis and myocardial infarction exhibit certain similarities, which stand in contrast to pulmonary thromboembolism. The most prominent evidence lies in Heart Rate, where in both diseases, the average value progressively decreases after admission, reaching its lowest point approximately 2 h after admission before beginning to rise again.

In this paper, we presented another valuable AI tool, which performed the prediction (forecast) of myocardial ischemia. Our literature review uncovered no relevant studies addressing the use of machine learning to assist physicians in evaluating the progression of patients' conditions post-diagnosis, showing the relevance of this study. If physicians were alerted 13 min in advance that a patient might experience myocardial ischemia, with an accuracy of around 90%, they could take proactive measures rather than reactive ones, and we believe our AI modeling tool can lead them in that direction. Upon refinement, this model may be further tested prospectively to predict ischemia and arrhythmia in monitored cardiac patients. We would like to point out, in addition, that we have shown that our machine learning model can be applied to any other disease, with the sole requirement being that the patient must be connected to a medical device that collects ST Segment Variables.

It is also important to mention that applying exploratory data analysis to other diseases could provide a better understanding of their progression, but it must be performed within a singular analysis.

Author Contributions: Conceptualization, J.C.F. and L.B.E.; methodology, L.B.E. and M.N.; Validation, L.B.R., M.S.D. and J.C.F.; formal analysis L.B.E., L.B.R., M.S.D. and J.C.F.; writing—original draft preparation, L.B.E. and M.N.; writing—review and editing, L.B.E., J.C.F., M.S.D., L.B.R.; supervision, J.C.F., M.S.D. and L.B.R. All authors have read and agreed to the published version of the manuscript.

Funding: This work was partially funded by national funds through FCT—Fundação para a Ciência e Tecnologia, I.P., under the projects FCT UIDB/04466/2020, and FCT DSAIPA/AI/0122/2020 AIMHealth—Mobile Applications Based on Artificial Intelligence. This research also received funding from ERAMUS+ project NEMM with grant 101083048. During the development of this work, Luís Elvas was a Ph.D. grant holder, funded by FCT with UI/BD/151494/2021.

Institutional Review Board Statement: Not applicable.

Informed Consent Statement: Not applicable.

Data Availability Statement: Not applicable.

Acknowledgments: We would like to acknowledge both João Ribeiro and Pilar Cardim from Hospital de Santa Maria, for the in-house data-collection process.

Conflicts of Interest: The authors declare no conflict of interest.

References

1. Mensah, G.A.; Roth, G.A.; Fuster, V. The Global Burden of Cardiovascular Diseases and Risk Factors. *J. Am. Coll. Cardiol.* **2019**, *74*, 2529–2532. [CrossRef] [PubMed]
2. Roth, G.A.; Mensah, G.A.; Johnson, C.O.; Addolorato, G.; Ammirati, E.; Baddour, L.M.; Barengo, N.C.; Beaton, A.Z.; Benjamin, E.J.; Benziger, C.P.; et al. Global Burden of Cardiovascular Diseases and Risk Factors, 1990–2019: Update From the GBD 2019 Study. *J. Am. Coll. Cardiol.* **2020**, *76*, 2982–3021. [CrossRef] [PubMed]
3. Cardiovascular Disease Cost the European Union Economy €282bn in 2021. Available online: https://www.ndph.ox.ac.uk/news/cardiovascular-disease-cost-the-european-union-economy-20ac282bn-in-2021 (accessed on 27 August 2023).
4. Capobianco, E. Data-driven clinical decision processes: It's time. *J. Transl. Med.* **2019**, *17*, 44. [CrossRef] [PubMed]
5. Kriegova, E.; Kudelka, M.; Radvansky, M.; Gallo, J. A theoretical model of health management using data-driven decision-making: The future of precision medicine and health. *J. Transl. Med.* **2021**, *19*, 68. [CrossRef]
6. Amal, S.; Safarnejad, L.; Omiye, J.A.; Ghanzouri, I.; Cabot, J.H.; Ross, E.G. Use of Multi-Modal Data and Machine Learning to Improve Cardiovascular Disease Care. *Front. Cardiovasc. Med.* **2022**, *9*, 840262. Available online: https://www.frontiersin.org/articles/10.3389/fcvm.2022.840262 (accessed on 16 August 2023). [CrossRef]
7. Celermajer, D.S.; Chow, C.K.; Marijon, E.; Anstey, N.M.; Woo, K.S. Cardiovascular Disease in the Developing World. *J. Am. Coll. Cardiol.* **2012**, *60*, 1207–1216. [CrossRef]
8. Sarker, I.H. Machine Learning: Algorithms, Real-World Applications and Research Directions. *SN Comput. Sci.* **2021**, *2*, 160. [CrossRef]
9. Islam, M.N.; Raiyan, K.R.; Mitra, S.; Mannan, M.R.; Tasnim, T.; Putul, A.O.; Mandol, A.B. Predictis: An IoT and machine learning-based system to predict risk level of cardio-vascular diseases. *BMC Health Serv. Res.* **2023**, *23*, 171. [CrossRef]
10. Elvas, L.B.; Ferreira, J.C.; Dias, M.S.; Rosário, L.B. Health Data Sharing towards Knowledge Creation. *Systems* **2023**, *11*, 435. [CrossRef]
11. Moher, D.; Liberati, A.; Tetzlaff, J.; Altman, D.G. Preferred reporting items for systematic reviews and meta-analyses: The PRISMA statement. *BMJ* **2009**, *339*, b2535. [CrossRef]
12. Ramkumar, G.; Seetha, J.; Priyadarshini, R.; Gopila, M.; Saranya, G. IoT-based patient monitoring system for predicting heart disease using deep learning. *Meas. J. Int. Meas. Confed.* **2023**, *218*, 113235. [CrossRef]
13. Yıldırım, E.; Çalhan, A.; Cicioğlu, M. Performance analysis of disease diagnostic system using IoMT and real-time data analytics. *Concurr. Comput. Pract. Exp.* **2022**, *34*, e6916. [CrossRef]
14. Bhagat, R.K.; Yadav, A.; Rajoria, Y.K.; Raj, S.; Boadh, R. Study of Fuzzy and Artificial Neural Network (ANN) Based Techniques to Diagnose Heart Disease. *J. Pharm. Negat. Results* **2022**, *13*, 1023–1029.
15. Krittanawong, C.; Aydar, M.; Virk, H.U.; Kumar, A.; Kaplin, S.; Guimaraes, L.; Wang, Z.; Halperin, J.L. Artificial Intelligence-Powered Blockchains for Cardiovascular Medicine. *Can. J. Cardiol.* **2022**, *38*, 185–195. [CrossRef]
16. So, S.; Khalaf, A.; Yi, X.; Herring, C.; Zhang, Y.; Simon, M.A.; Akcakaya, M.; Lee, S.; Yun, M. Induced bioresistance via BNP detection for machine learning-based risk assessment. *Biosens. Bioelectron.* **2021**, *175*, 112903. [CrossRef]
17. Panchavati, S.; Lam, C.; Zelin, N.S.; Pellegrini, E.; Barnes, G.; Hoffman, J.; Garikipati, A.; Calvert, J.; Mao, Q.; Das, R. Retrospective validation of a machine learning clinical decision support tool for myocardial infarction risk stratification. *Healthc. Technol. Lett.* **2021**, *8*, 139–147. [CrossRef]
18. Li, B.; Ding, S.; Song, G.; Li, J.; Zhang, Q. Computer-Aided Diagnosis and Clinical Trials of Cardiovascular Diseases Based on Artificial Intelligence Technologies for Risk-Early Warning Model. *J. Med. Syst.* **2019**, *43*, 228. [CrossRef]

19. Kartal, E.; Balaban, M.E. Machine learning techniques in cardiac risk assessment. *Turk. J. Thorac. Cardiovasc. Surg.* **2018**, *26*, 394–401. [CrossRef]
20. Senthil, R.; Narayanan, B.; Velmurugan, K. Develop the hybrid Adadelta Stochastic Gradient Classifier with optimized feature selection algorithm to predict the heart disease at earlier stage. *Meas. Sens.* **2023**, *25*, 100602. [CrossRef]
21. Almutairi, S.; Manimurugan, S.; Chilamkurti, N.; Aborokbah, M.M.; Narmatha, C.; Ganesan, S.; Alzaheb, R.A.; Almoamari, H. A Context-Aware MRIPPER Algorithm for Heart Disease Prediction. *J. Healthc. Eng.* **2022**, *2022*, 7853604. [CrossRef]
22. Desai, D.; Shende, P. Integration of internet of things with quantum dots: A state-of-the-art of medicine. *Curr. Pharm. Des.* **2021**, *27*, 2068–2075. [CrossRef] [PubMed]
23. Gearhart, A.; Gaffar, S.; Chang, A.C. A primer on artificial intelligence for the paediatric cardiologist. *Cardiol. Young* **2020**, *30*, 934–945. [CrossRef] [PubMed]
24. Wirth, R.; Hipp, J. CRISP-DM: Towards a standard process model for data mining. In Proceedings of the 4th International Conference on the Practical Applications of Knowledge Discovery and Data Miningjan, Manchester, UK, 11–13 April 2000.
25. Thygesen, K.; Alpert, J.S.; Jaffe, A.S.; Chaitman, B.R.; Bax, J.J.; Morrow, D.A.; White, H.D.; Executive Group on behalf of the Joint European Society of Cardiology (ESC)/American College of Cardiology (ACC)/American Heart Association (AHA)/World Heart Federation (WHF) Task Force for the Universal Definition of Myocardial Infarction. Fourth universal definition of myocardial infarction (2018). *Eur. Heart J.* **2019**, *40*, 237–269. [CrossRef]
26. Mustaqeem, A.; Anwar, S.M.; Majid, M. A modular cluster based collaborative recommender system for cardiac patients. *Artif. Intell. Med.* **2020**, *102*, 101761. [CrossRef] [PubMed]
27. Huang, M.; Han, H.; Wang, H.; Li, L.; Zhang, Y.; Bhatti, U.A. A Clinical Decision Support Framework for Heterogeneous Data Sources. *IEEE J. Biomed. Health Inform.* **2018**, *22*, 1824–1833. [CrossRef] [PubMed]
28. Fathima, M.D.; Samuel, S.J.; Natchadalingam, R.; Kaveri, V.V. Majority voting ensembled feature selection and customized deep neural network for the enhanced clinical decision support system. *Int. J. Comput. Appl.* **2022**, *44*, 991–1001. [CrossRef]
29. Mohammed, P.; Begum, S.J. Developing an Integrated Model for Heart Disease Diagnosis (IM-HDD) using ensemble classification methods. *J. Intell. Fuzzy Syst.* **2022**, *43*, 4161–4171. [CrossRef]

Disclaimer/Publisher's Note: The statements, opinions and data contained in all publications are solely those of the individual author(s) and contributor(s) and not of MDPI and/or the editor(s). MDPI and/or the editor(s) disclaim responsibility for any injury to people or property resulting from any ideas, methods, instructions or products referred to in the content.

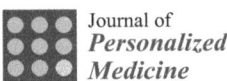

Journal of
Personalized
Medicine

Opinion

Redesigning Primary Care: The Emergence of Artificial-Intelligence-Driven Symptom Diagnostic Tools

Christian J. Wiedermann [1,2,*], Angelika Mahlknecht [1], Giuliano Piccoliori [1] and Adolf Engl [1]

1. Institute of General Practice and Public Health, Claudiana—College of Health Professions, 39100 Bolzano, Italy
2. Department of Public Health, Medical Decision Making and HTA, University of Health Sciences, Medical Informatics and Technology-Tyrol, 6060 Hall, Austria
* Correspondence: christian.wiedermann@am-mg.claudiana.bz.it

Abstract: Modern healthcare is facing a juxtaposition of increasing patient demands owing to an aging population and a decreasing general practitioner workforce, leading to strained access to primary care. The coronavirus disease 2019 pandemic has emphasized the potential for alternative consultation methods, highlighting opportunities to minimize unnecessary care. This article discusses the role of artificial-intelligence-driven symptom checkers, particularly their efficiency, utility, and challenges in primary care. Based on a study conducted in Italian general practices, insights from both physicians and patients were gathered regarding this emergent technology, highlighting differences in perceived utility, user satisfaction, and potential challenges. While symptom checkers are seen as potential tools for addressing healthcare challenges, concerns regarding their accuracy and the potential for misdiagnosis persist. Patients generally viewed them positively, valuing their ease of use and the empowerment they provide in managing health. However, some general practitioners perceive these tools as challenges to their expertise. This article proposes that artificial-intelligence-based symptom checkers can optimize medical-history taking for the benefit of both general practitioners and patients, with potential enhancements in complex diagnostic tasks rather than routine diagnoses. It underscores the importance of carefully integrating digital innovations while preserving the essential human touch in healthcare. Symptom checkers offer promising solutions; ensuring their accuracy, reliability, and effective integration into primary care requires rigorous research, clinical guidance, and an understanding of varied user perceptions. Collaboration among technologists, clinicians, and patients is paramount for the successful evolution of digital tools in healthcare.

Keywords: primary health care; artificial intelligence; symptom assessment; telemedicine; patient satisfaction

Citation: Wiedermann, C.J.; Mahlknecht, A.; Piccoliori, G.; Engl, A. Redesigning Primary Care: The Emergence of Artificial-Intelligence-Driven Symptom Diagnostic Tools. *J. Pers. Med.* **2023**, *13*, 1379. https://doi.org/10.3390/jpm13091379

Academic Editor: Daniele Giansanti

Received: 4 September 2023
Revised: 13 September 2023
Accepted: 14 September 2023
Published: 15 September 2023

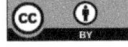

Copyright: © 2023 by the authors. Licensee MDPI, Basel, Switzerland. This article is an open access article distributed under the terms and conditions of the Creative Commons Attribution (CC BY) license (https://creativecommons.org/licenses/by/4.0/).

1. Introduction

Modern health care is critical. The convergence of burgeoning patient demands, primarily due to a progressively aging population and a diminishing general practitioner (GP) workforce, has rendered access to primary care increasingly challenging [1,2]. This situation is exacerbated by the prevalence of non-urgent medical consultations which unnecessarily strain the system. Consequently, we face a paradoxical situation in which an escalation in technological advancements is countered by decreasing patient satisfaction [3,4].

The COVID-19 pandemic has provided unexpected observations, highlighting the efficacy of alternative consultation methods. The pandemic-induced decline in face-to-face visits highlights the prospect that some treatments, which are now deemed superfluous, potentially carry the risk of iatrogenic harm. Such revelations underscored the opportunity to minimize unnecessary care, thereby safeguarding patient well-being and fortifying the sustainability of healthcare [5].

This article discusses the role and potential of AI-driven symptom checkers [6], particularly in light of the challenges confronting modern healthcare. We aimed to evaluate the efficiency, utility, and challenges of integrating these digital tools into primary care settings by drawing insights from a recent study conducted in Italian general practices [7]. The perspectives of both physicians and patients regarding this emergent technology were elucidated, shedding light on its potential advantages and pitfalls.

2. Symptom Checkers

Symptom checkers with chatbots are digital tools that use AI algorithms to engage users in a conversational interface that allows them to input and describe their medical symptoms. These tools then analyze the provided information to offer potential differential diagnoses, provide triage recommendations, and suggest appropriate next steps in care [8]. Designed to be user-friendly and accessible, they offer patients an initial point of contact for health concerns, helping to guide them towards appropriate medical care or self-management options [9].

In the evolving healthcare landscape, the role of AI is slowly gaining recognition [10]. AI-driven symptom checkers based on chatbots are being explored as potential tools for addressing ongoing challenges in the sector. These digital platforms, which merge algorithmic analyses with user interfaces, are seen as possible aids in complementing the work of GPs. Their tentative benefit may be to offer patients a preliminary platform for self-assessment, possibly assisting in their healthcare decisions. Such tools might offer GPs an additional layer of information, potentially allowing them to allocate more time to intricate cases [9]. However, recent studies have shed light on physicians' perceptions regarding the extensive use of AI in primary care [11]. A significant proportion of GPs perceive the potential of AI as somewhat constrained, a sentiment that contrasts with the optimism of biomedical informaticians. Furthermore, the sophisticated framework underlying symptom checkers has added to the allure of these digital tools. Not only are they designed to collect preliminary data, but they also possess the capability to provide differential diagnoses based on inputted symptoms. This feature becomes pivotal in guiding patients towards appropriate medical action, whether the tool recommends immediate medical attention or considers alternative treatment pathways [12]. Essentially, these tools may play a crucial role in the triage process, helping prioritize cases based on urgency and clinical relevance. Such functionalities could dramatically reshape the way primary care operates, optimize resource allocation, and ensure timely medical intervention.

However, each revolutionary tool presents challenges that cannot be ignored. Symptom checkers suggest potential causes and recommend courses of action based on symptoms. However, if their output does not align with the users' personal experiences or falls short of their expectations, it might lead to unwarranted healthcare-seeking behaviors [13,14]. The effectiveness and reliability of symptom checkers are subject to intense scrutiny [15,16]. Although they undoubtedly present a revolutionary approach to preliminary medical assessments, the crux of their value lies in their ability to provide accurate and safe advice.

Previous research has shed light on areas of concern. Causal reasoning remains a vital missing component for applying machine learning to medical diagnoses [17]. Some studies have highlighted the propensity of these tools to either misdiagnose or lean towards excessively cautious triage recommendations [9,16].

The diagnostic and triage capabilities of symptom checkers remain limited, especially in non-urgent primary care situations [9,18]. A study revealed that most laypersons performed better than symptom checkers when assessed using clinical vignettes, although the symptom checkers were more reliable in identifying emergency cases [19]. These potential pitfalls serve as cautionary notes, emphasizing the need for rigorous validation, continuous updates, and user education to ensure that symptom checkers realize their full potential without compromising patient safety.

Insights from the Italian Experience

Amid rapid advancements in AI, the Italian healthcare system has actively explored the integration of AI-driven symptom checkers into primary care. The study in question [7], conducted in northern Italian GP offices, particularly during the challenging times of the pandemic, is among the first of its kind. Specifically designed as a feasibility study, the research focused on ten general practitioners (GPs) and the patients visiting their offices.

The patients were prompted to use a chatbot-based symptom checker before their medical visits. This checker not only facilitated anamnestic screening for COVID-19 but also employed a medical history algorithm tailored to the patient's specific medical problem. The data entered were then relayed to the GP, serving as an auxiliary medical history aid. After their medical consultations, both the participating physicians and their patients were tasked with evaluating the symptom checker based on their experience. Of the 225 patients who participated in the study, 145 completed the post-visit survey; however, after excluding 29 patients due to a chatbot-estimated medium or high anamnestic risk for COVID-19, a total of 116 post-visit questionnaires were included in the final analysis. The patients were predominantly female (55%), with a median age of 47 years. Most had vocational schooling (39%) or were high school graduates (28%). A vast majority (87%) relied on their GP for health information, while 14% used online sources. Health assessments varied, with 44% considering their health 'very good' and 15% marking it 'average'. To ensure a comprehensive evaluation, the physicians also offered a final overarching review of the symptom checker upon completing the practice phase. Table 1 presents the main findings.

Table 1. Comparative perspectives on symptom checkers from patients and GPs in Italian primary care [7].

Variable	Patients' Perspectives	GPs' Perspectives
Experience with Symptom Checkers	Most had not previously used a symptom checker Positive feedback on the ease of use	Varied experiences and perspectives
Satisfaction	49% were 'rather' or 'very' satisfied	27% were 'rather' or 'very' satisfied
Usefulness	Precise questioning Time-saving potential Encourages self-reflection	Value as an auxiliary medical history aid
Willingness to Use	50% are willing to use it at home	Concerns about additional workload
Impact on Medical Visit Duration	75% felt no impact	84% felt no impact
Trust in AI	Surface-level interaction General guidance	AI suggestions should be scrutinized and evaluated more critically

Abbreviations: AI, artificial intelligence; GPs, general practitioners.

From the results, it became evident that while most patients had not previously engaged with symptom checkers, those who had regarded them positively. Specifically, almost half of the patients and a quarter of the doctors said they were 'fairly' or 'very' satisfied. When asked to provide reasons for their opinions, the patients applauded the checker's ease of use, precise questioning, time-saving potential, and the tool's capacity to encourage self-reflection. Interestingly, every second patient expressed a willingness to use the symptom checker at home, viewing it as a potential means of assessing initial health concerns, minimizing unnecessary medical visits, and assisting their physicians. Demographics such as age, sex, and education level did not play a significant role in shaping patients' attitudes towards the symptom checker. Notably, the vast majority of participants believed that the tool did not affect the duration of the medical visit. Only a marginal fraction felt that the tool might disrupt the quality or flow of the consultation [7].

An Italian study provided insights into the reception of symptom checkers, revealing varied perspectives between patients and doctors. While there is interest in such tools, it is still uncertain whether they will become standard in primary care. This study emphasizes that careful clinical guidance is crucial before considering wider adoption.

3. Discussion

Recent study results [9,18,20], further illuminated by an Italian publication [7], underscore the importance of meticulous clinical guidance in the evolution of symptom checkers. Symptom checkers have emerged as a potential avenue for addressing challenges in primary care, such as the growing workload due to an aging population and the declining number of GPs. Their adoption could increase healthcare efficiency and possibly relieve GPs; however, their broad implementation demands a robust, evidence-based evaluation of their efficacy, safety, and cost-effectiveness.

An Italian study [7] pointed out a dichotomy in attitudes towards symptom checkers: patients tend to view them positively, finding empowerment in controlling their health, whereas some GPs see them as rather unhelpful in relation to the patients' self-management or reducing unnecessary visits. This difference in perception stresses the importance of understanding both patients' and GPs' experiences with digital tools. Trust in symptom checkers might differ between patients and GPs based on their respective vulnerabilities, the anticipation of the AI's decisions, an understanding of the 'contract' with the AI, an evaluation of the AI's trustworthiness, and what is needed from explainable AI [21]. Patients might have more surface-level interactions, trusting the system to provide guidance, whereas GPs, with their deeper medical knowledge, might scrutinize and evaluate the AI's suggestions more critically. Interestingly, neither patients nor GPs perceived the use of symptom checkers as significantly time-averse during medical consultations. Moreover, the varied levels of satisfaction among GPs in the study, especially in relation to post-visit evaluations and the concluding survey, hint at external factors that influence GPs' opinions [7]. From the patient's standpoint, the use of symptom checkers adds an element of novelty without incurring significant effort. On the other hand, for GPs, especially during high-workload periods such as the COVID-19 pandemic, integrating these tools with their tasks potentially skewing their satisfaction rates.

However, one constant was persistent skepticism regarding the diagnostic accuracy of symptom checkers. The divergence in perceptions of the value of symptom checkers between GPs and patients hints at broader challenges in healthcare, particularly regarding the emphasis on human touch and the tactile aspects of the diagnostic process. While digital advancements in patient-GP communication are highly sought after, with patients voicing a strong desire for features such as direct messaging platforms, streamlined appointment scheduling, and efficient symptom tracking, it is imperative to note the irreplaceable value that patients place on face-to-face consultations and the significance of maintaining eye contact during visits [22]. The lack of consistent evidence regarding the workload-reducing potential of symptom checkers requires further research. Balancing digital innovations with human touch is important for optimizing patient care. The highlighted interest of about half of the patients in the chatbot's use for pre-visit preparations suggests a potential avenue for enhancing patient-GP interactions. The chatbot's positive effect on the patients' self-reflection and attentiveness during medical consultations is worth noting.

While patients appreciated the symptom checkers' speed and user-friendly interface in an Italian study, GPs reported observing technical and procedural challenges among patients. This discrepancy underscores the need to design tools that are both intuitive and user-centric. In addition, the data hinted at a possible age bias in the acceptance and usage of symptom checkers, suggesting that a more tailored approach for diverse populations might be beneficial. In light of the observed differences between the patients' and GPs' attitudes towards AI-based symptom checkers, strategies could be pursued to bridge this divide. Firstly, it is pertinent to emphasize the importance of iterative feedback. By establishing mechanisms that enable GPs to consistently convey their experiences and hurdles with these tools to AI developers, we can ensure that these symptom checkers are fine-tuned in real time to better serve clinical needs. On the patient front, refining the user interfaces of AI tools to be more intuitive can heighten their appeal and usability. A design centered around the patient experience ensures that the tools are more aligned with their expectations and comfort levels. Lastly, a clearer insight into the algorithms underpinning AI tools can dispel reservations and foster deeper trust. By elucidating how these systems arrive at specific conclusions, we can instill greater confidence in both patients and doctors. Implementing these strategies could prove instrumental in harmonizing perceptions and facilitating a smoother integration of AI-driven symptom checkers into primary care.

Our findings are consistent with a growing body of literature that examines the utility, efficacy, and challenges of using AI and decision support systems (DSSs) in primary care settings. Gottliebsen and Petersson [15] investigated the use of intelligent online triage tools in primary care and observed that the current systems might be underdeveloped, providing limited benefits. This resonates with our observations of the challenges of seamlessly integrating such tools into routine clinical practice. Moreover, Semigran et al. [9] conducted an audit on the diagnostic and triage accuracy of online symptom checkers. They found that these systems often lacked diagnostic accuracy albeit being risk-averse, thus potentially directing patients to seek unnecessary medical attention. Such findings echo concerns about overburdening healthcare infrastructures with avoidable patient visits. In addition, a systematic review [16] discussed the uncertainties surrounding digital symptom checkers and their potential impact on healthcare outcomes. These authors noted the specific preference of younger and more educated populations for online and digital services, emphasizing the implications for health equity.

There are studies examining the broader implications and potentials of differential diagnosis DSSs in primary care. McParland et al. [23] indicated potential roles for such DSS in assisting both clinicians and the public; however, the design and implementation considerations must cater to the specific needs of these groups. Kostopoulou et al. [24] highlighted the opportunity for DSSs to combat the incompleteness and biases prevalent in routine primary care data. Such findings underscore the importance of a holistic approach when designing and implementing these systems. Furthermore, while the utility of some online diagnostic systems like Isabel in general practice has been assessed, some have suggested the need for further modifications to ensure their suitability in primary care contexts [25]. This mirrors our study's emphasis on the customization and adaptability of AI tools for their intended clinical settings.

In conclusion, while there is interest and potential in the domain of AI and DSS in primary care, there are evident challenges and considerations. Our study, in light of others like those cited above, reinforces the importance of thorough evaluations, iterative design processes, and stakeholder engagement in this rapidly evolving landscape.

This opinion article offers an exploration of AI-driven symptom checkers in primary care, drawing insights primarily from a recent study [7]. Though it provides valuable perspectives, its limitations include the subjective nature of the content, potential biases from the focus on a specific demographic, and concerns about the generalizability of the findings, particularly given the rapidly evolving nature of AI. The highlighted value of face-to-face consultations and the diagnostic accuracy of symptom checkers require further exploration. Moreover, the unique circumstances of the COVID-19 pandemic may have influenced the observations, questioning their post-pandemic relevance. A broader empirical foundation and consideration of various settings can enhance the insights presented here.

A pivotal question surrounding symptom-checkers with chatbots revolves around their capacity to overcome present limitations. Specifically, can these tools, through continued development, successfully replicate the causal reasoning of a human expert? As AI evolves, there is a growing optimism that future iterations of AI systems will improve in emulating complex human reasoning processes. However, it remains uncertain whether technology can ever truly capture the nuanced and multifaceted nature of human cognitive abilities. Thus, while advancements are anticipated, the extent to which these tools can match human intuition and reasoning is still a topic of debate.

4. Conclusions

AI-driven symptom checkers have emerged as promising tools for addressing primary care challenges. Recent findings, especially from an Italian context, demonstrate a dichotomy in perspectives: while patients appreciate the empowerment and user-friendliness of these tools, some GPs voice concerns, particularly regarding the tools' diagnostic accuracy. Neither group perceived significant time-saving benefits during consultations. Emphasizing human touch remains paramount despite the push for digital innovations in patient-GP communication. Further, the highlighted interest of the patients in using chatbots for pre-visit preparations hints at enhancing patient-GP interactions.

The potential of AI-based symptom checkers becomes evident, especially when considering the optimization of medical-history taking. For GPs, these tools can streamline the process, making it more efficient and focused. For patients, they can be empowering, offering a sense of agency and participation. However, it is recognized that in routine general practice, the challenge is not so much diagnostic difficulty for common ailments but rather the increasing demands of rare diseases. Given this issue, while AI tools can aid in routine diagnostics, their real potential lies in assisting with the more complex and intricate diagnostic tasks. By concentrating on these challenging areas, AI can significantly complement the expertise of GPs, leading to more accurate and timely interventions.

The study underscores the need for symptom checkers to be intuitive and user-centric and the importance of rigorous validation to ensure patient safety. These observations warrant further exploration. Future research should aim for a broader empirical foundation across various settings to fully capture the potential challenges of AI in primary care.

Author Contributions: Conceptualization, C.J.W. and A.M.; writing—original draft preparation, C.J.W.; writing—review and editing, A.M., G.P. and A.E. The authors sought assistance from OpenAI's ChatGPT in content structuring and language clarification. While ChatGPT provided linguistic and formatting guidance, the authors formulated all the substantive content, interpretations, and conclusions drawn in the manuscript. The responsibility for the content and potential errors rests entirely on the authors. All authors have read and agreed to the published version of the manuscript.

Funding: This research received no external funding.

Data Availability Statement: No new data were created.

Conflicts of Interest: The authors declare no conflict of interest.

References

1. Jia, H.; Yu, X.; Jiang, H.; Yu, J.; Cao, P.; Gao, S.; Shang, P.; Qiang, B. Analysis of Factors Affecting Medical Personnel Seeking Employment at Primary Health Care Institutions: Developing Human Resources for Primary Health Care. *Int. J. Equity Health* **2022**, *21*, 37. [CrossRef] [PubMed]
2. Chada, B.V. Virtual Consultations in General Practice: Embracing Innovation, Carefully. *Br. J. Gen. Pract.* **2017**, *67*, 264. [CrossRef] [PubMed]
3. Pearl, R. Kaiser Permanente Northern California: Current Experiences with Internet, Mobile, and Video Technologies. *Health Aff.* **2014**, *33*, 251–257. [CrossRef] [PubMed]
4. Atherton, H.; Brant, H.; Ziebland, S.; Bikker, A.; Campbell, J.; Gibson, A.; McKinstry, B.; Porqueddu, T.; Salisbury, C. *The Potential of Alternatives to Face-to-Face Consultation in General Practice, and the Impact on Different Patient Groups: A Mixed-Methods Case Study*; Health Services and Delivery Research; NIHR Journals Library: Southampton, UK, 2018.
5. Moynihan, R.; Johansson, M.; Maybee, A.; Lang, E.; Légaré, F. Covid-19: An Opportunity to Reduce Unnecessary Healthcare. *BMJ* **2020**, *370*, m2752. [CrossRef]
6. You, Y.; Gui, X. Self-Diagnosis through AI-Enabled Chatbot-Based Symptom Checkers: User Experiences and Design Considerations. *AMIA Annu. Symp. Proc.* **2020**, *2020*, 1354–1363. [PubMed]
7. Mahlknecht, A.; Engl, A.; Piccoliori, G.; Wiedermann, C.J. Supporting Primary Care through Symptom Checking Artificial Intelligence: A Study of Patient and Physician Attitudes in Italian General Practice. *BMC Prim. Care* **2023**, *24*, 174. [CrossRef]
8. Munsch, N.; Martin, A.; Gruarin, S.; Nateqi, J.; Abdarahmane, I.; Weingartner-Ortner, R.; Knapp, B. Diagnostic Accuracy of Web-Based COVID-19 Symptom Checkers: Comparison Study. *J. Med. Internet Res.* **2020**, *22*, e21299. [CrossRef]

9. Semigran, H.L.; Linder, J.A.; Gidengil, C.; Mehrotra, A. Evaluation of Symptom Checkers for Self Diagnosis and Triage: Audit Study. *BMJ* **2015**, *351*, h3480. [CrossRef]
10. Asan, O.; Choi, E.; Wang, X. Artificial Intelligence-Based Consumer Health Informatics Application: Scoping Review. *J. Med. Internet Res.* **2023**, *25*, e47260. [CrossRef]
11. Blease, C.; Kaptchuk, T.J.; Bernstein, M.H.; Mandl, K.D.; Halamka, J.D.; DesRoches, C.M. Artificial Intelligence and the Future of Primary Care: Exploratory Qualitative Study of UK General Practitioners' Views. *J. Med. Internet Res.* **2019**, *21*, e12802. [CrossRef]
12. Perlman, A.; Zilberg, A.V.; Bak, P.; Dreyfuss, M.; Leventer-Roberts, M.; Vurembrand, Y.; Jeffries, H.E.; Fisher, E.; Steuerman, Y.; Namir, Y.; et al. Characteristics and Symptoms of App Users Seeking COVID-19–Related Digital Health Information and Remote Services: Retrospective Cohort Study. *J. Med. Internet Res.* **2020**, *22*, e23197. [CrossRef] [PubMed]
13. Winn, A.N.; Somai, M.; Fergestrom, N.; Crotty, B.H. Association of Use of Online Symptom Checkers With Patients' Plans for Seeking Care. *JAMA Netw. Open* **2019**, *2*, e1918561. [CrossRef] [PubMed]
14. Luger, T.M.; Houston, T.K.; Suls, J. Older Adult Experience of Online Diagnosis: Results from a Scenario-Based Think-Aloud Protocol. *J. Med. Internet Res.* **2014**, *16*, e16. [CrossRef] [PubMed]
15. Gottliebsen, K.; Petersson, G. Limited Evidence of Benefits of Patient Operated Intelligent Primary Care Triage Tools: Findings of a Literature Review. *BMJ Health Care Inform.* **2020**, *27*, e100114. [CrossRef] [PubMed]
16. Chambers, D.; Cantrell, A.J.; Johnson, M.; Preston, L.; Baxter, S.K.; Booth, A.; Turner, J. Digital and Online Symptom Checkers and Health Assessment/Triage Services for Urgent Health Problems: Systematic Review. *BMJ Open* **2019**, *9*, e027743. [CrossRef]
17. Richens, J.G.; Lee, C.M.; Johri, S. Improving the Accuracy of Medical Diagnosis with Causal Machine Learning. *Nat. Commun.* **2020**, *11*, 3923. [CrossRef]
18. Schmieding, M.L.; Kopka, M.; Schmidt, K.; Schulz-Niethammer, S.; Balzer, F.; Feufel, M.A. Triage Accuracy of Symptom Checker Apps: 5-Year Follow-up Evaluation. *J. Med. Internet Res.* **2022**, *24*, e31810. [CrossRef]
19. Schmieding, M.L.; Mörgeli, R.; Schmieding, M.A.L.; Feufel, M.A.; Balzer, F. Benchmarking Triage Capability of Symptom Checkers Against That of Medical Laypersons: Survey Study. *J. Med. Internet Res.* **2021**, *23*, e24475. [CrossRef]
20. Hill, M.G.; Sim, M.; Mills, B. The Quality of Diagnosis and Triage Advice Provided by Free Online Symptom Checkers and Apps in Australia. *Med. J. Aust.* **2021**, *214*, 143–143.e1. [CrossRef]
21. Jacovi, A.; Marasović, A.; Miller, T.; Goldberg, Y. Formalizing Trust in Artificial Intelligence: Prerequisites, Causes and Goals of Human Trust in AI. In Proceedings of the 2021 ACM Conference on Fairness, Accountability, and Transparency, Toronto, ON, Canada, 3–10 March 2021; pp. 624–635.
22. Van den Bos, A.L.F. Improving Communication between GPs and Patients within an eHealth app. Master's Thesis, Norwegian University of Science and Technology, Trondheim, Norway, 2023.
23. McParland, C.R.; Cooper, M.A.; Johnston, B. Differential Diagnosis Decision Support Systems in Primary and Out-of-Hours Care: A Qualitative Analysis of the Needs of Key Stakeholders in Scotland. *J. Prim. Care Community Health* **2019**, *10*, 2150132719829315. [CrossRef]
24. Kostopoulou, O.; Tracey, C.; Delaney, B.C. Can Decision Support Combat Incompleteness and Bias in Routine Primary Care Data? *J. Am. Med. Inform. Assoc.* **2021**, *28*, 1461–1467. [CrossRef] [PubMed]
25. Henderson, E.J.; Rubin, G.P. The Utility of an Online Diagnostic Decision Support System (Isabel) in General Practice: A Process Evaluation. *JRSM Short. Rep.* **2013**, *4*, 31. [CrossRef] [PubMed]

Disclaimer/Publisher's Note: The statements, opinions and data contained in all publications are solely those of the individual author(s) and contributor(s) and not of MDPI and/or the editor(s). MDPI and/or the editor(s) disclaim responsibility for any injury to people or property resulting from any ideas, methods, instructions or products referred to in the content.

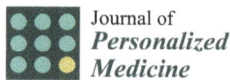

Journal of Personalized Medicine

Article

Intelligent Clinical Decision Support System for Managing COPD Patients

José Pereira [1,2], Nuno Antunes [1], Joana Rosa [1], João C. Ferreira [1,2,3,*], Sandra Mogo [4] and Manuel Pereira [5]

1. INOV Inesc Inovação—Instituto de Novas Tecnologias, 1000-029 Lisbon, Portugal; jose.pereira@inov.pt (J.P.); nuno.f.antunes@inov.pt (N.A.); joana.rosa@inov.pt (J.R.)
2. Instituto Universitário de Lisboa (ISCTE-IUL), ISTAR (Information Sciences, Technologies and Architecture Research Center), 1649-026 Lisboa, Portugal
3. Logistics, Molde University College, NO-6410 Molde, Norway
4. Departamento de Física, Universidade da Beira Interior, 6201-001 Covilhã, Portugal; sipmogo@gmail.com
5. Hope Care, S.A, 2510-216 Óbidos, Portugal; manuel.pereira@hope-care.pt
* Correspondence:jcafa@iscte.pt

Abstract: Chronic obstructive pulmonary disease (COPD) is the third leading cause of death worldwide. Health remote monitoring systems (HRMSs) play a crucial role in managing COPD patients by identifying anomalies in their biometric signs and alerting healthcare professionals. By analyzing the relationships between biometric signs and environmental factors, it is possible to develop artificial intelligence models that are capable of inferring patients' future health deterioration risks. In this research work, we review recent works in this area and develop an intelligent clinical decision support system (CIDSS) that is capable of providing early information concerning patient health evolution and risk analysis in order to support the treatment of COPD patients. The present work's CIDSS is composed of two main modules: the vital signs prediction module and the early warning score calculation module, which generate the patient health information and deterioration risks, respectively. Additionally, the CIDSS generates alerts whenever a biometric sign measurement falls outside the allowed range for a patient or in case a basal value changes significantly. Finally, the system was implemented and assessed in a real case and validated in clinical terms through an evaluation survey answered by healthcare professionals involved in the project. In conclusion, the CIDSS proves to be a useful and valuable tool for medical and healthcare professionals, enabling proactive intervention and facilitating adjustments to the medical treatment of patients.

Keywords: chronic obstructive pulmonary disease (COPD); decision support system (DSS); intelligent clinical decision support system (CIDSS); health remote monitoring system (HRMS); triage validation module (TVM)

Citation: Pereira, J.; Antunes, N.; Rosa, J.; Ferreira, J.C.; Mogo, S.; Pereira, M. Intelligent Clinical Decision Support System for Managing COPD Patients. *J. Pers. Med.* **2023**, *13*, 1359. https://doi.org/10.3390/jpm13091359

Academic Editor: Daniele Giansanti

Received: 10 August 2023
Revised: 30 August 2023
Accepted: 30 August 2023
Published: 6 September 2023

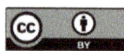

Copyright: © 2023 by the authors. Licensee MDPI, Basel, Switzerland. This article is an open access article distributed under the terms and conditions of the Creative Commons Attribution (CC BY) license (https:// creativecommons.org/licenses/by/ 4.0/).

1. Introduction

1.1. COPD Introduction and Definition

According to the World Health Organization (WHO), chronic obstructive pulmonary disease is one of the most deadly major lung diseases and the third leading cause of death worldwide [1]; the organization further indicates that COPD was responsible for about 3.24 million deaths in 2019. The Portuguese Society of Pulmonology [2] estimates that 5.42% of individuals in Portugal between the ages of 35 and 69 suffer from COPD. According to the Portuguese Lung Foundation [3], COPD was responsible for approximately 2834 fatalities in the country. The same organization calculates that in 2019, this illness cost the economy EUR 1.6 billion.

COPD is caused by airway obstruction. The most common symptoms of COPD are coughing, wheezing, and dyspnea (shortness of breath). Patients often seek medical attention only when the disease reaches an advanced stage, as it is a condition that progresses slowly.

Initially, the disease presents as a cough accompanied by increased sputum production. However, as it progresses, it can lead to repeated episodes of acute bronchitis and respiratory infections. As the disease develops further, shortness of breath becomes more frequent, even with seemingly minor tasks, such as talking and performing daily hygiene. Shortness of breath is most noticeable during activities that require physical effort.

1.2. Importance of COPD Management and Monitoring Systems

The integration of technology into healthcare has revolutionized patient care, with health remote monitoring systems (HRMSs) emerging as powerful tools. By storing data, such as heart rate (HR) and oxygen saturation (SPO2) levels, HRMSs help medical professionals to treat patients with COPD. These systems offer real-time monitoring and personalized treatment options. However, to maximize the potential of HRMSs, it is crucial to integrate them with well-defined clinical processes, therapeutics, and rules. This integration ensures that the collected measurements are correlated and directly linked to effective patient care, enabling proactive interventions and improving health outcomes.

The Internet of Things plays a crucial and influential role in the successful implementation of HRMSs. Wearable device sensors, videos, and images are essential to gathering valuable patient information. Daily physiological data of the patient is collected and stored by the HRMS through data processing tools, analytics, and artificial intelligence (AI). Recording daily physiological data provides healthcare providers with actionable insights, facilitating proactive and personalized care.

The use of AI by HRMSs to predict patient health deterioration is a significant benefit. AI algorithms examine historical patient data to find patterns that might point to higher risks of unfavorable events or health deterioration. These forecasts offer healthcare professionals with insightful information that enables them to intervene early and prevent complications. A more preventive model of care is promoted by this proactive approach, which also enhances patient safety and lowers hospital admissions.

1.3. Effect of External Variables (Climate, Humidity, Particles) in COPD Patients

Over the past decades, several epidemiological studies have demonstrated the adverse health impacts of exposure to particulate matter (PM), both in coarse and fine fractions [4–7]. The origin of this particulate matter can be natural, such as desert dust, or anthropogenic, such as aerosols generated by biomass burning or fossil fuel combustion processes. The concentration of particles in the atmosphere depends on the emission sources, meteorological variables, and transport processes, as aerosols can travel long distances (transported by air masses). Additionally, house activities can be relevant sources of fine particles. Particles resulting from cooking and heating can more deeply enter the respiratory system, especially when they are finer.

The household air pollution data from the World Health Organization pointed out that among the 3.2 million deaths from household air pollution exposure, 19% are from COPD, and 23% of all deaths from COPD in adults in low- and middle-income countries are due to exposure to household air pollution [8].

1.4. Research Questions and Problems

The research question addressed by this study is: "Is it possible to automatically monitor and analyse the risk of potential health deteriorations of COPD patients?". With this research question in mind, the defined objective is to develop a system that is capable of providing early information concerning patient health evolution and risk analysis in order to support the treatment of patients with COPD. Additionally, the system allows healthcare professionals to more efficiently manage their time by automatically providing said professionals with alerts, supported by a risk analysis of the patient's COPD health status.

1.5. Purpose and Description of the Present Work

The Hope Care Intelligent Services Platform (HC PSI) is a P2020 project that involves the participation of Hope Care SA, INOV—INESC Inovação and the University of Beira Interior. Its main objective is to research and develop an intelligent services platform that enables healthcare professionals to make more informed decisions regarding the health conditions of COPD patients, thereby increasing the efficiency of clinical entities.

The components of the HC PSI include a CIDSS, HCAlert platform, and environmental data sources, all geared toward automating the clinical treatment of COPD patients who are being remotely monitored.

This research work focuses on the CIDSS developed by INOV—INESC Inovação. The CIDSS assists in making decisions regarding patient treatment. This platform is composed of three modules: an HRMS that provides patients' health information through a mobile application to the CIDSS, a TVM that receives and processes patient risk information from the CIDSS, and a graphical user interface (GUI) that displays relevant clinical information to healthcare professionals.

Figure 1 presents the HC PSI architecture, which includes the CIDSS developed by INOV, the HCAlert platform, and other external data sources.

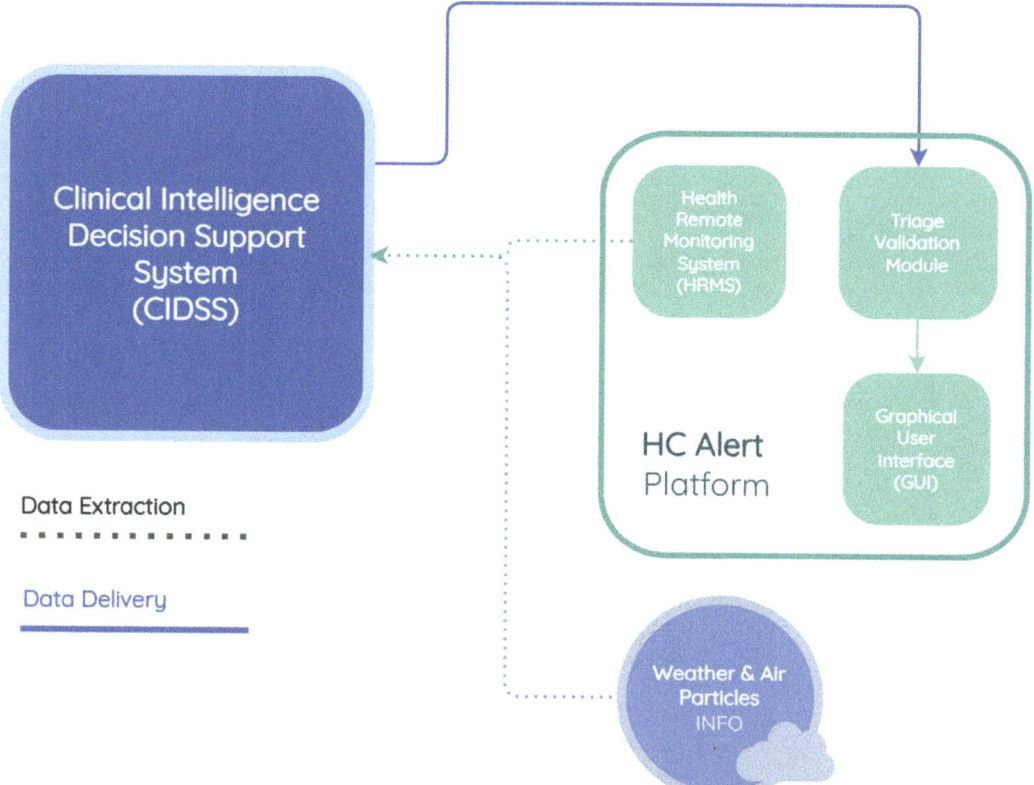

Figure 1. HC PSI architecture, including the CIDSS developed by INOV, the HCAlert platform, and other external data sources.

The HCAlert platform was developed by Hope Care SA and includes a mobile application that supports HRMSs and a set of backend services for clinical validation and triage.

In the scope of the HC PSI project, the requirements for the HCAlert mobile application include the collection of patient symptoms and residential data. For the clinical validation and triage backend services, the following requirements are defined:

- Capability to categorize alerts.
- Capability to provide early warning scores and other relevant metrics of patients to healthcare professionals.
- Capability to obtain information about hospital visits internally or from other sources.
- Enabling the clinical team to have an overview of new alerts for each patient, including the client's name, data type, and last measurement date.
- Allowing the clinical team to define what relevant health values to display on the dashboard.

1.6. Methodology

In this research work, since we focused on artifact development, we applied the design science research methodology.

The DSR methodology is a research methodology that is commonly used in the field of information systems; it focuses on the development and evaluation of innovative artifacts, which include cutting-edge framework prototypes, techniques, and algorithms that address present-day challenges. It consists of the following six phases: problem identification, definition of objectives, design and development, demonstration, evaluation, and communication. This methodology focuses on creating and evaluating artifacts based on their effectiveness, quality, and usefulness in addressing real-world problems [9].

Figure 2 presents the iterations within the design science research methodology (DSRM) process.

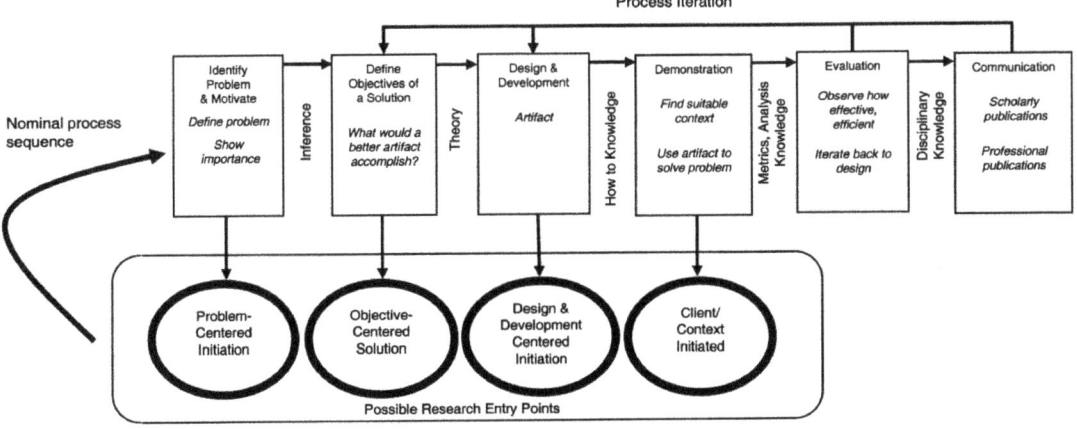

Figure 2. Iterations represented in the design science research methodology (DSRM) process model; Peffers et al. [10].

2. Related Work

In this section, we present an overview of the systematic review conducted in this article, which follows the PRISMA (preferred reporting items for systematic reviews and meta-analysis) methodology [11]. This section covers the latest advances in managing pulmonary disease patients, particularly COPD patients. We emphasize the augmented efficacy that remote health monitoring brings to patient treatment by providing real-time warnings to medical professionals; we also discuss the enhanced effectiveness of remote health monitoring supported by predictive analytics, which provides early warnings about the risk of patient deterioration.

This systematic review also covers factors and biometric signs associated with acute deterioration in COPD patients and how the prediction of biometric signs and subsequent early warning generation can indicate the risk of future patient deterioration. Table 1 presents the topics and the respective queries used to extract and filter related works.

Table 1. Topics of related work and their corresponding queries used to filter research papers related to each topic.

Subsection	Query
In-Home Healthcare for COPD	("Healthcare Management Systems" AND "Real-time Detection")
E-Healthcare supported by Predictive analytics	("Healthcare Management Systems" AND "Early Detection" AND ("Artificial Intelligence" AND "Machine Learning"))
Factors related with COPD deterioration	("Early Detection" AND "Vital Signs" AND "COPD")
Machine Learning for for Early Identification of a Deterioration	("Early Detection" AND "Vital Signs" AND "Machine Learning")

Table 2 presents the eligibility criteria used to filter documents in the related work.

Table 2. Eligibility criteria to filter research papers.

Eligibility Criteria	
Inclusion Criteria	**Exclusion Criteria**
Written in English or Portuguese	Not written in English or Portuguese
Publication date after/during 2010	Publication date before 2010

We identified 810 documents, with 10 documents removed due to duplication issues. A total of 400 articles not related to healthcare or artificial intelligence (AI) were excluded from further screening based on titles and abstracts. Moreover, 40 articles were excluded as we were unable to access their full versions, leaving 160 articles for full-text screening. A total of 82 articles were removed as they did not fit the eligibility criteria. Finally, 56 articles were excluded as they did not contain relevant information concerning vital signs, time series techniques, and health remote monitoring systems. The selection results, according to the PRISMA flow diagram, are shown in Figure 3.

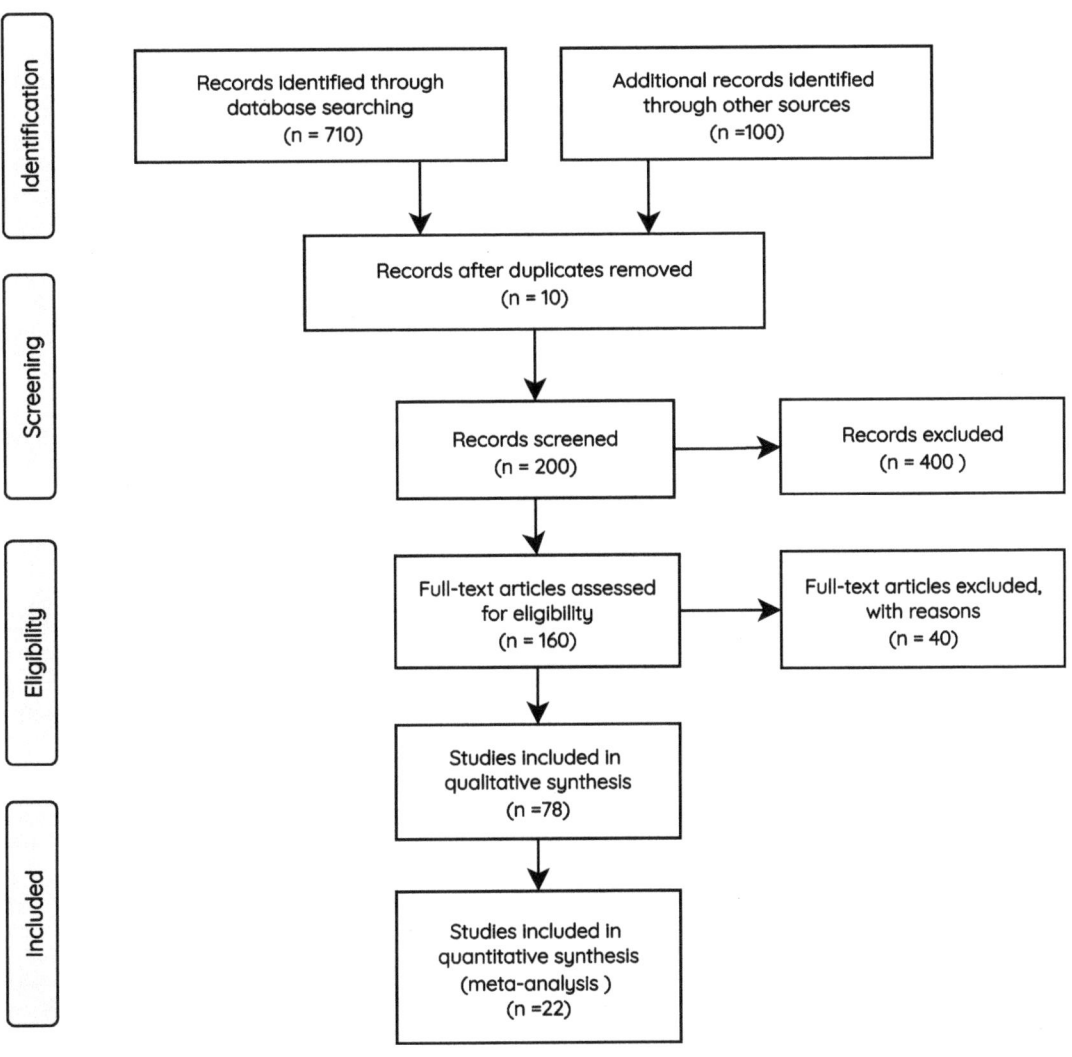

Figure 3. PRISMA methodology [11].

2.1. In-Home Healthcare for COPD

Home telemonitoring is a term used to describe the utilization of audio, video, and other telecommunication technologies for monitoring a patient's status from a distance [12]. This approach involves the remote monitoring of a patient's health parameters, typically within the framework of a larger chronic care model. In fact, telemonitoring is an essential component of telehealth and telemedicine [13]; it has the potential to help patients manage disease and predict complications [14]. Telemonitoring projects involving patients with pulmonary conditions have demonstrated the ability to identify early changes in the patient's condition, thus supporting immediate intervention and avoiding exacerbation. Patients have been very receptive to telemonitoring as a patient management approach and have shown very positive attitudes toward it [12]. A systematic review and meta-analysis found that telemonitoring interventions prevent unnecessary ER visits and may help to reduce severe COPD exacerbation to some extent. In 20 studies (90%) that carried out telemonitoring interventions for six months, a meta-analysis showed that the intervention effectively reduced the number of ER visits (pooled SMD = 0.14 corresponding to a small effect size; 95% CI (confidence interval): −0.28, −0.01) [13]. In a retrospective, population-based cohort study on 944 telemonitoring and 9838 control individuals, the total direct medical costs were significantly lower in the telemonitoring group (EUR −895.11, $p = 0.04$). The main driver for the total cost difference was the reduction in hospitalization costs by EUR −1056.04. ($p = 0.01$). A lower percentage of individuals died in the intervention group than in the control group (3.23 vs. 6.22%, $p < 0.0001$), translating into a mortality hazard ratio (HR) of 0.51 (95% CI: 0.30–0.86). Over the 12-month period, the proportion of patients hospitalized due to all causes (−15.16%, $p < 0.0001$), due to COPD (−20.27%, $p < 0.0001$), and for COPD-related emergency department (ED) visits (−17.00%, $p < 0.0001$) was consistently lower in telemonitoring patients, leading to fewer all-cause admissions (−0.21, $p < 0.0001$), fewer COPD-related admissions (−0.18, $p < 0.0001$), and fewer COPD-related ED admissions [15].

2.2. E-Healthcare Supported by Predictive Analytics

Telemonitoring has become indispensable in diagnosing and medically intervening for COPD patients. Nowadays, due to better storage of electronic health records and improved vital sign detection methods, large amounts of patient data are available daily in ICUs [16]. Medical equipment, ranging from hands-free monitors and portable devices to modern wristbands and watch-like monitors, have helped in the collection of biometric data, such as heart rate, blood pressure, physical activity, and sleep information [17].

A remote monitoring system, capable of gathering extensive data and backed by predictive analytics algorithms and techniques for effective data assessment and identifying underlying patterns, provides better efficiency in identifying declining patient health [18]. In the present COPD case study, such systems can reduce emergency room (ER) visits, acute deterioration-related readmissions, days spent in the hospital, and mortality in patients with COPD [19].

Predictive analytics refers to the systematic use of statistical or machine learning methods to make predictions and support decision-making. Predictive analytics applied to healthcare can be divided into two components: the data underlying the model, particularly predictors or features, and machine learning and statistical methods, both based on a set of mathematical techniques applied to data in order to generate an output [20].

Machine learning is a crucial methodology in predictive analytics. Conventional statistical analysis focuses on explaining data and relies on an expert (i.e., human) to formulate and discover cause–effect relationships, driven by a set of predefined assumptions. Machine learning is more data-focused and orientated toward generating hypotheses and building predictive models using algorithms. It has enabled clinical support research and applications to provide actionable insights by utilizing large amounts of intensive care unit patient datasets that are useful in many clinical scenarios [16]. Machine learning can predict in-hospital mortality and the risk of 30-day readmission due to COPD exacerbation [21].

2.3. Factors Associated with COPD Exacerbation

The prevention of acute exacerbation in COPD requires the identification of factors associated with exacerbation. Most studies have shown that oxygen saturation (SpO2) (p-value < 0.05), respiratory rate (RR), and heart rate (HR) (p-value < 0.05) influence exacerbation events, with SpO2 being the most predictive vital sign. The deterioration in COPD patients has been associated with a slight decrease in oxygen saturation and a slight increase in HR. One article suggested that using multiple vital signs as the inputs of a single classifier could provide better predictions, given that these multiple-input models showed the best AUC results [22].

Although some studies monitored blood pressure in order to determine whether there was a significant correlation with acute exacerbation, there was no sufficient evidence indicating that a change in blood pressure during a COPD exacerbation was a potent predictive factor for exacerbation (p-value > 0.05, i.e., not significant).

Body temperature with a p-value equal to 0.059 could be considered an exacerbation predictor. In the study conducted by Martin-Lesende, changes in body temperature had triggered 27.8% of alerts, of which, 5% were due to temperatures exceeding 37 °C [23].

Most studies have focused on vital signs and internal factors of COPD patients, rather than external ones, despite being equally relevant. Some meteorological data, such as humidity (p-value = 0.0137), variation of diurnal temperature (p-value = 0.0472), the cumulative lowest temperature 7 days prior to acute deterioration (p-value = 0.005), and total rainfall in the 7 days preceding an acute exacerbation (p-value = 0.0389) was associated with acute exacerbation in COPD. Lee J. [24] conducted a univariate analysis of air pollution and COPD exacerbations and identified a strong correlation between PM10 levels one day before a patient's condition worsened and acute exacerbation (p-value = 0.0260) [24].

The analysis of both internal and external factors with significant correlations to COPD exacerbation revealed that the frequency with which certain variables are measured must also be taken into consideration. The higher the frequency of a vital sign measurement, the better the perception of its association with an exacerbation occurrence. Daily or multi-daily vital sign monitoring improves the analysis of these signs. For example, Pépin J-L [17] mentions that overnight pulse oximetry increases sensitivity, allowing for early detection of deterioration [17].

2.4. Machine Learning for Early Identification of Deterioration

In recent literature, machine learning techniques have attracted attention for predicting the clinical conditions of patients. Time series forecasting models have been applied successfully in medical applications to predict disease progression, estimate mortality rates, and assess time-dependent risks. These models are able to identify patterns and trends from sequential data collected over time, such as health-related signals [25,26].

Some traditional machine learning techniques, such as random forest, SVM (support vector machine), Bayesian networks, and logistic regression, have been employed to improve predictive performance in identifying early clinical deterioration [27]. However, these traditional models are not optimized for handling the unique characteristics of time series data, such as autocorrelation, seasonality, and trend patterns [28,29].

With sufficient data, the development of deep learning models can reduce several preprocessing steps, emphasizing the relationships between the data, without the need to identify the best predictors, leading to better results [30]. For instance, long short-term memory network (LSTM) can learn extended time series dependencies, while a convolutional neural network can generate a compact latent representation.

Gradient boosting models are alternatives to specialized models, such as long short-term memory network (LSTM) and gated recurrent unit (GRU) [31,32]. Although these models are not ideal for time series forecasting, they are still generally better suited for handling sequential data compared to non-sequential algorithms (such as random forest, SVM, logistic regression, and naive Bayes) [29].

3. CIDSS Design

The CIDSS receives every patient's vital signs, which are remotely monitored by Hope Care SA as inputs. Additionally, it daily incorporates weather forecast conditions and air particle forecasts that are specific to each patient's location. In response, the system provides daily vital sign predictions and early warning scores for each patient for the following five days. It also provides the basal values of each patient and issues an alert whenever a vital sign measurement falls outside the expected parameter range, requiring a reevaluation.

Figure 4 illustrates the CIDSS developed by INOV—INESC Inovação, its interactions with weather and air pollution data providers, and the HCAlert platform. The CIDSS comprises five distinct modules, each serving a specific purpose. These modules are as follows:

Communication manager—this module assumes a crucial role within the system, and is responsible for the communication interactions among HC (Hope Care) Alert, weather, air particles API, and the clinical decision support system.

Vital sign prediction module—it is designed to generate forecasts for a five-day period regarding four essential vital signs: oxygen saturation level (SpO2), heart rate, systolic blood pressure (SBP), and body temperature. This module utilizes various machine learning algorithms to accomplish the predictions. The input data for these models are sourced from the stored vital sign records within the database. Subsequently, the predicted vital signs are stored back in the database for further reference and analysis.

Early warning score calculation module—within this module, the recorded vital sign predictions from the database play a crucial role in calculating the early warning score for each of the five predicted days. The early warning score is computed using the aforementioned vital sign data and the resulting early warning scores are subsequently stored in the database.

Biometric signal error detection module—the primary objective of this module is to thoroughly analyze and evaluate potential measurement errors and abnormal variations detected within the patient's historical data. The purpose is to promptly alert both the patients themselves and the attending nurse regarding the invalidity or questionable nature of the entered information. By diligently identifying such anomalies, this module serves as a critical mechanism for ensuring data accuracy and reliability within the system.

Basal value monitoring module—the main function is to monitor and continuously and intelligently adjust the patient's baseline values. This adjustment is based on the historical records of vital sign values measured by the patient and documented within the HCAlert platform. The module's purpose is to enhance the precision and effectiveness of the monitoring system by dynamically adapting the baseline values in accordance with the patient's specific health history.

3.1. Requirements

During the initial phase of the HC PSI project, we defined the functional requirements through an interactive and iterative process involving UBI and Hope Care SA. Certain clinical-oriented requirements were specifically delegated based on their domain of expertise. Subsequently, the remaining requirements served as the fundamental basis for the development of the CIDSS discussed in this article. All CIDSS functional requirements have been grouped into system modules, as shown in the following Table 3.

Table 3. Functional requirements associated with each module.

Requirements	Module
The predictive service should collect environmental data, such as air quality, seasonal infection incidences, and weather conditions	Vital Signs Prediction
The predictive service should correlate parameters and detect patterns	
The predictive service should reevaluate the weighting of each parameter, depending on the context (e.g., patient, clinical history, etc.)	
The collected data should undergo anonymization (if applicable), normalization, and data fusion	
The predictive service should consider the early warning score to generate alerts	Communication Manager
The predictive service should consider the alert classification to detect false positives	

Table 3. *Cont.*

Requirements	Module
The predictive service should advise the user to take a new measurement and launch inquiries to validate if it is a false positive	Biometric Sign Error Detection
The predictive system should apply the early warning score to the clinical protocol and suggest changes to the protocol based on the basal value	Early Warning Calculation
The predictive service should calculate the early warning score (define the correlation weighting of each parameter in the EWS calculation)	
The predictive system should recommend a reassessment of the basal value	Basal Value Monitoring
The predictive system should take into account changes made to the clinical protocol by the clinical team	
The predictive system should analyze the threshold for advising changes to the applied clinical protocol for the patient	

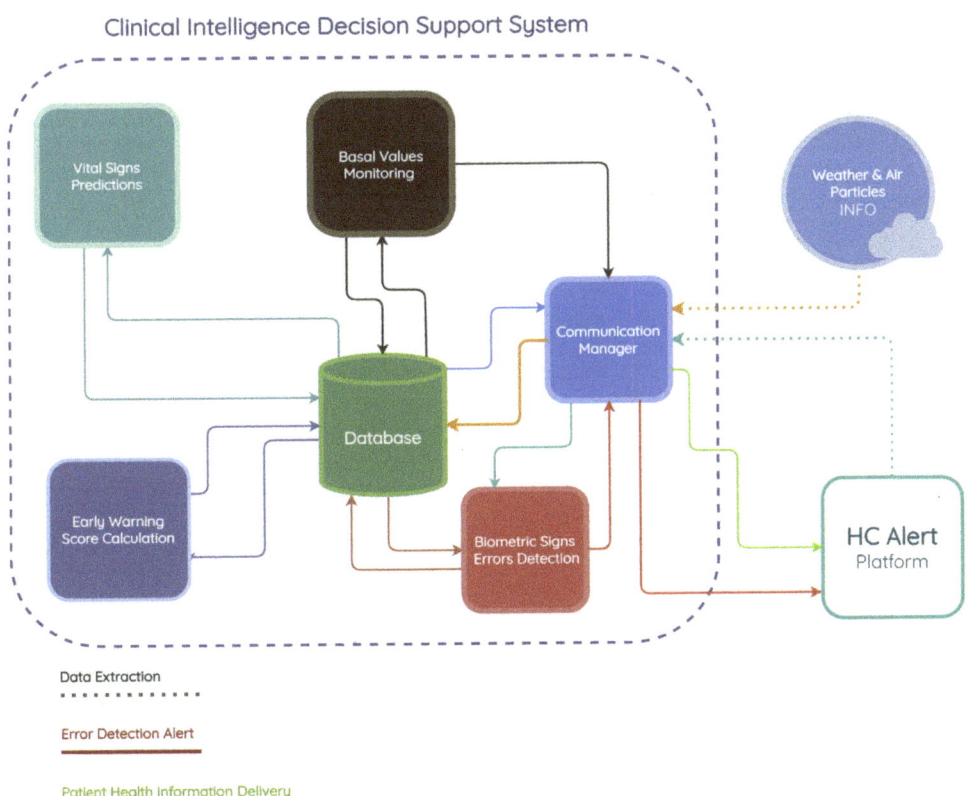

Figure 4. The CIDSS architecture and interactions with external modules.

3.2. Communication Manager

This module is composed of four submodules: data extraction, measurement error alert, basal values notification, and the patient's risk information delivery submodule, as is present in Figure 5.

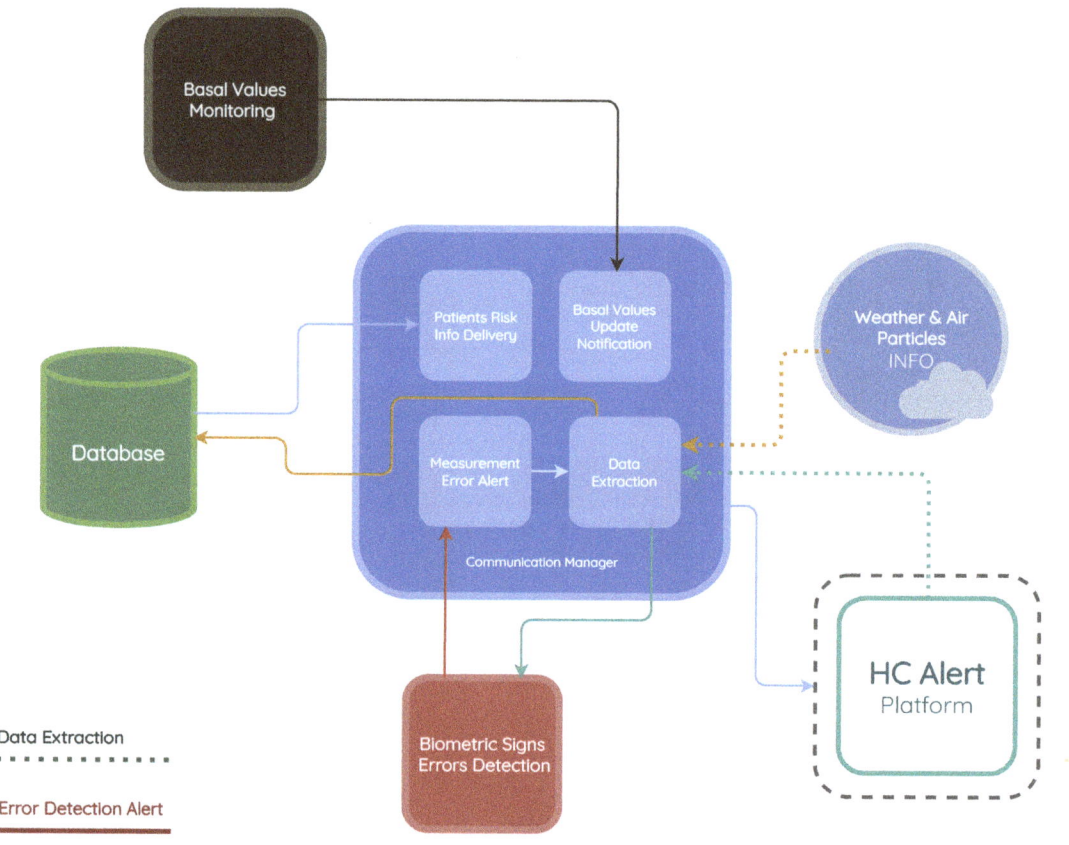

Figure 5. Communication manager module architecture.

3.2.1. Data Extraction

The medical records, which stored the vital signs used as input for the CIDSS, are presented in Table 4. Each record is formatted to have one entry per day per parameter. Each record had an ID (idRawMeasurement), the collection date (createdOn), the coordinates where it was collected (latitude and longitude), the measurement type (ProviderMNameStandard), measurement value (value), and the units representing the value (units).

The measurement type could address various factors, including vital signs, such as oxygen saturation level (SpO2), heart rate (HR), body temperature, systolic blood pressure

(SBP), and diastolic blood pressure (DBP), as well as other biometric indicators, like the number of steps, body fat, energy burned, weight, and height.

Table 4. Clinical information extracted from the Hope Care API.

idRawMeasurement	Measurement Identifier
createdOn	Measurement creation date
clientID	Identification of the patient to whom the measurement belongs
Latitude	Latitude of the patient
Longitude	Longitude of the patient
ProviderMNameStandard	Standard name of the type of measurement
Value	Measurement value
Unit	Units of measurement (in the dataset are available %, C, bpm, count, mmHg, NA, null, and percent)

The weather historical information used as input for the predictive models was provided by the Weatherbit API. Each record had an ID (idWeatherMeasurement), the coordinates of the station (latitude, longitude), date of measurement (columns year, month, day), mean daily temperature (T_MED), and mean relative humidity (HR_MED), as shown in Table 5.

Table 5. Weather historical information.

idWeatherMeasurement	Measurement Identifier
Station ID	Station identifier
Latitude	Latitude of the station
Longitude	Longitude of the station
Year	Year of the collected measurement
Month	Month of the collected measurement
Day	Day of the collected measurement
T_MED	Value of the daily mean temperature in Celsius
HR_MED	Value of the daily mean relative humidity in percent

The air pollution historical information used as input for the predictive models was provided by the OpenWeather API. Each record had an ID (idWeatherMeasurement), the coordinates of the station (latitude, longitude), date of the measurement, an average count of 10-micrometer particles (PM10), and an average count of 2.5-micrometer particles (PM2_5), as shown in Table 6.

Table 6. Historical information on air pollution.

idParticlesMeasurement	Measurement Identifier
Location	Location of the station
Latitude	Latitude of the station
Longitude	Longitude of the station
Date	Date of the collected measurement
PM10	Value of PM10
PM2_5	Value of PM2.5

3.2.2. Measurement Error Alert

This submodule was designed to receive alerts from the biometric sign error detection module and subsequently send alerts to the HCAlert platform. After a set short duration, it sends a notification to the data extraction submodule to execute the data extraction of biometric signs from HCAlert, concerning the specific patient dataset where the error was found.

3.2.3. Basal Value Monitoring Notification

The basal value update notification submodule was designed to receive notifications from the basal value monitoring module; it subsequently notifies the HCAlert platform with new basal value recommendations for a specific patient.

3.2.4. Patient Risk Information Delivery

The patient risk information delivery submodule extracts information regarding the last five days of vital sign predictions and the calculated early warning scores stored in the database. It then sends this information to the HCAlert platform.

3.3. Biometric Sign Error Detection

The HCAlert platform's operational efficiency is affected by the patients' inaccurate vital sign measurements, which can result in inaccurate clinical protocol adjustment alerts and future vital sign projections. It is necessary to guarantee that the system receives data that obey certain quality levels.

Prior to the implementation of the current project, measurements are validated by nurses who identified instances of anomalous readings, reporting potential causes, such as deterioration in the patient's condition, measurement errors, cold fingers during measurements, etc.

The biometric sign error detection module consists of three components:

- Validation of clinical rules: This component compares the measurements taken by the patient with a set of business rules defined according to Hope Care guidelines. For example, a measurement of oxygen saturation above 100 or below 20 cannot be correct since a percentage value cannot exceed 100, and a value below 20 corresponds to situations of compromised brain function and even comas. The medical team involved in this research work validated all ranges used to filter the vital signs.
- Patient pattern modeling: The objective of this component is to approximate a probability density function for each metric in the patient's measurements. These probability density models are then stored in the database, eliminating the need to repeat the function modeling each time a new inference is made. This module runs monthly to create a new probability function that captures the variability of the new measurements entered by the patient.
- Validation of atypical measurements based on the patient's history: This module uses the probability density models stored in the database, which are associated with each patient's vital signs, to determine whether a newly recorded measurement falls within the normal patterns for that specific patient. As these variations could be due to disease exacerbation, improvements from a new medication, or other factors, need to be validated by a nurse and, if necessary, by the patients themselves, to determine the true cause of the variation.

The operationalization of this module is presented in Figure 6. The system begins with the measurement and input of a vital signal by a patient in the HCAlert application. The measurement is compared and validated based on clinical rules, according to the type of measurement performed. The following clinical rules are defined, where the value is considered erroneous and discarded in the following cases:

- Oxygen saturation above 100 or below 20;
- Body temperature below 30 or above 40;

- Systolic blood pressure below 50 or above 350;
- Diastolic blood pressure below 40 or above 200;
- Pulse rate less than or equal to 30, or greater than 250.

Figure 7 presents the architecture of the Biometric sign error detection module.

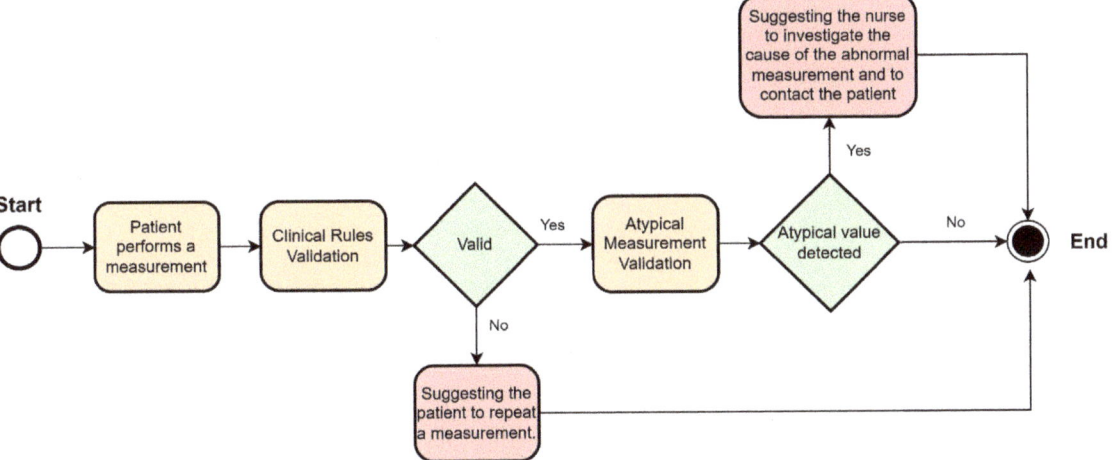

Figure 6. Biometric sign error detection implementation.

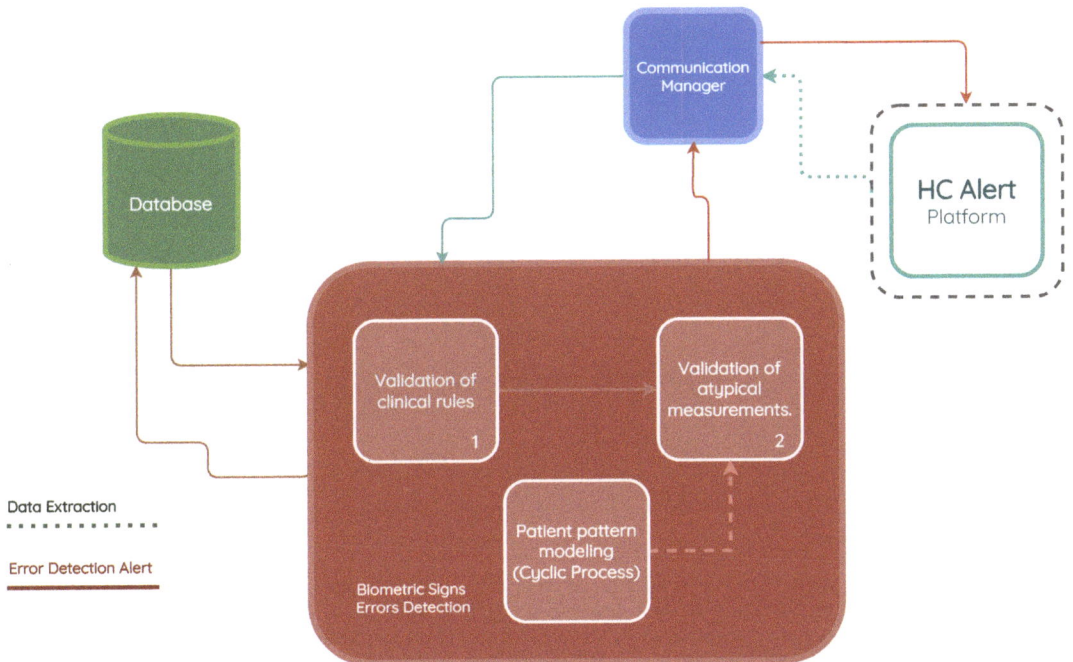

Figure 7. Biometric sign error detection module architecture.

In the event of an incorrect measurement, a type 1 alert is triggered, recommending a new measurement of the vital signal by the patient.

If there is no inconsistency with the rules, the system then determines if the measurement is atypical for a patient. If it is not considered atypical, the verification process is concluded without any identified errors. If an atypical value is recorded, a type 2 alert is triggered, and human verification of this alert is recommended to a nurse and the patient. This is done to verify whether this value corresponds to a health deterioration, an improvement in the clinical condition, or a measurement error.

Probability density functions were applied in order to model the pattern of vital signs of each patient and assess the probability that a newly measured value fits the distribution function computed for that specific patient's vital sign. The process of training a model for a given patient begins with the request for all the vital sign measurements made by this patient. From this request, as shown in Figure 8, a distribution function is trained and stored in the database for each vital sign recorded, with the following steps:

1. From all the measurements collected for the patient, only the measurements made for specific vital signs in training are used.
2. Existing outliers in the database, prior to modeling, are removed. Outliers are removed based on the standard deviation by calculating the standard score (z-score), which corresponds to the number of standard deviations by which a newly recorded value deviates from the mean of the observed measurements. If the z-score is greater than 3, which corresponds to a value that is three times the standard deviation away from the mean of the data, the value is not used in the modeling.
3. The following distributions are tested: normal, exponential, Pareto, double Weibull, t, generalized extreme value distribution, gamma, lognormal, beta, and uniform. For each distribution, the density and weights of the histogram are computed. Subsequently, an estimation of the function parameters is performed based on the data. The maximum likelihood estimation (MLE) is used to identify the values that best fit the data.
4. The goodness-of-fit is calculated with a test of the sum of squares of the residuals for each distribution found.
5. The model with the best goodness-of-fit, which implies a lower value in the sum of squares of the residuals, is stored for the vital signs of the patient under study.

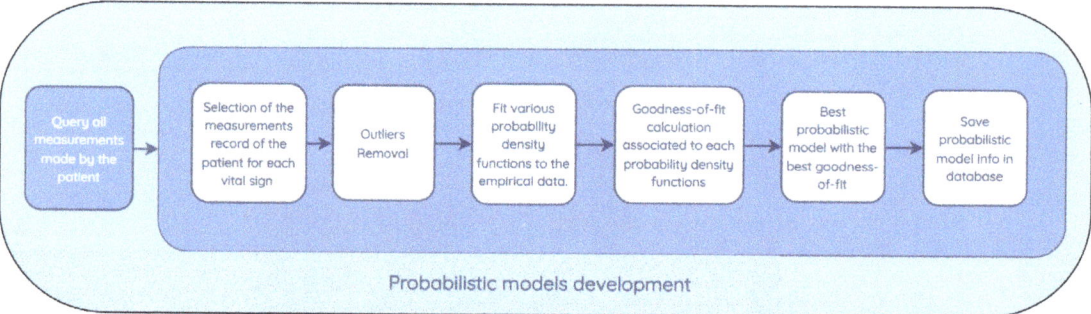

Figure 8. Biometric sign error detection model development.

The inference starts with the reception of a vital sign measurement taken by a patient and entered into the HCAlert system. The system selects the model corresponding to the probability density function that models the distribution of the vital signs measured for the patient who entered it into the system, as is present in Figure 9.

This model is then used to test the null hypothesis, which corresponds to checking whether the value that has been measured is outside the typical pattern of the patient, based on the selected distribution and the parameters adjusted according to the empirical distribution of the patient. If the *p*-value is less than 0.05, it implies that the null hypothesis is not rejected, which means that there is a probability that the measurement may correspond to an error, exacerbation, or improvement of the condition. A reminder should be sent to both the nurse and the patient to investigate the situation.

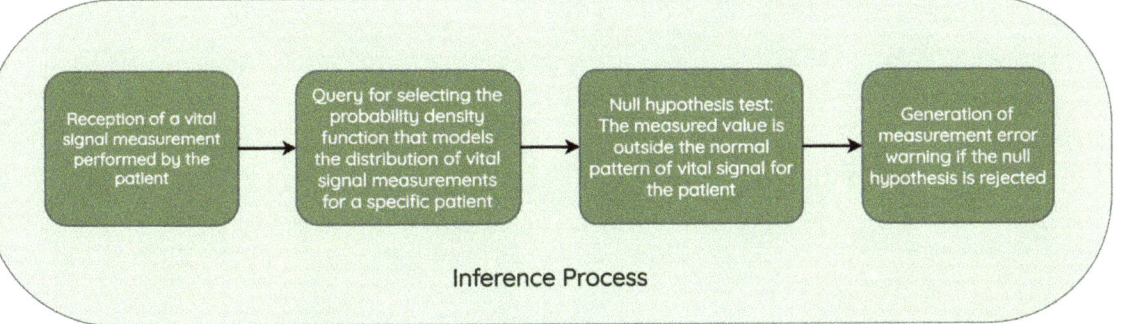

Figure 9. Biometric sign error detection inference process.

3.4. Basal Value Monitoring

The deterioration or improvement of COPD reflected in the negative or positive evolution of the patient's baseline values may be due to several explanatory factors, such as weather conditions, exposure to particulate matter, a change in medication or lifestyle, among others. The recorded baseline values are indicative of the severity of a condition, as outlined by the Global Initiative for Chronic Obstructive Lung Disease (GOLD) [33] strategy for the diagnosis, management, and prevention of COPD.

Values below or above the standards result in the patient's category changing into one of the GOLD I–GOLD IV [33] categories, depending on the severity of the patient's condition, with GOLD I being the most severe condition. It is important to identify and monitor any deterioration in a patient's baseline values in order to adjust the clinical protocol and treatment guidelines.

Figure 10 presents a clinical protocol defined by the Hope Care SA medical team; it is based on the GOLD strategy and addresses patients whose basal values are within a normal range and, thus, do not belong to categories GOLD I–GOLD IV. Consequently, the range of colors isn't associated with the GOLD categories. The color is associated with the severity of the COPD patient's condition: Category I (red) corresponds to a higher degree of deterioration in their health condition, while Category V (green) corresponds to the lowest or non-deterioration of their health condition. Some fields are filled with the expression "N/D" because there is no defined range of values for that specific category.

3.4.1. Basal Value Monitoring Module Architecture

This module, as shown in Figure 11, uses the list of metrics to be monitored and the history of vital signs recorded by each patient as input. Based on these measurements, the patient's current baseline value and the forecast of the evolution of the same value are determined. In case there is a substantial difference between the most recently recorded value and the historical baseline value, an alert should be triggered, containing the previous baseline value, the newly calculated value, and the difference. The newly calculated baseline value is suggested as a change to the clinical protocol.

Color	Systolic mm Hg	Diastolic mm Hg	Pulse bpm	Oximetry (with oxygen therapy) %	Oximetry (without oxygen therapy) %	Temperature °C	Weight kg	Steps # steps weekly average	FEV %
I	0 – 70	0 – 30	0 – 50	0 – 85	0 – 85	N/D		N/D	0 – 30
II	70 – 80	30 – 40	N/D	85 – 91	85 – 92	0 – 35		N/D	30 – 50
III	80 – 90	40 – 50	N/D	N/D	N/D	N/D		N/D	50 – 80
IV	N/D	N/D	N/D	N/D	N/D	N/D		N/D	N/D
V	90 – 140	50 – 90	50 – 100	91 – 100	92 – 100	35 – 37.6	Rules to be denied for each patient	N/D	80 – 100
IV	N/D	N/D	N/D	N/D	N/D	N/D		N/D	N/D
III	140 – 160	90 – 100	N/D	N/D	N/D	N/D		0 – 12000	N/D
II	160 – 180	100 – 110	N/D	N/D	N/D	N/D		N/D	N/D
I	180 – 250	110 – 250	100 – 250	N/D	N/D	37.6 – 50		N/D	N/D
Absence of measurements	28h	28h	28h	28h	28h	28h	28h	128h	28h

Figure 10. Clinical protocol defined by the Hope Care SA Medical Team and based on the GOLD clinical protocols.

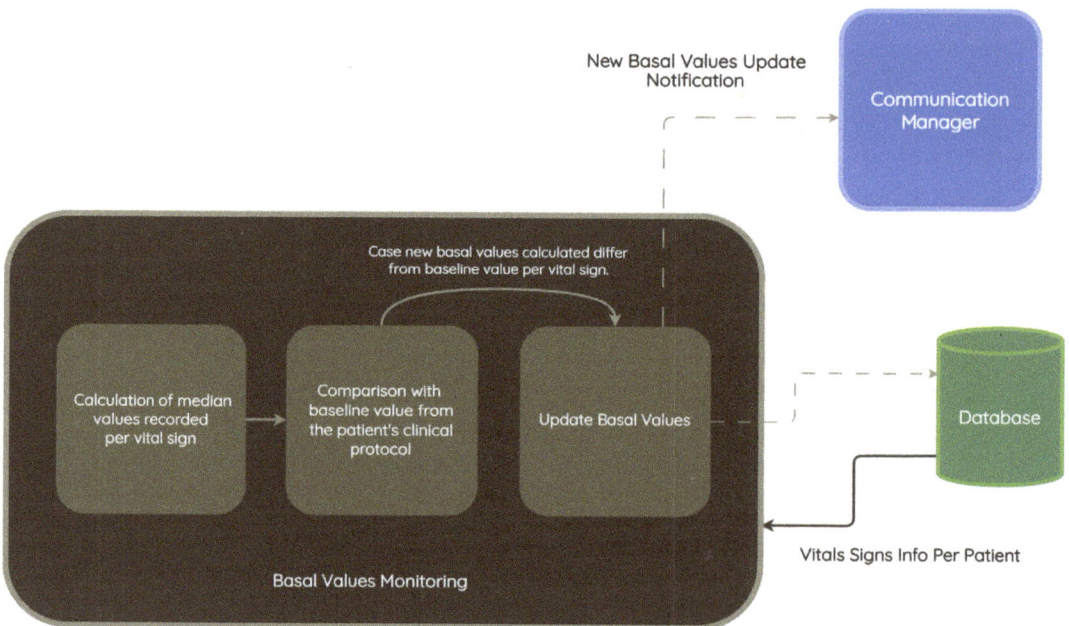

Figure 11. Basal value monitoring module architecture.

The following variables are also used as input to the module:

- Number of months considered: This indicates the past time window that is analyzed for the baseline calculation. The default value is 3 months, which indicates that when this module runs, the measurements taken from the last 3 months are extracted for the baseline calculation. This value can be configured by rules in the system.

- Minimum number of records: This corresponds to the minimum number of measurements taken by the patient, so that the calculated baseline information is considered reliable. If the patient does not have a satisfactory number of measurements in the time horizon under study, the module will not provide recommendations. For example, a patient with only five SpO2 measurements over 3 months will not be considered for updating the baseline value. This value is configurable by a rule, and value 50 is used by default in the system.
- Patience: In case the patient does not present enough measurements of a certain parameter in the defined time horizon, the system expands the time horizon of the search to include more months of history until it finds an acceptable amount of records. For example, with a patience of 3 months and a minimum of 50 required measurements, if the patient only has 30 measurements, an additional month will be incorporated into the analysis, and the module will be rerun using the past four months, reducing the patience counter by 1. In case patience reaches zero, and the minimum value of measurements defined is not reached, the system will not provide any recommendation for the given parameter due to the lack of consistency in the measurements. The default value for patience, which can be configurable by a rule, is 3.

The default values in the system are set and adjusted after testing with historical values recorded by patients in the HCAlert platform, provided by Hope Care SA.

3.4.2. Basal Value Monitoring Module Implementation

In this section, we present the implementation details of the basal value monitoring module. Figure 12 shows an activity diagram, which represents the operations performed by the module.

As presented and detailed in the previous section, the system inputs are the list of metrics under evaluation, the patient's vital signs history, the number of months to be considered, the minimum number of records, the baseline value of the patient's clinical protocol, and patience.

For each metric under evaluation, the system performs the following process:

1. A flag representing the current patience is initialized to zero.
2. The measurements are related to the period of months corresponding to the last X months from the date of execution of the module, where X is the sum between the system input "number of months to consider" and the current patience value.
3. The number of measurements performed by the patient is calculated.
   (a) In case the number of measurements is not sufficient, the current patience is incremented by 1.
      (i) If the current patience value is equal to the user-defined patience value, no recommendation is displayed, and the cycle continues to the next measurement in the list.
      (ii) If the current patience value is less than the set patience value, the system summarizes the run from step 2.
   (b) In case the measurements are sufficient, the system summarizes the run in step 4.
4. The median of the patient's measured values of a given vital sign is calculated.
5. The median value is compared with the baseline value recorded in the clinical protocol.
   (a) If the values are very different, a recommendation is made to update the baseline value to reflect the new median value recorded in the time interval under consideration. This recommendation should be evaluated by a medical professional.
   (b) If the values are similar, the baseline value is not adjusted, and the system summarizes in step 1, with a new iteration of a new metric under evaluation.
6. The cycle ends when all metrics in the list have been processed.

This process is run independently for each patient in the system. It is worth noting the use of the median as the metric calculated for the baseline value. This is due to the fact that it better handles extreme values outside of a patient's normal patterns, such as exacerbation, which should not be considered for the calculation of a baseline value, as it does not correspond to a normal patient pattern.

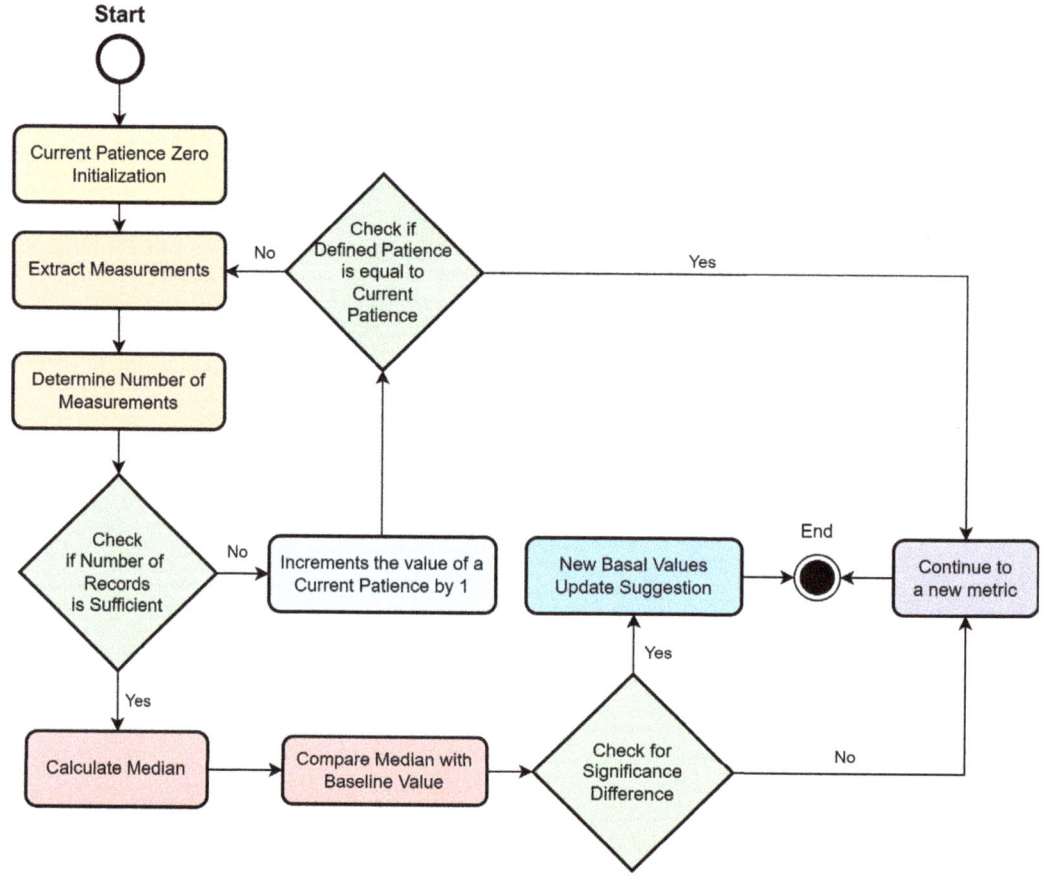

Figure 12. Basal value monitoring module implementation.

3.5. Vital Signs Prediction Module

3.5.1. Predictive Model Development

Data Treatment

For the predictive model development and evaluation, 91 patients who were flagged as having COPD were included. Each patient was monitored remotely and provided health status information for tracking their health status. The vital sign information was then gathered by each medical center. These patients were from different districts of the country, such as Aveiro (Anadia), Leiria (Óbidos, Pombal), Santarém (Ourém) Castelo Branco (Fundão), Coimbra (Cantanhede, Cernache, Assafarge, Antanhol, Condeixa-A-Nova, Mira, Almargem Bispo), Lisboa (Amadora, Rinchoa, Queluz, Algueirão, Tapada Das Merces, Rio de Mouro), and Faro (Quarteira, Albufeira, Tavira, Olhão, Loulé, Lagos, Portimão, and Castro Marim).

Meteorological variables (temperature, humidity, wind, and rain) and exterior particle matter concentrations (PM10, PM2.5) were obtained from the nearest IPMA and EPA stations. To analyze the source and transport pathways of the air masses and relate the air masses with aerosols, we used the NOAA HYSPLIT model [34,35].

Information about the weather, air quality, and vital signs was analyzed. The data processing module was divided into four sub-phases: data cleaning, data transformation, patient datasets selection, and environmental data integration, as is present in Figure 13.

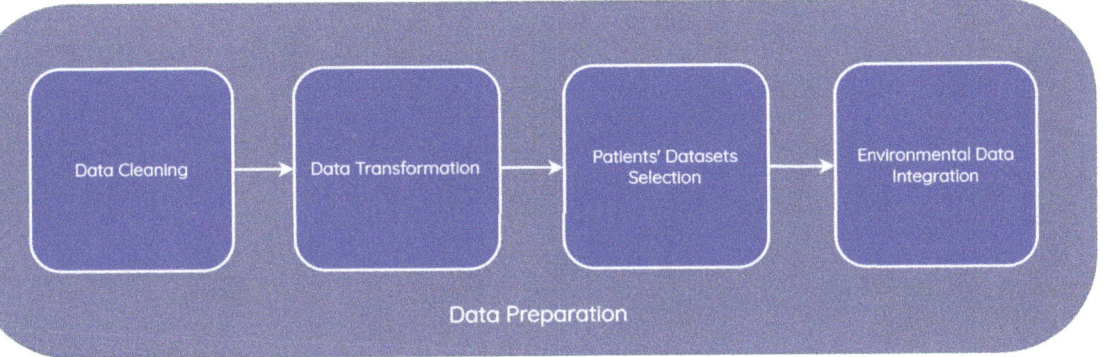

Figure 13. Data preparation pipeline.

During the data cleaning process, a thorough analysis was conducted on outliers (values that deviated significantly from the rest of the dataset and could potentially introduce anomalies in the results obtained from algorithms and analysis systems) based on the distribution of values in Figures 14–17, as well as on null values within the vital signs.

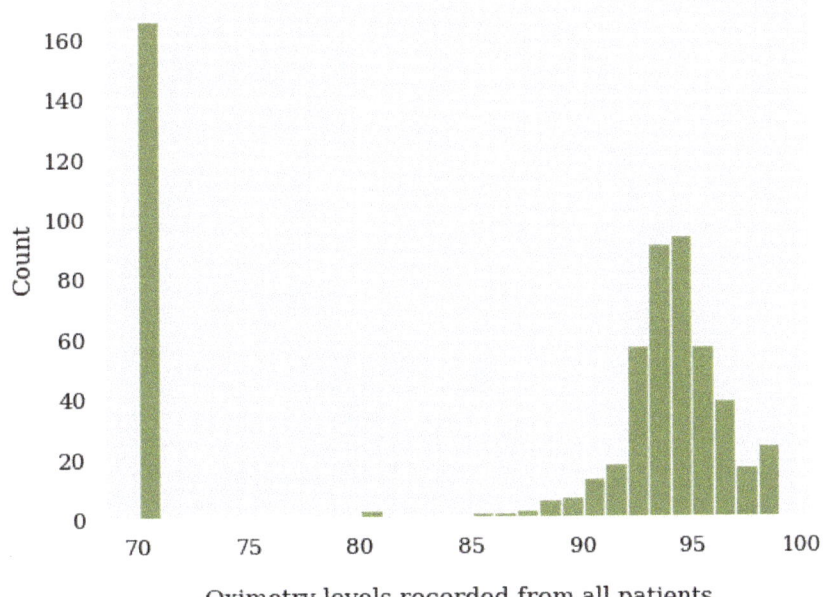

Figure 14. Oxygen saturation level value distribution of all patients analyzed.

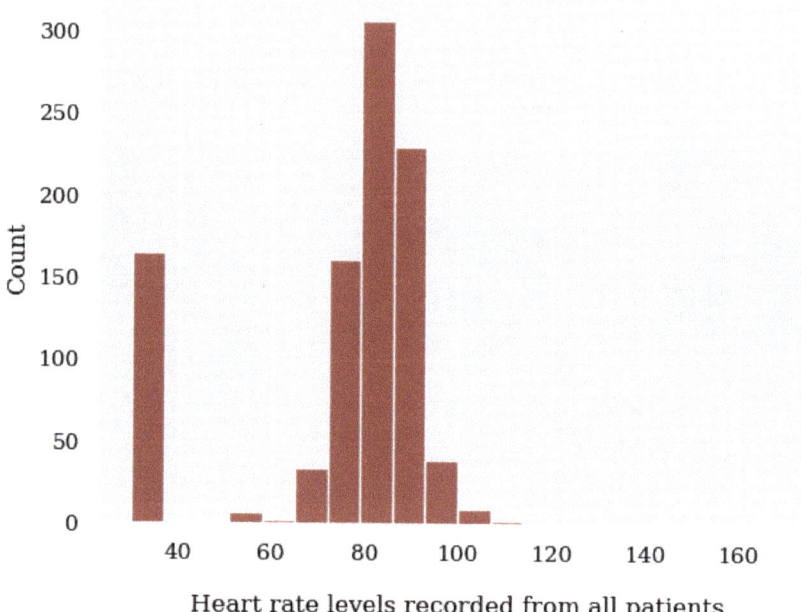

Figure 15. Heart rate level value distribution of all patients analyzed.

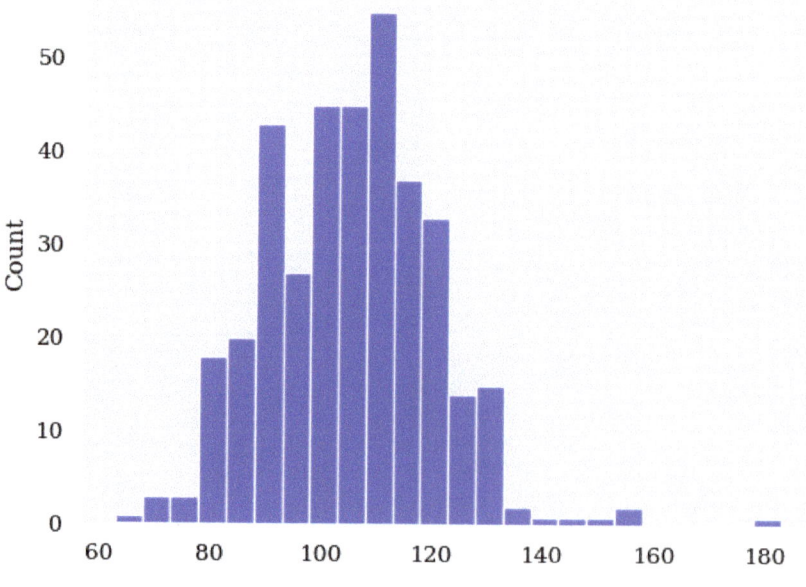

Figure 16. Systolic blood pressure value distribution of all patients analyzed.

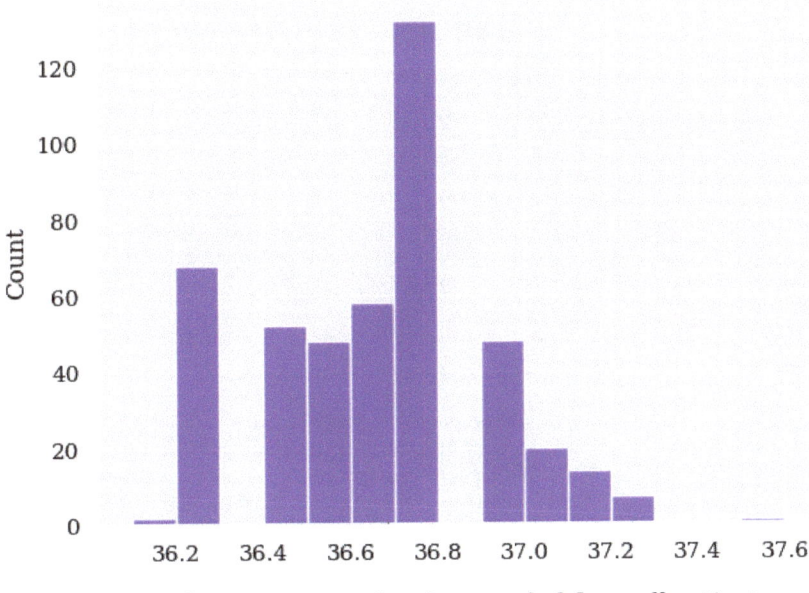

Figure 17. Body temperature value distribution of all patients analyzed.

Regarding vital signs, any values that met the following criteria were identified as outliers and subsequently removed:

- For oxygen saturation (SpO2), any values below or equal to 70% and above 100%. Since we have detected many measurements at exactly 70%, we suspect these are measurement errors;
- For body temperature, all values below 30 °C and above 40 °C;
- For systolic blood pressure (SBP), any values below 50 mmHg and above 350 mmHg;
- For heart rate (HR), any values below 39 BPM and above 250 BPM.
- For diastolic blood pressure (DBP), any values below 40 mmHg or above 200 mmHg.

In the data transformation process, we adjusted the format of historical records related to the vital sign data of patients. The data, initially in a format of one record per day per parameter, were converted to one record per day with all the collected vital sign values for that day. Specifically, there was a change in the granularity of each data row from one row per measurement of a specific vital sign at a specific moment in time for a specific patient to one row for each day of measurements taken for a specific patient, with columns representing the measured vital signs (data pivoting). After the format change, every time segment with over 10 consecutive days of missing data was removed and only patients with over 180 records whose vital sign data were fully complete were selected.

In the data integration process, the historical records of each patient's vital signs were supplemented with information regarding weather data (average daily temperature, average relative humidity, and amount of daily precipitation) and air particle data (10 μm particles and 2.5 μm particles, as these two dimensions have a greater impact on the patients' respiratory capacity).

Modeling and Evaluation

Following the data treatment, we modeled the development and evaluation. As a result of the data treatment phase, only 14 datasets were considered for the model training and evaluation phase. Since the CIDSS was designed to assist COPD patients with different health profiles, we developed models using 14 different datasets and incorporated the best models in the system. Figure 18 shows the steps of the development and evaluation phase.

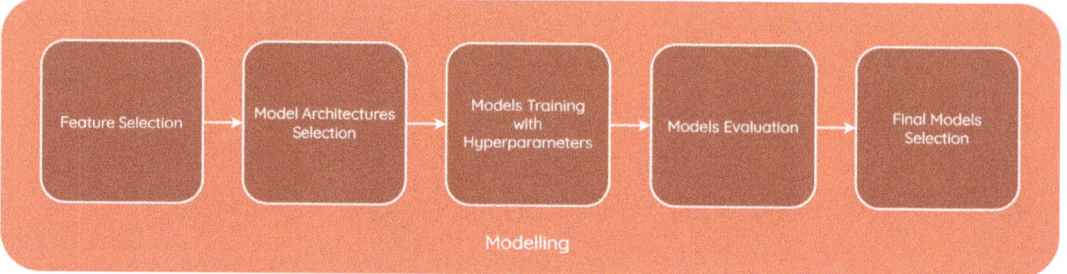

Figure 18. Modeling and evaluation pipeline.

We employed multivariate machine learning models capable of conducting the multi-step-ahead time series prediction of vital signs. Multi-step-ahead forecasting involves predicting multiple future time steps in a time series [36]. In our case, it would mean predicting the vital sign values for the following 5 days. The vital signs chosen for prediction include SpO2, heart rate, body temperature, and systolic blood pressure, which are utilized in the early warning score calculation module to assess the risk of deterioration.

During the feature selection process, we conducted a comprehensive correlation analysis between vital signs and clinical validation, resulting in the identification of the most relevant vital signs for predicting health variations in COPD patients.

Figure 19 shows an example of a correlation between SpO2 values (Spo2_1_day), the pm25 external parameter (PM25), relative humidity (HR_MED), and SpO2 values (SpO2) of the previous day, using the dataset for the patient with ID no. 156.

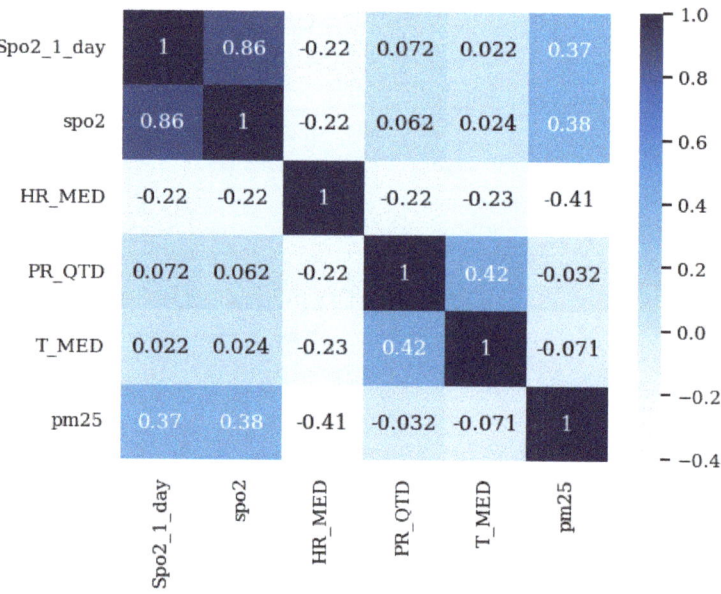

Figure 19. Correlation matrix of values of the SpO2 parameter with the relative humidity, the levels of precipitation, the pm25 concentration, the external temperature values, and SpO2 level from the previous day, using the dataset for the patient with ID no. 156.

For multi-step-ahead time series prediction, all vital signs receive the previous day's value (n − 1) as input to forecast the value for the current day (n). To predict the value of SpO2, we selected the following inputs: the SpO2 value of the previous day, the relative humidity value of the previous day, the levels of precipitation from the previous day, the pm25 value from the previous day, and the external temperature value from the previous day.

Regarding the other vital signs, based on the analysis of the correlation between the four vital signs analyzed in Figure 20, and the clinical insight provided by the Hope Care SA medical team suggesting that SpO2 influences heart rate, body temperature, and systolic blood pressure, we decided to use only the SpO2 value from the previous day and the specific vital sign in question from the previous day as inputs.

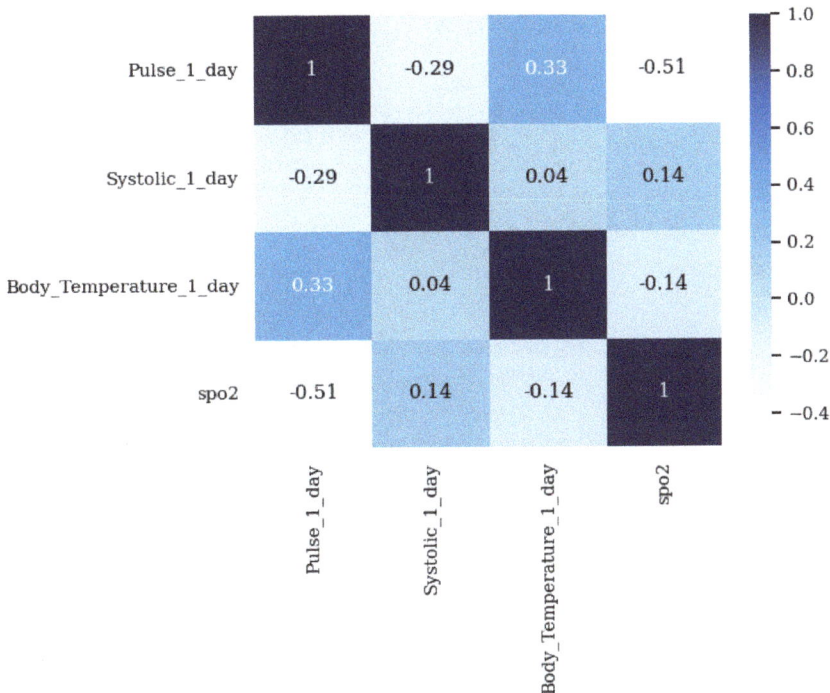

Figure 20. Correlation matrix of values of SpO2 parameter with the pulse rate, systolic blood pressure and body temperature values of the following day, using the dataset for the patient with ID no. 156.

To ensure the selection of the most optimal model architecture for predicting a specific vital sign, we trained and evaluated six distinct machine learning models. These models encompassed a diverse range of architectures, namely ARIMA (autoregressive integrated moving average), LSTM (long short-term memory), BILSTM (bidirectional long short-term memory), GRU (gated recurrent unit), LightGBM (light gradient boosting machine), and XGBoost (extreme gradient boosting).

The training process was preceded by essential hyperparameter tuning, which is a critical step in developing machine learning models. This tuning allowed us to optimize the models for the best possible performance. In our case, the models' performance was assessed using the root mean square error (RMSE), which measures the difference between prediction and the ground truth in the regression algorithm evaluation.

Table 7 presents an example of the RMSEs achieved for the fifth-day predictions via different machine learning model architectures for each vital sign prediction using the dataset for the patient with ID no. 156.

Table 7. Root mean square error values for the 5th-day predictions of different model architectures trained using the dataset for the patient with ID no. 156.

Model	SpO2	Heart Rate	Systolic Blood Pressure	Body Temperature
ARIMA	2.080718	7.089329	9.783878	0.247163
XGBoost	0.817778	0.96435	2.407083	0.302518
LightGBM	0.064668	0.380769	2.170715	0.058705
GRU	0.083168	0.110159	0.130179	0.131379
LSTM	0.092241	0.573169	0.135822	0.137075
BILSTM	0.084948	0.113384	0.132097	0.130094

As a result of our evaluation, we saved the models that demonstrated the lowest root mean square error (RMSE) for each vital sign. Consequently, we had 4 distinct models for each of the 14 patient-specific datasets, with each model specialized in predicting a specific vital sign.

Table 8 presents an example of the RMSEs for the 5th-day predictions achieved by the best machine learning model architectures for each vital sign prediction using the dataset for the patient with ID no. 156.

Table 8. Root mean square error values for the 5th-day predictions using the best model architectures trained on the dataset for the patient with ID no. 156.

Vital Sign Predicted	Type	RMSE
SpO2	LightGBM	0.064668
Heart Rate	GRU	0.110159
Systolic Blood Pressure	GRU	0.130179
Body Temperature	LightGBM	0.058705

3.5.2. Production

In this section, we present the incorporation of the previously described predictive models into the clinical information decision support system (CIDSS).

The vital signs prediction module presented in Figure 21 is composed of two sub-processes: a data pre-processing stage followed by the application of predictive models. The data pre-processing stage is essential to ensure that the data are in the correct format and that the vital sign measurements are appropriately integrated with the external measurements, as previously mentioned in Section 3.5.1.

The vital signs prediction process takes place daily, and the resulting predictions are stored in the database for future reference. Subsequently, the early warning module utilizes these data to assess and calculate the risk of a patient experiencing deterioration within the following five days.

When a new patient is integrated into the system, the prediction for each vital sign is calculated as the average of the predictions from all the models that predict the particular vital sign. After a period of 6 months, the error (root mean squared error—RMSE) of each predictive model is analyzed by measuring the distance between the values predicted by each model and the actual values of the vital signs for each patient. The model with the lowest error is the one associated with the patient.

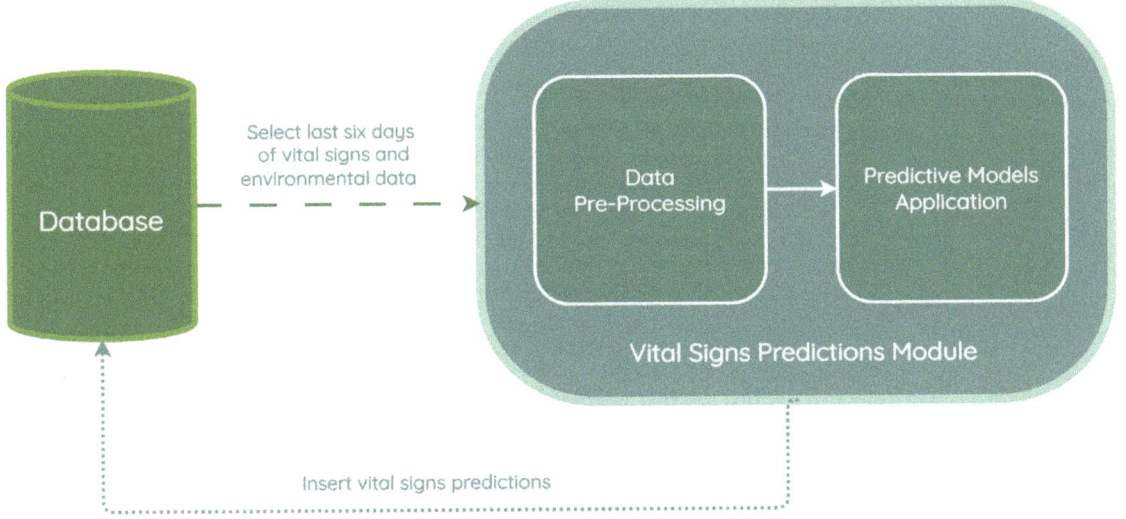

Figure 21. Vital signs prediction module architecture.

3.6. Early Warning Score Calculation Module

In this module, the risk of a patient experiencing deterioration is assessed using the early warning score (EWS) clinical protocol. The EWS is utilized for monitoring and detecting the risk of health deterioration in patients and it is calculated by combining vital signs and clinical data, such as heart rate, blood pressure, respiration rate, body temperature, oxygen saturation (SpO2), and degree of consciousness. Individual scores for each vital sign are then totaled up, resulting in a total EWS score.

The higher the overall EWS score, the more likely a patient is suffering from a health deterioration. This clinical protocol presented in Table 9 is indicated by Hope Care SA's medical team.

Table 9. Early warning score clinical protocol suggested by Hope Care SA's medical team.

	Description	0 Points	1 Point	2 Points	3 Points
SpO2	Difference between the predicted value for the day and the value from the previous day	<3%	3–5%	6–7%	>7%
Heart Rate	BPM Value	46–100	101–110	111–115	>115 or <46
Systolic Blood Pressure	Percentage difference between the predicted value for the day and the baseline value	<20%	≥20%	≥23%	≥25%
Body Temperature	Temperature value in Celsius	<37.5	37.5–37.9	38–38.4	>38.5

Similar to the vital signs prediction module, the early warning score calculation is performed daily, and the resulting scores are stored in the database.

4. Demonstration and Evaluation

To demonstrate how the CIDSS addresses the research question, we present a system trial with the incorporation of a new patient. We use the patient with ID no. 300. The patient health information used in this trial consists of historical information for a three-year period consisting of HRMS monitoring provided by Hope Care SA through the HCAlert platform.

The monitoring for the patient with ID no. 300 was initiated on 21 April, 2022. The CIDSS received a notification from the HCAlert platform, regarding the need to incorporate this new patient, leading to the creation of a new record in the database. All vital signs monitored for the patient with ID no. 300 were transmitted to the HCAlert platform and subsequently extracted by the CIDSS, starting from 21 April. These vital signs underwent analysis through the biometric sign error detection module. As no outliers were detected in the vital signs, they were seamlessly integrated into the database.

Table 10 presents the last five days of data extracted from the database for vital sign predictions on 25 April.

Table 10. Last 5 days of data extracted from the database for vital sign predictions on 25 April.

Date (yy-mm-dd)	Heart Rate (BPM)	Body Temperature (°C)	SpO2 (%)	Systolic Blood Pressure (mmHg)	T MED (°C)	HR MED (%)	PR QTD (mm)	pm25 (Count)
2022-04-20	60.0	37.1	96.0	92.0	9.68	51.30	0.11	0.82
2022-04-21	61.0	36.2	95.0	95.0	9.60	63.25	1.86	1.66
2022-04-22	63.0	36.0	95.0	93.0	7.53	82.97	23.25	0.93
2022-04-23	59.0	36.5	96.0	96.0	8.95	69.24	1.91	0.58
2022-04-24	65.0	36.2	96.0	100.0	10.79	67.82	0.29	1.14
2022-04-25	57.0	35.9	96.0	102.0	12.35	65.43	0.01	2.63

By 25 April 2022, a sufficient amount of vital sign data is available to provide insights into the patient's risk of health deterioration. The CIDSS proceeds with the prediction of vital signs and subsequently calculates the early warning score. Various models are employed to forecast the patient's vital signs for the initial 6 months of integration. The risk information regarding the patient's potential deterioration is provided to the HCAlert platform through a JSON file.

Table 11 presents the vital sign prediction values for 26 April. The predicted vital signs are then used to calculate the risk.

Table 11. Predicted vital sign values from 26 April to 30 April.

Date (yy-mm-dd)	SpO2 (%)	Heart Rate (BPM)	Systolic Blood Pressure (mmHg)	Body Temperature (Celsius)
2022-04-26	95.028053	63.863962	98.327346	36.244274
2022-04-27	94.801013	64.027884	98.783749	36.162657
2022-04-28	94.948091	64.413307	99.589877	36.218256
2022-04-29	95.127560	64.438053	99.516291	36.246443
2022-04-30	95.054558	64.429125	99.496265	36.196343

Table 12 presents the values of the early warning score calculated on 25 April.

Table 12. Calculated values of the early warning score from 26 April to 30 April.

Date (yy-mm-dd)	SpO2 (%)	Heart Rate	Systolic Blood Pressure	Body Temperature
2022-04-26	0	1	0	0
2022-04-27	0	1	0	0
2022-04-28	0	1	0	0
2022-04-29	0	1	0	0
2022-04-30	0	1	0	0

Listing 1 presents part of the structure of a part of the JSON file concerning the predicted vital signs and early warning score calculated from 26 April to 30 April.

Listing 1. Structure of the JSON file provided to HCAlert for patient risk information on 25 April.

```
1  {'predict_date': '2022-04-26',
2  'global_ews_score': 1,
3  'vitals':
4  '{``spo2'': {
5    ``predict_value'': ``95.02805293812013'',
6    ``predict_score'': ``0'', ``units'': ``{\%}''},
7  ``pulse'': {
8    ``predict_value'': ``63.86396198309728'',
9    ``predict_score'': ``1'', ``units'': ``BPM''},
10 ``systolic'': {
11   ``predict_value'': ``98.32734618907372'',
12   ``predict_score'': ``0'', ``units'': ``mmHg''},
13 ``body_temperature'': {
14   ``predict_value'': ``36.244273924492624'',
15   ``predict_score'': ``0'', ``units'': ``ºC''}}}
```

After an evaluation spanning over 6 months, we focused on identifying the most suitable models to enhance the care of patient 300. Our selection process prioritized models with the lowest root mean square error (RMSE), as shown in Table 13.

Table 13. Root mean square error (RMSE) values of the top selected models for predicting the vital signs of patient 300.

Dataset Used to Train the Model	Model	Parameter	Value (RMSE)
304	BILSTM	Spo2	0.285014
181	GRU	Heart Rate	1.520008
184	BILSTM	Systolic Blood Pressure	1.904305
181	GRU	Body Temperature	0.250580

We analyzed the patient's data from the previous 6 months; we provide a new basal value that reflects the patient's health condition, which is, consequently, used for the patient's clinical protocol adjustment, as shown in Listing 2.

Listing 2. Suggested new basal values for patient 300 to the HCAlert platform.

```
1  {
2  'spo2': {
3    'median_value': 96.0,
4    'number_of_months': 6},
5  'body_temperature': {
6    'median_value': 35.6,
7    'number_of_months': 6},
8  'pulse': {
9    'median_value': 73.0,
10   'number_of_months': 6},
11 'systolic': {
12   'median_value': 99.0,
13   'number_of_months': 6}
14 }
```

During the course of 6 months, while closely monitoring patient 300's health, we detected an error involving one of the SpO2 measurements. Initially, this measurement seemed to comply with the clinical rules and was considered valid. However, upon atypical measurement validation, it became evident that the probability of this value ($p = 0.01599$) belonging to the distribution of SpO2 values for patient 300 was relatively low, falling below the threshold of 0.05. Due to this fact, this measurement was discarded from the dataset.

Figure 22 presents the distribution of SpO2 values of patient 300 analyzed for the error alert validation.

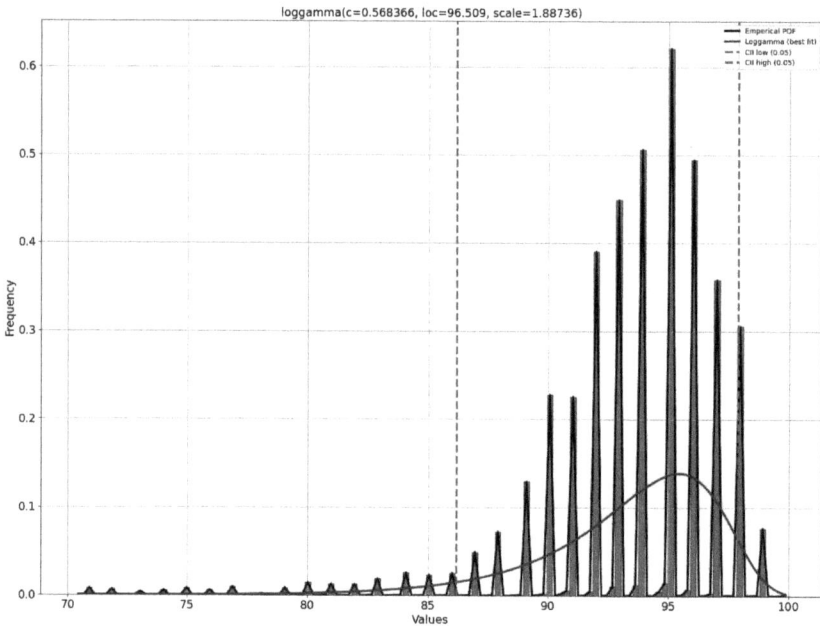

Figure 22. Distribution of SpO2 values analyzed of patient 300.

On 25 October, the CIDSS provided essential health information about the risk of patient deterioration. However, this risk was generated using predictions from the selected best models, as mentioned earlier.

Table 14 presents the last five days of extracted data from the database for vital sign predictions on 25 October.

Table 14. Last 5 days of data extracted from the database for vital sign predictions on 25 October.

Date (yy-mm-dd)	Heart Rate (BPM)	Body Temperature (°C)	SpO2 (%)	Systolic Blood Pressure (mmHg)	T MED (°C)	HR MED (%)	PR QTD (mm)	pm25 (Count)
2022-10-20	68.0	35.40	96.0	96.0	14.47	82.26	10.73	1.42
2022-10-21	68.0	35.60	96.0	96.0	15.05	79.13	3.94	1.94
2022-10-22	74.0	35.80	96.0	96.0	14.91	74.00	18.72	1.20
2022-10-23	70.0	35.90	95.0	94.0	14.15	67.11	5.45	2.91
2022-10-24	72.0	35.80	97.0	93.0	14.32	72.58	1.47	1.93
2022-10-25	76.0	35.00	95.0	98.0	16.13	64.89	7.87	1.94

Table 15 presents the vital sign prediction values from 25 October. The predicted vital signs are then used to calculate the risk.

Table 15. Predicted vital sign values from October 26 October to 30 October.

Date (yy-mm-dd)	SpO2 (%)	Heart Rate (BPM)	Systolic Blood Pressure (mmHg)	Body Temperature (°C)
2022-10-26	96.386055	70.779388	95.078346	35.292265
2022-10-27	96.228622	72.117355	94.664948	35.597720
2022-10-28	96.208916	72.186485	94.973228	35.796912
2022-10-29	96.297836	73.253487	95.260201	35.886715
2022-10-30	96.020462	72.828354	96.042572	35.796912
2022-10-31	96.320145	71.559845	95.059273	35.292265

Table 16 presents the early warning score values calculated on 25 October.

Table 16. Calculated early warning score values from 26 October to 30 October.

Date (yy-mm-dd)	SpO2 (%)	Heart Rate (BPM)	Systolic Blood Pressure (mmHg)	Body Temperature (°C)
2022-10-26	0	1	0	0
2022-10-27	0	1	0	0
2022-10-28	0	1	0	0
2022-10-29	0	1	0	0
2022-10-30	0	1	0	0
2022-10-31	0	1	0	0

Listing 3 presents the structure of a JSON file concerning the predicted vital signs and early warning score calculated from 26 October to 30 October.

Listing 3. Structure of the JSON file provided to HCAlert for patient risk information on 25 October.

```
{'predict_date': '2022-10-26',
  'global_ews_score': 1,
  'vitals': '{
  ``spo2'':{
    ``predict_value'': ``96.38605499267578'',
    ``predict_score'': ``0'', ``units'': ``\%''},
  ``pulse'': {
    ``predict_value'': ``70.85945892333984'',
    ``predict_score'': ``1'', ``units'': ``BPM''},
  ``systolic'': {
    ``predict_value'': ``94.98711395263672'',
    ``predict_score'': ``0'', ``units``: ''mmHg''},
  ``body_temperature'': {
    ``predict_value'': ``36.07156866129014'',
    ``predict_score'': ``0'', ``units'': ``ºC''}}'},
```

System Evaluation

We performed a set of white-box tests, evaluating each module for its functionality (unit tests) and integration with the related modules of the system (integrated tests). Afterward, we conducted a survey to gather feedback from the health professionals to evaluate the system based on a set of criteria inspired by Prat et al. [37]. Based on the positive feedback collected from the survey, it appears that the system was well-designed and valuable for managing the treatment of COPD patients.

Table 17 shows the evaluation given by the health professionals. They were asked to answer questions, indicating a number between 1 and 5, where 1 corresponds to not relevant or not useful and 5 corresponds to very relevant or very useful.

Table 17. Results of the evaluation of the system by health professionals.

Criteria	Questions	Objective Statement	Eval 1	Eval 2
Clinical impact on patient treatment	Indicates the importance of an smart clinical decision support system capable of provide 5-day early warning scores for monitoring patients with COPD.	Importance of the intelligent clinical decision support system for monitoring patients with COPD.	5	5
Patients Life Quality Impact	Indicates the impact of a smart clinical decision support system, providing a 5-day early warning score on the quality of life of a patient with COPD.	Impact of a clinical intelligence decision support system on the quality of life of a patient with COPD.	5	5
Utility	Indicates the usefulness of a system for healthcare professionals; generates information whenever there are changes in patients' baseline values.	Usefulness of a intelligent clinical decision support system that notifies about patient baseline value modifications.	4	5
Utility	Indicates the importance of a system that provides short-time horizon (in minutes) early warning scores for the clinical follow-up of patients with COPD.	Importance of an intelligent clinical decision support system on the clinical follow-up of patients with COPD.	5	5
Utility	Indicates the usefulness of a real-time alert system for healthcare professionals whenever an abnormal measurement occurs for a specific patient.	Usefulness of an intelligent clinical decision support system that notifies about abnormal measurement detections.	5	5
Consistency with the organization	Indicates the relevance of involving healthcare professionals in defining clinical intervals for abnormal measurements.	Clinical validation on the definition of intervals for abnormal measurements.	5	5
Consistency with the organization	Indicates the relevance of involving healthcare professionals in defining the formula for calculating the basal value.	Clinical validation on the definition of the basal value calculation formula.	4	5
Consistency with the organization	Indicates the relevance of involving healthcare professionals in selecting environmental and clinical parameters (e.g., vital signs) that most influence the clinical progression of patients with COPD.	Clinical validation on the selection of environmental and biometric signs that most influence the clinical progression of patients with COPD.	5	5
Integration with clinical protocols	Indicates the relevance of the adopted early warning score matrix for clinical decision-making and adjustment of therapeutic protocols for patients.	Relevance of the adoption of the early warning score matrix for the clinical decision-making and adjustment of therapeutic protocols for patients.	5	4

5. Conclusions

5.1. Work Conclusions

In this paper, we developed a system prototype that answers our research question: "Is it possible to automatically monitor and analyse the risk of a potential health deterioration of COPD patients?". This system aims to provide early information concerning a patients health status evolution in order to support the treatment of patients with COPD.

As mentioned in Section 3, the CIDSS comprises two primary components: the vital signs prediction module and the early warning score calculation module. These components specifically address the research question.

The vital signs prediction module, as mentioned in Section 3.5, generates vital sign predictions using different types of model architectures. These predictive models are optimized using a fine-tuning process, with each model corresponding to a specific patient with a specific health profile. As demonstrated in Section 3.5.2, the integration of predictive models developed using data from fourteen different patients shows that the CIDSS has the flexibility to predict vital signs and, in turn, calculate the patient deterioration risk for various health profiles. This system has the ability to evolve and adapt to every patient condition since the first stage corresponds to using an ensemble of models to predict vital signs and the second stage corresponds to only using models with the lowest RMSE.

The early warning score calculation module uses vital sign records and determines the patient health deterioration based on a clinical protocol.

The CIDSS is also composed of three other modules: biometric sign error detection, basal value monitoring, and the communication manager.

The biometric sign error detection ensures the quality of all information concerning vital signs by validating, in a two-phase process, whether the vital sign values fall within the normal range for general COPD patients and subsequently, within the specific patient's normal range using a probability density function.

The basal value monitoring analyzes the vital signs and suggests recommendations for new basal values to the patient if they deviate from the baseline provided by the HCAlert platform. The communication manager deals with all connections between the CIDSS modules, the HCAlert platform, and weather information sources.

The CIDSS system completed the white-box tests, including unit tests and integration tests.

All of these tests validate its functionality and contribution to preventing and potentially improving patient treatment by offering an early indication of the patient's risk for deterioration.

Despite our ability to employ real-time telemonitoring patient data, we employed clinical historical longitudinal data that were gathered over a substantial period of time (2–3 years) through a telemonitoring application. This extended time frame enabled us to formulate conclusions regarding the system's validity, supported by the early warning score implementation and the errors of the applied predictive models.

5.2. Limitations

The non-approval of the incorporation of new patients by the ethics committee associated with the HC PSI project made the testing and analysis of the CIDSS effectiveness in providing quality information regarding patient health deterioration risk difficult.

The scarcity of data was a limitation in our study, and two key aspects contributed to this challenge. Firstly, the measurements we had access to were not collected at hourly intervals, which restricted our ability to capture fine-grained variations in the data. The absence of hourly data points hindered our capacity to discern short-term patterns and trends, potentially hiding crucial insights that might have emerged with more frequent data collection.

Another significant data gap stemmed from the lack of information concerning home sensors, specifically data related to humidity levels. Humidity is a vital environmental factor that influences various aspects of indoor comfort, air quality, and overall well-being. The absence of the essential sensor data limited our ability to comprehensively assess the interplay between different environmental parameters, potentially leading to an incomplete understanding of the complex dynamics within the studied environment.

Despite the limitations, the system was validated, end-to-end, and clinically recognized as important for COPD monitoring, being adjustable enough to integrate these data sources if included in the project and handle a lower granularity of information to make predictions.

5.3. Future Work

As part of our future work, we will aim to identify some potential advancements to pursue. Firstly, we will aim to validate the effectiveness of the CIDSS (clinical deterioration surveillance system) by obtaining real-time patient data through the HCAlert platform. Analyzing these data over an extended period will help us assess the accuracy and quality of early information provided by the CIDSS, particularly regarding a patient's risk of deterioration.

To enhance the robustness of our research, we will seek to access a more extensive and diverse dataset that includes patient data from different countries. Expanding our data collection to the international stage will ensure that our findings are relevant to a broader population.

Adopting a more inclusive approach involves considering a broader range of age-related values. By including individuals across various age groups, we could reveal some patterns and trends that may be present within different life stages.

To achieve more precise and detailed analyses, we propose incorporating more daily frequent recordings. This higher data capture frequency will enable us to detect subtle fluctuations and temporal dynamics that might be missed in less frequent sampling, providing real-time insights into patients' vital signs.

Additionally, the integration of sensor technology to monitor indoor humidity levels would facilitate the extraction of valuable insights regarding the relationship between environmental factors and health deterioration.

By pursuing these advancements, we seek to increase the importance and reliability of our research, which could ultimately contribute to better patient treatment.

Author Contributions: J.P. software, validation, visualization, investigation, writing; N.A. investigation, software, writing, review, and editing; J.R. software; review and editing; M.P. writing and review; M.P. writing and review; S.M. writing and review; J.C.F. writing, review and editing. All authors have read and agreed to the published version of the manuscript.

Funding: This research was funded by the P2020 project, HC-PSI—Plataforma de Serviços Inteligentes, coordinated by INOV—Instituto de Engenharia de Sistemas e Computadores Inovação, Hope Care SA, and Universidade da Beira Interior. This work was also supported by national funds through FCT, Fundação para a Ciência e a Tecnologia, under the project code CENTRO-01-0247-FEDER-070275, in the scope of the Sistema de Apoio à Investigação Científica e Tecnológica Programas Integrados de IC& DT.

Data Availability Statement: Data are available upon request after approval from the Ethical Committee.

Conflicts of Interest: The authors declare no conflict of interest.

References

1. World Health Organization (WHO). Available online: www.who.int/data/global-health-estimates (accessed on 1 August 2023).
2. Portuguese Society of Pneumology. Available online: https://www.sppneumologia.pt/saudepublica/dpoc/ (accessed on 1 August 2023).
3. Portuguese Lung Foundation. Observatório Nacional Doenças Respiratórias 2022. Available online: https://ondr2022.fundacaoportuguesadopulmao.org/ (accessed on 1 August 2023).
4. Mogo, S.; Cachorro, V.E.; de Frutos, A.M. Morphological, chemical and optical absorbing characterization of aerosols in the urban atmosphere of Valladolid. *Atmos. Chem. Phys.* **2005**, *5*, 2739–2748. [CrossRef]
5. Arranz, M.C.; Moreno, M.F.M.; Medina, A.A.; Capitán, M.A.; Vaquer, F.C.; Gómez, A.A. Health impact assessment of air pollution in Valladolid, Spain. *BMJ Open* **2014**, *4*, e005999. [CrossRef] [PubMed]
6. Bayram, H. Effect of Global Climate Change-Related Factors on COPD Morbidity. *Tanaffos* **2017**, *16*, S24. [PubMed]
7. World Health Organization(WHO). Review of Evidence on Health Aspects of Air Pollution: REVIHAAP Project: Technical Report. Available online: https://apps.who.int/iris/handle/10665/341712 (accessed on 1 August 2021).
8. World Health Organization(WHO). Available online: https://www.who.int/news-room/fact-sheets/detail/household-air-pollution-and-health (accessed on 1 August 2023).
9. Gregório, J.; Reis, L.; Peyroteo, M.; Maia, M.; da Silva, M.M.; Lapão, L.V. The role of Design Science Research Methodology in developing pharmacy eHealth services. *Res. Soc. Adm. Pharm.* **2021**, *17*, 2089–2096. . [CrossRef] [PubMed]
10. Peffers, K.; Tuunanen, T.; Rothenberger, M.A.; Chatterjee, S. A design science research methodology for information systems research. *J. Manag. Inf. Syst.* **2007**, *24*, 45–77. [CrossRef]
11. Page, M.J.; McKenzie, J.E.; Bossuyt, P.M.; Boutron, I.; Hoffmann, T.C.; Mulrow, C.D.; Shamseer, L.; Tetzlaff, J.M.; Akl, E.A.; Brennan, S.E.; et al. The PRISMA 2020 statement: An updated guideline for reporting systematic reviews. *Int. J. Surg.* **2021**, *88*, 105906. [CrossRef]
12. Pare, G.; Jaana, M.; Sicotte, C. Systematic Review of Home Telemonitoring for Chronic Diseases: The Evidence Base. *J. Am. Med. Inform. Assoc.* **2007**, *14*, 269–277. [CrossRef]
13. Jang, S.; Kim, Y.; Cho, W.K. A Systematic Review and Meta-Analysis of Telemonitoring Interventions on Severe COPD Exacerbations. *Int. J. Environ. Res. Public Health* **2021**, *18*, 6757. [CrossRef]
14. Kruse, C.; Pesek, B.; Anderson, M.; Brennan, K.; Comfort, H. Telemonitoring to Manage Chronic Obstructive Pulmonary Disease: Systematic Literature Review. *JMIR Med. Inform.* **2019**, *7*, e11496. [CrossRef]
15. Achelrod, D.; Schreyögg, J.; Stargardt, T. Health-economic evaluation of home telemonitoring for COPD in Germany: Evidence from a large population-based cohort. *Eur. J. Health Econ.* **2016**, *18*, 869–882. [CrossRef]

16. Hong, N.; Liu, C.; Gao, J.; Han, L.; Chang, F.; Gong, M.; Su, L. State of the Art of Machine Learning–Enabled Clinical Decision Support in Intensive Care Units: Literature Review. *JMIR Med. Inform.* **2022**, *10*, e28781. [CrossRef]
17. Pépin, J.L.; Degano, B.; Tamisier, R.; Viglino, D. Remote Monitoring for Prediction and Management of Acute Exacerbations in Chronic Obstructive Pulmonary Disease (AECOPD). *Life* **2022**, *12*, 499. [CrossRef] [PubMed]
18. Exarchos, K.; Aggelopoulou, A.; Oikonomou, A.; Biniskou, T.; Beli, V.; Antoniadou, E.; Kostikas, K. Review of Artificial Intelligence Techniques in Chronic Obstructive Lung Disease. *IEEE J. Biomed. Health Inform.* **2022**, *26*, 2331–2338. [CrossRef] [PubMed]
19. Lu, J.-W.; Wang, Y.; Sun, Y.; Zhang, Q.; Yan, L.-M.; Wang, Y.-X.; Gao, J.-H.; Yin, Y.; Wang, Q.-Y.; Li, X.-L.; et al. Effectiveness of Telemonitoring for Reducing Exacerbation Occurrence in COPD Patients With Past Exacerbation History: A Systematic Review and Meta-Analysis. *Front. Med.* **2021**, *8*. [CrossRef] [PubMed]
20. Sanchez-Morillo, D.; Fernandez-Granero, M.A.; Leon-Jimenez, A. Use of predictive algorithms in-home monitoring of chronic obstructive pulmonary disease and asthma. *Chronic Respir. Dis.* **2016**, *13*, 264–283. [CrossRef]
21. Carlin, C.; Taylor, A.; van Loon, I.; McDowell, G.; Burns, S.; McGinness, P.; Lowe, D.J. Role for artificial intelligence in respiratory diseases—Chronic obstructive pulmonary disease. *J. Hosp. Manag. Health Policy* **2021**, *5*, 27–27. [CrossRef]
22. Rajeh, A.A.; Hurst, J. Monitoring of Physiological Parameters to Predict Exacerbations of Chronic Obstructive Pulmonary Disease (COPD): A Systematic Review. *J. Clin. Med.* **2016**, *5*, 108. [CrossRef]
23. Martín-Lesende, I.; Orruño, E.; Bilbao, A.; Vergara, I.; Cairo, M.C.; Bayón, J.C.; Reviriego, E.; Romo, M.I.; Larrañaga, J.; Asua, J.; et al. Impact of telemonitoring home care patients with heart failure or chronic lung disease from primary care on healthcare resource use (the TELBIL study randomised controlled trial). *BMC Health Serv. Res.* **2013**, *13*, 118. [CrossRef]
24. Lee, J.; Jung, H.M.; Kim, S.K.; Yoo, K.H.; Jung, K.S.; Lee, S.H.; Rhee, C.K. Factors associated with chronic obstructive pulmonary disease exacerbation, based on big data analysis. *Sci. Rep.* **2019**, *9*, 6679. [CrossRef]
25. Liu, Z.; Alavi, A.; Li, M.; Zhang, X. Self-Supervised Contrastive Learning for Medical Time Series: A Systematic Review. *Sensors* **2023**, *23*, 4221. [CrossRef]
26. Bui, C.; Pham, N.; Vo, A.; Tran, A.; Nguyen, A.; Le, T. Time Series Forecasting for Healthcare Diagnosis and Prognostics with the Focus on Cardiovascular Diseases. In Proceedings of the 6th International Conference on the Development of Biomedical Engineering in Vietnam (BME6), Ho Chi Minh City, Vietnam, June 2016; Springer: Singapore, 2017; pp. 809–818.
27. Kaieski, N.; da Costa, C.A.; da Rosa Righi, R.; Lora, P.S.; Eskofier, B. Application of artificial intelligence methods in vital signs analysis of hospitalized patients: A systematic literature review. *Appl. Soft Comput.* **2020**, *96*, 106612. [CrossRef]
28. Xie, J.; Wang, Z.; Yu, Z.; Guo, B. Enabling Timely Medical Intervention by Exploring Health-Related Multivariate Time Series with a Hybrid Attentive Model. *Sensors* **2022**, *22*, 6104. [CrossRef] [PubMed]
29. Sang, S.; Qu, F.; Nie, P. Ensembles of Gradient Boosting Recurrent Neural Network for Time Series Data Prediction. *IEEE Access* **2021**. [CrossRef]
30. da Silva, D.B.; Schmidt, D.; da Costa, C.A.; da Rosa Righi, R.; Eskofier, B. DeepSigns: A predictive model based on Deep Learning for the early detection of patient health deterioration. *Expert Syst. Appl.* **2021**, *165*, 113905. [CrossRef]
31. Haselbeck, F.; Killinger, J.; Menrad, K.; Hannus, T.; Grimm, D.G. Machine Learning Outperforms Classical Forecasting on Horticultural Sales Predictions. *Mach. Learn. Appl.* **2022**, *7*, 100239. [CrossRef]
32. Chacón, H.; Koppisetti, V.; Hardage, D.; Choo, K.K.R.; Rad, P. Forecasting call center arrivals using temporal memory networks and gradient boosting algorithm. *Expert Syst. Appl.* **2023**, *224*, 119983. [CrossRef]
33. Global Initiative for Chronic Obstructive Lung Disease (GOLD). Available online: https://goldcopd.org/2023-gold-report-2/ (accessed on 1 August 2023).
34. Draxler, R.; Hess, G. *Hybrid Single-Particle Lagrangian Integrated Trajectories (HY-SPLIT): Version 4.0-Description of the Hysplit_4 Modeling System*; NOAA Technical Memorandum ERL ARL-224; NOAA: Silver Spring, MD, USA, 2010; Volume 12.
35. Rolph, G.; Stein, A.; Stunder, B. Real-time Environmental Applications and Display sYstem: READY. *Environ. Model. Softw.* **2017**, *95*, 210–228. [CrossRef]
36. Chandra, R.; Goyal, S.; Gupta, R. Evaluation of deep learning models for multi-step ahead time series prediction. *IEEE Access* **2021**, *9*, 83105–83123. [CrossRef]
37. Prat, N.; Comyn-Wattiau, I.; Akoka, J. Artifact Evaluation in Information Systems Design-Science Research—A Holistic View. 2014. Available online: https://aisel.aisnet.org/pacis2014/23/ (accessed on 1 August 2023).

Disclaimer/Publisher's Note: The statements, opinions and data contained in all publications are solely those of the individual author(s) and contributor(s) and not of MDPI and/or the editor(s). MDPI and/or the editor(s) disclaim responsibility for any injury to people or property resulting from any ideas, methods, instructions or products referred to in the content.

MDPI
St. Alban-Anlage 66
4052 Basel
Switzerland
www.mdpi.com

Journal of Personalized Medicine Editorial Office
E-mail: jpm@mdpi.com
www.mdpi.com/journal/jpm

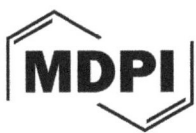

Disclaimer/Publisher's Note: The statements, opinions and data contained in all publications are solely those of the individual author(s) and contributor(s) and not of MDPI and/or the editor(s). MDPI and/or the editor(s) disclaim responsibility for any injury to people or property resulting from any ideas, methods, instructions or products referred to in the content.

www.ingramcontent.com/pod-product-compliance
Lightning Source LLC
LaVergne TN
LVHW070237100526
838202LV00015B/2143